NUTRITION AND DIET RESEARCH PROGRESS

FISH OIL

PRODUCTION, CONSUMPTION AND HEALTH BENEFITS

NUTRITION AND DIET RESEARCH PROGRESS

Additional books in this series can be found on Nova's website
under the Series tab.

Additional E-books in this series can be found on Nova's website
under the E-book tab.

NUTRITION AND DIET RESEARCH PROGRESS

FISH OIL

PRODUCTION, CONSUMPTION AND HEALTH BENEFITS

MATTHIAS VAN DIJK
AND
JÜRGEN VITEK
EDITORS

Nova Biomedical Books
New York

For permission to use material from this book please contact us:
Telephone 631-231-7269; Fax 631-231-8175
Web Site: http://www.novapublishers.com

Additional color graphics may be available in the e-book version of this book.

Library of Congress Cataloging-in-Publication Data

Fish oil : production, consumption, and health benefits / editors, Matthias van Dijk and J|rgen Vitek.
p. ; cm.
Includes bibliographical references and index.
ISBN 978-1-61470-963-3 (hardcover)
I. Dijk, Matthias van. II. Vitek, J|rgen.
[DNLM: 1. Fish Oils--therapeutic use. 2. Fatty Acids, Omega-3--therapeutic use. QU 86]
LC-classification not assigned
615.3'4--dc23

2011028898

Published by Nova Science Publishers, Inc. † New York

Contents

Preface

Fish oils contain the omega-3 fatty acids eicosapentaenoic acid (EPA) and docosahexaenoic acid (DHA), precursors of eicosanoids that are known to reduce inflammation throughout the body, and are thought to have many health benefits. In this book, the authors present topical research in the study of the production, consumption and health benefits of fish oil, including polyunsaturated fatty acids and their dietary implications during pregnancy; plant-derived antioxidants as potential omega-3 pufa stabilizers; stability and behavior of omega-3 food emulsions; the combined effects of omega-3 fatty acids and exercise on cardiovascular disease risk and mortality and fish oil and male fertility.

Chapter I- The annual production of fish body oil presented important fluctuations over the last two decades. These fluctuations, as mentioned by Barlow, have been due to El Niño phenomenon, which has greatly affected the fish oil production in Chile and Peru. This is particularly evident in 1998 where the total production of Peru and Chile only reached 130 thousand tons, which was 15 % of total annual production whereas it generally represented more than 40 %. The El Niño of 1991-1992 and 2002-2003 also caused reductions of fish oils production but they were not as strong as that of 1997-1998.

The changing uses of fish oil between 1970 and 2009 are shown. The most noticeable is the current importance of fish oil in the production of aquafeeds which is estimated as 81 % of total fish oil production. Only 6 % of fish oil is hydrogenated or has an industrial use whereas in 1970 it was totally used by these two types of oil processing. Another significant aspect is the increasing production of refined edible oil, which is related to the recognized health benefits associated with the fish oil consumption. The percentage of fish oil used in aquaculture has substantially increased but between 2000 and 2008 the amount to produce aquafeeds has been stationary despite the continuous growth of global aquaculture production. The authors show the percentage of of fish oil usage in aquaculture in 2009. The highest percentage went to salmon and trout production (68 %) but in 2000 it represented 40 % of total. This increase reflects the growing production of salmonids in Norway, Chile, Canada and various European countries

Chapter II- Fish oil is rich in the omega-3 fatty acids eicosapentaenoic acid (EPA) and docosahexaenoic acid (DHA). There is now extensive evidence that supports the cardiovascular benefits of these omega-3 polyunsaturated fatty acids (PUFAs). Both EPA and DHA cannot be made in sufficient quantities in the body and must therefore be obtained by a diet rich in oily fish or by consuming fish oil supplements. The mechanism by which these omega-3 PUFAs favorably impact cardiovascular disease is thought to be due to their anti-inflammatory, anti-platelet and anti-thrombotic effects and their favorable effects on arrhythmias, hypertriglyceridemia, endothelial function and telomere shortening which can preserve the genetic youth of individual cells.

The evidence for the cardiovascular benefits of omega-3 PUFAs comes from numerous epidemiological studies and several large randomized clinical studies conducted in patients with coronary artery disease, myocardial infarction and heart failure. These large randomized clinical trials have shown that modest doses of omega-3 PUFAs significantly reduce the risk of unstable angina, myocardial infarction, sudden cardiac death and death in coronary artery disease and heart failure patients. However, more recent studies have questioned the cardiovascular benefits of fish oil.

Based on the scientific evidence the American Heart Association (AHA) has recommended eating fish at least two times a week for all individuals to prevent cardiovascular disease. For individuals with coronary artery disease the recommended dose of omega-3 PUFAs is 1 g of EPA and DHA daily. To lower triglyceride levels much higher doses are needed and the AHA recommends a dose 2 to 4 g of EPA and DHA daily. To obtain the recommended dose of fish oil for individuals with coronary artery disease or to lower triglyceride levels, fish oil supplements are often needed. There are numerous over-the-counter fish oil supplements that contain varying doses of EPA and DHA and one high dose prescription formulation. The Food and Drug Administration (FDA) has approved this prescription omega-3 PUFA supplement at a dose of 4 g daily for the treatment of very high triglyceride levels.

Despite the compelling evidence for the cardiovascular benefits of omega-3 PUFAs and the AHA recommendations, most physicians to not recommend fish oil supplements for their high-risk patients. In addition there is confusion regarding the formulations of fish oil that are available and the doses of fish oil that should be used in clinical practice. The purpose of this review is to discuss the production of fish oil, the differences between available fish oil supplements and to summarize the current scientific evidence on the cardiovascular health benefits of fish oil consumption

Chapter III- Although animals can modify fatty acyl chains by introducing more than one double bond, certain limitations exist. Chain elongation alternates with desaturation, which together with peroxisomal retro-conversion reactions allow the synthesis of long-chain polyunsaturated fatty acids (LCPUFA) from linoleic acid (18:2ω6) and α-linolenic acid (18:3ω3), the only nutritionally essential fatty acids (EFA). Arachinonic acid and other C20 LCPUFA give rise to eicosanoids (prostaglandins, thromboxanes, leukotrienes and lipoxins), which are signaling molecules classified as local hormones. Polyunsaturated fatty acids (PUFA) are also biological regulators, and many of their effects relate to their abilities to regulate gene expression and downstream events. These effects are cell-specific and involve members of the super-family of nuclear receptors that function as transcription factors. PUFA are susceptible to autooxidation by a process that is especially complex in the cell membrane, where it increases the consumption of vitamin E – a chain-breaking antioxidant that prevents the propagation of free radical reactions. Other antioxidant defenses exist, in the form of certain enzymes (e.g., superoxide dismutases, catalase, gluthatione peroxidase and other peroxidases) and of compounds that protect against the oxidation process or repair the damage caused. Normal fetal development requires both EFA and LCPUFA, and the nutritional status of the mother during gestation has been related to fetal growth.

Supplementing diets with oils rich in LCPUFA during the last trimester of gestation has been advised; however, in excess, they may cause competitive inhibition of the Δ6 and Δ5 desaturases that control the conversion of EFA into LCPUFA by the ω-3 and ω-6 pathways, thus inhibiting the synthesis of certain LCPUFA that could be essential for fetal growth. Maternal dietary LCPUFA are taken up by adipose tissue during early pregnancy, where they are stored temporarily, before being released during late pregnancy to become available to the fetus in the last stages of its development. In maternal plasma most LCPUFA circulate in their esterified form in different lipoproteins, and around parturition they are diverted to mammary gland where – through the induction of lipoprotein lipase – they are used for milk synthesis and thus become available to the newborn. Efforts have been made to determine whether supplements with LCPUFA during different perinatal stages can improve the short- or long-term developmental outcome, but no definitive conclusion has been attained, and additional studies are required.

Chapter IV- The initial aim of the present chapter was to assess the suitability of a fish oil diet to correct the metabolic and hormonal defects otherwise encountered in rats deprived of a dietary supply of long-chain polyunsaturated ω3 fatty acids. For such a purpose, 8 groups of 4 rats each were first exposed from the 8th week after birth and for the ensuing 3 months to either a soya oil or sunflower oil diet and then examined at the end of this 3 months initial period or after a further period of one, two or 8 weeks exposure to a fish oil diet. The fatty acid profile of jejunum, caecum, liver, red blood cells and brain phospholipids, as well as liver triglycerides and visceral adipose tissue lipids, was analyzed. Changes in food intake, body weight and the HOMA index for insulin resistance were also monitored. The results document the efficiency of this procedure for the correction of both the ω3 deficiency and insulin resistance, without any undesirable increase in liver steatosis, visceral obesity, food intake or body weight. Emphasis is also placed on the dual regulation of the lipid fatty acid profile as attributable to either a direct link with the fatty acid content of the diet or the transfer of information from one organ to another.

Chapter V- Omega–3 and Omega–6 Fatty Acids are predominant in fish oils compared to other animal oils. Omega–3 polyunsaturated fatty acids (PUFA) such as Docosahexaenoic acid (DHA) and Eicosapentaenoic acid (EPA) have attracted considerable interest in both nutraceutical and pharmaceutical fields. The major beneficial role of omega – 3 fatty acids is to reduce the risk of coronary heart disease and help in brain, neural and retinal developments. Consumption of diet containing PUFA reduces blood pressure, plasma triglycerides and cholesterol levels, thereby increasing the blood coagulation time, which are responsible for maintenance of normal blood flow by preventing platelets from sticking to each other. PUFA not only alleviates blood vessel disorders and inflammatory diseases, but also controls immune functions resulting in alleviation of autoimmune diseases such as arthritis and certain types of dermatitis. Human diet deficient in DHA and EPA can cause several disorders such as restrictive growth, abnormality of skin and hair, damage of reproductive system and abnormal composition of serum and tissue fatty acids. Fish oil rich in PUFA, is also associated with decreased risk of Dementia and Alzheimer's disease. Increased levels of DHA in brain are believed to reduce ageing.

This chapter describes the beneficial effects of consumption of fish oil containing PUFA in protecting human health; besides addressing certain individual diseases

Chapter VI- The dietary intake of omega-3 fatty acids, which are long chain polyunsaturated fatty acids (PUFA), commonly found in fish or fish oil has numerous health benefits such as the prevention of heart diseases, cancer, dementia and several neurological and psychiatric diseases. The effect of omega-3 fatty acids, especially in the form of eicosapentaenoic acid (EPA) and docosahexaenoic acid (DHA) in the prevention of primary and secondary cardiovascular diseases is well addressed. Their cardioprotective mechanisms extend from antiartherosclerotic to antithrombotic, antiarrhythmic and anti-inflammatory activity including lowering of blood pressure and triglyceride levels. Moreover, omega-3 PUFA have been shown to inhibit the formation of various types of cancers and have also been implicated in the brain and eye development in infants and young children.

Due to many health benefits of omega-3 fatty acids, inclusion of these essential fatty acids in the diet has been recommended. The World Health Organization (WHO) has recommended one to two servings of fatty fish per week (each serving should provide the equivalent of 200 to 500 mg of EPA+DHA) and is generally being considered as a standard reference in terms of dietary intake of omega-3 fatty acids. However, various organizations worldwide have established their own recommendations for the consumption of omega-3 fatty acids for health promotion and prevention of various chronic diseases. Currently, the dietary recommendations for EPA and DHA are being met by the intake of omega-3 fatty acids rich fish, fish oil supplements as well as algal supplements. Unfortunately, the PUFA present in fish oil are vulnerable to oxidation which decreases the shelf life and nutritional value of the fish oil. In this chapter, the authors have briefly discussed about lipid oxidation in fish oil, synthetic antioxidants and plant-derived natural antioxidants.

Chapter VII- Dietary sources and Biosynthesis pathways represents the main suppliers for the fatty acids needed by the human body for construction of hydrophobic parts of Bio molecules . Various animal and vegetable lipids are ingested, hydrolyzed at least partially by digestive enzymes and absorbed through the intestinal wall to be distributed through the body, first in the lymphatic system and then in the blood stream . To some extent such dietary supply may adjust the composition of fatty acids in the body lipids.

On the other hand, metabolic processes in the tissues of the normal human body can modify the dietary fatty acids and or those that are synthesized in these tissues, to produce almost all the various structures that are needed .For this reason,with one exception the actual composition of the fatty acids supplied in the diet is relatively unimportant. This one exception involves the need for appropriate proportions of the relatively highly unsaturated fatty acids since many higher mammals; including humans are unable to produce fatty acids with double bonds very far towards the end of the molecule either during de novo synthesis or by modification of the dietary acids. Accordingly these fatty acids can provides essential fatty acids and acting also as carriers for oil soluble vitamins like A,D,E,K additionally their intestinal absorption . The oils derived from cold-water fish are unique among all the edible oils and fats. They are an important source of long chain ω-3 or n-3 polyunsaturates.

Fatty acids group referred to as conjugated Linoleic acid are receiving now greater interest due to having health promoting properties. The liver oils from fish such as cod and halibut have an added feature as natural source of highly importance for oil soluble vitamins like A and D.

Two forms of polyunsaturates are considered essential, known as n-3 and n-6, average intake of the former have fallen considerably as compared to the second. This induced more emphasis regarding the need for an adequate intake of performed long chain ω-3 polyunsaturated fatty acids from fish. Dietary 18 c fatty acids (essential fatty acids) were previously referred to as vitamins F1 and F2. These 18 c fatty acids (Linoleic and α linoleic) are converted by a common enzyme system into 20, 22 carbon derivatives. Since the conversion enzymes are the same for both n-3 and n-6 the phenomenon of competitive inhibition occurs. Accordingly, the predominance of one family may deviate the other away from enzyme sites and the conversion process favor the first one. As a result an excess of the dietary ω-6 will inhibit ω-3 conversion to 20, 22 carbons from specifically eicosapentaenoic and Docosahexenoic acids.

Chapter VIII- N-3 Polyunsaturated fatty acids have been shown to have potential beneficial effects for chronic diseases including cancer, insulin resistance and cardiovascular disease. Eicosapentaenoic acid (EPA) and docosahexaenoic acid (DHA) in particular have been studied extensively. In some diets, such as the typical North American diet, intakes of EPA and DHA are typically very low. The fish oil used in this study is a commercial ingredient for the food industry. It is a concentrate from fish oil, mainly salmon, which is recommended for formulation of functional foods such as chocolate, yogurt, jam, pastry filling, salad oil, mayonnaise and dressings. The use of this oil permits food manufacturers to ensure a controlled content of omega-3, EPA, DPA and DHA fatty acids, in the final products and supplies vitamin E. Thus, regarding some of these applications it is very interesting to study its behavior in emulsion systems. In the food industry, stabilization of emulsions is obtained by the addition of proteins. Sodium caseinate is a well-used ingredient because of its functional properties: good solubility and emulsifying properties, high stability during heating, water and fat binding, thickening and gelation. The addition of this protein has a double stabilizing effect since it provokes together with other added surfactants an increase of both viscosity of the continuous phase and stability of the interface. The physicochemical properties of emulsions play an important role in food systems as they directly contribute to texture, sensory and nutritional properties of food. One of the main properties is stability, which refers to the ability of an emulsion to resist changes in its properties over time. Physical instability results in an alteration in the spatial distribution or structural organization of the molecules. Creaming, flocculation, coalescence, partial coalescence, phase inversion, and Ostwald ripening are examples of physical instability. It is important for food scientists to identify the relative importance of each mechanism, the relationship between them, and the factors that influence them, so that effective means of controlling the stability and physicochemical properties of emulsions can be established. Turbiscan MA 2000 is one of the methods used to study emulsion stability. It is a vertical scan analyzer, which allows the optical characterization of any type of dispersion. The reading head is composed of a pulsed near-IR light source and two synchronous detectors: the transmission and the backscattering detectors. The backscattering and transmission profiles as a function of the sample height allow following the physical evolution of this process without disturbing the original system and with good accuracy and reproducibility. Thus, by repeating the scan of a sample at different time intervals, the stability or the instability of dispersions can be studied in detail. The profiles allow calculation of creaming, sedimentation, or phase separation rates, as well as flocculation, and the mechanism making the dispersion unstable can be deduced from the transmission or the backscattering data. The aim of the present work is to investigate the effect of oil-to-protein ratio, sugar concentration on the stability of emulsions formulated with concentrated fish oil as fat phase. Creaming and flocculation kinetics were quantified analyzing the samples with a Turbiscan MA 2000.

Chapter IX- The Omega 3 polyunsaturated fatty acids (w-3 PUFA or n-6 PUFA) from fish oil are known not only because its essentiality, but because their unquestionable anti-inflammatory effect. This effect has put the fish oil on the top of the list of the most studied oil in the world. The anti-inflammatory effect of fish oil has been observed in a variety of inflammatory diseases, such as colitis, asthma and cardiovascular disease. Fatty acids are components of cell membranes, which are important for maintaining cellular homeostasis and intercellular communication. Several studies have shown that changes in diet composition may alter the lipid composition of membrane phospholipids, altering their functionality (Calder 2002).

The relationship between inflammatory response and fatty acids (FAs), especially in regard to polyunsaturated fatty acids (PUFA), has been investigated on the last years. One reason for this interest, comes from the fact that arachidonic acid (AA), n-6 PUFA, which is a precursor of eicosanoids, substances that have important and inflammatory properties, is derived directly from dietetic vegetable oils sources such as soybean, corn and sunflower or indirectly formed from linoleic acid (18:2 n-6) or gamma-linolenic acid (18:3 n-6).

On the other hand, epidemiological studies have shown that the Eskimos population, large consumers of eicosapentaenoic acid (EPA) and docosahexaenoic acid (DHA), both polyunsaturated n-3, have low incidence of inflammatory and immunological diseases (Kromman & Green 1980). Since the report of this finding, a number of researchers have documented the beneficial effects of n-3 PUFA (rich in EPA and DHA) on acute and chronic inflammatory conditions (Wu & Meydani 1998, Harbidge 1998). These effects were considered to result mainly from a modification in the production of inflammatory mediators (cytokines, chemokines, and costimulatory molecules) and the suppression of inflammatory leukocytes (neutrophils, lymphocytes, macrophages, and dendritic cells).

Chapter X- Myocardial infarction associated with atherosclerosis is the leading cause of death globally. Novel therapies are needed to reduce the rates of mortality and morbidity associated with cardiovascular disease (CVD). Previous study findings suggest omega-3 fatty acids (FO) may have a beneficial effect on risk for CVD and its associated morbidity and mortality rates. Both docosahexaenoic acid (DHA) and eicosapentaenoic acid (EPA) have demonstrated positive effects on cholesterol levels, inflammatory markers, blood pressure, endothelial dysfunction, resting hear rate, and arrhythmia. Study authors have reported positive effects on low-density lipoprotein cholesterol (LDL), high-density lipoprotein cholesterol (HDL), triglycerides, and emerging risk factors of LDL particle number and LDL size. Additionally, various study outcomes have demonstrated an effect of n-3 on inflammatory markers such as Interleukin-6 (IL-6), Interleukin-1beta (IL-1β), and Tumor Necrosis Factor-alpha (TNF-α). Many of these same effects have been reported for individuals who regularly engage in aerobic exercise including a decreased heart rate and additional improvements in heart rate variability. The primary inflammatory markers associated with exercise have been improved levels of IL-6, IL-1 β, TNF-α, and C-reactive protein (CRP). Therefore exercise may contribute to the reduction of vascular and inflammatory diseases, more specifically CVD. Recently, studies have emerged attempting to understand the effects of combining exercise and supplementing FO on mortality and morbidity associated with CVD. Findings have ranged from increased performance during exercise to improving heart function or heart rate variability, decreasing resting heart rates, and improving lipid and inflammatory profiles. Most importantly there has been emerging evidence that the combination of exercise and FO supplementation may have a synergistic effect when combined. Though little is known among the general public and health practitioners about this combination of therapy on the reduction in heart disease, a growing body of research has addressed this issue. Therefore the purpose of this chapter will be to explore the literature to address what effects combining exercise and FO supplementation have on CVD. Specifically the authors will address issues of cholesterol, inflammation, heart rate variability, blood pressure, and general health markers of CVD.

Chapter XI- Richard Dawkins has written "The evolution of the capacity to simulate seems to have culminated in subjective consciousness. Why this should have happened is, to me, the most profound mystery facing modern biology." In writing this review of recent research on fish oil, I invite you to consider another exciting mystery of modern science that depends upon fish oil, consciousness. Omega-3 (n-3) fatty acids are essential in the human diet for the brain to function. From a biochemical perspective, it is clear how DHA, the longest omega-3 fatty acid, which is found in FO (fish oil found in cold water fish), plays an essential role in brain function. Using epidemiological studies of people, scientists have discovered that those who consume FO have a lower risk for dementia. In biochemical analyses of molecules that are necessary for the brain, researchers have elucidated how FO provides flexibility for dendritic mobility. We now know that dietary nutrients produce metabolic signals similar to hormones. This review provides vocabulary and structures necessary to understand some important fatty acids, and presents fats in the brain related to FO. It describes the origin of those fatty acids in algae and their functions in fish and humans. DHA in FO activates at least two areas in the brain that reduce appetite and increase basic metabolic rate. I review other nutrition studies done during recent years that demonstrate that FO is important for both brain function and weight regulation. These studies demonstrate the benefit for humans of a daily intake of FO from before conception through senescence to maintain optimal health.

Chapter XII- In the collective mind, terms such as "omega-3", "DHA", "EPA" and "fish/fish oil" are generally associated with health benefits. Oily cold-water fish are the main dietary source of omega-3 fatty acids eicosapentaenoic acid (EPA) and docosahexaenoic acid (DHA). These fatty acids have important biological functions including primary roles in cell membranes and in eicosanoid metabolism. Indeed, there are evidences that omega-3 polyunsaturated fatty acids are essential nutrients for infant development. Also their positive roles in reducing cardiovascular risk, arthritis, cancer as well as improving mental health have been widely documented in human and animals studies for the last three decades. Furthermore, omega-3 fatty acids may have specific health benefits in female reproduction. A little less is known about the roles of omega-3 fatty acids in male reproduction. This review based on animal models and human studies will focus on the potential benefits as well as harmful effects of fish oil supplementation on male fertility.

Chapter XIII- Since, at the end of the ′80s, epidemiological studies began to establish a certain relationship between a high fatty fish consumption and a low incidence of cardiovascular diseases in Nordic people, the amount clinical and biological essays about polyunsaturated fatty acids (PUFA), especially omega-3 fatty acids, has greatly increased, being voluminous the current available information related to their biochemical mechanisms of action, biological effects and health implications. Nowadays, nobody doubts about the importance of omega-3 fatty acids, especially EPA and DHA, in human diet, which recommended daily intakes have been established by several nutritionist committees all over the world. As a consequence, the demand of omega-3 enriched products and nutraceuticals has grown up noticeably, especially in those societies with a diet based a on high consumption of seed oils and meat, which has promoted the development of plenty of novel strategies and competitive methods for producing, on large scale, the high quality omega-3 concentrates requested for both food and pharmaceutical industries.

This chapter is proposed as an overview of the current situation of omega-3 fatty acids. Firstly, a brief introduction about essential fatty acids, focusing on the most relevant clinical studies published in the last 10 years about their role in human health. The last part of the chapter reviews the state-of-the-art of fish oil and omega-3 production processes on large scale, with an emphasis on the scientific articles and patents published from 2000 to 2010 and distinguishing two main groups: conventional methods based on physical and chemical processes and alternative methods based on the use of supercritical fluid technologies. In addition, a short compilation of different fish oil and omega-3 concentrates currently available in the market is presented

Chapter XIV- The last decades of human history saw an expressive modification in both the amount and the composition of dietary fat, with increased intake of saturated, trans, and omega-6 polyunsaturated fats, and a concomitant substantial reduction in the consumption of omega-3 sources. Intake of saturated and trans fatty acids have long been recognized to impair metabolic control while polyunsaturated fatty acids (PUFAs) in general have been thought to be less harmful (Albuquerque et al. 2006; Buettner et al. 2007; Innis 2007).

The importance of intake of adequate amounts of the essential fatty acids linoleic acid (LA, 18:2ω-6) and α-linolenic acid (ALA, 18:3ω-3) is well established. The long-chain ω-3 fatty acids, particularly eicosapentaenoic acid (EPA, 20:5ω-3) and docosahexaenoic acid (DHA, 22:6ω-3), are essential constituents of cell membranes and are highly concentrated in neuronal membrane phospholipids, playing important roles in aspects as relevant as membrane stability, neuroplasticity, neurotransmission and signal transduction (Innis 2007).

The current ratio of ω-6 to ω-3 total intake is estimated to be in the range of 10-25 to 1, an imbalance that has been suggested to contribute to the deleterious health consequences culminating in the current worldwide epidemic of obesity and co-morbidities (Connor 2000; Simopoulos 2011). There have been reports linking high intake of ω-6 PUFAs to increased adipogenesis rate in children and adults. Studies conducted in either experimental animals or human subjects have shown high ω-6 PUFA intake to be positively linked to insulin resistance and obesity. On the other hand, intake of ω-3 PUFA, which are highly enriched in fish oils, have been inversely related with body adiposity and have thus been ascribed a protective role (Ruzickova et al. 2004; Ailhaud et al. 2006; Kabir et al. 2007; Phillips 2010; Oliver et al. 2010).

Obesity results from the disequilibrium between energy intake and expenditure, parameters that are regulated by complex central nervous system mechanisms. Disruption of this control results in hyperphagia and/or inadequation of food intake to energy requirements. Food intake is a complex behavior controlled by the interaction of homeostatic and hedonic influences, mainly processed in hypothalamic and mesocorticolimbic sites, respectively. While the homeostatic component of this control system aims at promoting body energy and nutrient equilibrium, the hedonic pathway operates under the command of motivational and reward aspects associated with eating.

The hypothalamus is a key site in the central nervous system control of energy balance. Under the influence of the peripheral adiposity and satiety signals, the activity of anabolic and catabolic neurons of various hypothalamic nuclei modulates food intake and energy expenditure. Several hypothalamic sites are implicated in the feeding regulatory circuitry, mainly the arcuate nucleus (ARC), the ventromedial nucleus (VMH), the paraventricular nucleus (PVN), the dorsomedial nucleus (DMH) and the lateral area (LHA). The proper balance between the orexigenic and the anorexigenic influences exerted by the mediators produced in these nuclei is essential for energy homeostasis and the disruption of this equilibrium plays a prominent role in the pathogenesis of obesity (Ribeiro et al. 2006; Velloso et al. 2006; Ribeiro 2009).

The hypothalamus is importantly impacted by the hedonic influences as the LHA receives inputs from the nucleus accumbens (NAc), an important center of the hedonic component of feeding control, whose dopaminergic, opioid, and endocannabinoid innervations are stimulated by motivation- and reward- related signals. Orexigenic mediators at the LHA are thus influenced by these signals (Erlanson-Albertsson et al. 2005).

Fish oil intake has been shown to be able to interact with the central control of food intake and some potential mechanisms underlying the fish oil effects have been examined. The purpose of the present review is to summarize recent findings linking dietary consumption of fish oil, or of its ω-3 fatty acid constituents, to the central control of feeding. Although the majority of studies focusing on the mechanisms targeted by fish oil have been performed in animals, their examination provide valuable insights into the processes by which these nutrients may modify food intake in the context of feeding disorders like obesity and anorexia.

Chapter XV- Due to the weight of prior evidence, the American Heart Association has endorsed the use of omega-3 fatty acids for the secondary prevention of cardiovascular(CV) events in patients with known coronary artery disease. This recommendation was based on a large number of epidemiologic studies as well as a few large randomized control studies. In particular, the GISSI-Prevenzione illustrating significant reductions in both sudden cardiac death and CV events and the JELIS trial illustrating significant reductions in CV events contributed to these recommendations. However, more recent trials such as the OMEGA trial, the Alpha Omega Trial, and Kowey et al.'s study of omega-3 supplementation in atrial fibrillation(AF) patients have shown some conflicting results. The OMEGA trial evaluated supplementing 1g/d for one year and was unable to show a significant difference in CV outcomes in post myocardial infarction patients. This discrepancy could have potentially been from the improvements in medical therapy from the decade older trials which resulted in a lower number of events. The Alpha Omega trial investigated the supplementation of omega-3 in the form of 18.8 g of margarine per day and also showed no significant differences in CV events in patients with a history of myocardial infarctions. The patients in this trial were also on a modern regimen of CV medications and only received a small supplement of omega-3 which may have not been enough to exert an effect. In Kower et al.'s trial of AF patients, omega-3 supplementation did not reduce the recurrence of AF in the 6 month study period. On the other hand, the omega-3 arm of the GISSI heart failure (HF) trial showed an 8% reduction of mortality and CV admissions in patients supplemented with omega-3 fatty acids. Although more recent trials have not shown the robust benefits that were seen in the earlier ones, the balance of evidence still favor the beneficial effects of omega-3 fatty acids. We would recommend the continuation of omega-3 fatty acids in patients with CV disease and in particular HF.

Chapter XVI- Important benefits exists in the human health associated with the ingestion of fish and his oil, such as the prevention of cardiovascular diseases, immunological diseases, diabetes mellitus, colon´s cancer, beside serving like helpingly in the treatment of arthritis and taking part in the development of the brain and retina. The origin of marine oils perform at the present great importance in the supplies and in the human nutrition, due to it contained high place of polyunsaturated fatty acids (PUFA) specially, omega 3. The fished ones of deep and sweets waters called of meat blue or fished blue they are a source of omega-3 fatty acids as alpha - linolenic acid (ALA), eicosapentanoic acid (EPA) and docosahexaenoic acid (DHA). According to the database FAOSTAT 2007, in many countries such as China, Japan, United States and Mexico, per capita intake of fresh water fish was of 12.3, 4.9, 4.5 and 1.2 Kg respectively. It recommends to increase the consumption frequency of fish in quantities adapted in the populations with low ingestion, as the Mexican one, since this food constitutes a nutritional practical and cheap form to incorporate in the supply omega-3 fatty acids. The aim of the present work is to give updated information about the benefits in the human health that offers the consumption of fish oil.

Chapter XVII- The n-6 or omega 6 series [i.e. arachidonic acid (AA)] and the n-3 or omega-3 polyunsaturated fatty acids (n-3 PUFA), and particularly the long chain highly unsaturated ones (LC PUFA) [i.e. eicosapentaenoic and docosahexaenoic acid (EPA and DHA)], are essential for humans and work sometimes in synergy and sometimes in competition. Today, their role has been recognized as not only mere caloric, but with effects in cell differentiation and communication through a deep modulation to the cell core involved in gene regulation. These effects occur in all of the body systems and organs, but with different outcomes depending on local or systemic inputs. Therefore, during fetal and neonatal development, LC PUFA contribute to growth and evolution, while, during inflammation, they orchestrate various functions of cells. Many disease conditions develop from inflammation. Obesity and metabolic syndrome are two examples in which diet and the hormonal milieu may disrupt multiple cells with the release of cytokines. In the case of chronic stimuli, body metabolism changes. LC PUFA again, prove to be a potent tool to reverse or enhance these changes. In this chapter, we want to focus on the effects of n-3 PUFA with regard to brain development and obesity.

Chapter XVIII- The marine environment represents largely an untapped reservoir of novel and valuable bioactive compounds including lipids and lipid-soluble substance such as fatty acids, pigments, fat-soluble vitamins, terpenes, saponins, sterols, and glycolipids. Among them, marine long-chained polyunsaturated fatty acids fatty acids (LC-PUFA), specifically, docosahexaenoic acid [DHA, 22:6(n-3)] and eicosapentaenoic acid [EPA, 20:5(n-3)], have received considerable attention of researchers because of their beneficial biochemical and pharmacological effects on human health. With growing public awareness of the clinical benefits of EPA and DHA, sale of marine oil supplements have grown almost ten folds over the last decade. Most of these represent fish oil capsules made from various seafood sources including fish byproducts. In comparison with LC-PUFA, the other natural lipids from marine sources such as squalene and wax esters have received much less attention in spite of their proven potential as bioactive resources in promoting the human health and industrial applications. In addition, marine oils of inferior quality, which are not suitable for human consumption can also be used as a starter material for biodiesel production to manage the eminent energy crisis of the world. This chapter mainly deals with composition of marine lipids and the different techniques for the production of LC-PUFA, squalene, wax esters and biodiesel from marine oils.

In: Fish Oil: Production, Consumption and Health Benefits ISBN: 978-1-61470-963-3
Editors: Matthias Van Dijk and Jürgen Vitek

Chapter I

Fish Oil: Production, Consumption and Health Benefits

***Narcisa Maria Bandarra**[*1]**, Irineu Batista**[1]**, Paulo Bispo**[1]**, Maria Leonor Nunes**[1]**, Elena Venegas-Venegas**[2]**, Miguel Ángel Rincón-Cervera**[2] **and José Luis Guil-Guerrero**[2]*

[1] INRB/IPIMAR, Lisboa, Portugal

[2] Universidad de Almería, Almería, Spain

1. Fish Oil Production

The annual production of fish body oil presented important fluctuations over the last two decades (Fig. 1). These fluctuations, as mentioned by Barlow [1], have been due to El Niño phenomenon, which has greatly affected the fish oil production in Chile and Peru. This is particularly evident in 1998 where the total production of Peru and Chile only reached 130 thousand tons, which was 15 % of total annual production whereas it generally represented more than 40 %. The El Niño of 1991-1992 and 2002-2003 also caused reductions of fish oils production but they were not as strong as that of 1997-1998.

The changing uses of fish oil between 1970 and 2009 are shown in figure 2. The most noticeable is the current importance of fish oil in the production of aquafeeds which is estimated as 81 % of total fish oil production [2]. Only 6 % of fish oil is hydrogenated or has an industrial use whereas in 1970 it was totally used by these two types of oil processing. Another significant aspect is the increasing production of refined edible oil, which is related to the recognized health benefits associated with the fish oil consumption. The percentage of fish oil used in aquaculture has substantially increased but between 2000 and 2008 the amount to produce aquafeeds has been stationary despite the continuous growth of global aquaculture production [2]. In figure 3 is shown the percentage of of fish oil usage in

[*] INRB/IPIMAR Av. Brasília 1449-006 Lisboa Portugal, narcisa@ipimar.pt

aquaculture in 2009. The highest percentage went to salmon and trout production (68 %) but in 2000 it represented 40 % of total [3]. This increase reflects the growing production of salmonids in Norway, Chile, Canada and various European countries.

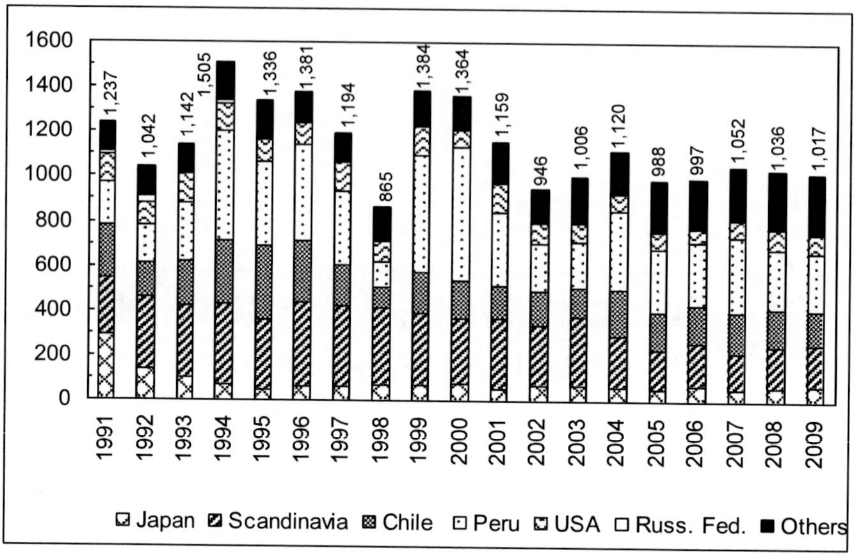

Figure 1. Major worldwide producers of fish body oil between 1991 and 2009.

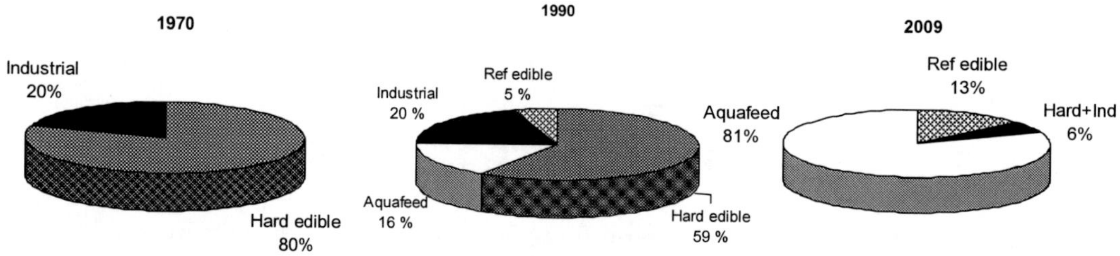

Figure 2. Evolution of fish oil usage in the period between 1970 and 2009.

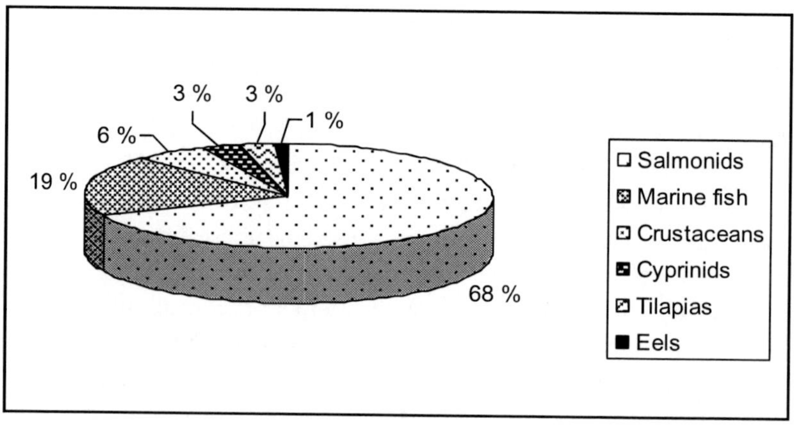

Figure 3. Percentage of fish oil used in aquaculture in 2009.

1.1. Fish Oil Recovery

Fish body oil is almost exclusively produced from small pelagic species, such as anchovy, sardine and jack mackerel in South America and sandeel, capelin, sprat, herring and horse mackerel in Europe [3]. In these species the lipids are deposited under the skin, distributed in their muscle tissue and also located in the tissues of the intestine and mesentery. The oil may be also produced from the liver of white lean fish and blubber of marine mammals [4].

Fish oil composition varies markedly depending on a variety of factors including species, sex and season. As reported [5], commercial fish oil is usually composed of over 90 % triacylglycerols (TAGs), about 8 % of mono-, and di-acylglycerols and other lipids such as phospholipids. The unsaponifiable fraction accounts for thc remaining 2 % and includes sterols (mainly cholesterol), glyceryl ethers, hydrocarbons, fatty alcohols and fat-soluble vitamins (A, D, and E).

1.1.1. Traditional Methods for Oil Recovery

Fish oil is a coproduct of fish meal production, which could be produced by two general types of processes: wet-reduction and dry-rendering. The wet-reduction process applies to the processing of fatty species and consists of the following main operations: (1) heating or cooking small whole fish or ground fish offal with live steam under pressure, (2) pressing the cooked fish to release the liquid fraction, the press liquor, and retaining the semi-dry portion, the press cake, (3) screening out the suspended fish solids from the press liquor and returning the wet solids to the press cake, (4) drying the press cake, which was previously fluffed, (5) grinding and sacking the dried meal, (6) heating and centrifuging the screened press liquor to obtain the oil and a aqueous phase, the stickwater, (7) oil purification by centrifuging, (8) recovery of the stickwater, which involves concentration and returning to the press cake.

The dry-rendering process is mainly applied to the production of fish meal from fish or fish offal from nonoily fish. The main steps involved in this process are: (1) coarse grinding of fish offal and (2) treatment of the ground material in a steam-jacketed cooker drier. Sometimes the residual oil may be extracted by pressing.

Thus, the wet-reduction method is particularly suited for the extraction of oil from fatty species and dry rendering is preferred when small quantities of nonoily fish are available [6]. The latter process yields much darker oil than that obtained by the wet-reduction process.

Several other processes for oil extraction involving protein coagulation at temperatures higher than 95 °C were patented [7, 8, 9]. More recently the wet rendering method was used to separate the oil from precooked and non-precooked tuna heads [10]. Higher yields of crude oil were obtained from precooked tuna heads but the oil from non-precooked raw material had higher quality than that from precooked samples. However, crude oil from precooked samples had high DHA (25.5 %) than oil from non-precooked samples (18.8 %).

1.1.2. A Modified Conkix Process for Oil Extraction

A new method based on the Conkix process from Alfa Laval for the oil recovery from fish by-products was investigated. This process involves fish mincing, pumping of minced material to a heat exchanger where the fish oil is released and the proteins denaturated, centrifugation in a three-phase decanter, and collection of fish oil. It was used for upgrading by-products from salmon slaughtering [11]. The salmon oil obtained in this process was not rancid and according to the authors well suited for human consumption or usage. The same process was used for the extraction of herring oil from the by-products resulting from the production of maatjes herring [12].

1.1.3. Oil Recovery from The Washing Mince Process

Small fatty fish species represent a significant resource and their utilization for the production of fish minces or surimi has been considered as an alternative to fish meal production. However, the high fat content of these species constitute an important drawback, which led to the development of different approaches to remove fat. One of these processes was tried with capelin [13], which involved cutting the fish into small pieces, washing out the depot fat, dark pigments and viscera under acid (pH 4) or neutral conditions and heating at 40 – 45 °C and bone separation. The maximum release of lipids (*ca.* 80 % of total lipids) at pH 4 was obtained in approximately 60 min. The same amount of lipids was also removed after the same stirring period under neutral conditions when the temperature was adjusted to 40 – 45 °C. This process was also applied in the preparation of snipefish and boar-fish [14].

The process currently used in commercial plants to produce surimi from sardine is similar to the conventional one for lean fish species. However, it presents a difference in the leaching cycle, which involves a first washing step with a cold diluted alkaline solution (0.15 % NaCl, 0.2 % $NaHCO_3$ with an ionic strength of 0.05 and a final pH between 6.8 and 7.3) [15]. The material recovered from this washing step may be leached one or two times in water or 0.2-0.3 % NaCl. Hirata [16] described a method to recover fish oil from highly nutritional fish meat. In this process the sardine mince was ground with diluted alkaline solution (0.125 % $NaHCO_3$, 0.125 % NaCl, water/fish ratio 4:1). The slurry was centrifuged, water added to the floating oil layer resulting from centrifugation and heated up to 40 °C. The mixture was then centrifuged at 10,000xg and collected the oil released. According to the authors, this oil presented a light yellow colour and the amount of volatile compounds was much smaller than that of sardine oil prepared by conventional method at a fish meal plant.

In an alternative processing method to produce surimi from dark-fleshed fatty species [17], the fish muscle is disintegrated into very small particles prior to leaching. The particle reduction is carried out under vacuum to reduce lipid and protein oxidation and also to promote a ready separation of lipids. These authors also used a mixture of sodium pyrophosphate (0.05 – 0.1 %) and bicarbonate (0.1 %) as the leaching medium. The leaching process was done under vacuum, which facilitated the release of water-soluble compounds and lipids. Nishioka *et al.* [18] studied the effect of different vacuum levels, particle size and suction time at 5 mmHg on the fat removal from fish mince. The highest oil removal was achieved in the material with the finest particles (1 mm) at a pressure of 5 mmHg and after 20 min of suction time. The vacuum leaching permitted to remove fat more completely, rapidly and consistently than other methods [19]. Mendes *et al.* [20] reported that the use of vacuum leaching for short time periods was highly efficient and produced a 50 % decrease in fat content of European sardine washed mince when compared with the washing process at atmospheric pressure. The triacylglycerols were extracted the most [21] mainly at intermediate pressure values and increase washing periods. Polyunsaturated fatty acids were the major groups of fatty acids, mainly EPA and DHA, extracted at low pressure levels (4 mmHg) and increased periods of washing. The recovery of sardine by centrifugation of surimi wastewater was described [22]. The wastewater resulting from the surimi preparation was centrifuged continuously by two types of three-phase nozzle centrifuge at 8 – 15 °C and the oil phase was further dewatered by high-speed continuous centrifuge. The recovered oil showed light yellow colour and a peroxide value less than 1.0 meq/kg. The oil quality indicated that it could be directly used as food materials without further purification.

1.1.4. Oil Recovery from Acid and Alkaline Protein Solubilization

The application of acid and alkaline digestion methods for the extraction of oil from low oil content fish liver was early described in 1955 [23]. In this type of fish livers the oil is more closely held by the proteins and steaming methods traditionally used for oil extraction from livers with high oil content are not effective. An acid digestion method for oil extraction was reported [6], which is based on a patent by Van Deurs [24]. Later on an alkaline process for fish liver oil recovery was described [25], which intended to yield high vitamin potency oils. In a more recent patented method [26] for the protein recovery involving acid solubilization followed by protein precipitation it is claimed that neutral lipids are also separated during the process. These authors reporting the utilisation of this process to the recovery of proteins from mackerel light muscle referred that 97 % of the initial lipid content were removed [27]. A method for isolation edible protein from animal muscle by solubilizing the proteins in an alkaline aqueous solution was also described [28]. In this process it is claimed that neutral lipids can be separated from the aqueous phase by centrifugation. Kristinsson and Demir [29] using the acid- and alkali-aided processing to prepare protein isolates obtained higher lipid reduction than the conventional surimi processing. The lipid reduction depends on the fish species as well as on the processing alternatives followed in these methods. It was also referred [30] that acid and alkali processes led to a great reduction of membrane and neutral lipids in the protein isolate obtained, which clearly distinguishes from other available processes. In another work [31] was also achieved around 70 % reduction in neutral lipids and about 50 % reduction in membrane phospholipids in the recovery of proteins from herring light muscle by acid or alkaline solubilization processes. Hultin [32] reported that the oil released is richer in saturated fatty acids whereas most of the unsaturated membrane phospholipids are sedimented during centrifugation. Another oil extraction method for sardine (*Sardinops sagax*) involving pH adjustment was developed [33]. The pH of sardine muscle was adjusted to the isoelectric point (5.5) with either HCl or tartaric or citric acid (with and without calcium) followed by centrifugation. The highest oil recovery was achieved with citric acid plus calcium and the oil extracted showed the best quality and the highest □3 PUFA content. The oil extracted by pH adjustment was more stable against oxidation than the oil extracted by the traditional heat extraction method. The beneficial effect of calcium addition in terms of lipid oxidation stability and oil colour was also observed.

1.1.5. Solvent Oil Extraction

The production of fish protein concentrates (FPC) for human consumption requires the presence of very low oil content (below 1 %, frequently in the vicinity of 0.1 %) in order to make the product palatable for humans. The process of FPC production generally involved an oil extraction step with a solvent. Such as reported [34] this process could be done by employing a standard cycling of a solvent through homogenized fish or using a solvent in an azeotropic distillation-solvent extraction technique. The solvents most successfully used in conventional liquid extraction process are alcohols such as ethanol, propanol or isopropanol [35, 36, 37]. The two-step VioBin process [38] is an azeotropic extraction technique where the first extraction is done with ethylene dichloride and in the second extraction is used isopropanol. In general, organic solvent extraction is effective for lipid removal but it causes protein denaturation and loss of functional properties [39]. On the other hand, the production of FPC requires massive inputs of capital, energy, and expertise [40]. The quality of the recovered oil was not generally mentioned in the many works published on the preparation of FPC because proteins were the main objective. However, it was referred [6] that the oil recovered by solvent extraction was darker than that produced by the wet reduction process and was pointed out [34] that oil recovered in the second extraction in the VioBin process is highly polymerized.

1.1.6. Enzymatic Methods for Oil Recovery

The enzymatic oil extraction from the starting material (whole fish or parts) using food-grade proteases has been indicated as an alternative method because it takes place at moderate temperatures and for a short duration, thus limiting the negative chemical changes occurring in fatty acids during oil recovery by the traditional methods. Proteases are used to disrupt tissues and cell membranes leading to the release of oil.

One of the earliest references to the utilization of enzymatic hydrolysis for oil extraction dates back to the 1930's [41]. The hydrolysis was done with pepsin at pH between 1.2 and 1.5 followed by an alkaline digestion at approximately pH 9. This process was considered advantageous because it minimized the difficulty of separating the oil from the emulsion formed during the alkaline digestion and reduced the oil acidity due to the inactivation of lipases. However, the need of suitable equipment, of process control and the relatively high costs involved were pointed out as the main disadvantages of the method [23]. Bailey [42] also used proteolytic enzymes under acid conditions to release oil from fish livers with low oil content. The process reduced the oil hydrolysis by lipases and emulsification and allowed to higher oil recovery.

Fish ensiling is a preservation technique first developed in the Nordic countries [43]. In this process the fish liquefaction is due to the activity of endogenous proteases, mainly present in the digestive organs. This autolytic process permitted the oil release, which is removed by centrifugation after heating the autolysate to facilitate oil separation from sludge and dissolved matter [44]. However, it was concluded [45] that the oil recovered from acid medium results in high free fatty acid (FFA) values due to the dissociation of fatty acids salts and breakdown of the oil by a low pH optimum lipase present in some fish species. Moreover, the oil from fish silage is very dark and presents a reduced iodine value [43]. The pigmentation of the oil during ensiling was shown to be caused by the release of haemin, a product resulting from acid hydrolysis of haemoglobin [46]. This author also showed that a 2 % addition of 20 volume hydrogen peroxide inhibit oil pigmentation and reduced FFA content in the recovered oil.

A method to prepare fish muscle tissue with very low lipid content based on the autolysis of skin and belly line was patented [47]. In this process chopped fish is suspended in acidified water which is slowly heated and gently stirred. According to the authors, skin and belly line dissolve completely and the oil released floats to the surface. The enzymic hydrolysis of salmon frames was studied [48] using the commercial protease mixture Protamex^{TM}, which has been referred to produce non-bitter hydrolysates. The authors recovered approximately 77 % of total lipids present in the salmon frames, which had 9.3 % EPA and 11.3 % DHA.

The use of enzymatic extraction of fish oil from by-products by Linder *et al.* [49] was patented. These authors [50] also reported the application of three commercial proteases (Alcalase®, Neutrase®, and Flavourzyme™) to extract the oil from salmon heads under mild conditions (below 55 ºC). The amount of oil released after two hours of hydrolysis was about 17 % regardless of the enzyme used and was close (20 %) to that obtained by the Bligh and Dyer method [51].

With the objective of obtaining the highest possible amount of valuable products from farmed cod by-products (backbones and liver), it was studied the effect of different hydrolysis conditions on the yield, functional properties and lipid distribution in the various fractions obtained [52]. The enzymatic hydrolysis was performed with Alcalase and it was concluded that centrifugation forces were important for separation of oily fractions, but not to separate the protein fractions. The results indicated that a two step separation process could be designed, one using low centrifugation speed and a second step at high speed centrifugation to separate oil and emulsion. The major lipid class in the oil and emulsion fractions was triacylglycerols, while phospholipids were found mostly in the protein containing fractions (protein hydrolysate and sludge).

The utilization of various proteases (papain, chymotrypsin, Protamex™, and Flavourzyme®) for the fat extraction of cod by-products (head, backbones, viscera, roes, milt, skin, and cut-offs) was reported in another work [53]. The authors concluded that the use of proteolytic enzymes had generally enhanced the fat extraction, particularly phospholipids.

A number of papers were published in 2005 on the preparation of protein hydrolysates from cod by-products. Thus, it was obtained [54] the highest lipid recovery in the enzymatic hydrolysis (with Flavourzyme or Neutrase) cod by-products when water was not added. The amount of oil fraction obtained with Neutrase was up to 10 % higher compared to Flavourzyme. Similarly, using the same type of raw material and the same enzymes obtained higher oil recovery in the trials without addition of water [55]. They also obtained higher amount of oil released in autolysates with added water than in hydrolysates prepared with commercial enzymes. The highest yields of oil fraction were also obtained in the hydrolysates where Neutrase was used. The presence of digestive tract in the raw material increased the amount of free fatty acids and gave darker colours. The oil fraction contained mostly triacylglycerols and monounsaturated fatty acids. In a last paper [56], was concluded that initial heating of cod by-products causes formation of protein-lipid complexes, which were found in all protein containing fractions being phospholipids and other polar lipids the main part of lipids. The highest amount of separated oil was obtained in the experiments without added water and after initial heating. It was also concluded that the maximum oil and protein hydrolysate yield and the minimum emulsion and sludge yield were achieved in the hydrolysis of unheated raw material with Alcalase and water added.

In another work [57] was reported the use of commercial proteases to extract oil from salmon heads. The oil recovery by the enzymatic method attained 19.6 % whereas the heat treatment led to 14.5 % and the oil released had about 35 % of polyunsaturated fatty acids (PUFA) (7.7 % EPA and 11.9 % DHA). Industrial proteases were also used by Dumay *et al.* [58] to improve lipid and phospholipid recovery from European sardine viscera. The total lipid content in the oily phase and aqueous phases represented 85 % of lipids presented in the raw material indicating that wide-spectrum proteases enhance lipid recovery. It was also concluded that a pre-hydrolysis step led to an increase of total lipids content when compared with the classic organic solvent extraction methods. In another study [59] on the oil recovery from sardine by-products the highest percentage of oil recovery was obtained from the raw by-products sing Alcalase or Protamex. The latter protease was tested in the hydrolysis of black scabbardfish (*Aphanopus carbo*) [60]. About 36 % of oil was released and 50 - 60 % remained in and emulsion.

1.1.7. Supercritical Fluid Extraction

The specificity of physicochemical properties of supercritical fluids led to the development of a new process for the extraction of different substances. Supercritical fluids behave as intermediates between liquid and gases, which allow them to dissolving large quantities of natural substances. Such as mentioned [61], the relatively high gas density gives good solvent power, while the relatively low viscosity and high diffusivity provide appreciably higher gas permeability into the solute matrix. Several advantages have been pointed out to this process: (i) gentle treatment of heat-sensitive materials, (ii) solvent-free products covering all legal requirements, (iii) fragrances and aromas remain unchanged, (iv) selective extraction and fractionated separation, and (v) simple solvent recovery. The supercritical fluid extraction (SFE) technique was tested to extract oil from oilseeds and later on for removing lipids from fish muscle proteins. In 1984, Eisenbach [62] reported the effectiveness of the SFE process for fractionating fish oil esters. This technique was also studied for the concentration of n-3 fatty acids [63-69]. The use of this technique for the oil extraction and concentration of n-3-PUFA from fish oil was reviewed [70-73].

The coupled process allowed keeping a high solvent power for SFE-CO2 and also reaching high selectivity levels due to the filtration of supercritical mixtures through a nanofiltration membrane. It was also stated that the coupled separation permitted the concentration of EPA and DHA in the retentate stream and short-chained fatty acids in the permeate.

The supercritical extraction technique has been also used for oil extraction directly from fish muscle although less extensively. This methodology was tested for the removal of lipids from freeze-dried Antarctic krill [74]. As working conditions they used a pressure of 25 MPa at 40 °C, 60 °C and 80 °C. The oil recovered was composed solely by nonpolar lipids, largely triglycerides and presented a relatively high proportion of EPA (11 %). SFE-CO_2 at 4.9 – 24.5 MPa and 40 °C was applied to the lipid extraction of freeze-dried mackerel (*Scomber japonicus*) powder [75]. The yield achieved in the oil extraction increased with pressure and was comparable to that from hot hexane extraction.

The application of SFE-CO_2 for lipid and cholesterol extraction from rainbow trout muscle allow to concluding that: (i) the increase of oil removal with increasing the extraction time from 3 h to 9 h; (ii) the use of ethanol as an entrainer significantly enhanced lipid extraction attaining 97 % but coextraction of polar lipids occurred [61].

This technique was used for the oil removal from freeze-dried Atlantic mackerel (*Scomber scombrus*) muscle [76]. These authors optimized the extraction temperature and pressure. The highest oil yield and concentration of n-3 PUFA was achieved for the temperature range between 35 °C and 55 °C and pressure in the interval 20.7 MPa and 34.5 MPa. According to these authors the high lipid removal and retention of protein functionality in the residue may make this technique useful for future food applications.

This technique was used for the extraction of sardine (*Sardina pilchardus*) oil from freeze-dried muscle [77, 78]. The extraction experiments were done under pressures of 12.6 to 108.0 MPa and temperatures ranging from 40 °C to 48 °C. The loading of sardine oil in

CO_2 (kg oil/kg CO_2) increased with increasing pressure, but diminished with increasing temperature. A slight increase in PUFA content of the oil extracted by SFE-CO_2 was observed throughout the extraction.

In a study [79] on the SFE-CO_2 lipid extraction from freeze-dried salmon roe was found that triacylglycerols were not completely extracted and phospholipids PLs not at all. However, the SFE-CO_2 with 10, 15 or 20 % of ethanol as an entrainer was effective in extracting PLs from the above raw material [80]. These authors reported that the extraction with SFE-CO_2 and 20 % ethanol mixture allowed to extracting more than 80 % of the PLs.

The previously reported studies were done in dried fish samples but moisture of the materials may interfere with SFE-CO_2 extraction [81]. Thus, the effect of moisture content on the SFE-CO_2 extractability of oil from Atlantic mackerel was studied [82]. They reported that dehydration of the muscle to 10.2 % (w/w) resulted in high oil yield with minimum changes in protein content and composition.

A mathematical model based on the interaction between oil and water in the fluid phase was developed [83]. This study was done in Atlantic mackerel fillets with different moisture levels prior to extraction at 35 °C and 34.5 MPa. The model developed simulated the extraction behaviour of both oil and water in the initial solubility-controlled region.

The SFE-CO_2 conditions of sardine oil extraction from canning by-products was optimized by Létisse *et al.* [84]. The optimal conditions for pressure, temperature and CO_2 rate were, respectively, 300 bar, 75 °C and 2.5 ml/min during 45 min extraction. The yield of 10.36 % of extracted oil was achieved with an amount of 10.95 % of EPA and 13.01 % of DHA. According to these authors, this technique presented the advantages of a shorter extraction time, prevention of heating and a better organoleptic aspect of the oil by excluding the use of not legally allowed organic solvents.

The extraction of phospholipids from tuna shavings by SFE-CO_2/ethanol was also tried [85]. It was performed at 17.7 MPa and 33 °C and ethanol concentrations higher than 5 % were used. In order to reduce the amount of consumed ethanol in the process, the tuna shavings were previously soaked in the same volume of ethanol before extraction with neat SFE-CO_2. The extraction was done both at laboratorial and industrial scale and it was concluded that the amount of consumed CO_2 per g tuna shavings decreased with increase in reactor-scale.

This technique was applied to the extraction of squalene from shark liver oil containing around 50 % squalene. Squalene of 95 % purity was obtained without using external reflux [86]. However, the purity could be increased to a maximum of 99 % at fractionation conditions of 250 bar and 60 °C and using reflux of squalene. The extraction and fractionation of a range of crude fish oils (orange roughy oil, deep sea shark and spiny dogfish liver oil and commercial cod liver) using SFE-CO_2 and CO_2+ethanol mixtures was reported [87].

The use of extremely high pressures and high capital costs have been the main disadvantages pointed out [88], which may limit the widespread use of supercritical fluid technique for the oil extraction or PUFA concentration.

2. Oil Refining Process

The composition and characteristics of crude fish oils depend very much on process and raw material (Table 1). This intermediate product contains a wide range of undesirable compounds, which have to be removed to make the oil meet the quality standards in regard to the obligatory properties for edible or technical applications [89]. Thus, the quality of raw material has to fit the adequate requirements [90] and the process has to be done in a way that essential fish oil components are not being damaged, e.g. polymerisation should be avoided. Within intrinsic materials, small amounts of proteins, water, pigments, free fatty acids (FFAs), phospholipids, and lipid oxidation products are the most significant. Trace components related to environmental pollutants can also be present.

Table 1. Crude fish oil properties and physical characteristics (Adapted from [90])

Properties	
Moisture and impurities	Usually 0.5 up to 1 %
FAs	Range 1-7 % oleic acid (usually 2-5)
Peroxide value	3-20 meq O_2/kg
Anisidine value	4-60
Totox value	10-60
Iodine value	Capelin (95-160); Herring (115-160); Menhaden (120-200); Sardine (160-200); Anchovy (180-200)
Iron	0.5-7.0 mg/kg
Copper	Less than 0.3 mg/kg
Phosphorus	5-100 mg/kg
Physical characteristics	
Colour (Gardner scale)	Up to 14
Slip melting point	10-15 °C
Boiling point	Greater than 250 °C
Specific gravity	About 0.92 (at 15 °C),
Viscosity	About 60-90 cp (at 20 °C), 20-30 cp (at 50 °C), 10cp (at 90 °C)

The common oil refining is usually made by chemical methods, which include namely settling, and degumming, de-acidification, bleaching, deodorization, and storage and antioxidant addition. In the frame of this purpose hydrogenation is not included.

Settling is made with or without heating, allowing the aqueous phase separation, which is further withdrawn, and in such way part of water, proteinaceous material and phospholipids are purged. Degumming, considered in some circumstances an optional stage, consists of a treatment with water or aqueous solutions of acids or salts (at 30 – 100 °C) to remove soluble and insoluble impurities that are then separated either by centrifugation or decantation. De-acidification or alkali refining is typically performed with an aqueous alkaline solution to remove FFAs and reduce oil acidity. In addition to the use of alkali substances, supercritical fluid technology, jointly with membrane and enzymatic processes, and thin film deodorisation technologies may be alternatives to the classical procedure [91, 92]. The oil is then heated to 80-85°C and mixed with an activated bleaching clay and/or activated carbon. Sulphurous compounds, soaps, trace metals, and part of the most stable pigments and pigment-breakdown products are separated. Physical adsorption on activated carbon is necessary when the removal of organic contaminants such as dioxins/furans and dioxin-like PCBs is required [93, 94]. This step also converts hydroperoxides to their respective aldehydes, ketones and other products [95].

The deodorisation step, intended to remove FFAs, aldehydes and ketones, which give unpleasant smell and flavour characteristics to the oil, is conventionally based on the application of high temperatures [96, 97]. The volatile materials are stripped by means of a stripping gas, normally steam at high temperature (190-200 ºC) and low pressure (2-5 mbar). However, the application of such temperatures has to be carefully considered since for temperatures higher than 180 ºC the degradation of n-3 PUFA take place, involving the formation of polymers, isomers, cyclic FAs monomers and other undesirable compounds [98]. Optional methods, such as vacuum steam distillation at low temperatures followed by a treatment in a silica gel column [99], adsorption with a resin [100], or treatment with diatomaceous earth [101] have been considered.

After leaving the deodoriser equipment and be cooled, the fish oil is dosed with the suitable amounts of selected antioxidant(s) and then transferred to appropriate storage tanks; preferably, stainless steel tanks under nitrogen blanketing and at low temperature. To avoid oxidation, improve the stability and extend the fish oil shelf-life, a great number of antioxidants (natural and synthetic compounds) have been proposed [102, 103, 104]. The adequate concentration of antioxidant depends on the chosen substance, the storage conditions and the intended applications. The oxidation of fish oils may also be delayed by encapsulation or microencapsulation with a coating material [105]. For this purpose, various physical and chemical processes using several wall materials have been developed [106], being spray-drying the most common and cheaper method [107]. Other processes such as freeze drying [108], ultrasonic atomization [109] or coacervation [110] have also been proposed recently as alternative to reduce n-3 PUFA oxidation. Oil-in-water emulsions are increasingly being used as delivery systems for fish oils for functional foods. If properly designed such emulsions can protect the fish oil from lipid oxidation before the addition to foods [111, 112] and in some cases it may also improve the oxidative stability of the fish oil enriched food [113].

2.1. Characteristics of Refined Fish Oils

The chemical and physical characteristics of refined fish, which are influenced by the refining process itself and by the raw material, are quite variable and influence the potential uses and price. Based on information disseminated by [95, 114, 115] and the Codex Standard (1981) some guidelines are given in Table 2.

Table 2. Some quality guidelines for refined fish oils [95, 114, 115]

Parameter	Quality guidelines
Colour	<3.0 Red, 30 Yellow
Odour and taste	Bland
Matter volatile at 105°C	<0.2 %
Insoluble impurities	<0.05 %
Soap content	<0.005 %
Iron	<0.12 mg/kg
Free FAs	<0.10 % (as oleic acid)
Copper	<0.05 mg/kg
Peroxide value	<0.1 meq O_2/kg
Nickel	<0.20 mg/kg

3. n-3 PUFA Concentrates

The preparation of n-3 PUFA concentrates usually comprises five steps: de-acidification (optional), transesterification, concentration, deodorisation/earth treatment, and antioxidant addition and fill off. The raw material must have previously undergone a meticulous refining process, including the removal of contaminants [92]. These concentrates may be in different forms: FFAs, methyl and ethyl esters or acylglycerols.

De-acidification is typically the first step, when such operation was not included in the refining strategy. For the most common industrial process, transesterification is the following step, which may be carried out by a chemical catalyst (usually sodium ethoxide at 80-90 °C) or by non-selective lipases [88, 92, 116]. For concentration numerous methods have been anticipated, but only a few are suitable for large-scale production, being the most widespread process the concentration of n-3 PUFA by molecular distillation. Other available methods less frequently used include: adsorption or partitioning chromatography, enzymatic splitting, low-temperature crystallization, supercritical fluid extraction, and urea complexation. Each methodology has its own advantages and drawbacks, and all present important shortcomings that limit their use by the industry. The decision for one specific technology or the combination of two or more must depend on the required final characteristics of n-3 PUFA concentrates and on the costs associated to each choice.

Fractional distillation has been extensively used for partial separation of mixtures of fatty acid esters. Separation is done by asset of their different boiling points. The method applies lower temperatures and shorter heating intervals than conventional distillation methods. Moreover, the use of high vacuum is very common with temperatures ranging from 100-200 °C typically being used during processing in order to minimise heat damage to the oils. Nevertheless, fractionation of marine oil esters has some problems; namely, separation of components becomes less effective with increasing molecular weight, as happens with n-3 PUFA. Moreover, concentration in the natural TAG form (without previous transesterification) presents very important practical difficulties [117].

Adsorption chromatography is based on the potential of some appropriate adsorbents to separate fatty acids (FAs) according to their carbon number or degree of unsaturation. High performance liquid chromatography [118] and silver resin chromatography [119] have been used for the production of n-3 PUFA concentrates. Counter current chromatography and centrifugal partition chromatography have gained much attention in last two decades for isolation of PUFA [120]. In what concerns enzymatic methods, lipases are utilized to catalyze esterification, hydrolysis or exchange of FAs in esters [121]. Accordingly, this technology may enable the performance of the transesterification and concentration phases in a single step. The direction and efficiency of the reaction can be influenced by the choice of experimental conditions and the source of lipase [122]. Low-temperature crystallization is based on the fact that solubility of fats in organic solvents decreases with increasing molecular weight and increases with higher levels of unsaturation [123]. Consequently, at low temperature, long chain saturated FAs which have higher melting points crystallize out and n-3 PUFA remain in the liquid fraction. The low-temperature crystallization process may be carried out in the absence of a solvent or in a selected solvent mixture [88]. The frequently used solvents are methanol and acetone, which pose problems in products for human consumption. Crystallization in the absence of a solvent occurs by using the Tirtiaux process, which involves slow cooling and slow agitation, and in the hydrophilisation process. SFE-CO_2 is another alternative method for the preparation of n-3 PUFA concentrates [70]. SFE-CO_2 fractionation of fish oil fatty acid ethyl esters was investigated to obtaining enriched n-3 PUFA and a suitable EPA/DHA ratio [72]. The results obtained by these authors indicated that optimizing the extraction conditions could modify the original fatty acid ethyl esters concentrations.

Coupled SFE-CO_2 with nanofiltration separation was used for the concentration of PUFA [73]. Urea complexation by itself or complexation after an enzymatic reaction offers important technical possibilities [49, 124, 125, 126, 127]. This methodology is based on the crystallization of urea in hexagonal structures within the hexagonal crystals, provided the presence of long straight-chain molecules in the medium [128]. The formed channels are sufficiently large to accommodate aliphatic chains. However, whereas straight-chain saturated FAs fit easily in the channels, the presence of double bonds in the carbon chain increases the bulk of the molecule, thereby reducing the likelihood of its complexation with urea [129]. FAs must be previously converted to free FAs (FFAs) or ethyl esters. These forms of the FAs are mixed with an ethanolic solution of urea with some moderate heating. Afterwards, the mixture is allowed to cool down to a particular temperature, depending on the degree of concentration desired [88]. The saturated, monounsaturated and, to a lesser extent, the dienoic FAs are crystallized with urea and the other FAs remain non-crystallized in the solution, being separated by filtration. Among these, a high concentration of n-3 PUFA is found.

Having in mind that concentration may lead to the formation of small amounts of off-odours and leave trace amounts of some impurities, a thorough deodorisation/purification (removal of impurities) process of the oil may be carried out. For this purpose, the concentrated material is heated to 80-85 °C and mixed with an activated bleaching clay and/or activated carbon. The bleaching clay removes any oxidation products which may be present in the oil along with heavy metals. The addition of activated carbon is required when the removal of organic contaminants such as dioxins/furans and dioxin-like PCB's is still necessary. Another possibility is to promote the contact with powdered or granulated diatomaceous earth [130].

Then, the concentrates have to be stored and stabilized by using similar procedures to those described previously for the refined fish oils.

3.1. Characteristics of N-3 PUFA Concentrates

The intensive use of n-3 PUFA concentrates for human health and well-being purposes obliges their characteristics to fulfil a high number of requirements. Thus, all the processing steps must reduce exposure to factors that accelerate oxidation, such as heat, intense light or oxygen. Peroxide values must be kept low throughout all the concentration process. The levels of off-flavours and impurities must be below human sensory perception [92. FFAs must be limited to a minimum because hydrolysis and acidity represent a major loss of quality for n-3 PUFA concentrates. According to the GRAS notifications, concerning food-grade specifications accepted by FDA for different omega-3 concentrates, some quality guideline can be viewed in Table 3 [131, 132].

The form in which concentrates are present is of utmost importance. Effectively, some studies have reported that n-3 PUFA concentrates are better absorbed by human organism and more stable against oxidation when they are in triacylglycerols (TAGs) form than as esters [133, 134]. Moreover, stability is also higher when n-3 PUFA are bound to *sn*-2 position of the glycerol structure than to the *sn*-1,3 position [135]. Therefore, the production of TAGs concentrates with n-3 PUFA in *sn*-2 position and the development of viable technological solutions for this purpose have been acknowledged as a wishful outcome [92].

Table 3. Some quality guidelines for omega-3 FAs concentrates [131, 132].(FDA GRAS Notification 2002; 2006)

Parameter	Quality guidelines
Appearance	Light yellow to yellow at room temperature
Triglycerides	>50 %
Odour and taste	At worst, a slightly fishy odour and taste
Acid value	<1.0 %
Peroxide value	<2.5 meq O_2/kg
p-Anisidine value	<20
Totox value	<25
Density	0.85-1.00 g/ml
Tocopherols	>2.0 mg/g
Moisture	<0.1 %
Unsaponifiables	<2.35 %

4. Structured Triacylglycerols

Most of TAGs found in fish oils has a LLL-type structure, which symbolizes three long-chain fatty acids (LCFAs) (16 or more carbon atoms) esterified in the three carbon atoms in the glycerol backbone (named *sn*-1, *sn*-2 and *sn*-3). Once ingested, dietary TAGs are hydrolyzed in the small intestine to *sn*-2 monoacylglycerols (*sn*-2 MAGs) and FFAs released from the *sn*-1,3 positions of the original TAGs due to the action of the human pancreatic lipase, which is *sn*-1,3 specific [136] (Fig. 4).

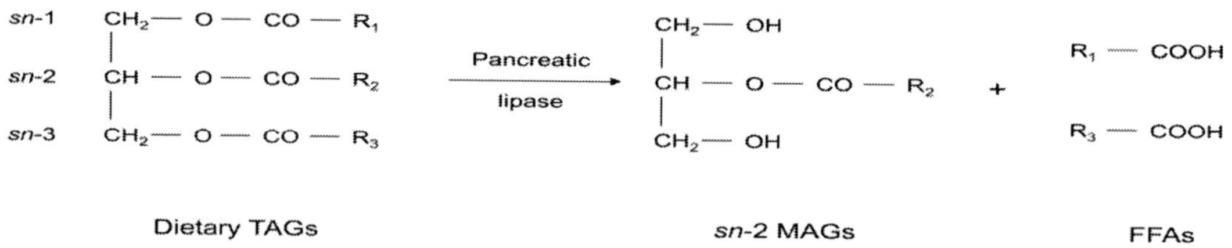

Figure 4. Enzymatic hydrolysis of dietary TAGs by pancreatic lipase. Hydrocarbon chains of FAs esterified in *sn*-1, *sn*-2 and *sn*-3 are represented by R_1, R_2 and R_3 respectively.

Sn-2 MAGs are the most favorable structure for LCFAs to be absorbed by the intestinal mucosa. Thus, allowing these FAs to be used in biosynthetic processes [137]. On the other hand, LCFAs released from *sn*-1 and *sn*-3 positions are mainly transported to the large intestine to form calcium soaps, which are removed with stools. This way, the metabolic use of these FAs is usually impaired.

The hydrolytic activity of pancreatic lipase is higher towards medium-chain FAs (MCFAs) (from 8 to 14 carbon atoms) than for LCFAs, especially PUFA [138]. Therefore, a structured triacylglycerols (STAGs) having a MLM structure (in which "M" refers to a MCFA esterified in *sn*-1,3 positions of the glycerol backbone and "L" refers to a LCFA esterified in *sn*-2 position) offer the most favorable case for the metabolic bioavailability of LCPUFAs, and also is a suitable source of MCFAs, which are transported to the liver to be used as a quick energy source; thus, improved absorption of MLM-type TAGs has been reported [139, 140]. Unfortunately, no natural sources containing MLM-TAGs have been found until now. However, MLM-TAGs can be achieved by means of chemical or enzymatic reactions.

STAGs, generally named structured lipids (SLs), are synthesized molecules, where MCFAs and LCFAs are esterified in the three carbons in the glycerol backbone. MLM-STAGs can be used with alimentary or pharmaceutical purposes. The most employed MCFAs for the STAG synthesis are caprylic acid (8:0) and capric acid (10:0) [141-144]. Most of the experimental designs to obtain STAGs are based in enzymatic reactions, due to its several advantages when compared with chemical synthesis, such as mild reaction conditions, more biocompatible and safer operative procedures, and the possibility of a more effective control of the FA positional distribution in the final product, due to the use of regiospecific enzymes.

Fish oil constitutes a raw material for STAGs synthesis due to its high content in n-3 PUFA mainly EPA and DHA. The properties of both n-3 PUFAs in the treatment and prevention of a number of pathologies such as coronary heart disease, retinal and brain development, hypertension, rheumatoid arthritis and some types of cancers has been widely reported [145, 146]. Although EPA and DHA are reported to be mainly located in the *sn*-1,3 positions of TAGs of marine mammals, they are usually located in the *sn*-2 position in the TAGs of fish oil [140]. This way, fish oil is a suitable source to be used as a starting material in the synthesis of STAGs containing EPA and DHA in *sn*-2 position. In addition, fish oil has a competitive price compared to other *sn*-2 PUFA rich oils, as single cell oils from algae. Moreover, it seems to be an appropriate way to add value to the by-products generated in the fishery industry.

4.1. Enzymatic Synthesis of Stags

The synthesis of STAGs containing n-3 PUFA located in the *sn*-2 position, like EPA or DHA, and MCFAs in *sn*-1,3 positions, have received increasing attention in the last years. Thus, as explained above, PUFAs from STAGs can be directly absorbed as *sn*-2 MAGs after lipase pancreatic digestion, resulting in increasing absorption rates and becoming in a target product for alimentary and pharmaceutical industry.

The designing of STAGs with a particular structure requires specific modifications at the desired positions in the glycerol backbone [142]. Although some commercial STAGs have been produced by chemical methods [147], the random nature of the reactions usually limits the possibilities of such procedures. In contrast, the use of *sn*-1,3 regioespecific lipases allows to a positionally specific modification of TAGs. Lipases belong to the hydrolase family, although their physiologic role is the AG hydrolysis, can also operate "in reverse" under low water activity conditions, synthesizing an ester bond. This property has been widely exploited in the production of STAGs, allowing the catalysis of different types of reactions such as interesterification, acydolysis, alcoholisis or esterification (Fig. 5).

$$R_1COOR_2 + H_2O \xrightarrow{\text{Hydrolysis}} R_1COOH + R_2OH$$

$$R_1COOH + R_2OH \xrightarrow{\text{Esterification}} R_1COOR_2 + H_2O$$

$$R_1COOR_2 + R_3COOR_4 \xrightarrow{\text{Interesterification}} R_3COOR_2 + R_1COOR_4$$

$$R_1COOR_2 + R_3COOH \xrightarrow{\text{Acidolysis}} R_3COOR_2 + R_1COOH$$

$$R_1COOR_2 + R_3OH \xrightarrow{\text{Alcoholysis}} R_1COOR_3 + R_2OH$$

Figure 5. Different reactions catalyzed by lipases (adapted from Houde et al. [148]).

Actually, there is a wide supply of regioespecific lipases which show specificity for one or more individual FAs and also present different degrees of regioespecifity. Immobilization supports modify lipase properties, confer thermostability and allow an easy recovery of the biocatalyst, but can also influence a non-desired process of acyl-migration [149], so the choice of a suitable lipase becomes in a great importance step in the design of a STAG synthesis reaction. These processes can be composed of one or more reactions:

4.1.1. One-Step Processes

Interesterification reaction is indeed an ester exchange where FAs from different TAGs are relocated. Thus, employing a *sn*-1,3 regiospecific lipase, FAs in the extreme positions of the glycerol backbone of an *sn*-2 PUFA rich oil can be replaced by a MCFA, resulting in a mixture of MLM-type STAGs. This kind of reaction has been employed by Xu and coworkers [150], who obtained different products by interesterification of fish oil and a caprylic and capric acid mixture of TAGs, although a percentage of the original PUFAs remained at *sn*-1,3 positions (3.7% of EPA+DHA from total FAs in *sn*-1,3 position).

Acydolisis has been commonly applied looking for a modification of fish oil. In this process, the acyl exchange takes places between an ester and a FA. With this objective, a wide number of works have been reported. Shimada et al. [151] achieved a modified tuna oil with nearly 45% incorporation of caprylic acid mainly located in *sn*-1,3 position (0.5% mol of total FAs in *sn*-2 position) and 14.5% of EPA+DHA in *sn*-2 position, although DHA bounded at *sn*-1,3 position was not exchanged. Similar results were obtained by Zhou et al. [152], who reported a 45.2% incorporation of caprylic acid. Hita el al. [149] indicates an increase in caprylic acid incorporation up to 56% and 26.7% mol EPA+DHA of total FAs in *sn*-2 position when acidolysis of tuna oil was performed, parallel to an increase in the caprylic acid content in *sn*-2 position. Results were improved in a later work [137], when acidolysis of tuna oil in a continuous mode was performed. A 39.3% incorporation of caprylic acid and 42.1% mol of DHA of total *sn*-2 FAs was achieved with an optimal distribution.

4.1.2 Two-Step Processes

In order to obtain high purity MLM-STAGs from fish oil, two-step enzymatic methods have been developed, involving *sn*-2 MAG production by alcoholysis prior to the final esterification step.

Alcoholysis has been applied by Schmid et al. [153] to different fish oils, performing MAGs with 70% (EPA+DHA), 75% (EPA+DHA) and 50% (EPA) PUFAs. The controversial issue of this method is that purification procedures developed to purify *sn*-2 MAGs used could produce acyl-migration processes.

Muñío et al. [154] reported the production and purification of *sn*-2 MAGs from tuna oil, obtaining a purified fraction of MAGs with 31.8% EPA+DHA, but no regiospecific data were provided. By applying solvent extraction to purify *sn*-2 MAGs, and later an esterification reaction with caprylic acid, acyl-migration seems to be avoided, since PUFA content in *sn*-2 position of STAGs agrees with PUFA content in MAGs, resulting in 39.9% of EPA+DHA of total FAs in *sn*-2 position and 64% incorporation of caprylic acid [155].

Irimescu et al. [156] developed a method for the synthesis of STAG involving ethanolysis of bonito oil and a reesterification of *sn*-2 MAGs with ethyl caprylate. They achieved a final STAG mixture: 85.3% STAGs with two caprylic acid residues, 13% with two original FA residues and 1.7% of tricapryloylglycerol. The calculated 1,3-dicapryloyl-2-docosahexaenoylglycerol to 1,2(2,3)-dicapryloyl-3(1)-docosahexaenoylglycerol ratio was greater than 50:1, showing a good regiospecifity in the whole method.

4.2. Stags Quality and Safety

Lipid oxidation is one of the major causes of quality deterioration in lipid-containing foods. Despite their health benefits, all oils containing PUFA are highly susceptible to rapid oxidative deterioration and thus experience problems with storage stability [157]. Therefore, is important to prevent oxidation of any edible oil and foods that contain them in order to maintain their quality and safety.

Oxidation of oils may be initiated by light, heat, and in the presence of metal ions. Oil oxidation occurs via a free-radical chain reaction mechanism involving initiation, propagation, and termination steps [158]. Oxidative deterioration of edible oils involves autoxidation accompanied by both oxidative and nonoxidative reactions [159]. The oxidation products from oils, which include hydroperoxides, decompose to produce a variety of volatile compounds that result in off-flavor and offodor in oils [160].

Peroxidation can be measured by a great number of methods, which include oxygen consumption of PUFAs, lipid hydroperoxide formation, thiobarbituric acid (TBA) trials of malonaldehyde (MDA), gas chromatography/mass spectrometry (GC/MS) of volatile compounds and sensory evolution, and diene conjugation [161].

Rancidity of lipids can be retarded by several procedures. Among them, phenolic compounds, such as butylated hydroxyanisole (BHA), butylated hydroxytoluene (BHT) and organic esters of gallic acid (gallates) have been widely used as antioxidants in foods containing oils [159].

Several authors discuss the oxidizability of STAGs. The most interesting results among literature are shown below. The oxidative stability of STAGs based on γ-linolenic acid (18:*3n*-6; GLA)-rich borage oil (BO) and evening primrose oil (EPO), modified with DHA was compared with unmodified borago oil and evening primrose oil as controls [160]. It was probed that STAGs gave rise to higher quantities of conjugated dienes, TBARS, and headspace volatiles as compared to their unmodified counterparts, and results indicated that modified oils were less stable than their unmodified counterparts.

Other work about STAGs pointed in the same direction. This way, after the incorporation of capric acid (CA) into the DHA single cell oil DHASCO, the oxidative stability of the modified DHASCO in comparison with the original DHASCO, as indicated in the conjugated diene values, showed that the unmodified oil remained relatively unchanged during storage for 72 h, but DHASCO-based structured lipid was oxidized to a much higher level than the original oil. It was argued that removal of antioxidants during the process is primarily responsible for the compromised stability of the modified oil [162].

Other studies about STAGs made for infant milk formulation founded that the oxidative stability index, after purification by distillation and addition of antioxidants, was similar between STAGs and the starting oil blends, and also that oxidative stability of the STAGs can be improved with tocopherol addition as antioxidants [163].

After the literature, and taking into account that STAGs may contain FAs with a high degree of unsaturation, to prevent its oxidation it seems advisable to keep the maximum precautions that are usual for PUFAs: the addition of antioxidants, the performing enzymatic synthesis processes in an inert atmosphere, and its preservation at low temperatures.

To conclude STAGs having MLM structure is the best source of *sn*-2 MAGs, which are the most favorable structure for LCFAs, allowing these to be used in biosynthetic processes. Unfortunately, no natural sources containing MLM have been found until now. However, MLM-TAGs can be achieved by means of chemical or enzymatic reactions.

Although some commercial STAGs have been produced by chemical methods, the random nature of the reactions usually limits the possibilities of such procedures. In contrast, the use of *sn*-1,3 regioespecific lipases allows to a positionally specific modification of TAGs. These processes can be composed of one or more reactions. Among one-step processes, acydolisis has been commonly applied looking for a modification of fish oil, while for two-step processes ethanolysis of bonito oil and a reesterification of the obtained *sn*-2 MAGs with ethyl caprylate showed good results.

Considering that STAGs may contain FAs with a high degree of unsaturation, to prevent its oxidation it seems advisable to keep the maximum precautions that are usual for PUFAs.

5. Fish Oil Health Benefits

Epidemiological studies later confirmed that the marine oil consumed by the Inuit population rich in EPA and DHA, was directly correlated with a cardioprotective role on the risk of cardiovascular disease in healthy individuals [164-168]. Over the years the number of studies in this area has increased, emphasizing the importance of fish oil consumption mainly supported by two important intervention studies that found a cardioprotective effect of these n-3 PUFA, the DART and GISSI studies: (i) DART - Diet and reinfarction trial: a secondary prevention study in which male individuals who had previously suffered a myocardial infarction, ingested over 2 years fish oil capsules, results showed a 29% reduction in overall mortality, and a 33% decrease of deaths caused by heart disease [169]; (ii) The GISSI-Gruppo Italiano per Studio della Sopravvivenza nell it 'miocardico infarction –a secondary prevention study with 11,324 patients surviving a myocardial infarction, receiving for 42 months fish oil capsules with 850 mg of EPA + DHA/day. Results pointed out that there was a 15% reduction in death from heart attack or stroke. The overall mortality decreased 21% and sudden death caused by heart disease decreased 45% [170]. Among the possible mechanisms of intake of n-3 PUFA in reducing cardiovascular disease and platelet stability, is described its effect in decreasing the total lipids in plasma, decreased by approximately 25-30% of TAGs in plasma decreased very low density lipoprotein (VLDL) production [165, 171].

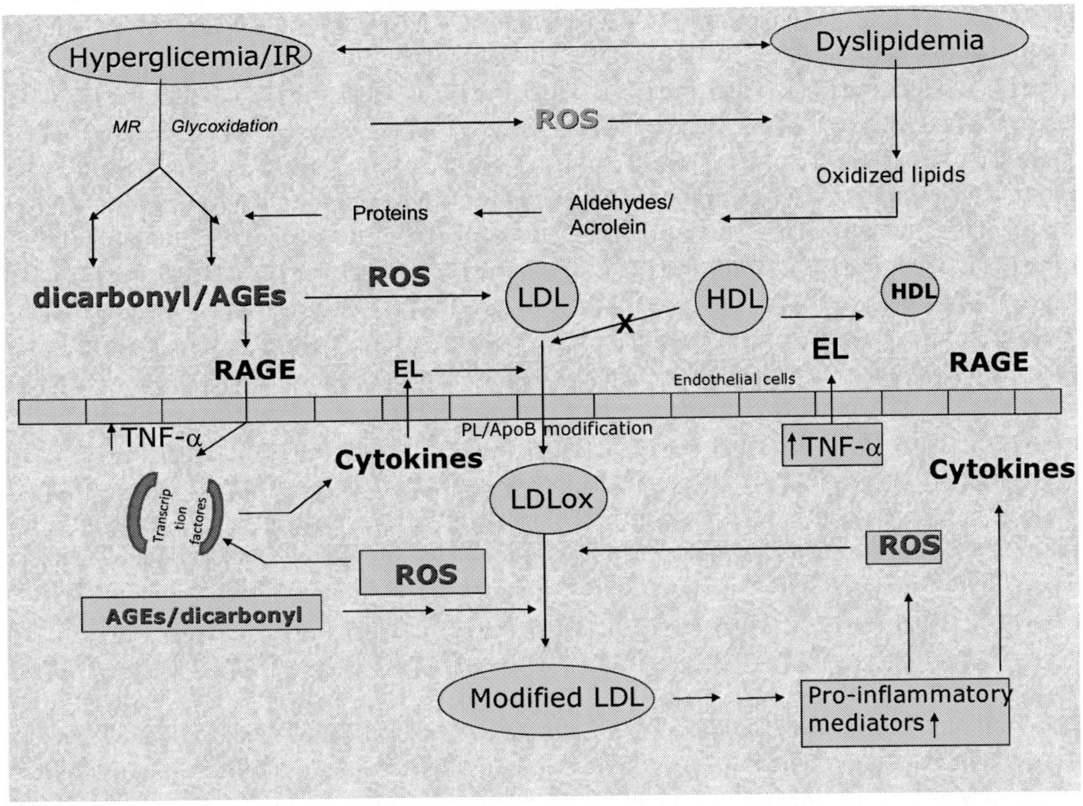

Figure 6. Hyperglicemia and dyslipidemia can lead to increase production of ROS, reactive carbonyl compounds and AGEs, which, by several mechanisms, can impair lipoprotein metabolism and endothelial function. IR: Insulin Resistance; MR: Maillard Reactions; AGEs: Advanced Glycation End Products; RAGE: AGE Receptor; ROS: Reactive Oxygen Species; PL: Phospholipids; EL: Endothelial Lipase.

Metabolic disorders, like obesity, metabolic syndrome (Met Synd) and diabetes, are characterized by increasing TAG production and impair of TAG metabolism, contributing for VLDL and chylomicron (QM) particle accumulation. Combined, these metabolic features contributed for LDL clearance delay, by LDL-receptor (LDL-R) competition with TAG-rich lipoproteins, lead to long-time LDL circulation. This can take to LDL modified particles towards a small and dense LDL (sdLDL). n-3 PUFA, mainly EPA, enhances β-oxidation, and decreases the substrate available for *neo* TAG synthesis *in vivo*. Both, EPA and DHA, can significantly decrease the VLDL production, by several mechanisms, and n-3-TAG-enriched lipoproteins are more rapidly metabolized by TAG lipases [172-174]. sdLDL, by itself, has less affinity for LDL-R and are more prone to oxidation. Metabolic disorders can also be characterized by an increase in the lipid oxidation, the Maillard reaction and glycoxidation. These effects increase radical-mediated reaction, ROS production, and the accumulation of very reactive aldehydes and dicarbonyl compounds. This scenario can lead to increasing susceptibility of LDL particles for modifications and oxidation (LDLox), an important biomarker of cardimetabolic risk (Figure 6).

LDL modified particles also favour the expression of adhesion molecules, increasing macrophages activation and the release of pro-inflammatory mediators, like TNF-α. The later can stimulate transcriptional factors that amplify the production of pro-inflammatory mediators, leading to endothelial cells dysfunction [175-178]. Fish oils ingestion can contribute to a beneficial lipoprotein profile. Moreover, the decrease of TAG-rich lipoproteins effect is well known. However, more accurate evidences of n-3 PUFA mediate lipoprotein effect are needed based on molecular mechanisms. In fact, the majority of studies showed no significant changes in both, total LDL-C and HDL-C. A regular ingestion of fish oil promotes significant changes on HDL2/HDL3 ratio, as well in their phospholipid (PL) composition. The beneficial effects of n-3 PUFA, on lipoprotein profile, can be related with their ability to change the composition, the size or the properties (e.g, antioxidant or cholesterol scavenger capacity) of HDL, and also for LDL particles [179-184]. A shift toward a large HDL and LDL subfractions seems to be beneficial in respect to n-3 PUFA cardioprotective effect, and part of this effect is obtained independently of the changes in the total HDL-C or LDL-C [179, 181, 184]. A more favourable n-3 PUFA mediated lipoprotein profile is achieved even in those individuals that do not significantly alter the total HDL-C or LDL-C. The role of HDL particles on reverse cholesterol transport is partially dependent of PL composition of these lipoproteins. Likewise, the role of HDL particles in ceramide pathway (inhibiting the sphingosine kinase) seems to be, at least in part, mediated by the type of fatty acids in PL of these lipoproteins [185]. These features support the pivotal role of HDL, and justify the indication for HDL increase/changes (in quantity and/or quality), even in the subjects that achieved a normal LDL-C range [186]. n-3 PUFA can lead to changes in HDL subfractions, increasing large HDL particles and/or reducing small HDL particles. The later seems to be less cardioprotective than large HDL. Some of the effects attributed to n-3 PUFA on lipoproteins can be related to the TAG- and PL-lipase activity. Both, activity and/or expression of LPL (liproteic lipase) and HL (hepatic lipase) can be modulated by n-3 PUFA [187]. However, phospholipase activity might be the key feature in this process. EL (endothelial lipase) is predominantly a phospholipase enzyme, compared with HL and LPL, and has a pronounced effect on HDL metabolism *in vivo*. EL is related to the total HDL-C and with changes of the profile of HDL particles and size [188, 189]. The effect of n-3 PUFA on EL activity and expression can be an important mechanism to understand the effect of n-3 PUFA on HDL (and LDL) subfractions. EPA and DHA can alter the biosynthetic pathways of PL, changing the composition of lipoproteins and EL activity. Moreover, EL showed to possess specificity for different PL and, within the same class, a preference for DHA at *sn*-2 position of PL [190]. The effect of pro-inflammatory mediators on both EL activity and expression seems to be an important mechanism for over-expression of EL that is related with the decrease of the total HDL-C and remodelling of HDL particles molecular composition

[189, 191, 192] (Figure 6). EPA and DHA can directly regulate the activity and/or expression of EL; and indirectly, by down-regulating the production of inflammatory mediators [193]. EL has a dual role on lipoprotein metabolism. Despite the effect on HDL remodelling (e.g. PL) and catabolism (Apo A1), the lipase also acts on Apolipoprotein B [189]. HDL Apo A1 catabolism can reduce the protection of LDL particles from oxidation mediated by those apolipoproteins. The effect of n-3 PUFA on ApoAI/ApoB ratio, an important cardiovascular biomarker [194], as well HDL/ApoA1 ratio, can bring some light on the action of these fatty acids related to EL. Future work may explain the potential benefit of n-3 PUFA on lipoprotein metabolism, mediated by direct/indirect effect on EL expression and/or activity.

Studies also pointed out that consumption of n-3 PUFA is related to the relaxation of the endothelium, since the path is vasodilatation dependently enhanced by increased production of NO (nitric oxide), and independently by suppression of the influx of calcium ion through the channel activated by transmembrane potential differences in smooth muscle cells and endothelium. Inhibition of these channels also contributes to reducing the large and rapid fluctuations in the concentration of free calcium, which contributes to the reduction of ventricular arrhythmias (seen with supplementation with fish oil capsules [195, 196]. Thus, the intake of fish oil (EPA and DHA) is associated with the decrease of blood pressure, this decrease could be related to the inhibition of the renin-angiotensin system, including angiotensin converting enzyme, thereby inhibiting the release of the hormone aldosterone, which is responsible for the increase in blood pressure [197, 198]. Intake of fish oil is also associated with improvements in processes and reduction of atherosclerotic platelet aggregation as well as decreased production of clotting factors and fibrinolytic factors [199-202]. The participation of EPA and DHA in the autonomic nervous system is also evident, since they are associated with decreased activation of the sympathetic system, increasing the activity of the parasympathetic system, thereby reducing cardiovascular risk [203].

Another important effect of fish oil ingestion is related with the impact of n-3 PUFA in membrane fluidity, flexibility, permeability essential for the proper functioning of tissues and organs [204,205]. In fact, n-3 PUFA, particularly EPA and DHA are important structural components of membrane phospholipids, serving as biosynthetic and cellular mediators. DHA is selectively concentrated in the synaptic membrane and retinal membranes and is thought to be related to visual function, brain development, behavior and learning. More recent studies indicate the beneficial effect of n-3 PUFA the neurological level, anti-depressive and mental health [206-208].

n-3 PUFA also act as autacoids, doing regulation of gene expression, the factors of non-nuclear (SREBP-1c_sterol regulatory element binding protein, isoform 1, subform c) and nuclear transcription (PPARα PPARγ, LXR, and HNF-4α, NF-κ B). The SREBP-1c is a binding protein, which participates in the activation of the transcription of genes involved in fatty acid synthesis (acetyl-CoA enzyme, acyl-CoA and Δ6, Δ9 and Δ5 desaturases). In the presence of PUFA, the transcription of SREBP-1c is suppressed, and no interference in the activation process of SRBP-1c precursor, which occurs in the membrane of the reticulum endoplasmic reducing the activity of this protein in binding to genes encoding the enzymes of fatty acid synthesis [209]. Moreover, the PPARα (peroxisome proliferator activated receptor isoform α), induces the genes for enzymes involved in β-oxidation, and liver desaturases, establishing a direct link to PUFA. When in excess PUFA inhibit the transcription of the desaturase and activate the transcription of the enzymes of β-oxidation of fatty acids [209]. The fatty acid profile of erythrocyte as a biomarker of several pathologic situations has been receiving increasing attention. Dietary intake, digestion, absorption, metabolism, storage and exchange amongst compartments, greatly influence the fatty acid composition in several blood cells, plasma and tissues [210]. Erythrocytes provide a good model for study fatty acid metabolism [211] and plasma exchanges explains the enrichment of n-3 PUFA in PL-membrane of erythrocytes [212] (Figure 7).

Eicosanoid biosynthesis is also a central mechanism in regulating the anti-inflammatory process in body, modulating the intensity and duration of immune response. n-3 PUFA becomes the substrate for the synthesis of prostaglandins, thromboxanes and leukotrienes, responsible for increased vascular permeability, vasodilation and increased production of anti-inflammatory cytokines such as IL-4, IL-10 and TNF-β and regulation eliminating the production of inflammatory cytokines such as IL-1, IL-2, IL-6, IL-8, TNF-α and CRP. Therefore, fish oils seem to have a beneficial effect in diseases such as rheumatoid arthritis, Crohn's disease, cystic fibrosis, obesity, atherosclerosis, among others [197, 214-218].

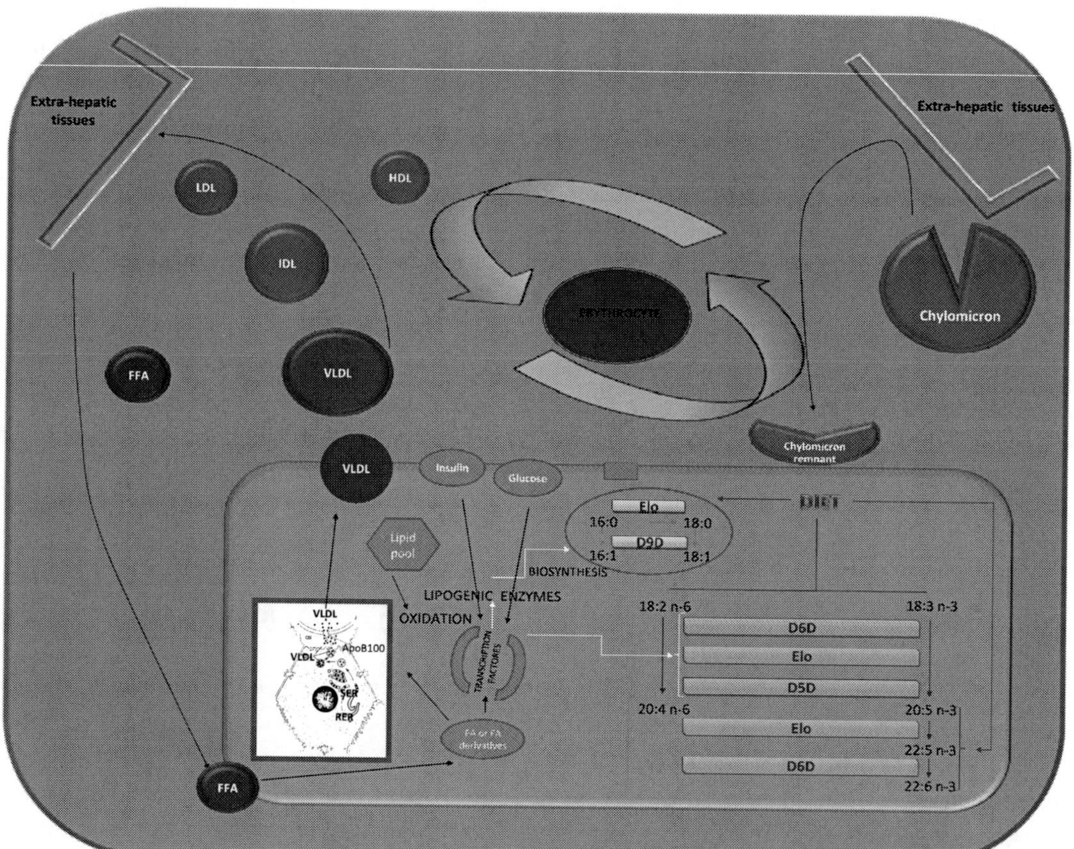

Figure 7. Fatty acids could be incorporated into erythrocytes by exchanges with plasma, as a function of dietary intake, metabolism, and storage and exchange amongst different compartments (adapted for [213]).

At normal physiologic conditions a correct balance between inflammatory mediators is the usual situation. The immunomodelation of pro and anti-inflammatory mediators increased in importance in the cases of bowel inflammatory disease, asthma, diabetes, autoimmune diseases or in cancer [219, 220], as well as in obesity and cardiometabolic disorders. The activation of $CD4^+$ T cells can lead to differentiation of T-helper cells and amplified immune system response. The $CD4^+$ T cells can polarize between the Th1 and Th2 subset as function of different internal and external stimulus. Th1 and Th2 cells release specific cytokines, the first produces mainly IFN-γ, IL-2 and TNF-α [221, 222], that can enhance the pro-inflammatory response by activating the macrophages and increasing the citotoxic capacity of $CD8^+$ T cells. The IFN-γ stimulates B cells to produce antibodies and IL-12, produced by $CD8^+$, DC, and macrophages promote more polarization to Th1 cells by activating STAT4 (signal transducer and activator of transcription 4) [222]. Th2 cells produce mainly IL-4, IL-5, IL-9, IL-10 and IL-13 [219, 222]. IL-4 promotes Th2 cells differentiation, by activation of STAT6, and IL-13, which enhance production of IgG1 and IgE, are related with asthma and allergic reaction. T cells can also differentiate to Th3 cells, that produce TGF-β (transforming growth factor-beta) [222] and have an important role in antigen immunotolerance. The TGF-β can modulate Th1/Th2 balance, macrophages, NK and B cells. This means that TGF-β could have an important role in immunomodelation and inflammation. Dietary components, like n-3 PUFA, can modulate the polarization of T cells by different mechanisms, in both human and animal studies. EPA, DHA and fish oils can 1) reduce the Th1 polarization [219] and provide a better Th1/Th2 balance [223]; 2) decrease IL-1, IL-2, IFN-γ, and TNF-α production [219, 223]; 3) create a more favourable eicosanoids profile; 4) EPA and DHA, or their derivatives, can inhibit transcriptional factor that is involved in pro-inflammatory cascade; and 5) possibly by the increase of TGF-β secretion [224]. This means that n-3 PUFA can produce, locally or systematically a proper environmental by changing Th1/Th2 polarizations, increasing Th3 differentiation, and decreasing pro-inflammatory mediators. The consumption of higher levels of n-3 PUFA, leads to the replacement of ARA in membranes by EPA, including the inflammatory cells. In these cells the incorporation of EPA and DHA is made in a dose-response. This replacement results in decreased inflammatory response due to the formation of eicosanoids 10-100 times less potent than those derived from ARA, increased formation of resolvins E Series with anti-inflammatory action, decreased production of inflammatory cytokines, decreased leukocyte signaling, decreased expression of adhesion molecules like ICAM- 1 and VCAM-1 [214]. Despite the unique properties of EPA and DHA (or derivatives), some of the above mentioned mechanisms could bee integrated in light of n-3/n-6 fatty acids ratio. In addition, immunomodelation of n-3 PUFA can be explained by the capacity to change cellular membrane properties, as a function of their capacity to altering conformation, organization and cellular signalling pathways [219, 223, 225]. Conformational organization of n-3 PUFA acyl chains (Figure 8) alters the properties of the membrane. The change in lipid rafts, constituted mainly by saturated fatty acids, seems to be an important mechanism for anti-inflammatory and immunomodelation properties of n-3 PUFA [223, 226]. DHA and EPA, modulation of cellular signalling pathways could been explained, at least in partially, by the modification of membrane microdomain organization; reducing NF-κB activation and IL-2 secretion, in $CD4^+$ T cells, by inhibitions of the protein kinase C [227], and of the JNK activity and nuclear factor of activated T cells [228], respectively. The (micro) environmental perpetuation of T cells is an important feature in inflammation and cancer development. Activation of caspase 8, via Fas ligand [226] or TNFRI, induced apoptosis, and is closely related with membrane properties and lipid rafts [229].

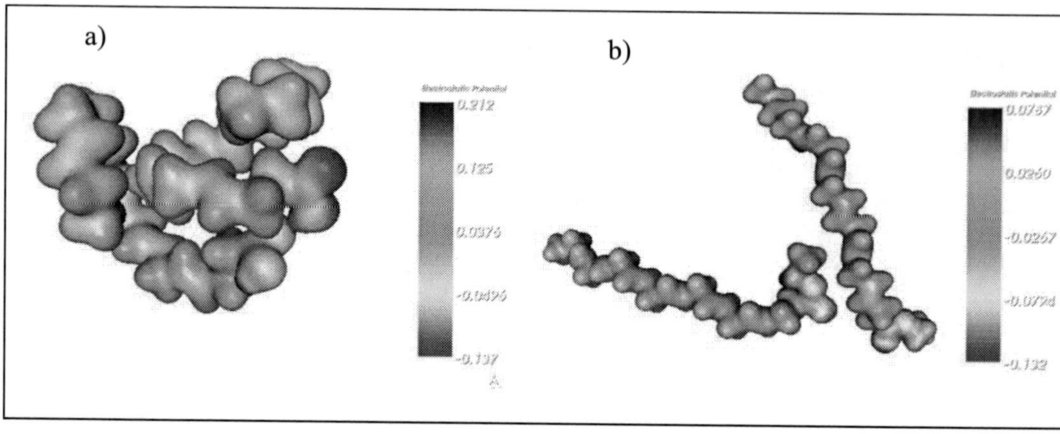

Figure 8. Electrostatic potential for DHA and derivatives. The electrostatic potential (in a.u.) is represented over a constant electronic isodensity ρ (in Å^{-3}) surfaces of volume V_s (in Å^{-3}). All figures correspond to $\rho = 0.05$ Å^{-3}. (a) DHA dimer, (b) DHA ester dimer.

6. Recommended Intake Levels of N-3 PUFA and N-3 Sources in the Diet VER Refs

Current recommendations for the intake of n-3 PUFA (18:3n-3 including, EPA and DHA) were established for the prevention of deficiency in EFA, and the prevention and treatment of CVD. Thus, the WHO recommended for the prevention of CHD and stroke ischaemia, the PUFA in the diet should represent 60-10% of total energy intake, being 5-8% n-6 PUFA and 1-2% n-3 PUFA, as well as a regular consumption of 1-2 servings of oily fish per week, representing 400-1000 mg of EPA + DHA / day [230]. The ISSFAL (International Society for the Study of Fatty Acids and Lipids) recommended that the maintenance of cardiovascular health that LA represents 2% of energy, LNA 0.7% of the energy and 0.5 g of EPA + DHA / day [231]. The AHA (American Heart Association) recommended in 2006 that the American people should eat two portions (85 g) of oily fish a week, about 400-500 mg of EPA + DHA/day, and to secondary prevention should use 1g of EPA + DHA /day [232, 233].

However the intake of more than 3 g of n-3 PUFA / day appear to be responsible for gastrointestinal disorders [234]. Supplementation with very high n-3 PUFA levels (> 7g/dia) may generate excessive bleeding when the level of n-6 PUFA in the diet is low (ARA, EPA 4:1), suppress certain immune responses, increase cholesterol (especially in individuals with familial combined hyperlipidemia) or cause damage oxidative they contain low levels of vitamin E [235, 236], and can transiently increased glycemia, by enhancing neoglucogenic subtracts [237] and/or increased β-oxidation.

References

[1] Barlow, S. (2003). World market overview of fish meal and fish oil. In Peter J. Bechtel (Ed.), *Advances in Seafood Byproducts: 2002 Conference Proceedings* (pp. 11-25). Alaska Sea Grant College Program, University of Alaska Fairbanks, Fairbanks.

[2] Chamberlain, A. (2011). Fishmeal and fish oil – The facts, figures, trends, and IFFO's responsible supply standard. International Fishmeal & Fish Oil Organisation. *http://www.iffo.net/downloads/Datasheets%20Publications%20SP/FMFOF2011.pdf (5th April 2011)*

[3] Bergé, J.-P. & Barnathan, G. (2005). Fatty acids from lipids of marine organisms: Molecular biodiversity, roles as biomarkers, biologically active compounds, and economical aspects. In Y. Le Gal and R. Ulber (Eds.), *Marine Biotechnology I* (pp. 49-125). Springer-Verlag Berlin.

[4] Shahidi, F. (2007). Maximizing the value of marine by-products: an overview. In F. Shahidi (Ed.), *Maximising the value of marine by-products* (pp. xxi-xxv). Woodhead Publishing Limited, Cambridge, England.

[5] Hjaltason, B. (1990). New products, processing possibilities and market for fish oil. *In Proceedings of the International By-products Conference, Anchorage, Alaska, USA,* 131.

[6] Brody, J. (1965). *Fishery By-Products Technology*. The Avi Publishing Company, Inc. 232 p.

[7] Takahashi, C. & Mitsui, K. (1923). *Improvements relating to the extraction of oils from fish.* British Patent GB199054.

[8] Fawcett, E. W. (1935). *Process of refining crude fats and fatty oils.* British Patent GB438056.

[9] Fosse, J. (1947). *Improved apparatus for the heat treatment of animal material, especially from whale, herring or other fishes for the production of oil and dry stuff.* British Patent GB590638.

[10] Chantachum, S., Benjakul, S. & Sriwirat, N. (2000). Separation and quality of fish oil from precooked and non-precooked tuna heads. *Food Chemistry*, 69: 289-294.

[11] Skåra, T. & Cripps, S. (1997). Upgrading of waste from salmon slaughteries using a three phase separation process. In Luten, J. B., Børrensen, T., Oehlenschläger, J. (Eds.), *Seafood From Producer to Consumer, Integrated Approach to Quality*. Elsevier Science, B. V.: Amsterdam, The Netherlands, p. 103-111.

[12] Aidos, I. (2002). *Production of high-quality fish oil from herring byproducts*. Ph. D. Thesis, Wageningen University, The Netherlands, 205 p.

[13] Eide, O., Børresen, T. & Strøm, T. (1982). Minced fish production from capelin (*Mallotus villosus*). A new method for gutting, skinning and removal of fat from small fatty fish species. *J. Food Sci.*, 47, 347-349, 354.

[14] Nunes, M. L. (1983). *Minces from snipefish Macroramphosus spp and boar-fish Capros aper gutted and cleaned by a chemical and physical method.* XVII International Congress of Refrigeration, Commission C2. Paris

[15] Shimizu, Y., Toyohara, H. & Lanier, T. C. (1992). Surimi Production from Fatty and Dark-Fleshed Fish Species. In T. C. Lanier and C. M. Lee (eds), *Surimi Technology* (pp. 181-207), Marcel Dekker, Inc., New York.

[16] Hirata, F., Saeki, H., Nonaka, M., Kawasaki, K., Ooizumi T. & Motoe, K. (1993). *Recovery of fish oil from the manufacturing process of highly nutritional fish meat for foodstuffs from sardine.* Nippon Suisan Gakkaishi, 59, 111-116.

[17] Tokunaga, T. & Nishioka, F. (1988). Surimi production from fatty Japanese sardines. *In Proc. Intl. Conf. Fatty Fish Utilization: Upgrading from Feed to Food* (p. 143). Raleigh NC, UNC Sea Grant Publ. 88-04.

[18] Nishioka, F., Tokunaga, T., Fujiwara, T. & Yoshioka, S. (1990). Development of new leaching technology and a system to manufacture high quality frozen surimi. *In Chilling and freezing of new products* (pp. 73-80). International Institute of Refrigeration Commission C2, Aberdeen.

[19] Lanier, T. C. (1994). Functional fod protein ingredients from fish. In Z. E. Sikorski, B. S. Pan, and F. Shahidi (Eds) *Seafood proteins* (pp. 127-159). Chapman and Hall, New York.

[20] Mendes, R., Gómez-Guillén, C. & Montero, P. (1997). *Effect of a new vacuum leaching technology on the textural characteristics of sardine mince.* Z Lebens Unters Forsch A, 204, 113-120.

[21] Mendes, R., Vital, R., Bandarra, N. M., 2000. Effect of a vacuum-leaching technology on the proteins and lipids of lean sardine (*Sardina pilchardus*) mince. *Eur Food Res Techol,* 212, 31-38.

[22] Toyoshima, K., Noguchi, R., Hosokawa, M., Fukunaga, K., Nishiyama, T., Takahashi, R. & Miyashita, K. (2004). Separation of sardine oil without heating from surimi waste and its effect on lipid metabolism in rats. *J. Agric. Food Chem.*, 52, 2372–2375.

[23] Butler, C. (1955). The fish liver oil industry. U. S. Fish and Wildlife Service. *Fishery Leaflet* 233.

[24] Van Deurs, J. A. S. (1931). *Process for treating fatty raw materials.* U. S. Pat. No. 1,833,061.

[25] Aure, L. (1967). Manufacture of fish-liver oil. In M. E. Stansby (Ed.) *Fish oils. Their chemistry, Technology, Stability, Nutritional Properties, and Uses* (pp. 193-205). The AVI Publishing Company, Inc.

[26] Hultin, H. O. & Kelleher, S. D. (1999). *Process for isolating a protein composition from a muscle source and protein composition.* US Patent 6,005,073.

[27] Hultin, H. O. & Kelleher, S. D. (2000). *High efficiency alkaline protein extraction.* U. S. Patent 6,136,959.

[28] Hultin, H. O.& Kelleher, S. D. (2000). Surimi processing from dark muscle fish. In Jae W. Park (Ed.), *Surimi and Surimi Seafood* (pp. 59-77). Marcel Dekker, Inc., New York.

[29] Kristinsson, H. G. & Demir, N. (2003). Functional protein isolates from underutilized tropical and subtropical fish species and byproducts. In P. Bechtel (Ed.), *Advances in Seafood Byproducts* (pp. 277-298). Alaska Sea Grant College Program, University of Alaska, Anchorage.

[30] Kristinsson H. G., Theodore, A. E. & Ingadottir, B. (2007). Chemical processing methods for protein recovery from marine by-products and underutilized species. In F. Shahidi (Ed.*), Maximising the value of marine by-products* (pp. 144–168). Woodhead Publishing Limited, Cambridge, England.

[31] Undeland, I., Kelleher, S. D. & Hultin, H. O. (2002). Recovery of functional proteins from herring (*Clupea harengus*) light muscle by an acid or alkaline solubilization process. *J. Agric. Food Chem.*, 50, 7371-7379.

[32] Hultin, H. O. (2002). Recent Advances in Surimi Technology. In M. Fingerman and R. Nagabhushanan (Eds.) *Recent Advances in Marine Biotechnology* (pp. 241-251). Volume 7. Seafood Safety and Human Health, Science Publishers, Inc., Enfield (NH), USA.

[33] Okada, T. & Morrissey, M. T. (2007). Recovery and characterization of sardine oil extracted by pH adjustment. *J. Agric. Food Chem.*, 55, 1808–1813.

[34] Pigott, G. M. (1967). Production of fish oil. In M. E. Stansby (Ed.), *Fish oils. Their chemistry, Tecnohology, stability, nutritional properties, and uses* (pp. 183–192). The Avi Publishing Company, Inc.

[35] Anon. (1966a). Extraction process wins protein from fish. *Chem. Eng.*, 73, 98–99.

[36] Anon. (1966b). Marine protein concentrate. *Fishery Leaflet* 584. U.S. Fish & Wildlife Service, Washington, D. C.

[37] Windsor, M. L. (1977). *Fish protein concentrate.* Torry Advisory Note No. 39. Torry Research Station, 10 p.

[38] Levin, E. & Finn, R. K. (1955). A process for dehydrating and defatting tissues at low temperature. *Chem. Eng. Progr.*, 51, 223–226.

[39] Pariser, E. R., Wallerstein, M. B., Corkery, C. J. & Brown, N. L. (1978*). In Fish protein concentrate Panacea for Protein Malnutrition?* MIT Press, Cambridge, Mass. 296 pp.

[40] Pariser, E. R. & Wallerstein, M. B. (1980). Fish protein concentrate - lessons for future food supplementation. *Food Policy*, 5, 298–305.

[41] Brocklesby, H. N. & Green, K. (1937). Variations in vitamin A content of liver oils in the grayfish. Fisheries Res. Board Can., Ottawa.

[42] Bailey, B. E. (1952). Digestion methods in the production of marine oils. *Marine Oils Fish*. Res. Bd Canada, Bulletin No. 89, pp. 195–197.

[43] Tatterson, I. N. & Windsor, M. L. (1974). Fish silage. *J. Sci. Fd Agric.*, 25, 369–379.

[44] Raa, J., Gildberg, A. & Strøm, T. (1983). Silage production – theory and practice. In D. A. Ledward, A. J. Taylor & R. A. Lawrie (Eds), *Upgrading waste for Feeds and Food* (pp. 117–132). Butterworths, London.

[45] Reece, P. (1980). Control and reduction of free fatty acid concentration in oil recovered from fish silage prepared from sprat. *J. Sci. Food Agric.*, 31, 147–155.

[46] Reece, P. (1981). Recovery of high quality oil from mackerel and sprat by the silage process. *J. Sci. Food Agric.*, 32, 531–538.

[47] Eide, O., Raa, J., Strøm, T. & Tiedemann, E. (1979). *Norwegian Patent 791481.*

[48] Liaset, B., Julshamn, K. & Espe, M. (2003). Chemical composition and theoretical evaluation of the produced fractions from enzymic hydrolysis of salmon frames with Protamex^{TM}. Process Biochemistry, 38, 1747-1759.

[49] Linder, M., Fanni, J. & Parmentier, M. (2002). Procédé d'extraction d'huile par voie enzymatique et obtention d'hydrolysats protéiques à fonctionnalités dirigées. *Brevet FR* 2.835.703.

[50] Linder, M., Fanni, J. & Parmentier, M. (2005). Proteolytic extraction of salmon oil and PUFA concentration by lipases. *Marine Biotechnology*, 15, 70-76.

[51] Bligh, E. G. & Dyer, W. J. (1959). A rapid method of total lipid extraction and purification. *Can. J. Biochem. Physiol.*, 37, 911-917.

[52] Šližytė, R., Nguyen, J. V., Rustad, T. & Storrø, I. (2004). Hydrolysis of cod (*Gadus morhua*) by-products: Influence of initial heat inactivation, concentration and separation conditions. *J. Aquatic Food Prod. Technol.*, 13, 31-48.

[53] Dumay, J., Barthomeuf, C. & Bergé, J. P. (2004). How enzymes may be helpful for upgrading fish by-products: Enhancement of fat extraction. *J. Aquatic Food Prod. Technol.*, 13: 69-84.

[54] Šližytė, R., Daukšas, E., Falch, E., Storrø, I. & Rustad, T. (2005). Yield and composition of different fractions obtained after enzymatic hydrolysis of cod (*Gadus morhua*) by-products. *Process Biochemistry*, 40, 1415–1424.

[55] Daukšas, E., Falch, E., Šližytė, R. & Rustad, T. (2005). Composition of fatty acids and lipid classes in bulk products generated during enzymic hydrolysis of cod (*Gadus morhua*) by-products. *Process Biochemistry*, 40, 2659-2670.

[56] Šližytė, R., Rustad, T. & Storrø, I. (2005). Enzymatic hydrolysis of cod (*Gadus morhua*) by-products. Optimization of yield and properties of lipid and protein fractions. *Process Biochemistry*, 40, 3680 – 3692.

[57] Gbogouri, G. A., Linder, M., Fanni, J. & Parmentier, M. (2006). Analysis of lipids extracted from salmon (*Salmo salar*) heads by commercial proteolytic enzymes. *Eur. J. Lipid Sci. Technol.*, 766-775.

[58] Dumay, J., Donnay-Moreno, C., Barnathan, G., Jaouen, P. & Bergé, J.P. (2006). Improvement of lipid and phospholipid recoveries from sardine (*Sardina pilchardus*) viscera using industrial proteases. *Process Biochemistry*, 41, 2327–2332.

[59] Batista, I., Ramos, C., Mendonça, R. & Nunes, M. L. (2009). Enzymatic hydrolysis of sardine (*Sardina pilchardus*) by-products and lipid recovery. *Journal of Aquatic Food Product Technology* 18, 120-134.

[60] Batista, I., Ramos, C., Coutinho, J., Bandarra, N. M. & Nunes, M. L. (2010). Characterization of protein hydrolysates and lipids obtained from black scabbardfish (*Aphanopus carbo*) by-products and antioxidative activity of the hydrolysates produced. *Process Biochemistry*, 45: 18–24.

[61] Hardardottir, I. & Kinsella, J. E. (1988). Extraction of lipid and cholesterol from fish muscle with supercritical fluids. *J. Food. Sci.*, 53, 1656-1658, 1661.

[62] Eisenbach, W. (1984). Supercritical fluid extraction: a film demonstration. Ber. Bunsenges. *Phys. Chem.,* 88: 882-887.

[63] Krukonis, V. J. (1988). Processing with supercritical fluids: overview and applications. In B. A. Charpentier and M. R. Sevenants (Eds.), Supercritical Fluid Extraction and Chromatography: Techniques and Applications (pp. 26–43), B. A., *ACS Symp. Series No. 366*, American Chemical Society, Washington, DC.

[64] Rizvi, S. S. H., Chao, R. R. & Liew, Y. J. (1988). Concentration of omega-3 fatty acids from fish oil using supercritical carbon dioxide. In B. A. Charpentier and M. R. Sevenants (Eds.), Supercritical Fluid Extraction and Chromatography: Techniques and Applications (pp. 89–108). *ACS Symp. Series No. 366,* American Chemical Society, Washington, DC.

[65] Nilsson, W. B., Gauglitz, E. J. & Hudson, J. K. (1989). Supercritical fluid fractionation of oil esters using incremental pressure programming and temperature gradient supercritical fluid CO_2. *J. Am. Oil Chem. Soc.*, 66, 1596-1600.

[66] Nilsson, W. B., Gauglitz, E. J., Hudson, J. K., Stout, V. F. & Spinelli, J. (1988). Fractionation of menhaden oil ethyl esters using supercritical fluid CO_2. *J. Am. Oil Chem. Soc.*, 65, 109-117.

[67] Nilsson, W. B., Seaborn, G. T. & Hudson, J. K. (1992). Partition coefficients for fatty acid esters in supercritical CO_2 with and without ethanol. *J. Am. Oil Chem. Soc.,* 69, 305-308.

[68] Higashidate, S., Yamauchi, Y. & Saito, M. (1990). Enrichment of eicosapentaenoic acid and docosahexaenoic acid esters fro esterified fish oil by programmed extraction-elution with supercritical carbon dioxide. *J. Chromatogr.*, 515: 295–303.

[69] Staby, A. & Mollerup, J. (1993). Solubility of fish oil fatty acid ethyl esters in sub- and supercritical carbon dioxide. *J. Am. Oil Chem. Soc.*, 70, 583-588.

[70] Mishra, V. K., Temelli, F. & Ooraikul, B., 1993. Extraction and purification of □3-fatty acids with an emphasis on supercritical fluid extraction, a review. *Food Res. Intern.*, 26, 217-226.

[71] Riha, V., G. Brunner, G., 2000. Separation of fish oil ethyl esters with supercritical carbon dioxide. *J. of Supercritical Fluids*, 17: 55-64.

[72] Perretti, G., Motori, A., Bravi, E., Favatic, F., Montanari, L. & Fantozzi, P. (2007). Supercritical carbon dioxide fractionation of fish oil fatty acid ethyl esters. *J. of Supercritical Fluids*, 40: 349-353.

[73] Sarrade, S. J., Rios, G. M. & Carlès, M. (1998). Supercritical CO_2 extraction coupled with nanofiltration separation. Applications to natural products. *Separation and Purification Technology*, 14: 19 – 25.

[74] Yamaguchi, K., Murakami, M., Nakano, H., Konosu, S., Kokura, T., Yamamoto, H., Kosaka, M. & Hata, K. (1986). Supercritical carbon dioxide extraction of oils from Antarctic krill. *J. Agric. Food Chem.,* 34, 904-907.

[75] Ikushima, Y., Saito, N., Hatakeda, K., Ito, S., Asano, T. & Goto, T. (1986). A supercritical carbon dioxide extraction from mackerel (*Scomber japonicus*) powder: Experiment and modelling. *Bull. Chem. Soc. Jpn.*, 59: 3709–3713.

[76] Temelli, F., LeBlanc, E. & Fu, L. (1995). Supercritical CO_2 extraction of oil from Atlantic mackerel (*Scomber scombrus*) and protein functionality. *J. Food. Sci.*, 60, 703-706.

[77] Bandarra, N. M., Fontan, I., Esquível, M. M., Bernardo-Gil, M. G., Batista, I., Nunes, M. L. & Empis, J. M. A. (1995). Characterisation of sardine oil extracted by supercritical carbon dioxide and classical methods. Proceedings of the Conference "Current Status and Future Trends in Analytical Food Chemistry" *EURO FOOD VII,* Vienna, 18-20 September 1995. p. 219-223.

[78] Esquível, M. M., Bandarra, N. M., Fontan, I., Bernardo-Gil, M. G., Batista, I., Nunes, M. L. & Empis, J. A. (1997). Supercritical carbon dioxide extraction of sardine *Sardina pilchardus* oil. *Lebensm.-Wiss. u.-Technol.*, 30, 715-720.

[79] Tanaka, Y. & Ohkubo, T. (2003). Extraction of lipids from salmon roe with supercritical carbon dioxide. *Journal of Oleo Science*, 52, 295-301.

[80] Tanaka, Y., Sakaki, I. & Ohkubo, T. (2004). Extraction of phospholipids from salmon roe with supercritical carbon dioxide and an entrainer. *Journal of Oleo Science,* 53, 417-424.

[81] King, J.W., Johnson, H.J., Friedrich, J.P., 1989. Extraction of fat tissue from meat products with supercritical carbon dioxide. *Journal of Agricultural Food Chemistry* 37, 951–954.

[82] Dunford, N. T., Temmeli, F. & LeBlanc, E. (1997). Supercritical CO_2 extraction of oil and residual proteins from Atlantic mackerel (*Scomber scombrus*) as affected by moisture content. *J. Food Sci.*, 62, 289-294.

[83] Dunford, N.T.; Goto, M.; Temmeli, F. (1998). Modelling of oil extraction with supercritical CO_2 from Atlantic mackerel (*Scomber scombrus*) at different moisture content. *J. of Supercritical Fluids*, 13: 303-309.

[84] Létisse, M., Rozières, M., Hiol, A., Sergent, M. & Comeau, L. (2006). Enrichment of EPA and DHA from sardine by supercritical fluid extraction without organic modifier. I. Optimization of extraction conditions. *J. of Supercritical Fluids*, 38: 27-36.

[85] Tanaka, Y. & Sakaki, I. (2005). Extraction of phospholipids from unused natural resources with supercritical carbon dioxide and an entrainer. Journal of Oleo Science, 54, 569-576.

[86] Catchpole, O. J., von Kamp, J.-C. & Grey, J. B. (1997). Extraction of squalene from shark liver oil in a packed column using supercritical carbon dioxide. *Ind. Eng. Chem.* Res., 36: 4318-4324.

[87] Catchpole, O. J., Grey, J. B. & Noermark, K. A. (2000). Fractionation of fish oils using supercritical CO_2 and CO_2+ethanol mixtures. *J. of Supercritical Fluids*, 19: 25-37.

[88] Shaihidi, F. & Wanasundara U. N. (1998). Omega-3 fatty acid concentrates: nutritional aspects and production technologies. *Trends in Food Science & Technology,* 9, 230-240.

[89] FAO (1986). The production of fish meal and oil. *FAO Fisheries Technical Paper,* vol. 142. FAO, Rome (Italy), 61 p.

[90] EFSA (BIOHAZ - Working Group on fish oil for human consumption: Sava Buncic, Charlotte Jacobsen, Maria Leonor Nunes, Jörg Oehlenschläger and Miguel Prieto Maradona) 2010. Scientific Opinion on Fish Oil for Human Consumption. Food Hygiene, including Rancidity. Panel on Biological Hazards. *EFSA Journal*, 8, 1874-1922.

[91] Bhosle, B. M. & Subramanian, R. (2005). New approaches in deacification of edible oils-A review. *J. Food Eng*, 69, 481−494.

[92] Rubio-Rodríguez, N., Beltrán, S., Jaime, I., de Diego, S. M., Sanz, M. T. & Carballido, J. R. (2010). Production of omega-3 polyunsaturated fatty acid concentrates: a review. *Innov Food Sci Emerg Technol,* 11, 1-12.

[93] Maes, J., de-Meulenaer. B., van-Heerswhyngels, P., de-Greyt, W., de-Pauw, E. & Huyghebaert, A. (2005). Removal of dioxins and PCB from fish oil by activated carbon and its influence on the nutritional quality of the oil. *J Am Oil Chem Soc*, 82, 593-597.

[94] Oterhals, A., Solvang, M., Nortvedt, R. & Berntssen, M. H.G. (2007). Optimization of activated carbon-based decontamination of fish oil by response surface methodology. European *J Lipid Sci Technol*, 109, 691-705.

[95] Hamm. W. (2009). Processing of fish oil. In B. Rossell (Ed.), *Fish oils,* pp. pp. 81-98). UK: Wiley-Blackwell.

[96] Čmolik, J. & Pokorný, J. (2000). Physical refining of edible oils. *European J Lipid Sci Technol*, 102, 472-486.

[97] Aidos, I., van-der-Padt, A., Boom, R. M., & Luten, J. B. (2003). Quality of crude fish oil extracted from herring by-products of varying states of freshness. *J Food Sci,* 68, 458-465.

[98] Fournier, V., Destaillats, F., Juanéda, P., Dionisi, F., Lambelet, P., Sébédio, J. L. & Berdeaux, O. (2006). Thermal degradation of long-chain polyunsaturated FAs during deodorization of fish oil. *European J Lipid Sci Technol*, 108, 33-42.

[99] Chang, S. S., Bao, Y. & Pelura, T. J. (1989). *Purification of fish oil.* Patent U.S. 4.874.629.

[100] Nishimoto, Y. & Nagagawa, M. (1996). *Method for refining fish oil.* Patent JP 08311481.

[101] Yoshikazu, T., Hirosi, Y., Kazuko, H. & Satoru, K. (1997). *Method for refining and manufacturing fats and oils containing polyunsaturated FAs.* European Patent 0773283.

[102] Kamal-Eldin, A. & Yanishlieva, N. V. (2002). N-3 FAs for human nutrition: stability considerations. European *J Lipid Sci Technol*, 104, 825-836.

[103] Jacobsen, C., Let, M.B., Nielsen, N.S. & Meyer, A.S. (2008). Antioxidant strategies for preventing oxidative flavour deterioration of foods enriched with n-3 polyunsaturated lipids: A comparative evaluation. *Trends Food Sci Technol*, 19/2: 76-93.

[104] Jiménez-Alvárez, D., Giuffrida, F., Golay, P. A., Cotting, C., Lardeau, A. & Keely, B. J. (2008). Antioxidant activity of oregano, parsley, and olive mill wastewaters in bulk oils and oil-in-water emulsions enriched in fish oil. *J Agri Food Chem*, 56, 7151-7159.

[105] Matsuno, R. & Adachi, S. (1993). Lipid encapsulation technology – Techniques and applications to food. *Trends Food Sci Technol,* 4, 256-261.

[106] Desai, K. & Park, H. J. (2005). Recent developments in microencapsulation of food ingredients. *Drying Technol*, 23, 1361-1394.

[107] Gharsallaoui, A., Roudaut, G., Chambin, O., Voilley, A. & Saurel, R. (2007). Applications of spray-drying in microencapsulation of food ingredients: an overview. *Food Res Internat*, 40, 1107-1121.

[108] Heinzelmann, K., Franke, K., Velasco, J., & Márquez-Ruíz, G. (2000). Microencapsulation of fish oil by freeze-drying techniques and influence of process parameters on oxidative stability during storage. *European Food Research and Technol,* 211, 234-239.

[109] Klaypradit, W. & Huang, Y. W. (2008). Fish oil encapsulation with chitosan using ultrasonic atomizer. *Lebensmittel-Wissenschaft Technologie*, 41, 1133-1139.

[110] Barrow, C. J., Nolan, C. & Holub, B. J. (2009). Bioequivalence of encapsulated and microencapsulated fishoil supplementation. *J Functional Foods*, 1:38-43.

[111] Day, L., Xu, M., Hoobin, P., Burgar, I. & Augustin, M. A. (2007). Characterisation of fish oil emulsions stabilised by sodium caseinate, *Food Chem*, 105, 469–479.

[112] McClements, D. J., Decker, E. A., & Weiss, J. (2007). Emulsion-based delivery systems for lipophilic bioactive components, *J. Food Sci*, 72, 109–124.

[113] Let, M. B., Jacobsen, C. & Meyer, A. S. (2007). Lipid oxidation in milk, yoghurt and salad dressing enriched with neat fish oil or pre-emulsified fish oil. *J Agric Food Chem,* 55, 7802-7809.

[114] Bimbo, A. P. (1998). *Guidelines for characterizing food-grade fish oils.* Inform, 9, 473-483.

[115] Codex Standard nº 19, (1981). Codex Standard for edible fats and oils not covered by individual standards. P. 1-5 *(http://www.codexalimentarius.net/web/standard_list.jsp, retrieved in May 2011.*

[116] Akoh, C. C. (1993). Lipase-catalysed synthesis of partial glyceride. *Biotechnol Lett,* 15, 949.

[117] Stout, V. F., Niisson, W. B., Krzynowek, J. & Schlenk, H. (1990). Fractionation of Fish Oil and Their FAs. In M. E. Stansby (Ed.), *Fish Oils In Nutrition* (pp. 73-119). New York (USA): Van Nostrand Reinhold.

[118] Beebe, L. M., Brown, P. R. & Turcotte, L. G. (1988). Preparative-scale-high-performance liquid chromatography of omega-3 polyunsaturated fatty acid esters derived from fish oil. *J Chromatography*, 495, 369-378.

[119] Adlof, R. O. & Emiken, E. A. (1985). The Isolation of omega-3 polyunsaturated FAs and methyl esters of fish oils by silver resin chromatography. *J Am Oil Chem Soc*, 62, 1592-1595.

[120] Goffic, F.L., (1997). Countercurrent and centrifugal partition chromatography as new tools for preparative-scale lipid purification. *Lipid Technol,* 9:148-150.

[121] Marangoni, A. & Rousseau, D., (1995). Engineering Triacylglycerol: the Role of Interesterification. *Trends Food Sci Technol*, 6, 329-335.

[122] Yadwad, V. B., Ward, O. P. & Noronha, L. C. (1991). Application of lipase to concentrate the docosahexaenoic acid fraction of fish oil. *Biotech Bioeng*, 38, 956-959.

[123] Chawla, P. & deMan, J. M. 1990. Measurement of the size distribution of fat crystals using a laser particle counter. *J Am Oil Chem Soc*, 76, 329-332.

[124] Kojima, Y., Sakuradani, E. & Shimizu, S. (2006). Different specificity of two types of *Pseudomonas lipases* to C20 FAs with Δ5 unsaturated double bond and their application for selective concentration of FAs. *J Biosci Bioeng*, 101, 496–500.

[125] LeGoffic, F., Nguyen, A., & Khayat-Frydman, C. (2000). *Concentration and purification of polyunsaturated fatty acid esters by distillation enzymatic transesterification coupling*. WO 00/73254.

[126] Lin, T.J., Chen, S. W. & Chang, A. C. (2006). Enrichment of n−3 PUFA contents on triglycerides of fish oil by lipase-catalyzed trans-esterification under supercritical conditions. *Biochem Eng J,* 29, 27–34.

[127] Liu, S., Zhang, C., Hong, P. & Ji, H. (2006). Concentration of docosahexaenoic acid (DHA) and eicosapentaenoic acid (EPA) of tuna oil by urea complexation: Optimization of process parameters. *J Food Eng*, 73, 203–209.

[128] Smith, A. E. (1952). Crystal Structure of the Urea-Hydrogen Complexes. *Acta Cryst,* 5, 224-235.

[129] Schlenk, H. & Holman, R.T. (1950). Separation and stabilization of FAs by urea complexes. *J Am Oil Chem Soc*, 27, 5001-5004.

[130] Yoshikazu, T., Hirosi, Y., Kazuko, H. & Satoru, K. (1997). Method for refining and manufacturing fats and oils containing polyunsaturated FAs. European Patent 0773283.

[131] FDA GRAS Notification (2002). GRAS Notice 000105: eicosapentaenoic and docosahexaenoic acid concentrates. *www.accessdata.fda.gov/scripts/fcn/gras_notices/211666A.PDF* (retrieved on May 2011)

[132] FDA GRAS Notification (2006). GRAS Notice 000200. Eicosapentaenoic and docosahexaenoic acid concentrates. *www.accessdata.fda.gov/scripts/fcn/gras_notices/701521A.PDF* (retrieved on May 2011).

[133] Lawson, L. D. & Hughes, B. G. (1988). Human absorption of fish oil FAs as triacylglycerols free FAs or ethyl esters. *Biochem Biophys Res Communications*, 152, 328–335.

[134] Boyd, L. C., King, M. F. & Sheldon, B. (1992). A rapid method for determining the oxidation of n−3 FAs. *J Am Oil Chem* Soc 69, 4, 325−330.

[135] Wijesundera, C., Ceccato, C., Watkins, P., Fagan, P., Fraser, B., Thienthong, N. & Perlmutter, P. (2008). Docosahexaenoic acid is more stable to oxidation when located at the sn−2 position of triacylglycerol compared to sn−1(3). *J Am Oil Chem Soc*, 85, 6, 543−548.

[136] Mu, H. & Porsgaard, T. (2005). The metabolism of structured triacylglycerols. *Progress in Lipid Research*, 44, 430-48.

[137] Hita, E., Robles, A., Camacho, B., González, P. A., Esteban, L., Jiménez, M. J., Muñío, M. M. & Molina, E. (2009). Production of structured triacylglycerols by acidolysis catalyzed by lipases immobilized in a packed bed reactor. *Biochemical Engineering Journal,* 46, 257-64.

[138] Bottino, N. R., Vandenburg, G. A. & Reiser, R. (1967). Resistance of certain long-chain polyunsaturated fatty acids of marine oils to pancreatic lipase hydrolysis. *Lipids*, 2, 489-93.

[139] Christensen, M. S., Hoy, C. E., Becker, C. C. & Redgrave, T. G. (1995). Intestinal absorption and lymphatic transport of eicosapentaenoic (EPA), docosahexaenoic (DHA) and decanoic acids: dependence on intramolecular triacylglycerol structure. *American Journal of Clinical Nutrition*, 61, 56-61.

[140] Mu, H. (2006). Absorption of structured lipids and their applications in the diet. *Lipid Technology*, 12, 271-74.

[141] Torres, C. F., Lin, B., Moeljadi, M., Hill Jr, D. G. (2003). Lipase-catalyzed synthesis of designer acyl-glycerols rich in residues of eicosapentaenoic, docosahexaenoic, conjugated linoleic, and/or stearic acids. *European Journal of Lipid Science and Technology,* 105, 614-23.

[142] Iwasaki, Y. & Yamane, T. (2000). Enzymatic synthesis of structured lipids. *Journal of Molecular Catalysis B: Enzymatic*, 10, 129-40.

[143] González Moreno, P. A., Robles Medina, A., Camacho Rubio, F., Camacho Páez, B. & Molina Grima, E. (2004). Production of structured lipids by acidolysis of an EPA-enriched fish oil and caprylic acid in a packed bed reactor: analysis of three different operation modes. *Biotechnology Progress,* 20, 1044-52.

[144] Irimescu, R., Furihata, K., Hata, K., Iwasaki, Y. & Yamane, T. (2001). Utilization of reaction medium-dependent regiospecificity of *Candida antarctica* lipase (Novozym 435) for the synthesis of 1,3-dicapryloyl-2-docosahexanoyl (or eicosapentaenoyl) glycerol. *Journal of the American Oil Chemists' Society,* 78, 285-90.

[145] Connor, W. E. (2000). Importance of n-3 fatty acids in health and disease. *American Journal of Clinical Nutrition,* 71, 171-75.

[146] Simopoulos, A. P. (1999). Essential fatty acids in health and chronic disease. *American Journal of Clinical Nutrition*, 70, 560-69.

[147] Xu, X. (2000). Production of specific-structured triacylglycerols by lipase-catalyzed reactions: a review. *European Journal of Lipid Science and Technology*, 287-303.

[148] Houde, A., Kademi, A., Leblanc, D. (2003). Lipases and Their Industrial Applications. *An Overview. Applied Biochemistry and Biotechnology*, 118, 155-70.

[149] Hita, E., Robles, A., Camacho, B., Ramírez, A., Esteban, L., Jiménez, M. J., Muñío, M. M., González, P. A., Molina, E. (2007). Production of structured triacylglycerols

(STAG) rich in docosahexaenoic acid (DHA) in position 2 by acidolysis of tuna oil catalyzed by lipases. *Process Biochemistry*, 42, 415-22.

[150] Xu, X., Porsgaard, T., Zhang, H., Adler-Nissen, J., Høy, C.E. (2002). Production of structured lipids in a packed-bed reactor with *Thermomyces lanuginose* lipase. Journal of the American Oil Chemists′ Society, 79, 561-65.

[151] Shimada, Y., Sugihara, A., Maruyama, K., Nagao, T., Nakayama, S., Nakanno, H., Tominaga, Y. (1996). Production of Structured Lipid Containing Docosahexaenoic and Caprylic Acids Using Immobilized *Rhizopus delemar* Lipase. *Journal of Fermentation and Bioengineering*, 81, 299-303.

[152] Zhou, D., Xu, X., Mu, H., Høy, C.E., Adler-Nissen, J. (2000). Lipase-catalyzed production of structured lipids via acidolysis of fish oil with caprylic acid. *Journal of Food Lipids*, 7, 263-74.

[153] Schmid, U., Bornscheuer, U.T., Soumanou, M.M., McNeill, G.P., Schmid, R.D. (1998). Optimization of the Reaction Conditions in the Lipase-Catalyzed Synthesis of Structured Triglycerides. *Journal of the American Oil Chemists′ Society*, 75, 1527-31.

[154] Muñío, M. M., Esteban, L., Robles, A., Hita, E., Jiménez, M. J., P.A. González, Camacho, B., Molina, E. (2008). Synthesis of 2-monoacylglycerols rich in polyunsaturated fatty acids by ethanolysis of fish oil catalyzed by 1,3 specific lipases. *Process Biochemistry,* 43, 1033-39.

[155] Muñío, M. M., Robles, A., Esteban, L., González, P. A., Molina, E. (2009). Synthesis of structured lipids by two enzymatic steps: Ethanolysis of fish oils and esterification of 2-monoacylglycerols. *Process Biochemistry*, 44, 723-30.

[156] Irimescu, R., Furihata, K., Hata, K., Iwasaki, Y., Yamane, T. (2001). Two-Step Enzymatic Synthesis of Docosahexaenoic Acid-Rich Symmetrically Structured Triacylglycerols *via* 2-Monoacylglycerols. *Journal of the American Oil Chemists′ Society,* 78, 743-48.

[157] Senanayake, S. P. J. N. & Shahidi, F. (2001). Modified Oils Containing Highly Unsaturated Fatty Acids and Their Stability. In F. Shahidi and J.W. Finley (Eds.), Omega-3 Fatty Acids: Chemistry, Nutrition and Health Effects. *American Chemical Society Symposium Series* 788 (pp. 162–173). Washington, DC: American Chemical Society.

[158] Shahidi, F. & Wanasundara U.N. (1997). Measurement of Lipid Oxidation and Evaluation of Antioxidant Activity. In F. Shahidi (Ed.), *Natural Antioxidants: Chemistry, Health Effects, and Application* (pp. 379–395.) Champaign, IL: AOCS Press.

[159] Gray, J.I. (1978). Measurement of Lipid Oxidation: A Review. *Journal of the American Oil Chemists' Society*, 55, 539–546.

[160] Namal Senanayake, S. P. J. & Shahidi. F. (2002). Oxidative Stability of Structured Lipids Produced from Borage (*Borago officinalis* L.) and Evening Primrose (*Oenothera biennis* L.) Oils with Docosahexaenoic Acid. *Journal of the American Oil Chemical Society*, 79, 1003-1013.

[161] Guil-Guerrero, J. L., Giménez-Giménez, A., Robles-Medina, A., Rebolloso-Fuentes, M. M., Belarbi, H., Esteban-Cerdán, L. & Molina-Grima, E. (2001). Hexane reduces peroxidation of fatty acids during storage. *European Journal of Lipid Science and Technology*, 103, 271–278.

[162] Hamam, F. & Shahid, F. (2004). Synthesis of Structured Lipids via Acidolysis of Docosahexaenoic Acid Single Cell Oil (DHASCO) with Capric Acid. *Journal of Agricultural and Food Chemistry*, 52, 2900-2906.

[163] Maduko, C. O., Park, Y. W. & Akoh, C. C. (2008). Characterization and Oxidative Stability of Structured Lipids: Infant Milk Fat Analog. *Journal of the American Oil Chemists' Society,* 85, 197-204.

[164] Albert, C. M., Oh, K., Whang, W., Manson, J. E., Chae, C., Stampfer, M. J., Willet, W. C. & Hu, F. (2005). Dietary alpha-linolenic acid intake and risk of sudden cardiac death and coronary heart disease. *Circulation*, 112, 3232-38.

[165] Barrow, C. J., Nolan, C. & Holub, B. J. (2009). Bioequivalence of encapsulated and microencapsulated fish-oil supplementation. *Journal of Functional Foods*, 1, 38-43.

[166] Kurowska, E. M., Dresser, G. K., Deutsch, L., Vachon, D. & Khalil, W. (2003). Bioavailability of omega-3 essential fatty acids from perilla seed oil. Prostaglandins, Leukotrienes and Essential Fatty Acids, 68, 207–12.

[167] Shidhu, S. (2003). Health benefits and potential risks related to consumption of fish or fish oil. *Regulatory Toxicology and Pharmacology,* 38, 336-44.

[168] Wijendran, V. & Hayes, C. (2004). Dietary n-6 and n-3 fatty acid balance and cardiovascular health. *Annual Review of Nutrition*, 24, 597-615.

[169] Burr, M. L., Fehily, M., Rogers, S., Welsby, E., King, S. & Sandham, S. (1989). Diet and reinfarction trial (DART): design, recruitment, and compliance. *European Heart Journal,* 10, 558-67.

[170] GISSI - Prevenzione Investigators (1999). Dietary supplementation with n-3 polyunsaturated fatty acids and vitamin E in 11,324 patients with myocardial infarction: results of the GISSI. Prevenzione trial. *Lancet*, 354, 447–55.

[171] Morris, M. C., Sacks, F. & Rosner, B. (1993). Does fish oil lower blood pressure? A meta-analysis of controlled trials. *Circulation*, 88, 523-33.

[172] Bordin, P., Bodamer, O. A., Venkatesan, S., Gary, R. M., Bannister, P. A. & Halliday, D. (1998). Effects of fish oil supplementation on apoliprotein B 100 production and lipoprotein metabolism in normolipidaemic males. *Eur. J. Clin. Nutr.,* 52(2), 104.

[173] Willunsen, N., Vaagenes, H., Lie, O., Ustan, A. C. & Berge, R. G. (1996). Eicosapentaenoic acid, but not docosahexaenoic acid, increases mitochondrial fatty acid oxidation and upregulates 2,4-dienoyl- CoA reductase gene expression in rats. *Lipids*, 31(6), 579.

[174] Halminski, M. A., Marsh, J. B. & Harrison, E. H. (1991). Comparative effects of dietary fish oil (FO), safflower oil (SO) and palm oil (PO) on selected enzymes of hepatic lipid metabolism. In Simopoulos, A.P., Kiefer, R.R., Martin, R.E., Barlow, S.M. (Ed.), Textbook of Health effects of ω-3 polyunsaturated fatty acids in seafood (552). *World Rev. Nutr. Diet.* Basel, Karger.

[175] Roberts, C. K & Sindhu, K. K. (2009). Oxidative stress and metabolic syndrome. *Life Sciences*, 84, 705-12.

[176] Mertens, A, & Holvoet, P. (2001). Oxidized LDL and HDL: antagonists in atherothrombosis. *FASEB Journal*, 15, 2073-84.

[177] Griffin, B. A., Minihane, A.M., Furlonger, N., Chapman, C., Murphy, M., Willians, D., Wright, J. J. & Williams, C. M. (1999). Inter-relationships between small, dense low-density lipoprotein (LDL), plasma triacylglycerol and LDL apoprotein B in an atherogenic lipoprotein phenotype in free-living subjects. *Clinical Science*, 97, 269-76.

[178] Steinberg, D. (1997). Low density lipoprotein oxidation and its pathobiological significance. *The Journal of Biological Chemistry*, 272, 20963-966.

[179] Blonk, M. C., Bilo, H. G., Nauta, J. P, Popp-Snijders, C., Mulder, C. & Donker, A. M. (1990). Dose-response effects of fish-oil supplementation in healthy volunteers. *Am J Clin Nutr*, 52, 120-27.

[180] Sanders, T. A. B., Oakley, F. R., Miller, G. J., Mitropoulos, K. A., Crook, D. & Oliver, M. F. (1997). Influence of n-6 versus n-3 polyunsaturated fatty acids in diets low in saturated acids on plasma lipoproteins and hemostatic factors. *Arteriosclerosis, Thrombosis, and Vascular Biology*, 17, 3449-460.

[181] Mori, T. A., Burke, V., Puddey, I. B., Watts, G. F., O'Neal, D. N., Best, J. D. & Beilin, L. J. (2000). Purified eicosapentaenoic and docosahexaenoic acids have different effects on serum lipids and lipoproteins, LDL particles size, glucose, and insulin in mildly hyperlipidemic men. *Am J Clin Nutr*, 71, 1084-94.

[182] Gerasimova, E., Perova, N., Ozerova, I., Polessky, V., Metelskaya, V., Sherbakova, I., Lavachev, M., Kulakova, S., Nikitin, Y. & Astakhova, T (1991). *The effect of dietary polyunsaturated fatty acids on HDL cholesterol in Chukot residents vs Muscovites. Lipids,* 26(4), 261.

[183] Wilkinson, P., Leach, C., Ah-Sing, E. E., Hussain, N., Miller, G. J., Millward, D. J. & Griffin, B. A. (2005). Influence of α-linolenic acid and fish-oil on markers of cardiovascular risk in subjects with an therogenic lipoprotein phenotype. *Atherosclerosis*, 115-24.

[184] Satoh, N., Shimatsu, A., Kotani, K., Skane, N., Yamada, K, Suganami, T., Kusuya, H. & Ogawa, Y. (2007). *Purified eicosapentaenoic acid reduces small dense LDL; remnant lipoprotein particles, and C-rective protein in metabolic syndrome*, 30,144-46.

[185] Xia, P., Vadas, M. A., Rye, K-A, Barter, P. J. & Gamble, J. R. (1999). High density lipoproteins (HDL) interrupt the sphingosine kinase signaling pathway. *The Journal of Biological Chemistry,* 274, 33143-147.

[186] Sethi, A. A., Sampson, M., Warnick, R, Muniz, N., Vaisman, B., Nordestgaard, B. G., Tybjaerg-Hansen, A. & Remaley, A. T. (2010). High Pre-β1 HDL concentrations and low lecithin: cholesterol acyltransferase are strong positive risk markers for ischemic heart disease and independent of HDL-Cholesterol. *Clinical Chemistry*, 56, 1128-137.

[187] Harris, W.S., Lu, G., Rambjør, G.S, Wålen, A.I., Ontko, J.A., Cheng, Q. E & Windsor, S.H. (1997). Influence of n-3 fatty acid supplementation on the endogenous activities of plasma lipases. *Am. J. Clin. Nutr.*, 66, 254

[188] Badellino, K. O., Wolfe, M. L., reilly, M. P. & Rader, D. J. (2006). Endothelial lipase concentrations are increased in metabolic syndrome and associated with coronary atherosclerosis. *PLoS.Medicine*, 3, 245-52.

[189] Yasuda, T., Ishida, T, & Rader, D. J. (2010). Update on the role of endothelial lipase in high-density lipoprotein metabolism, reverse cholesterol transport and atherosclerosis. *Circulation Journal*, 74, 2263-70

[190] Chen, S & Subbaiah, P. V. (2007). Phospholipid and fatty acid specificity of endothelial lipase: potential role of the enzyme in the delivery of docosahexaenoic acid (DHA) to tissues. *Biochim Biophys Acta*, 1771, 1319-28.

[191] Shiu, S. W. M., Tan, K. C. B., Huang, Y., & Wong, Y. (2008). Type 2 diabetes mellitus and endothelial lipase. *Atherosclerosis*, 198, 441-47.

[192] Huang, J., Qian, H-Y, Li, Z-Z, Zhang, J-M, Wang, S., Tao, Y., Gao, Y-L, Yin, C-Q; Que, B., Sun, T., Zhao, Z-Y & Li, Z. (2010). Role of endothelial lipase in atherosclerosis. *Translational Research*, 156, 1-6.

[193] Klein-Platat, C., Drai, J., Oujaa, M., Schlienger, J-L,.& Simon, C. (2005). Plasma fatty acids composition is associated with the metabolic syndrome and low-grade inflammation in overweight adolescents. *Am J Clin Nutr,* 82, 1178-84.

[194] Barter, P. J., Ballantyne, C. M., Carmena, R., Castro Cabezas, M., Chapman, M. J., Couture, P., de Graaf, J., Durrington, P.N., Faergeman, O., Frohlich, J., Furberg, C. D., Gagne, C., Haffner, S. M., Humphries, S. E., Jungner, I., Krauss, R. M., Kwiterovich, P., Marcovina, S., Packard, C. J., Pearson, T. A., Reddy, K. S., Rosenson, R., Sarrafzadegan, N., Sniderman, A. D., Stalenhoef, A. F., Stein, E., Talmud, P. J., Tonkin, A. M., Walldius, G., Williams, K. M. (2006). Apo B versus cholesterol in estimating cardiovascular risk and in guiding therapy: report of the thirty-person/ten-country panel. *Journal of Internal Medicine*; 259, 247-58.

[195] Doughman, S. D., Srirama Krupanidhi, S. and Sanjeevi, C. B. (2007). Omega-3 fatty acids for nutrition and medicine: considering microalgae oil as a vegetarian source of EPA and DHA. *Current Diabetes Reviews*, 3, 198-203.

[196] Hooper, L., Thompson, R. I. & Harrison, R. A. (2006). Risks and benefits of omega 3 fats for mortality, cardiovascular disease, and cancer: systematic review. *BMJ,* 332, 752-755.

[197] Das, U. (2000). Beneficial effects of n-3 fatty acids in cardiovascular diseases: but, why and how?, *Prostaglandins, Leukotrienes and Essential Fatty Acids*, 63, 351-62.

[198] Engler, M. M., Engler, M. B. & Kroetz, D. L. (1999). The effects of a diet rich in docosahexaenoic acid on organ and vascular fatty acid composition in spontaneously hypertensive rats. *Prostaglandins, Leukotrienes and Essential Fatty Acids*, 61, 289-95.

[199] Harris W. & Schacky C. (2004). The Omega-3 Index: a new risk factor for death from coronary heart disease?. *Preventive Medicine*, 39, 212– 20.

[200] Morris, M. C., Sacks, F. & Rosner, B. (1993). Does fish oil lower blood pressure? A meta-analysis of controlled trials. *Circulation*, 88, 523-33.

[201] Nordoy, A., Hatcher, L. F., Ullmann, D. L. & Connor, W. E. (1993). Individual effects of dietary saturated fatty acids and fish oil on plasma lipids and lipoproteins in normal men. *American Journal of Clinical Nutrition*, 57, 634-39.

[202] Thies, F., Garry, J. M., Yaqoob, P., Rerkasem, K., Williams, J., Shearman, C. P., Gallagher, P.J., Calder, P. C. & Grimble, R. F. (2003). Association of n-3 polyunsaturated fatty acids with stability of atherosclerotic plaques: a randomized controlled trial. *Lancet*, 361, 477-85.

[203] Mazza, M., Pomponi, M. & Janiri, L. (2007). Omega-3 fatty acids and antioxidants in neurological and psychiatric diseases: An overview. *Progress in Neuro-Psychopharmacology and Biological Psychiatry,* 31, 12-26.

[204] Simopoulos, A. P. (2002). Omega-3 fatty acids in inflammation and autoimmune diseases. *J. Am. Coll. Nutr.*, 21, 495-505.

[205] Schmitz, G. & Ecker, J. (2008). The opposing effects of n-3 and n-6 fatty acids. *Progress in Lipid Research*, 47, 147–51.

[206] Dyall, S. C. & Michael-Titus, A. T. (2008). Neurological benefits of omega-3 fatty acids. *Neuromolecular Medicine*, 4, 219-35.

[207] Kimura, F., Endo, Y., Fujimoto, K., Doisaki, N. & Koriyama, T. (2005). Administration of two oils rich in n-3 long-chain polyunsaturated fatty acids to rat pups of dams fed a diet high in fat and low in n-3 polyunsaturated fatty acids. *Fisheries Science*, 71, 431–40.

[208] Ward, O. & Singh, A. (2005). Omega-3/6 fatty acids: Alternative sources of production. *Process Biochemistry*, 40, 3627–52.

[209] Pegorier, S., Wagner, L. A., Gleich, G. J. & Pretolani, M. (2006). Eosinophil-derived cationic proteins activate the synthesis of remodeling factors by airway epithelial cells, *Journal of Immunology*, 177: 4861–4869.

[210] Risé, P., Eligini, S., Ghezzi, S., Colli, S. & Galli, C. (2007). Fatty acid composition of plasma, blood cells and whole blood: Relevance for the assessment of the fatty acid status in humans. *Prostaglandins, Leukotrienes and Essential Fatty Acids*, 76: 363-69.

[211] Russo, C., Olivieri, O., Girelli, D., Guarini, P., Pasqualini, R., Azzini, M. & Corrocher, R. (1997). Increased membrane ratios of metabolite to precursor fatty acids in essential hypertension. *Hypertension*, 29: 1058-63.

[212] Harris, W.S. (2008). The omega-3 index as a risk factor for coronary heart disease. *Am J Clinical Nutrition*, 87 (6): 1997S-2002S.

[213] Shapiro, H., Tehilla, M., Attal-Singer, J., Bruck, R. & Luzzatti, R. (2010). The therapeutic potential of long-chain omega-3 fatty acids in non-alcoholic fatty liver disease. *Clinical Nutrition*, 30, 6-19.

[214] Calder, P. C. (2006). Polyunsaturated fatty acids and inflammation. *Prostaglandins, Leukotrienes and Essential Fatty Acids, 75*, 197-202.

[215] Garofolo, A. & Petrilli, S. (2006). Omega-3 and 6 fatty acids balance in inflammatory response in patients with cancer and cachexia. *Rev. Nutr. Campinas*, 19, 611-21.

[216] He, X., Yang, X. & Guo, Y. (2007). Effects of different dietary oil sources on immune function in cyclophosphamide immunosuppressed chickens. *Animal Feed Science and Technnology*, 139, 186-200.

[217] Medina, A. R., Cerdán, L. E., Giménez, A. G., Páez, B. C., González, M. J. I. & Grima, E. M. (1999). Lipase-catalyzed esterification of glycerol and polyunsaturated fatty acids from fish and microalgae oils. *Journal of Biotechnology*, 70, 379-91.

[218] Moyad, M. (2005). *An introduction to dietary/supplemental omega-3 fatty acids for general health and prevention: Part I; Urologic Oncology: Seminars and Original Investigations*, 23, 28-35.

[219] Chapkin, R. S., Davidson, L. A., Ly, L., Weeks, B. R & Lupton, J. (2007). Immunomodulatory effects of (n-3) fatty acids: putative link to inflamatio and colon cancer. *The Journal of Nutrition*, 200S-203S.

[220] Liblau, R. S., Singer, S. M. & McDevitt, H. O. (1995). Th1 and th2 $CD4^{+}$ T cells in the pathogenesis of organ-specific autoimmune diseases. *Immunology Today*, 16, 34-38.

[221] Abbas, A. K, Murphy, K. M. & Sher, A. (1996). Functional diversity of helper T lymphocytes. *Nature*, 383, 787-93.

[222] Neurath, M. F., Finotto, S. & Glimcher, L. H. (2002). The role of Th1/Th2 polarization in mucosal immunity. *Nature Medicine*, 8, 567-73.

[223] Zhang, P., Smith, R., Chapkin, R. S. & McMurray, D. N. (2005). Dietary (n-3) polyunsaturated fatty acids modulate murine Th1/Th2 balance toward the Th2 pole by suppression of Th1 development. *The Journal of Nutrition*, 1745-51.

[224] Krauss-Etschmann, S., Harti, D. & Rzehak, P. (2008). Decreased cord blood IL-4, IL-13, and CCR4 and increased TGF-β levels after fish oil supplementation of pregnant women. *J Allergy Clin Immunol*, 121, 464-70.

[225] Shaikh, S. R. & Edidin, M. (2006). Polyunsaturated fatty acids, membrane organization, T cells, and antigen presentation. *Am J Clin Nutr*, 8, 1277-89.

[226] Switzer, K. C., Fan, Y-Y., Wang, N., McMurray, D. N. & Chapkin, R. S. (2004). Dietary polyunsaturated fatty acids promote activation-induced cell death in Th1-polarized murine $CD4^+$ T-cells. *Journal of Lipid Research*, 45, 1482-92.

[227] Fan, Y-Y., Ly, L. H., Barhoumi, R., McMurray, D. N. & Chapkin, R. S. (2004). Dietary docosahexaenoic acid suppresses T cell protein kinase C theta lipid raft recruitment and IL-2 production. *Journal Immunol*, 173, 6151-60.

[228] Zeyda, M., Watchaust, W. & Stulnig, T. M. (2003). Suppression on T cell signalling by polyunsaturated fatty acids: selectivity in inhibition of mitogen-activated protein Kinase and nuclear factor activation. *Journal Immunol*, 170, 6033-39.

[229] Muppidi, J. R., Tschopp, J. & Siegel, R. M. (2004). Life and death decisions: secondary complexes and lipid rafts in TNF receptor family signal transduction. *Immunity*, 21, 461-65.

[230] WHO / FAO, 2003. World Health Organization/Food and Agriculture Organization (2003). Diet, nutrition and the prevention of chronic diseases. *Report of a joint WHO/FAO expert consultation.* Genebra, *WHO/FAO, WHO Technical Report Series* 916.

[231] ISSFAL, 2004. ISSFAL International Society for the Study of Fatty Acids and Lipids (2004) *Recommendations for intake of polyunsaturated fatty acids in healthy adults*, p 22

[232] Lichtenstein, A. H., Appel, L. J., Brands, M., Carnethon, M., Daniels, S., Franch, H. A., Franklin, B., Kris-Etherton, P., Harris, W. S., Howard, B., Karanja N., Lefevre M., Rudel L., Sacks F., Van Horn L., Winston M., Wylie-Rosett J. (2006) Diet and lifestyle recommendations revisions. A scientific statement from the American Heart Association Nutrition Committee. *Circulation* 114, 82-96.

[233] Kris-Etherthon PM, Harris WS & Appel LJ (2002). Fish consumption, fish oil, omega-3 fatty acids and cardiovascular disease. *Circulation*.; 106,2747-57. [Erratum, *Circulation.* 2003; 107:512.]

[234] Conquer, J. and Holub, B. (1996). Supplementation with an Algae Source of Docosahexaenoic Acid Increases (n-3) Fatty Acid Status and Alters Selected Risk Factors for Heart Disease inVegetarian Subjects. *Human and Clinical Nutrition*, 126, 3032-3039.

[235] Hooper L., Thompson R. I. &Harrison R. A. (2006). Risks and benefits of omega 3 fats for mortality, cardiovascular disease, and cancer: systematic review. *BMJ,* 332, 752-755.

[236] Schmitz, H. H., Poor, C. L., Wellman, R. B. & Erdman, J. W., Jr (1991) Concentrations of selected carotenoids and vitamin A in human liver, kidney and lung tissue. *J. Nutr.* 121,1613-1621.

[237] Puhakainen, I., Ahola, I. & Yri-Järvinen, H. (1995). Dietary supplementation with n-3 fatty acids increases gluconeogenesis from glycerol but not hepatic glucose production in patients with non-insulin-dependent diabetes mellitus. *Am J Clin Nutr,* 61, 121-26.

In: Fish Oil: Production, Consumption and Health Benefits ISBN: 978-1-61470-963-3
Editors: Matthias Van Dijk and Jürgen Vitek ©2012 Nova Science Publishers, Inc.

Chapter II

Cardiovascular Health Benefits of Fish Oil

Dean G. Karalis*
Drexel University College of Medicine, Philadelphia, Pennsylvania, U. S.

Abstract

Fish oil is rich in the omega-3 fatty acids eicosapentaenoic acid (EPA) and docosahexaenoic acid (DHA). There is now extensive evidence that supports the cardiovascular benefits of these omega-3 polyunsaturated fatty acids (PUFAs). Both EPA and DHA cannot be made in sufficient quantities in the body and must therefore be obtained by a diet rich in oily fish or by consuming fish oil supplements. The mechanism by which these omega-3 PUFAs favorably impact cardiovascular disease is thought to be due to their anti-inflammatory, anti-platelet and anti-thrombotic effects and their favorable effects on arrhythmias, hypertriglyceridemia, endothelial function and telomere shortening which can preserve the genetic youth of individual cells.

The evidence for the cardiovascular benefits of omega-3 PUFAs comes from numerous epidemiological studies and several large randomized clinical studies conducted in patients with coronary artery disease, myocardial infarction and heart failure. These large randomized clinical trials have shown that modest doses of omega-3 PUFAs significantly reduce the risk of unstable angina, myocardial infarction, sudden cardiac death and death in coronary artery disease and heart failure patients. However, more recent studies have questioned the cardiovascular benefits of fish oil.

Based on the scientific evidence the American Heart Association (AHA) has recommended eating fish at least two times a week for all individuals to prevent cardiovascular disease. For individuals with coronary artery disease the recommended dose of omega-3 PUFAs is 1 g of EPA and DHA daily. To lower triglyceride levels much higher doses are needed and the AHA recommends a dose 2 to 4 g of EPA and DHA daily. To obtain the recommended dose of fish oil for individuals with coronary artery disease or to lower triglyceride levels, fish oil supplements are often needed. There are

* Corresponding Author: Dean G. Karalis, MD, 227 N. Broad Street, Suite 200, Philadelphia, PA 19107, Phone: (215) 564-3050, Fax: (215) 564-3398, E-mail: dean.karalis@drexelmed.edu

numerous over-the-counter fish oil supplements that contain varying doses of EPA and DHA and one high dose prescription formulation. The Food and Drug Administration (FDA) has approved this prescription omega-3 PUFA supplement at a dose of 4 g daily for the treatment of very high triglyceride levels.

Despite the compelling evidence for the cardiovascular benefits of omega-3 PUFAs and the AHA recommendations, most physicians to not recommend fish oil supplements for their high-risk patients. In addition there is confusion regarding the formulations of fish oil that are available and the doses of fish oil that should be used in clinical practice. The purpose of this review is to discuss the production of fish oil, the differences between available fish oil supplements and to summarize the current scientific evidence on the cardiovascular health benefits of fish oil consumption.

Omega-3 polyunsaturated fatty acids (PUFAs) found in fish oils have been shown to have significant cardiovascular health benefits. The American Heart Association currently recommends that all Americans eat at least two servings of fish, preferably oily fish a week; while for individuals with coronary artery disease a higher dose of omega-3 PUFAs is recommended. For individuals with coronary artery disease 1 g of combined eicosapentaenoic acid (EPA) and docosahexaenoic acid (DHA) daily is recommended either by eating more oily fish or by using nutritional supplements (1). To understand the cardiovascular benefits of omega-3 PUFAs it is important to first review the chemistry of fatty acid and triglyceride metabolism in the human body.

Fatty acids are a major source of fuel, especially for cardiac and skeletal muscle and play an important role in the synthesis of cell membranes and in maintaining normal cell and tissue function. Fatty acids are made up of a long chain of hydrocarbons with a terminal carboxylate group. The long hydrocarbon chains of fatty acids can be either saturated or unsaturated and this in turn imparts important biological consequences onto the fatty acid. Saturated fatty acids have no double carbon bonds, so each carbon atom is attached to 2 hydrogen atoms, such that is each carbon atom is saturated with hydrogen atoms. Saturated fats are associated with a higher risk of cardiovascular disease than mono- or polyunsaturated fats. Foods that are high in saturated fats include dairy products, animal fats, coconut oil, palm oil and chocolate. Trans fats have been created by the food industry by adding hydrogen ions to polyunsaturated fats through a process called hydrogenation and like saturated fats, trans fats have been associated with a high risk for cardiovascular disease (2,3). Current public health recommendations are to keep saturated fat intake as low as possible and to avoid trans fats while maintaining a nutritionally adequate diet.

Monounsaturated fatty acids have one carbon-to-carbon double bond while polyunsaturated fatty acids have more than one carbon-to-carbon double bond. Polyunsaturated fatty acids are further classified into 2 groups, omega-3 or omega-6 based on the position within the fatty acid of the first double bond from the last omega-carbon atom. The most common omega-6 PUFAs are arachidonic acid, found in animal meat and linoleic acid, found in vegetable oils, seeds and nuts. The most common omega-3 PUFAs are eicosapentaenoic acid (EPA) and docosahexaenoic acid (DHA) from oily fish (Figure 1) and alpha-linolenic acid (ALA) from canola oil, soybeans, walnuts and flaxseed. Fish and other seafood contain all three types of fatty acids, while oily fish such as tuna, salmon, trout, mackerel, herring and sardines have high concentrations of omega-3 PUFAs. In the absence of sufficient dietary fat, the body is able to synthesize most fatty acids from carbohydrates.

Those fatty acids that cannot be produced in the body yet are necessary to maintain normal cell and tissue health are termed "essential" fatty acids. Essential fatty acids play an important role in many metabolic processes and are "essential" for good health. For humans there are only two essential fatty acids, the omega-3 PUFA alpha-linolenic acid and the omega-6 PUFA, linoleic acid. In humans alpha-linolenic acid can be converted to EPA and DHA, but in most people that conversion is inefficient. Hence both EPA and DHA are in essence also essential fatty acids. The omega-3 PUFAs EPA and DHA can only be obtained in sufficient quantity by eating a diet rich in oily fish or by taking fish oil supplements.

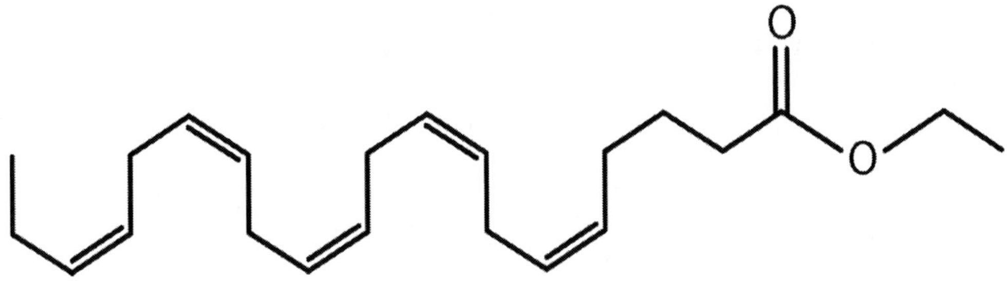

Eicosapentaenoic acid (EPA) (20:5 n-3)

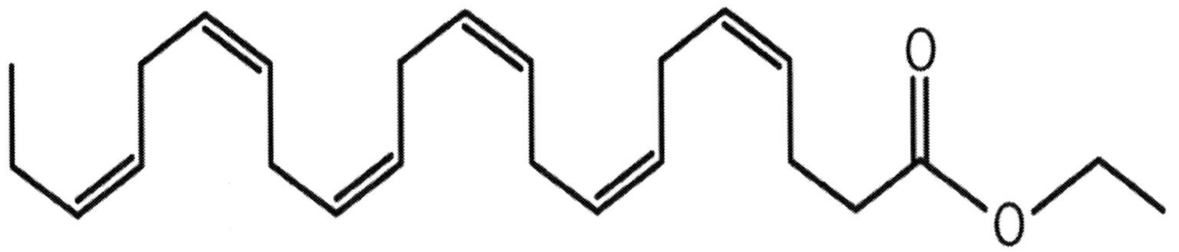

Docosahexaenoic acid (DHA) (22:6 n-3)

Figure 1. Chemical structures of the marine omega-3 polyunsaturated fatty acids (PUFAs). Eicosapentaenoic acid (EPA) has 20 carbons and 5 double bonds, it's name being derived from the Greek words "eicosa" meaning 20 and "penta" meaning 5. Docosahexaenoic acid (DHA) has 22 carbons and 6 double bonds, derived from the Greek words "docosa" meaning 22 and "hexa" meaning 6. For both EPA and DHA, the first double bond is three carbon atoms from the methyl or "omega" end (omega-3).

In contrast to the strong evidence for the cardiovascular benefits of omega-3 PUFAs, there is controversy as to whether omega-6 PUFAs reduce cardiovascular risk and there is some evidence to suggest that an excess intake of arachidonic acid is associated with an increased risk of cardiovascular disease. This is based on a number of studies that have found a positive relationship between the amount of arachidonic acid in adipose tissue and the risk of ischemic heart disease (4,5). Arachidonic acid is metabolized to prostaglandins and leukotrienes, which can lead to a proinflammatory and prothrombotic state. Although linoleic acid may have no direct adverse metabolic effects it can be metabolized to arachidonic acid. In addition an excess of omega-6 PUFAs may interfere with the cardiovascular benefits of omega-3 PUFAs (6). For these reasons many experts have argued that the high ratio of omega-6 to omega-3 PUFAs common in the diet of most Americans is a significant risk factor for coronary artery disease and have recommended significant reductions in the intake of omega-6 PUFAs. However other studies have shown that both arachidonic acid and linoleic acid do not lead to a proinflammatory state and do not interfere with the beneficial effects of omega-3 PUFAs. In the CHIANTI study by Ferrucci and colleagues (7), plasma levels of omega-6 PUFAs, mainly arachidonic acid were inversely associated with levels of several proinflammatory markers. In 2009 an American Heart Association Science Advisory Statement found no evidence to support a change in the dietary guidelines for omega-6 PUFAs and recommended an intake of omega-6 PUFAs of at least 5 to 10% of energy intake (8). However, these recommendations have been recently brought into question based on a meta-analysis of nine randomized controlled studies in over 11,000 patients evaluating omega-6 PUFAs and cardiovascular risk (9). In this meta-analysis there was a 28% increase in the relative risk of cardiovascular death as well as an increase of all relevant cardiovascular outcomes in those patients randomized to an omega-6 PUFA specific diet. In contrast, among patients randomized to a diet mixed with both omega-6 and omega-3 PUFAs there was an 8% reduction in all-cause mortality and a 22% reduction in the risk for cardiovascular death. The authors concluded that there was possible harm in a diet enriched with omega-6 PUFAs. Based on the current evidence the most practical advice a practitioner can give to his patients to reduce their risk for coronary heart disease is to focus on increasing their intake of omega-3 PUFAs, instead of reducing their omega-6 PUFA intake (10).

Fatty Acid and Triglyceride Metabolism

Fatty acids are derived from triglycerides either endogenously from hepatic production or exogenously from the food we ingest. After a meal, fat from animal, fish or vegetable oil is digested in the small intestine by pancreatic lipase and mixed with bile salts. These emulsified fat particles are further hydrolyzed, breaking down the triglycerides into free fatty acids and monoglyceride. Short and medium-chain fatty acids are directed into the portal circulation while long-chain fatty acids are re-esterified into triglycerides within intestinal epithelial cells. To carry these re-esterified triglycerides in plasma they are incorporated into chylomicrons of which ApoB 48 is the predominate apolipoprotein. Chylomicrons are secreted into the thoracic duct where they gain access to the peripheral circulation. Chylomicrons consist almost exclusively of triglycerides with a small amount of cholesterol ester. Chylomicrons are too large to cross the endothelial lining of blood vessels and undergo hydrolysis by lipoprotein lipase (LPL). The free fatty acids that are released are taken up by muscle cells for energy or by adipocytes for fat storage. Under normal physiologic conditions the liver rapidly takes up any remaining chylomicron remnants.

Within the liver, triglycerides and cholesterol esters are assembled with apoB-100 to form very-low density lipoprotein (VLDL) particles. In the fasting state the majority of triglycerides are transported in the bloodstream by VLDL particles. VLDL is hydrolyzed by hepatic lipase and the free fatty acids released can be taken up by muscle cells for energy use, taken up and stored in adipocytes as fat, or returned back to the liver. The remaining particles, intermediate-density lipoprotein (IDL) or small remnant VLDL can be taken back up by the liver or converted by hepatic lipase into low-density lipoprotein (LDL) particles.

Foods differ in their fat content and in the types of fatty acids they provide. Foods with a high concentration of saturated fatty acids and trans fats are associated with an increased risk of atherosclerosis and cardiovascular events. The increased cardiovascular risk associated with saturated and trans fat intake is thought to be primarily due their effect on increasing the concentration of LDL cholesterol. In addition, a diet high in saturated fats and carbohydrates can lead to hypertriglyceridemia. Increased intestinal absorption of fat leads to an overproduction of chylomicrons that exceeds the liver's ability to handle the excess free fatty acids and there is an accumulation of triglyceride rich lipoproteins in adipose tissue and other organs, which adversely affects insulin function (11). This inhibitory effect on insulin action further increases triglyceride and cholesterol synthesis. Increased triglyceride synthesis leads to large triglyceride rich VLDL particles, which activate cholesteryl ester transfer protein, leading to triglyceride enrichment of LDL and high density lipoprotein (HDL) particles (12). Subsequent hydrolysis of these triglyceride enriched particles by LPL results in small LDL and HDL particles (Figure 2). Small dense LDL particles are more atherogenic because they are more easily retained in the intima of blood vessels, are more easily oxidized and remain in circulation longer than larger LDL particles (13, 14). Small HDL particles are more easily filtered through the kidney leading to lower HDL levels. Additional evidence suggests that these triglyceride enriched HDL particles may be dysfunctional as well (15).

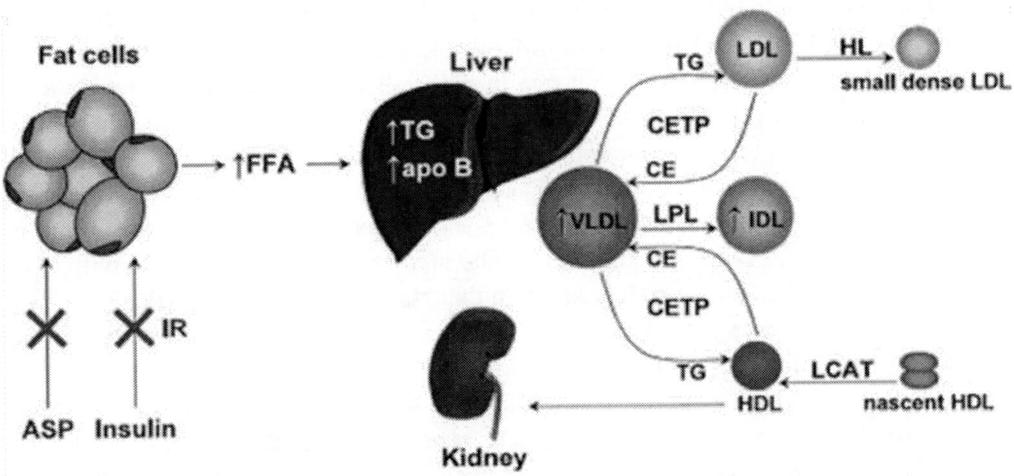

Figure 2. Mechanisms by which elevated triglyceride levels cause mixed dyslipidemia. An increased flux of FFA from adipose tissue increases the production of TG, apo B and VLDL cholesterol. Incomplete hydrolysis of large VLDL particles leads to increased concentrations of TG rich remnant lipoproteins such as IDL cholesterol. In addition TG in VLDL are exchanged for CE in LDL and HDL particles by CETP. As these TG rich LDL and HDL particles undergo hydrolysis by HL small LDL and HDL particles are produced. Small LDL particles are particularly atherogenic, and are more easily excreted by the kidney leading to low levels of HDL cholesterol. Apo B = apolipoprotein B; ASP = acylation stimulatory protein; CE = cholesterol esters; CETP = cholesterol ester transfer protein; FFA = free fatty acids; HDL = high-density lipoprotein; HL = hepatic lipase; IR = insulin resistance; IDL = intermediate density lipoprotein; LCAT = lecithin-cholesterol acyltransferase; LDL = low-density lipoprotein; LPL = lipoprotein lipase; TG = triglycerides. (Reprinted from Mudd et al. (12) with permission.)

Omega-3 PUFAs lower triglycerides and triglyceride rich lipoproteins. A diet rich in oily fish has been associated with a reduced risk of atherosclerosis and cardiovascular events (1). Although fish contains variable amounts of all types of fatty acids, oily fish such as tuna, salmon, mackerel, herring and sardines have high concentrations of the omega-3 PUFAs, EPA and DHA. The favorable impact on cardiovascular risk of a diet rich in omega-3 PUFAs are due to the anti-inflammatory, anti-platelet and anti-thrombotic effects of EPA and DHA and to their favorable effects on arrhythmias, hypertriglyceridemia, endothelial function and telomere shortening which can preserve the genetic youth of individual cells.

Evidence That Fish Oil Reduces Cardiovascular Risk

Over the last several decades there have been numerous epidemiological, observational and randomized clinical trials that have demonstrated the cardiovascular benefits of omega-3 PUFAs. Early observational studies described the low rate of coronary heart disease in the Greenland Eskimos and attributed their low cardiovascular risk to their diet of whale and seal blubber and fish rich in omega-3 PUFAs (16). These observations that a diet rich in omega-3 PUFAs is associated with a low risk of coronary heart disease has been extended to other populations from around the world whose diet is rich in oily fish; including the Alaskan Native Eskimos and people in Japan (17, 18). The typical Western European and American diet is low in omega-3 PUFAs, however individuals in these countries who consume a large amount of oily fish have also been shown to have a lower rate of coronary heart disease (19-21). The cardiovascular benefits of a diet rich in omega-3 PUFAs extends to women as well. In the Nurses Health Study (22) there was a direct relationship with increased intake of fish and omega-3 PUFAs and a lower rate of coronary heart disease death. The rate for coronary heart disease death among women who ate fish more than 5 times a week was 34% lower compared to women who rarely ate fish. Even a small consumption of fish was found to be beneficial. Women in the Nurses Health Study who ate fish only 1 to 3 times a month still had a 21% lower risk of coronary heart disease death than women who rarely ate fish.

The cardiovascular benefits of omega-3 PUFAs can be lost when individuals who have consumed a diet rich in omega-3 PUFAs immigrate to other countries and adopt a diet low in omega-3 PUFAs and high in saturated and trans fatty acids. In the Seven Countries Study an inverse relationship was found between fish consumption and coronary heart disease mortality, however this association was no longer significant when the effects of saturated fatty acids and cigarette smoking were considered (23). Japan has the lowest rate of coronary heart disease mortality among developed countries (24). This is in part attributed to their high intake of oily fish, with their fish intake being one of the highest in the world (25). Yet Japanese Americans have a higher risk of coronary heart disease than their Japanese ancestors (26) and this is thought to be due to changing their diet to one that is less rich in oily fish. In a study by Sekikawa and colleagues (27) Japanese men living in Japan had a 2 fold higher level of serum omega-3 PUFAs and lower carotid intimal-medial thickness (IMT) and less burden of coronary artery calcium (CAC) than white men or Japanese men living in the United States. Furthermore, although omega-3 PUFAs in fish reduce cardiovascular risk, environmental contaminants such as methyl mercury in certain fish may offset the beneficial effects of omega-3 PUFAs (1).

Randomized Clinical Trial with Omega-3 PUFAs

It has now been over 2 decades since the first randomized trial of omega-3 PUFAs was completed. Since then there have been numerous randomized clinical trials that have evaluated the cardiovascular benefits of omega-3 PUFAs from either fish or fish oil supplements (Table 1). Most have shown a positive outcome, though more recent trials have called into question the benefit of omega-3 PUFA supplements in patients with stable coronary artery disease.

Table 1. Large randomized clinical trials with omega-3 PUFAs. CAD = coronary artery disease, CV = cardiovascular, DHA = docosahexaenoic acid, EPA = eicosapentaenoic acid, MI = myocardial infarction, SCD = sudden cardiac death

Study	Patient Number	Patient Type	Daily Omega-3 PUFA Dose	Study Duration	Outcomes
DART (28)	2033 men	Recent MI	350 mg EPA	2 years	29% reduction in all-cause mortality ($p < 0.05$)
GISSI Prevenzione (30)	11,324 patients; 1665 (15%) were women	Recent MI	850 mg EPA and DHA	3.5 years	20% reduction in major CV events ($p = 0.008$); 30% reduction in CV death ($p = 0.02$); 45% reduction in SCD ($p = 0.01$)
JELIS (31)	18, 645 patients; 12,786 (69%) were women	CAD (20% of patients) and primary prevention patients	1800 mg EPA	4.6 years	19% reduction in major CV events ($p = 0.01$)
GISSI-HF (36)	6976 patients; 1516 (22%) were women	Chronic HF	850 mg EPA and DHA	3.9 years	6% reduction in CV death or hospitalization ($p = 0.04$)
Alpha Omega (37)	4837 patient; 1054 (22%) were women	Previous MI	400 mg EPA and DHA	3.4 years	No reduction in major CV events for all patients; non-significant 22% reduction in major CV events for diabetics ($p=0.11$)
OMEGA (38)	3851 patients; 1010 (26%) were women	Recent MI	840 mg EPA and DHA	1 year	No reduction in SCD, total mortality or major CV events ($p = 0.34$)

The first of such trials was the Diet and Reinfarction Trial (DART). In this study 2033 men who had been admitted to the hospital with a recent myocardial infarction were randomized to receive or not receive advise on several dietary factors including eating at least two weekly portions of fatty fish (28). The amount of fish that was recommended in DART was small and corresponded to only about 2.5 g of EPA weekly or about 350 mg of EPA daily. Those subjects advised to eat fatty fish had a 29% reduction in all-cause mortality as compared to those patients who were not so advised. The benefit of increased oily fish intake occurred early in the trial and the greatest benefit was in the reduction of fatal myocardial infarction. The reduction in all-cause mortality was entirely attributable to a reduction in ischemic heart disease deaths. Singh and colleagues reported the first small study of omega-3 fatty acid supplements for the secondary prevention of coronary heart disease (29). In this study, 120 patients admitted to the hospital with a suspected myocardial infarction were randomized to supplemental fish oil capsules that provided 1.8 g of EPA and DHA daily, 20 g of mustard oil providing 2.9 g of alpha-linolenic acid daily or placebo. After one year, total cardiovascular events were significantly less in the fish oil group compared with the placebo group (25% vs. 35%; $p < 0.01$). In addition there were significantly less nonfatal myocardial infarctions, total cardiac deaths, total cardiac arrhythmias, left ventricular enlargement and angina pectoris in the fish oil group compared to the placebo patients.

The first large randomized clinical trial to assess the role of omega-3 PUFA supplements for the secondary prevention of coronary heart disease was the GISSI-Prevenzione trial (30). The GISSI-Prevenzione trial randomized 11,324 recent survivors of a myocardial infarction (< 3 months) to 1 g daily of omega-3 PUFAs containing approximately 850 mg of EPA and DHA, 300 mg of vitamin E, both supplements, or no supplements for 3.5 years. Triglyceride levels were lowered by only 3 to 4% with fish oil therapy. Treatment with omega-3 PUFAs, but not vitamin E reduced the primary combined endpoint of death, nonfatal myocardial infarction and stroke by 15% ($p = 0.02$) and reduced cardiovascular death, nonfatal myocardial infarction and nonfatal stroke by 20% ($p = 0008$). When the individual components of the combined endpoint were analyzed, the 20% decrease in all-cause mortality, the 30% reduction in cardiovascular death and the 45% reduction is sudden cardiac death accounted for all the benefit seen in the combined endpoint. There was no difference between the treatment groups for nonfatal cardiovascular events.

The JELIS trial was the first large randomized trial of fish oil supplements to enroll a large population of primary prevention patients (31). This Japanese trial randomized 18,645 patients with and without a history of coronary artery disease and a total cholesterol > 250 mg/dL to statin therapy along with 1800 mg of EPA daily or statin therapy alone for 5 years. Just over 80% of the patients enrolled in this study (14,981 patients) had no history of coronary heart disease and women accounted for over two-thirds of the entire study population. The baseline LDL cholesterol and triglyceride levels in this study were 170 mg/dL and on average 151 mg/dL respectively. LDL-cholesterol was lowered by 25% in both groups and in the EPA group triglyceride levels were about 5% lower than in the placebo group. The primary endpoint was any major cardiovascular event (sudden death or nonfatal and fatal myocardial infarction) and any other nonfatal cardiovascular event (unstable angina or coronary revascularization). At a mean follow-up of 4.6 years, 262 patients (2.8%) met the primary endpoint in the EPA group compared to 324 patients (3.5%) in the control group, a 19% reduction ($p = 0.01$). Unstable angina and nonfatal myocardial infarction were significantly reduced, while sudden death and coronary death were not. Among the 3664 patients with coronary disease (secondary prevention), major coronary events were reduced by 19%, ($p < 0.05$) while in primary prevention patients, although major coronary events were reduced by a similar 18% this reduction did not reach statistical significance ($p = 0.13$). These results are even more impressive when one factors in the high intake of oily fish in the diet of the normal Japanese population. The placebo group in the JELIS trial likely had one of the highest intakes of oily fish in the world (25). Comparing JELIS to the GISSI Prevenzione trial, patients in JELIS were given a higher dose of omega-3 PUFAs and had a greater reduction in nonfatal cardiovascular events. In the GISSI Prevenzione trial, although patients randomized to omega-3 PUFAs had a lower cardiovascular mortality rate, the incidence of nonfatal cardiovascular events was no different in those patients randomized to low dose omega-3 PUFA supplements compared to patients in the placebo group. The authors concluded that low dose of omega-3 PUFAs can reduce cardiovascular mortality and sudden death while higher doses of omega-3 PUFAs, more than 1 g daily can reduce the risk on nonfatal cardiovascular events. Subsequent substudies from JELIS have expanded our understanding of the benefits of omega-3 PUFAs in reducing cardiovascular risk (32-35). The beneficial effects in reducing cardiovascular events from EPA were also seen in patients with a history of stroke, coronary artery disease, myocardial infarction, and in those patients with evidence of the metabolic syndrome. EPA had no adverse effects on glycemic control and did not increase the risk of bleeding.

The GISSI-HF trial extended the benefits of omega-3 PUFAs to patients with heart failure (36). In this study, 6,975 chronic heart failure patients (NYHA class II to IV) were randomized to omega-3 PUFAs (1 g daily) or placebo for 3.9 years. Patients were also randomized to rosuvastatin 10 mg daily or placebo. Heart failure patients could be enrolled in this study irrespective of their cause of left ventricular dysfunction, although most had systolic dysfunction as the cause or their heart failure. Almost one-half of patients had non-ischemic causes for their heart failure and over 90% had a left ventricular ejection fraction of less than 40%. The primary endpoint was time to death and time to death or any admission to the hospital for any cardiovascular reason. A total of 955 patients (27%) died from any cause in the omega-3 PUFAs group compared to 1014 patients (29%) in the placebo group ($p = 0.04$). A total of 1981 patients (57%) died or were admitted to the hospital for any cardiovascular reason compared to 2053 (59%) in the placebo group ($p=0.009$). In absolute terms 56 patients had to be treated for 3.9 years to prevent one death and 44 treated to prevent one death or admission to the hospital. Of the absolute risk reduction on total mortality, the greatest proportion was attributed to suspected sudden cardiac death and almost half of the absolute risk reduction for the first hospital admission for any cardiovascular reason was due to a reduction in admission for ventricular arrhythmias. In contrast to the benefits seen with omega-3 PUFAs, rosuvastatin had no effect on any of the primary endpoints. The authors concluded that treatment with omega-3 PUFAs is safe and well tolerated and can provide a small advantage in terms of mortality and admission to the hospital in chronic heart failure patients. Although the benefit was smaller than expected most of these patients were treated with recommended therapies for heart failure. On study admission 94% of patients were being treated with blockers of the renin-angiotensin system, 65% were being treated with beta-blockers, and 39% with spironolactone. Better heart failure treatment may explain the less than expected benefit of omega-3 PUFAs in this population of heart failure patients.

Each of these prior randomized studies showed a benefit of omega-3 PUFA supplementation in either reducing the risk of cardiovascular events or cardiovascular death in patients with coronary heart disease. Two more recent secondary prevention trials, the Alpha Omega trial (37) and OMEGA (38) failed to show an added benefit of omega-3 PUFA supplementation over standard therapy for the secondary prevention of coronary heart disease. The Alpha Omega trial randomized 4,837 patients aged 60 to 80 years old with a previous myocardial infarction to one of four treatment arms; a combination of EPA and DHA (400 mg daily), alpha-linolenic acid (2 g daily), a combination of EPA, DHA and alpha-linolenic acid or placebo. The omega-3 PUFAs were in margarine spread the patients consumed daily and patients were followed for on average 3.7 years. The primary endpoint of the study was the incidence of major cardiovascular events, comprising fatal and nonfatal cardiovascular events and any cardiovascular intervention, including percutaneous intervention or coronary artery bypass surgery. Low dose supplementation of EPA and DHA in this study failed to reduce the primary endpoint of fatal and nonfatal cardiovascular events or interventions, compared to patients treated with alpha-linolenic acid or placebo. In addition there was no benefit of fish oil supplements in any of the secondary endpoints, including death from ventricular arrhythmias. Among patients receiving alpha-linolenic acid alone there was a 9% nonsignificant reduction in cardiovascular events compared with placebo or omega-3 fatty acid patients and in subgroup analysis there was a 27% reduction in cardiovascular events in women taking alpha-linolenic acid and also a 22% lower event rate in diabetic patients taking EPA and DHA, though these reductions failed to reach statistical significance. The overall negative findings in this study contrast with the findings from the GISSI Prevenzione trial. The discordant findings of these two trials may be due to the fact that the number of deaths in the Alpha Omega trial was much less than anticipated. This may have been due to improved treatment of the patient's coronary heart disease. In the Alpha Omega trial 86% of patients were receiving lipid-lowering therapy in contrast to only 5% of patients in the GISSI Prevenzione trial at the outset of the study. In addition the dose of EPA and DHA used in the Alpha Omega trial (400 mg daily) was much lower than the dose used in those studies that showed a benefit of omega-3 fatty acid supplements, such as GISSI Prevenzione (850 mg of EPA and DHA daily), JELIS (1.8 g of EPA daily) and GISSI-HF (850 mg of EPA and DHA daily).

The OMEGA trial was the most recently published trial to test the efficacy of omega-3 PUFAs in the secondary prevention of coronary heart disease (38). As with the Alpha Omega trial this study failed to show any benefit of omega-3 PUFA supplements in patients with a history of myocardial infarction. This trial enrolled 3,851 patients within 2 weeks of a myocardial infarction to about 850 mg of EPA and DHA daily or placebo in addition to optimal medical care. The primary endpoint of the study was sudden death or the incidence of other secondary cardiovascular endpoints. After one year of follow-up no benefit was seen in the patients assigned to omega-3 PUFA supplements compared to placebo. However the event rate in this trial was very low. The rate of sudden cardiac death was only 1.5%, total mortality 4.6%, and the rate of all major cardiovascular events only 10.4%. There are several reasons to explain the different results seen in this trial compared to the GISSI-Prevenzione trial. First, the OMEGA trial may have been inadequately powered, second patients in the trial were better treated for their coronary heart disease and, third the trial follow-up was shorter compared to the GISSI Prevenzione trial. There are two ongoing studies that should help better determine the role for omega-3 PUFA supplements in the prevention of coronary heart disease, VITAL (39) and ASCEND (40). VITAL (Vitamin D and Omega-3 Trial) is recruiting 20,000 men over the age of 60 and women over the age 65 with no history of cardiac disease. Patients will be randomized to vitamin D (2000 IU daily) and/or omega-3 PUFA supplements (1 g daily). The primary outcome is cancer and cardiovascular disease events. The ASCEND trial is funded by the British Heart Foundation and is enrolling 10,000 diabetic patients without clinical manifestations of atherosclerotic disease to either low dose aspirin and/or 1g of prescription omega-3 PUFA supplements. The primary endpoint is major cardiovascular and cerebrovascular disease events. Both studies are currently ongoing.

Mechanisms by with Fish Oil Reduce Cardiovascular Risk

1. Anti-Inflammatory Effects

Systemic inflammation plays a key role in the development and progression of atherosclerosis (41) and clinical studies have shown that circulating inflammatory biomarkers are independent risk factors for coronary heart disease (42). Omega-3 PUFAs have been shown to have anti-inflammatory properties. In populations with a low intake of oily fish, arachidonic acid is the predominate PUFA present in tissue. (43-45). The oxidative metabolism of arachidonic acid by the cyclooxygenase and 5-lipooxygenase pathways leads to the production of eicosanoids, which are a class of bioactive molecules that include prostaglandins, leukotrienes and thromboxanes. The eicosanoids derived from omega-6 PUFAs, such as arachidonic acid are generally pro-inflammatory and promote platelet aggregation, while the eicosanoids derived from omega-3 PUFA are predominately anti-inflammatory and inhibit platelet aggregation. When diets are rich in oily fish or supplemented with fish oil capsules, the content of omega-3 PUFAs in tissue increases and omega-3 PUFA (predominately EPA) compete with arachidonic acid for prostaglandin and leukotriene synthesis. This leads to a reduction in the pro-inflammatory eicosanoids from arachidonic acid metabolism and a reduction in circulating biomarkers (46).

In the Heart and Soul Study (47) patients with stable coronary artery disease patients had blood levels of EPA and DHA examined to determine their relationship with the inflammatory biomarkers, C-reactive protein (CRP) and interleukin-6 (IL-6). After multivariate adjustment, the levels of EPA and DHA were inversely related to the levels of CRP and IL-6. Demographic factors including body-mass index, smoking, LDL cholesterol or statin use did, not modify the relationship between higher levels of omega-3 PUFAs and lower levels of these inflammatory biomarkers. In the Multi-Ethnic Study of Atherosclerosis (MESA) the intake of omega-3 PUFAs was inversely associated with plasma concentrations of IL-6, CRP and matrix metalloproteinase-3 (48). Metalloproteinases are thought to play a key role in plaque stability (49). As in the Heart and Soul Study, after adjustment for multiple covariates the inverse relationship between these inflammatory biomarkers and fish intake remained significant. In a small study, 14 patients with severe heart failure were randomized to high dose omega-3 PUFAs (8 g daily) or placebo and followed for 18 weeks (50). High dose omega-3 PUFA supplements resulted in a 59% reduction in tumor necrosis factor-alpha (TNF-α) and a 39% reduction in interleukin-1 (IL-1). In another study 30 healthy post-menopausal women on hormone replacement therapy were randomly assigned to one of three treatment groups, safflower oil, low dose fish oil, about 1 g of EPA and DHA daily or high dose fish oil, about 2 g of EPA and DHA daily (51). In both fish oil groups the levels of CRP were significantly lower compared to the safflower oil group. There was no difference in the reduction of CRP between the low and higher dose fish oil groups. IL-6 concentrations decreased in all three groups and plasma triglyceride levels and the triglyceride to HDL cholesterol ratio was significantly lower in the high dose fish oil group compared to those patients randomized to safflower oil. Triglyceride levels were lower in the high dose fish oil group compared to the low dose fish oil group, however this difference did not reach statistical significance. The authors concluded that fish oil supplementation might reduce some of the undesirable effects of hormone replacement therapy.

2. Anti-Platelet and Anti-Thrombotic Effects

The prostaglandin thromboxane A_2 is a major stimulant of platelet aggregation and thrombosis. Thromboxane is produced by oxidative metabolism of the omega-6 PUFA, arachidonic acid on cell membranes. Omega-3 PUFAs can displace omega-6 PUFA stores in cell membranes that are needed to produce thromboxane A_2, hence reducing their levels. Fish oil contains the omega-3 PUFA EPA. Fish oil supplementation markedly increases the eicosapentaenoate content of phospholipids from red blood cells and platelets and alters their pattern of thromboxane and prostacyclin synthesis (52). Previous studies have shown that omega-3 fatty acids can reduce platelet aggregability and the response of platelets to thromboxane (53). These effects are thought to be responsible for the anti-platelet and anti-thrombotic properties of omega-3 PUFAs. In a placebo controlled randomized clinical study, 63 patients who had undergone percutaneous intervention (PCI) and were receiving standard dual anti-platelet therapy (aspirin 75 mg and clopidogrel 75 mg daily) were randomized to 1 g of omega-3 ethyl ester containing 460 mg of EPA and 380 mg of DHA (54). After one month, the platelet reactivity index and maximal platelet aggregation were significantly lower (22% and 13% respectively) in those patients taking omega-3 PUFAs compared with placebo. In addition, adding omega-3 PUFAs to standard therapy in stable patients undergoing PCI significantly decreased thrombin formation and oxidative stress and favorably altered fibrin-clotting properties (54). There were no cases of major bleeding reported and the incidence of minor bruising was no different between the study groups. These effects of omega-3 PUFAs may lead to a decreased risk of thrombotic events after PCI, however a larger study is needed to determine the clinical benefits of adding omega-3 PUFAs to standard therapy after PCI. In another study, 485 patients with stable coronary artery disease taking low dose aspirin (75 to 162 mg daily) were screened for aspirin resistance. Thirty patients (6%) were found to be aspirin resistant and they were randomized to receive low dose aspirin and 4 omega-3 PUFA capsules daily (360 mg of EPA and 240 mg of DHA per capsule) or to a higher dose of aspirin, 325 mg daily (56). After one month of treatment 12 patients (80%) who received low dose aspirin along with omega-3 PUFAs and 11 patients (73%) taking 325 mg of aspirin alone were no longer aspirin resistant. Omega-3 PUFAs potentiate the anti-platelet effects of aspirin and clopidogrel in patients with coronary artery disease.

3. Anti-Arrhythmic Effects

Omega-3 PUFAs have anti-arrhythmic effects and several large randomized clinical trials have shown that omega-3 PUFAs can reduce the risk of ventricular arrhythmias and sudden cardiac death in patients with structural heart disease (30, 36, 57). Omega-3 PUFAs have also been shown to reduce the risk of atrial fibrillation (58, 59).

There are several mechanisms by which omega-3 PUFAs exert their anti-arrhythmic effects. In clinical studies omega-3 PUFAs have been shown to have significant effects on improving autonomic function. Omega-3 PUFAs have been shown to reduce heart rate variability and resting heart rate, slow atrial ventricular conduction and lessen the likelihood of QT prolongation (60). In addition omega-3 PUFAs have effects on ventricular repolarization by inhibiting both the fast voltage-dependent sodium channels and the L-type calcium channel (61). These latter effects may be the most important mechanisms by which omega-3 PUFAs prevent fatal ventricular arrhythmias and sudden cardiac death.

The GISSI Prevenzione trial was the first large randomized clinical study to suggest the potential anti-arrhythmic effects of fish oil (30). In this study a mixture of the omega-3 PUFAs, EPA and DHA showed a significant reduction in all-cause and cardiovascular mortality that was driven primarily by a reduction in sudden cardiac death. In contrast to the findings in the GISSI Prevenzione trial, coronary artery disease patients in JELIS (31) who were taking fish oil had a significant reduction in unstable angina and nonfatal myocardial infarction, but not in sudden cardiac death. In addition studies of omega-3 PUFAs in patients with implantable cardioverter defibrillators (ICD) have not shown beneficial effects in reducing the risk of ventricular tachycardia or ICD shocks (62, 63). In a meta-analysis of 12 studies of fish oil totaling over 32,000 coronary artery disease patients, which included GISSI Prevenzione and JELIS no anti-arrhythmic protection with fish oil was found (64). In this meta-analysis there was a 20% reduction in the risk of cardiac death. There was also a trend towards a reduction in the risk of ICD firings and a reduction in the risk of sudden cardiac death, however these results failed to achieve statistical significance. Since the publication of this meta-analysis there have been 3 additional large randomized clinical studies published. The GISSI-HF trial showed a modest but significant reduction in death and admission to the hospital with fish oil supplementation (36). Of the risk reduction in total mortality, the greatest proportion was attributed to suspected sudden death and almost half of the risk reduction for the first hospital admission for any cardiovascular reason was due to a reduction in admission for ventricular arrhythmias. In contrast to the findings of the GISSI Prevenzione and the GISSI-HF studies, the recent Alpha Omega (37) and Omega (38) trials failed to show any benefit of omega-3 PUFAs in reducing the risk of sudden death. The differences between these trials may be explained by the dose and type of omega-3 PUFAs used, the severity of cardiac disease at baseline and the improved cardiac therapies that patients received in the most recent trials. In the Omega trial less than one-quarter of patients had moderate to severe left ventricular systolic dysfunction, while in GISSI-HF over 90% of patients had a left ventricular ejection fraction of < 40%. In a post-hoc analysis of the GISSI Prevenzione trial the reduction in sudden cardiac death was concentrated in patients with left ventricular systolic dysfunction and those patients whose left ventricular ejection fraction was > 50%, no significant reduction in sudden death was seen (65). The current evidence does not support a role for omega-3 PUFAs in the prevention of sudden cardiac death for all patients with coronary artery disease. However, the evidence that fish oil can prevent life-threatening ventricular arrhythmias is strongest in patients with a history of myocardial infarction and left ventricular dysfunction or heart failure.

Omega-3 PUFAs also have significant effects in atrial fibrillation. Fish intake and the incidence of atrial fibrillation were assessed in participants from the Cardiovascular Health Study (CHS), a population-based, prospective study among older adults (58). Over a 12-year period there was a 30% lower risk of atrial fibrillation in those older adults who consumed high quantities of tuna or other broiled or baked fish. This benefit did not extend to those patients who ate fried fish or fish sandwiches. In another study 160 patients undergoing coronary artery bypass surgery (CABG) were randomized to a control group or to 2 g of omega-3 PUFAs started 5 days before undergoing elective CABG (59). The incidence of post-operative atrial fibrillation was reduced by more than half from 33.3 to 15.2% ($p = 0.013$) and post-operative hospital days were significantly less in those patients who had started taking omega-3 PUFA supplements prior to their CABG surgery. In a recent prospective randomized clinical study, Kowey and colleagues (66) randomized 663 patients with symptomatic or persistent atrial fibrillation but no structural heart disease to 8 g a day of prescription formulation omega-3 PUFA supplement for one week and then 4 g daily for a 24-week period or placebo. Each capsule of the prescription omega-3 PUFA formulation contained approximately 465 mg of EPA and 375 mg of DHA. About one-half of patients in both groups had recurrent symptomatic atrial fibrillation and omega-3 PUFA supplementation did not reduce the frequency of recurrent atrial fibrillation over the 6-month study period. However, in the prescription omega-3 PUFA group there was a reduction in the average ventricular rate of the first atrial fibrillation recurrence as compared to placebo patients. This suggests some positive biologic effect of omega-3 PUFA on atrial fibrillation. There are several reasons why the findings from this study were different from the findings of other previous studies. First, the recurrent atrial fibrillation events occurred most often within 2 weeks of follow-up and there may not have been enough time for the omega-3 PUFAs effects to take place. Second, patients in the study by Kowey and colleagues were younger and had no structural heart disease and the effects of fish oil on atrial fibrillation may be more prominent in older patients or patients with coronary artery disease and third, the anti-arrhythmic effects of omega-3 PUFAs on atrial fibrillation may be weak and not effective in patients who have already demonstrated a propensity towards recurrent atrial fibrillation.

4. Triglyceride Lowering Effects

Previous epidemiological studies have identified high triglycerides as a strong and independent risk factor for coronary heart disease (67-71). A meta-analysis of 29 prospective studies involving more than 260,000 participants found a strong correlation between triglyceride levels and coronary heart disease risk (72). The odds ratio for coronary heart disease was 1.72 after adjusting for multiple variables including age, gender, smoking and lipid concentrations in the top compared to the bottom tertile of triglyceride levels. Studies of genetic variants that specifically affect triglyceride levels provide further evidence for a causal relationship between high triglyceride levels and coronary heart disease. Apolipoprotein A5 (APOA5) is a recently discovered apolipoprotein that is primarily involved with triglyceride metabolism and polymorphisms at or near the APOA5 gene are associated with increased triglyceride levels. The Triglyceride Coronary Disease Genetics

Consortium and Emerging Risk Factors Collaboration identified 101 studies with over 70,000 individuals in whom data was available for the APOA5-1131T>C polymorphism (73). Carriers of two C alleles had 32.6% higher mean triglyceride levels (95% CI 26.7-39.0) than did non-carriers and an odds ratio for coronary artery disease of 1.40 (95% CI 1.12-1.75) compared with non-carriers. The increased risk for coronary heart disease associated with high levels of triglycerides are not due to triglycerides themselves, but to the presence of other atherogenic lipoproteins commonly associated with elevated triglyceride levels. As discussed earlier in this chapter, elevated triglyceride levels are commonly associated with increased concentrations of triglyceride rich remnant lipoproteins such as small VLDL and IDL particles, a high concentration of small dense LDL cholesterol particles and low levels of HDL cholesterol. In addition when triglyceride levels are very high, in excess of 1000 mg/dL there is an increased risk for pancreatitis.

The National Cholesterol Education Program Adult Treatment Panel (ATP) III guidelines (74) classify fasting triglyceride levels as normal (<150 mg/dL), borderline high (150 to 199 mg/dL), high (200 to 499 mg/dL) and very high (≥ 500 mg/dL). A recent statement from the American Heart Association recommended that optimal fasting triglyceride levels be defined as < 100 mg/dL (75). When triglycerides are elevated the current guidelines focus on LDL-cholesterol as the primary target and non-HDL cholesterol as a secondary target or therapy. However, when triglyceride levels are very high (> 500 mg/dL), triglyceride lowering becomes the primary target of therapy to reduce the risk of pancreatitis (74). An individual's LDL and non-HDL cholesterol target is based on a patient's risk factor profile. For individuals with coronary artery disease, type II diabetes mellitus or for coronary heart disease risk equivalents the optimal goal for LDL cholesterol is < 70 mg/dL and for non-HDL cholesterol < 100 mg/dL. For individuals with 2 or more major risk factors for coronary heart disease the optimal LDL cholesterol goal is < 100 mg/dL and for non-HDL cholesterol < 130 mg/dL (76, 77). Data from the National Health and Nutrition Examination Survey (78) from 2001 to 2006 identified that 1.7% of adult American, equating to roughly 3.4 million people had very high triglyceride levels (> 500 mg/dL). Less than 20% of these individuals were on medications known to lower triglycerides. Many patients with coronary artery disease are not achieving optimal lipid goals. We recently published data on over 10,000 coronary artery disease patients whose lipids were managed by a cardiologist (79). Only 35% of patients achieved an LDL cholesterol goal of < 70 mg/dL and only 44% achieved a non-HDL cholesterol goal of < 100 mg/dL. Overall, only 69% of patients achieved normal triglyceride levels and women were less likely to achieve normal triglyceride levels as compared to men. Few of these patients with elevated triglyceride levels were on drugs known to lower triglycerides.

The treatment for elevated triglyceride levels focuses on intensive therapeutic lifestyle changes (TLC). When TLC, do not achieve optimal triglyceride levels, pharmacologic therapy should be considered. Omega-3 PUFAs lower triglycerides and triglyceride rich lipoproteins in a dose dependent manner. The American Heart Association recommends 2 to 4 g of EPA and DHA daily for patients with elevated triglyceride levels (1). In a comprehensive review Harris reported that 3 to 4 g of marine-derived PUFAs lowered triglyceride levels by 25 to 30% and raised HDL cholesterol by 1 to 3%, while LDL cholesterol increased by 5 to 10% (80). There is a dose-response relationship between fish oil and triglyceride lowering with an approximate 5 to 10% reduction in triglyceride levels for every 1 g of EPA and DHA given. In addition, the higher the baseline triglyceride levels the greater the reduction in triglyceride achieved with omega-3 PUFAs (75). The Food and Drug Administration has approved a prescription omega-3 fish oil formulation (Lovaza) for the treatment of very high triglyceride levels (>500 mg/dL) (81). In patients with very high triglyceride levels Lovaza at a dose of 4 g daily lowered triglycerides by 45%, lowered non-HDL cholesterol by 14% and raised HDL cholesterol by 9% (82). High dose omega-3 PUFAs not only lower triglycerides and non-HDL cholesterol but also lower VLDL and triglyceride rich remnant lipoproteins. When fish oil supplements are used to lower triglyceride levels LDL cholesterol rises as it does with fibrate therapy. By normalizing VLDL particle size conversion to LDL cholesterol increases, hence increasing the concentration of LDL cholesterol. Although LDL cholesterol increases somewhat with fish oil supplements, the number of small dense LDL particles decrease as do levels of apolipoprotein B and LDL particles become larger and fluffier and potentially less atherogenic.

The mechanisms by with omega-3 PUFAs reduce triglyceride levels are not completely understood. Omega-3 PUFAs reduce the hepatic synthesis of triglycerides and increase hepatic fatty acid beta-oxidation. The mechanism of these actions seems to involve activators of peroxisome proliferator-activator receptor (PPAR)-alpha (60). Omega-3 fatty acids also inhibit acyl CoA: 1,2-diacylglycerol acyltransferase (DGAT2) a key enzyme in triglyceride synthesis and increase LPL activity, which results in increased conversion of VLDL cholesterol to LDL cholesterol.

Several studies have compared the triglyceride lowering effects of high doses of omega-3 PUFAs to gemfibrozil. In one small study gemfibrozil lowered triglycerides and raised HDL cholesterol more than did 4 g daily of Lovaza (83). In this study patients had very high triglycerides, and Lovaza only lowered triglycerides by 29%. The reduction in triglycerides in this study with Lovaza was less than expected based on other studies. In 2 other studies of patients with very high triglyceride levels no difference was seen between Lovaza and gemfibrozil in regards to their triglyceride lowering and HDL cholesterol raising effects (84, 85). Few studies have compared fenofibrate to Lovaza in patients with high levels of triglycerides. In one study, Gerber and colleagues (86) randomized 100 HIV infected patients on highly active antiviral therapy with very high triglyceride levels to 3 g of EPA and DHA daily or fenofibrate 160 mg daily for 8 weeks. The median baseline triglyceride level in the fish oil group was 662 mg/dL and 694 mg/dL in the fenofibrate group. Fish oil reduced triglyceride levels by 46% compared to a 58% with fenofibrate ($p = 04$). Although in this study, fenofibrate lowered triglyceride levels more than did fish oil, higher doses of fish oil would have led to greater reductions in triglyceride levels. For each additional gram of EPA and DHA given, triglyceride levels will fall an additional 5 to 10% (75). Had 4 g of fish oil (EPA and DHA) been given, then the triglyceride lowering seen in this trial with fish oil therapy would have been comparable with fenofibrate therapy. In general high dose fish oil (about 4 g of EPA and DHA daily) lower triglyceride levels comparably compared to fibrate therapy.

In patients with very high triglyceride levels, fish oil can be used in combination with other lipid lowering therapy including statins, niacin and fibrates. In a study of coronary heart disease patients with elevated triglyceride levels (> 200 mg/dL) receiving a stable dose of statin, Lovaza at a dose of 2 g two times a day significantly reduced serum triglyceride levels by 20 to 30% (87). Additional studies have shown that this prescription formulation fish oil supplement when used in combination with a statin is well tolerated and provides sustained reductions in triglyceride and non-HDL cholesterol levels (88). Using a statin in combination with high dose fish oil supplements can offset the rise in LDL cholesterol that is seen when fish oil alone is used to treat high triglyceride levels.

Other studies have evaluated omega-3 fatty acids in combination with other lipid lowering drugs. In one study, patients with very high triglycerides who were receiving fenofibrate were given Lovaza 4 g daily or placebo (89). After 8 weeks of combination therapy, Lovaza added to fenofibrate therapy provided an additional 18% lowering of triglycerides ($p = 0.003$) and an additional 15% lowering of VLDL cholesterol ($p = 0.03$) compared to placebo. The combination of high dose omega-3 PUFAs and fenofibrate was well tolerated and lowered triglycerides more than either drug alone. However, due to similarity in their mechanisms of action, the triglyceride lowering effects of combining these two drugs was not additive. In a small pilot study 29 patients with mixed dyslipidemia with high triglyceride levels (150 to 500 mg/dL) were given placebo, 3000 mg of immediate release niacin, Lovaza (4 g daily) or Lovaza and niacin in combination (90). The combination of Lovaza and niacin lowered triglyceride levels by 52%, lowered VLDL cholesterol by 60% and raised HDL cholesterol by 33%.

5. Blood Pressure Lowering Effects

It is well recognized that dietary intervention can lower blood pressure. Previous studies have suggested that fish oil exerts an anti-hypertensive effect (91, 92). In a meta-analysis of 36 randomized clinical trials of fish oil and blood pressure, omega-3 PUFAs at a mean dose of 4.1 g daily lowered systolic blood pressure on average by 1.5 mm Hg and diastolic blood pressure by 2.3 mm Hg (93). Systolic and diastolic blood pressure reductions were significantly greater in older compared to younger patients and in hypertensive compared to normotensive patients. The blood pressure lowering effects of fish oil were independent of the dose of fish oil used.

6. Effects on Cardiac Function

The GISSI Prevenzione Trial demonstrated that taking 1 g of omega-3 PUFAs after a myocardial infarction led to a significant reduction in the risk of death. This benefit was due primarily to a reduction in sudden cardiac death (30). In a post-hoc analysis the reduction in sudden cardiac death was isolated to those patients with systolic dysfunction (65). Other studies have shown that omega-3 fatty acids can prevent the development of heart failure and that the risk reduction was inversely proportional to the amount of omega-3 PUFAs taken (58, 94). In the GISSI-HF Trial only omega-3 PUFAs, not statin therapy was associated with improved outcomes (36). Although the benefit in clinical outcomes with omega-3 PUFA supplementation in GISSI-HF was only modest, the benefits were additive to other therapies that are considered standard of care for heart failure patients. New data may provide evidence for the mechanisms by which omega-3 PUFAs benefit patients with heart failure. Nodari and colleagues randomized 133 patients with a nonischemic cardiomyopathy and stable heart failure to high dose omega-3 PUFAs or placebo (95). All patients had a left ventricular ejection fraction of less than 45%, took 5 capsules a day (each omega-3 PUFA capsule contained 850 to 882 mg of EPA and DHA) for the first month and then 2 capsules daily for the next 11 months. All patients were well treated with standard therapies for heart failure. Ventricular diameters and volumes, left ventricular ejection fraction, and other echocardiographic markers of remodeling were significantly improved at 12 months in those patients randomized to omega-3 PUFAs compared to placebo. In addition exercise duration, peak VO_2, and mean NYHA functional class were better in the omega-3 PUFA treated group. Although the study was underpowered for clinical outcomes, there was a significant decrease in cardiovascular hospitalizations ($p = 0.003$), heart failure hospitalizations ($p = 0.0002$) and a trend for decreased all-cause hospitalization ($p = 0.06$) in those patients taking fish oil supplements. Compared to GISSI-HF, patients in the study by Nodari and colleagues were given a significantly higher dose of omega-3 PUFAs and treated earlier in their course of heart failure. Hence higher doses of omega-3 PUFAs and earlier treatment may provide even more benefit in patients with systolic heart failure.

7. Effects on Telomere Shortening

A telomere is a region of repeating DNA sequences at the end of a chromosome, which protects the chromosome from deterioration or coupling with adjacent chromosomes (96). During cell division the chromosome cannot fully replicate to the end of the chromosome and there is progressive degradation and loss of these telomeric repeats. This process of telomere shortening can lead to replicative senescence or apoptosis (97). Several studies have shown an association with telomere shortening and an increased risk of cardiovascular disease and cancer (98, 99). In an analysis from the Heart and Soul Study, baseline levels of omega-3 PUFAs were inversely related to telomere shortening over 5 years of follow-up in patients with stable coronary artery disease (100). For each one standard deviation increase in EPA and DHA levels there was a 32% reduction in the odds of telomere shortening. The authors of this study hypothesized that the mechanism by which omega-3 PUFAs lead to decelerated telomere attrition may be due to reduced oxidative stress and an increase in telomerase activity, an enzyme that replenishes telomeres on the ends of chromosomes.

Fish Oil Production

Fish oil is processed from whole fish, most often sardines, anchovies, herring, mackerel, salmon and tuna. The raw fish is cut into pieces and then cooked by steam. The cooked mass of fish is then pressed or centrifuged to separate the dry solids from the liquid, which consists of oil and water. The liquid called press liquor is processed to separate the oil from the water. The oil is further processed to remove impurities and toxins and in some cases antioxidants such as vitamin E are added to the fish oil, to maintain the fish oils freshness. The amount of omega-3 PUFAs and specifically the amount of EPA and DHA in a fish oil capsule vary depending on the brand and manufacturer. Most common non-prescription fish oil capsules contain between 250 to 500 mg of EPA and DHA per capsule.

The FDA has approved a prescription formulation fish oil capsule (Lovaza) for the treatment of very high triglyceride levels. Unlike other fish oil preparations, the complex multi-step refinement process by which Lovaza is manufactured leads to a more purified and concentrated fish oil capsule (82). This prescription fish oil is formulated as an ethyl ester and each 1 g capsule of Lovaza contains approximately 465 mg of EPA, 375 mg of DHA and 60 mg of other omega-3 fatty acids for a total of almost 900 mg of omega-3 fatty acids. Each Lovaza capsule contains almost 3 to 4 times more EPA and DHA then does the average over-the-counter fish oil capsule. Ethyl ester formulations allow for a high concentration of omega-3 PUFAs within one capsule, reducing the number of capsules that a patient needs to take to effectively lower triglycerides. Although triglyceride formulations of fish oil have lower concentrations of EPA and DHA per capsule, some studies have suggested that the triglyceride formulation fish oil provides more rapid absorption of EPA and DHA than an ethyl ester formulation (101, 102). However, other studies have shown that EPA and DHA are rapidly absorbed into the bloodstream whether given as ethyl esters or triglycerides (103). The triglyceride lowering effects of omega-3 PUFAs are due to their EPA and DHA content, not whether they are formulated as a triglyceride or ethyl ester (104). In addition, each large outcome study that demonstrated a significant cardiovascular benefit of fish oil used an ethyl ester, not a triglyceride omega-3 PUFA formulation. The primary difference between one fish oil product and another is the concentration of EPA and DHA per capsule. When using omega-3 PUFAs to lower triglycerides, physicians must use higher doses of approximately 4 g daily of EPA and DHA and physicians should choose the most concentrated formulation of fish oil available.

There is a semi-synthetic ethyl ester derivative of the omega-3 PUFA EPA that is in clinical trials. In the MARINE trial, 229 patients with triglyceride levels > 500 mg/dL were randomized to placebo or to 2 g or 4 g of AMR101, as the ethyl EPA is currently known (105). Triglyceride levels were reduced by 20% and 33% respectively, and all without an increase in LDL cholesterol. In follow-up to this trial, the ANCHOR trial enrolled 702 patients with somewhat lower, but still high triglyceride levels (200 to 499 mg/dL) to placebo or to 2 g or 4 g or AMR101 (106). All patients were being treated with statin therapy to achieve an LDL cholesterol level < 100 mg/dL. At the end of 12 weeks, treatment with both doses of AMR101 significantly lowered levels of triglycerides, non-HDL cholesterol, VLDL cholesterol, apolipoprotein B, and lipoprotein phospholipase A_2 (Lp-PLA$_2$). As in the MARINE trial, ethyl EPA did not increase LDL cholesterol levels as occurs with other omega-3 PUFA supplements that contain DHA. However, neither of these studies has been published in a peer-reviewed journal and the FDA has not yet approved this drug for the treatment of high triglycerides.

Safety of Fish Oil

Overall fish oil, even at high doses is safe and well tolerated. The most common sides effect from fish oil supplements are gastrointestinal and include a "fishy" aftertaste or smell, eructations, nausea and gastrointestinal upset (107). These side effects are due to oxidation and rancid conversion that occurs commonly with most fish oil preparations. Fish oils are naturally unstable and are highly susceptible to oxidation. To reduce fish oil oxidation and hence fish oil rancidity, manufacturers have added vitamin E to the fish oil preparation to extend its shelf life. Another way to reduce the "fishy" aftertaste seen with fish oil supplements is to refrigerate the fish oil, which maintains its freshness. The more purified a fish oil supplement is the less likely that these gastrointestinal side effects will occur, especially the strong and unpleasant rancid "fishy" taste and smell that may occur with less purified formulations. Due to its manufacturing process, the prescription formulation Lovaza is associated with much lower gastrointestinal side effects and "fishy" taste than other over-the-counter fish oil supplements (82).

Another concern among physicians is that fish oil, especially at high doses can increase the risk of bleeding. Fish oil contains the N-3 PUFA eicosapentaenoate. Fish oil supplementation markedly increases the eicosapentaenoate content of phospholipids from red blood cells and platelets and alters their pattern of thromboxane and prostacyclin synthesis. These effects are thought to be responsible for the anti-platelet and anti-thrombotic properties of omega-3 PUFAs (52). Although, omega 3-PUFAs at higher doses modestly prolong the bleeding time (108), there is little evidence to suggest that omega-3 PUFAs, even in high doses cause clinically significant bleeding. Aspirin inhibits platelet aggregation by inhibition of cyclooxygenase while clopidogrel reduces platelet activation via ADP receptor-dependent pathways. These findings raise concern that high dose fish oil could further increase the risk of bleeding in patients already taking aspirin and clopidogrel. Similarly fish oil may increase the risk of bleeding in patients taking warfain. However several reviews including an expert opinion report by Harris have concluded that there in no increased risk of clinically significant bleeding with omega-3 fatty acid doses up to 7 g daily, even when combined with anti-platelet therapy or warfarin (109).

Previous studies found no increased risk of bleeding when omega-3 fatty acids were prescribed in combination with either aspirin or warfarin. Eritsland and colleagues randomized 610 patients already taking either 300 mg of aspirin daily or warfarin following coronary artery bypass surgery to 4 g of prescription formulation omega-3 fatty acids or placebo (110). They reported no significant difference in the number of bleeding episodes at one year in those patients taking high dose fish oil compared to the placebo group. Leaf and colleagues randomized 551 patients on 325 mg aspirin a day following PCI to an even a higher dose of fish oil, 8 g of omega-3 PUFAs (providing a total of 6.9 g of EPA and DHA) daily or placebo (111). At 6 month follow-up the incidence of bleeding was low at 3 % and no difference in bleeding episodes was detected between groups. In another small study there was no difference in bleeding episodes in patients on chronic warfarin therapy randomized to up to 6 g of fish oil daily (112). We have published data on patients prescribed high dose omega-3 PUFAs in combination with aspirin and clopidogrel (113). We found no increased risk of bleeding when patients were on all 3 drugs compared to aspirin and clopidogrel alone. These studies support the safety of high dose omega-3 fatty acids when used in combination with anti-platelet or anti-thrombotic therapies.

Another major concern for physicians is the risk of contaminants and toxins, particularly methyl mercury in patients whose diet is rich in oily fish. This is less of a concern in fish oil supplements since mercury is water-soluble and protein bound and is hence present in the flesh of the fish and not in the oil. Therefore fish oil supplements contain very low levels of mercury (107). In addition certain fish oil supplements undergo an extensive purification process to remove contaminants and toxins. The prescription formulation fish oil, Lovaza undergoes an even more rigorous purification process compared to over-the-counter fish oil supplements to meet the requirements of the FDA as a prescription pharmaceutical. In several clinical trials this prescription formulation fish oil supplement was found to have no detectable concentrations of heavy metals nor other contaminants or toxins and in clinical studies with Lovaza no cases of illness related to environmental toxins have been reported (82).

However an individual who consumes a large amount of oil fish, may be at risk of environmental toxin exposure. It is for this reason that the FDA advises that children and pregnant women avoid those fish that have a potentially high concentration of mercury. Such fish include swordfish, tilefish, king mackerel and shark. Other fish still high in omega-3 fatty acids, such as salmon, sardines, trout, oysters and herring are very low in mercury and safe to eat. Overall the benefit of eating oily fish several times a week outweighs the small potential risk associated with exposure to environmental contaminants and toxins (114).

The low intake of omega-3 PUFAs especially compared to the intake of omega-6 PUFAs in Western diets is thought to contribute to an increased risk of cancer. Animal studies and experiments in tissue culture have shown a protective effect of omega-3 PUFAs and cancer risk. However, human studies have not shown consistently positive results (115). Several observational studies have shown that an increased consumption of fish is associated with a lower risk of many cancers, including colon, prostate and breast cancer (116-118). It is thought that the anti-inflammatory effects as well as the inhibitory effect on omega-6 eicosanoid biosynthesis may explain the beneficial effects of omega-3 PUFAs in reducing cancer risk. However, other studies have failed to show a definite link between increased fish consumption and a reduced risk for cancer and some studies have suggested that an increased intake of fish may increase tumor burden in men with prostate cancer (119, 120). In a recent study Brasky and colleagues performed a nested case-control analysis from participants in the Prostate Cancer Prevention Trial (120). Phospholipid fatty acids were extracted from serum and the concentration of fatty acids determined to assess their concentration of diet derived omega-3 PUFA and patients were followed for 7 years. Levels of DHA were positively associated with high grade prostate cancer, while levels of trans fatty acids were significantly lower among high grade cases of prostate cancer compared to controls. The findings from this study are in contrast to most previously published studies and not the results the authors had expected. These studies illustrate the complexity of research on nutrition and cancer risk. Despite these findings the benefit in reducing cardiovascular risk of a diet rich in marine omega-3 PUFAs outweighs any potential adverse risks.

Conclusions

The current American Heart Association guidelines recommend that Americans eat at least 2 to 3 helpings of oil fish a week to maintain good health and reduce cardiovascular risk. This is especially important given the low consumption of fish in most American diets. Although the American Heart Association also recommends 1 g of combined EPA and DHA for individuals with coronary artery disease, this recommendation has now been challenged by recent large randomized trials that have shown no benefit of low dose omega-3 PUFA supplementation in patients with a history of myocardial infarction. However, the evidence is strongest for a protective effect of omega-3 PUFA supplements in those patients with coronary artery disease who have heart failure or a low ejection fraction and physicians should consider using omega-3 PUFA supplements in these patients, especially if they have elevated levels of triglycerides.

Higher doses of omega-3 PUFA of approximately 4 g of EPA and DHA daily can lead to significant reductions in triglyceride levels and should be an important therapeutic option for patients with high and very high levels of triglycerides. When physicians use omega-3 PUFA supplements in their patients it is the dose of EPA and DHA per capsule that is most important. When high doses of EPA and DHA are needed to significantly lower triglyceride levels the most potent omega-3 PUFA formulation available should be prescribed.

We need to inform our patients about the benefits of omega-3 PUFAs and recommend that they increase their dietary intake of oily fish. For those patients where higher doses of omega-3 PUFAs are needed supplements should be used. The "fish tale" is not over and as we await further research and clinical trials evaluating the benefits of omega-3 PUFAs in reducing cardiovascular risk, the hope is that this tale will not end with the fish that got away.

References

[1] Kris-Etherton PM, Harris WS, Appel LJ; for the Nutrition Committee. AHA Scientific Statement: Fish consumption, fish oil, omega-3 fatty acids and cardiovascular disease. *Circulation* 2002; 106: 2747-2757.

[2] Siri-Tarino PW, Sun Q, Hu FB, Krauss, RM. Saturated fat, carbohydrate, and cardiovascular disease. *Am J Clin Nutr* 2010; 91: 502-509.

[3] Mozzaffarian D, Katan MB, Ascherio A, Stampfer MJ, Willet WC. Trans fatty acids and cardiovascular disease. *N Engl J Med* 2006; 354: 1601-1613.

[4] Kark JD, Kaufmann NA, Binka F, Goldberger N, Berry EM. Adipose tissue n-6 fatty acids and acute myocardial infarction in a population consuming a diet high in polyunsaturated fatty acids. *Am J Clin Nutr* 2008; 77: 796-802.

[5] Lang PD, Degott M, Heuck CC, Opherk D, Vollmar J. Fatty acid composition of adipose tissue, blood, lipids, and glucose tolerance in patients with different degrees of angiographically documented coronary arteriosclerosis. *Res Exp Med* 1982: 180: 161-168.

[6] Sachs FM, Campos H. Polyunsaturated fatty acids, inflammation, and cardiovascular disease: time to widen our view of the mechanisms. *J Clin Endocrinol Metab* 2006; 91: 398-400.

[7] Ferrucci L, Cherubini A, Bandinelli S, Bartali B, Corsi A, Lauretani F, Martin A, Andres-Lacueva C, Senin U, Guralnik JM. Relationship of plasma unsaturated fatty acids to circulating inflammatory markers. *J Clin Endocrinol Metab* 2006; 91: 439-446.

[8] Harris WS, Mozaffarian D, Rimm E, Kris-Etherton P, PhD, Rudel LL, Appel LJ, Engler MM, Engler MB, Sacks F. Omega-6 fatty acids and risk for cardiovascular disease. A science advisory from the American Heart Association Nutrition Subcommittee of the Council on Nutrition, Physical Activity, and Metabolism; Council on Cardiovascular Nursing; and Council on Epidemiology and Prevention. *Circulation* 2009; 119: 902-907.

[9] Ramsden CE, Hibbeln JR, Majchrzak SF, Davis JM. N-6 fatty acid-specific and mixed polyunsaturated dietary interventions have different effects on CHD risk: a meta-analysis of randomized controlled trials. *Br J Nutr* 2010; 104: 1586-1600.

[10] Harris WS, Poston WC, Haddock CK. Tissue n-3 and n-6 fatty acids and risk for coronary heart disease events. *Atherosclerosis* 2007; 193: 1-10.

[11] Lewis GF, Carpentier A, Adeli K, Giacca A. Disordered fat storage and mobilization in the pathogenesis of insulin resistance and type 2 diabetes. *Endocrine Reviews* 2002; 23: 201-229.

[12] Mudd JO, Borlaug BA, Johnston PV, Kral BG, Rouf R, Blumenthal RS, Kwiterovich PO. Beyond low-density lipoprotein cholesterol: defining the role of low-density lipoprotein heterogeneity in coronary artery disease. *J Am Coll Cardiol* 2007; 50: 1735-1741.

[13] Chait A, Brazg RL, Tribble DL, Krauss RM. Susceptibility of small, dense, low-density lipoproteins to oxidative modification in subjects with the atherogenic lipoprotein phenotype, pattern B. *Am J Med* 1993; 94: 350-356.

[14] Ip S, Lichtenstein AH, Chung M, Lau J, Balk EM. Systemic review: association of low-density lipoprotein subfractions with cardiovascular outcomes. *Ann Intern Med* 2009; 150: 474-484.

[15] Greene DJ, Skeggs JW, Morton RE. Elevated triglyceride content diminishes the capacity of high density lipoprotein to deliver cholesteryl esters via the scavenger receptor class B type I (SR-BI). *J Biol Chem* 2001; 276: 4804-4811.

[16] Bang HO, Dyerberg J, Nielsen AB. Plasma lipid and lipoprotein pattern in Greenlandic West-Coast Eskimos. Lancet 1971; 1: 1143-1146.

[17] Kromann N, Green A. Epidemiologic studies in the Upernavik District, Greenland. *Acta Med Scand* 1980; 208: 401-406.

[18] Iso H, Kobayashi M, Ishihara J, Sasaki S, Okada K, Kita Y, Kokubo Y, Tsugane S for the JPHC Study Group. Intake of fish and n3 fatty acids and risk of coronary heart disease among Japanese: the Japan Public Health Center-Based (JPHC) Study Cohort I. *Circulation* 2006; 113: 195-202.

[19] Stone NJ. Fish consumption, fish oil, lipids, and coronary heart disease. *Circulation* 1996; 94: 2337-2340.

[20] Daviglus ML, Stamler J, Orencia AJ, Dyer AR, Liu K, Greenland P, Walsh MK, Morris D, Shekelle RB. Fish consumption and the 30-year risk of fatal myocardial infarction. *N Engl J Med* 1997; 336: 1046-1053.

[21] Zhang J, Sasaki S, Amano K, Kesteloot H. Fish consumption and mortality from all causes; ischemic heart disease, and stroke: an ecological study. *Prev Med* 1999; 28: 520-529.

[22] Hu FB, Bronner L, Willett WC, Stampfer MJ, Rexrode KM, Albert CM, Hunter D, Manson JE. Fish and omega-3 fatty acid intake and risk of coronary heart disease in women. *JAMA* 22001; 287: 1815-1821.

[23] Kromhout D, Bloemberg BP, Feskens EJ, Hertog MG, Menotti A, Blackburn H. Alcohol, fish, fibre and antioxidant vitamins intake do not explain population differences in coronary heart disease mortality. *Int J Epidemiol* 1996; 25: 753-759.

[24] Verschuren WH, Jacobs DR, Bloemberg BP, Kromhout D, Menotti A, Aravanis C, Blackburn H, Buzina R, Dontas AS, Fidanza F, Karvonen MJ, Nedelijković S, Nissinen P, Toshima H. Serum total cholesterol and long-term coronary heart disease mortality in different cultures: Twenty-five-year follow-up of the seven countries study. *JAMA* 1995; 274: 131-136.

[25] Sekikawa A, Ueshima H, Kadowaki T, El-Saed A, Okamura T, Takamiya T, Kashiwagi A, Edmundowicz D, Murata K, Sutton-Tyrrell K, Maegawa H, Evans RW, Kita Y, Kuller LH, for the ERA JUMP Study Group. Less subclinical atherosclerosis in Japanese men in Japan than in white men in the United States in the post-World War II birth cohort. *Am J Epidemiol* 2001; 165: 617-624.

[26] D'Agostino SR, Grundy S, Sullivan LM, Wilson P, for the CHDRPG. Validation of the Framingham Coronary Heart Disease Prediction Scores: results of a multiple ethnic group investigation. *JAMA* 2001; 286: 180-187.

[27] Sekikawa A, Curb D, Ueshima H, El-Saed A, Kadowaki T, Abbott RD, Evans RW, Rodriguez BL, Okamura T, Sutton-Tyrrell K, Nakamura Y, Masaki K, Edmundowicz D, Kashiwagi A, Willcox BJ, Takamiya T, Mitsunami K, Seto TB, Murata K, White RL, Kuller LH, for the ERA JUMP Study Group. Marine-derived n-3 fatty acids and atherosclerosis in Japanese, Japanese-American and white men. *J Am Coll Cardiol* 2008; 52: 417-424.

[28] Burr ML, Gilbert JF, Holliday RM, Elwood PC, Fehily AM, Rogers S, Sweetnam PM, Deadman NM. Effects of changes in fat, fish, and fibre intakes on death and myocardial infarction and reinfarction trial (DART). *Lancet* 1989; 2: 757-761.

[29] Singh RM, Mohammad AN, Sharma JP, Kumar R, Rastogi V, Moshiri M. Randomized, double-blind, placebo-controlled trial of fish oil and mustard oil in patients with suspected myocardial infarction: the Indian experiment of infarct survival-4. *Cardiovasc Drugs Ther* 1997; 11: 485-491.

[30] GISSI-Prevenzione Investigators. Dietary supplementation with n-3 polyunsaturated fatty acids and vitamin E after myocardial infarction: results of the GISSI-Prevenzione trial. *Lancet* 1999; 354: 447-455.

[31] Yokoyama M, Origasa H, Matsuzaki M, Matsuzawa Y, Saito Y, Ishikawa Y, Oikawa S, Sasaki J, Hishida H, Itakura H, Kita T, Kitabatake A, Nakaya N, Sakata T, Shimada K, Shirato K, for the Japan EPA lipid intervention study (JELIS) investigators. Effects of eicosapentaenoic acid on major coronary events in hypercholesterolemic patients (JELIS): a randomized open-label, blinded, end-point analysis. *Lancet* 2007; 369: 1090-1098.

[32] Oikawa S. Yokoyama M. Origasa H. Matsuzaki M. Matsuzawa Y. Saito Y. Ishikawa Y. Sasaki J. Hishida H. Itakura H. Kita T. Kitabatake A. Nakaya N. Sakata T. Shimada K. Shirato K, for the Japan EPA lipid intervention study (JELIS) investigators. Suppression effects of EPA on the incidence of coronary events in hypercholesterolemia with impaired glucose metabolism: Sub-analysis of the Japan EPA lipid intervention study (JELIS). *Atherosclerosis* 2009; 206: 535-539.

[33] Tanaka K, Ishikawa Y, Yokoyama M, Origasa H, Matsuzaki M, Saito Y, Matsuzawa Y, Sasaki J, Oikawa S, Hishida H, Itakura H, Kita T, Kitabatake A, Nakaya N, Sakata T, Shimada K, Shirato K for the Japan EPA lipid intervention study (JELIS) investigators. Reduction in the recurrence of stroke by eicosapentaenoic acid for hypercholesterolemic patients: Subanalysis of the JELIS trial. *Stroke* 2008; 39: 2052-2058.

[34] Saito Y, Yokoyama M, Origasa H, Matsuzaki M, Matsuzawa Y, Ishikawa Y, Oikawa S, Sasaki J, Hishida H, Itakura H, Kita T, Kitabatake A, Nakaya N, Sakata T, Shimada K, Shirato K for Japan EPA lipid intervention study (JELIS) investigators. Effects of EPA on coronary artery disease in hypercholesterolemic patients with multiple risk factors:

sub-analysis of primary prevention cases from the Japan EPA Lipid Intervention Study (JELIS). *Atherosclerosis* 2008; 200: 135-140.

[35] Matsuzaki M, Yokoyama M, Saito Y, Origasa H, Ishikawan Y, Oikawa S, Sasaki J, Hishida H, Itakura I, Kita T, Kitabatake A, Nakaya N, Sakata T. Shimada K, Shirato K, Matsuzawa Y, for Japan EPA lipid intervention study (JELIS) investigators. Incremental effects of eicosapentaenoic acid on cardiovascular events in statin-treated patients with coronary artery disease secondary prevention analysis from JELIS. *Circ J* 2009; 73: 1283-1290.

[36] GISSI-HF Investigators. Effect of n-3 polyunsaturated fatty acids in patients with chronic heart failure (the GISSI-HF trial): a randomized, double-blind, placebo controlled trial. *Lancet* 2008; 372: 1223-1230.

[37] Kromhout D, Giltay EJ, Geleijnse JM, for the Alpha-Omega Trial Group. n-3 fatty acids and cardiovascular events after myocardial infarction. *N Engl J Med* 2010; 363: 2015-2026.

[38] Rauch B, Schiele R, Schneider S, Diller F, Victor N, Gohlke H, Gottwik M, Steinbeck G, Del Castillo U, Sack R, Worth H, Katus H, Spitzer W, Sabin G, Senges J, for the OMEGA Study Group. OMEGA, a randomized, placebo-controlled trial to test the effect of highly purified omega-3 fatty acids on top of modern guideline-adjusted therapy after myocardial infarction. *Circulation* 2010; 122: 2152-2159.

[39] Vitamin D and Omega-3 Trial (VITAL). Sponsored by the National Cancer Institute and the National, Heart, Lung, and Blood Institute. Information available at *http://www.ClinicalTrials.gov*.

[40] ASCEND: A study of cardiovascular events in diabetes. Sponsored by the British Heart Foundation. Information available at *http://www.ctsu.ox.ac.uk*.

[41] Tsimikas S, Willerson JT, Ridker PM. C-reactive protein and other emerging blood biomarkers to optimize risk stratification of vulnerable patients. *J Am Coll Cardiol* 2006; 47(8S): C19-31.

[42] Blake GJ, Ridker PM. C-reactive protein and other inflammatory risk markers in acute coronary syndromes. J Am Coll Cardiol 2003; 41(4S): 37S-42S.

[43] Luostarinen R, Boberg M, Saldeen T. Fatty acid composition in total phospholipids of human coronary arteries in sudden cardiac death. *Atherosclerosis* 1993; 99: 187-193.

[44] Lemaitre RN, King IB, Raghunathan TE, Pearce RM, Weinmann S, Knopp RH, Copass MK, Cobb LA, Siscovick DS. Cell membrane trans-fatty acids and the risk of primary cardiac arrest. *Circulation* 2002; 105: 697-701.

[45] Geppert J, Kraft V, Demmelmair H, and Koletzko B. Docosahexaenoic acid supplementation in vegetarians effectively increases omega-3 index: a randomized trial. *Lipids* 2005; 40: 807-814.

[46] Simopoulos AP. Omega-3 fatty acids in inflammation and autoimmune diseases. J *Am Coll Nutr*. 2002; 21: 495-505.

[47] Farzaneh-Far R, Harris W, Garg S, Whooley MA. Inverse association of erythrocyte n-3 fatty acid levels with inflammatory biomarkers in patients with stable coronary artery disease: The Heart and Soul Study. *Atherosclerosis* 2009; 205: 538-543.

[48] He K, Liu K, Daviglus ML, Jenny NS, Mayer-Davis E, Jiang R, Steffen L, Siscovick D, Tsai M, Herrington D. Associations of dietary long-chain n-3 polyunsaturated fatty acids and fish with biomarkers of inflammation and endothelial activation (from the Multi-Ethnic Study of Atherosclerosis [MESA]). *Am J Cardiol* 2009; 103: 1238-1243.

[49] Nanni S, Melandri G, Hanemaaijer R, Cervi V, Tomasi L, Altimari A, Van Lent N, Tricoci P, Bacchi L, Branzi A. Matrix metalloproteinases in premature coronary atherosclerosis: influence of inhibitors, inflammation, and genetic polymorphisms. *Transl Res* 2007; 149: 137-144.

[50] Mehra MR, Lavie CJ, Ventura HO, Milani RV. Fish oils produce anti-inflammatory effects and improve body weight in severe heart failure. *J Heart Lung Transplant* 2006; 25: 834-838.

[51] Ciubotaru I, Lee YS, Wander RC. Dietary fish oil decreases C-reactive protein, interleukin-6, and triacylglycerol to HDL-cholesterol ratio in postmenopausal women on HRT. *J Nutr Biochem* 2003; 14: 513-521.

[52] Knapp HR, Reilly IA, Alessandrini P, FitzGerald GA. In vivo indexes of platelet and vascular function during fish-oil administration in patients with atherosclerosis. *N Engl J Med* 1986; 314: 937-942.

[53] Mori TA, Beilin LJ, Burke V, Morris J, Ritchie J. Interactions between dietary fat, fish, and fish oils and their effects of platelet function in men at risk for cardiovascular disease. *Arterioscler Thromb Vasc Biol* 1997; 17: 279-286.

[54] Gajos G, Rostoff P, Undas A, Piwowarska W. Effects of polyunsaturated omega-3 fatty acids on responsiveness to dual antiplatelet therapy in patients undergoing percutaneous coronary intervention. *J Am Coll Cardiol* 2010; 55: 1671-1678.

[55] Gajos G, Zalewski J, Rostoff P, Nessler J, Piwowarska W, Undus A. Reduced thrombin formation and altered clot properties induced by polyunsaturated omega-3 fatty acids on top on dual antiplatelet therapy in patients undergoing percutaneous coronary intervention (OMEGA- PCI Clot). *Arterioscler Thromb Vasc Biol* 2011; available at http://atub.ahajournals.org.

[56] Lev EI, Solodky A, Harel N, Mager A, Brosh D, Assali A, Roller M, Battler A, Kleiman NS, Kornowski R. Treatment of aspirin-resistant patients with omega-3 fatty acids versus aspirin dose escalation. *J Am Coll Cardiol* 2010; 55: 114-121.

[57] Marchioli R, Barzi F, Bomba E, Chieffo C, Di Gregorio D, Di Mascio R, Franzosi MG, Geraci E, Levantesi G, Maggioni AP, Mantini L, Marfisi RM, Mastrogiuseppe G, Mininni N, Nicolosi GL, Santini M, Schweiger C, Tavazzi L, Tognoni G, Tucci C, Valagussa F, GISSI-Prevenzione Investigators. Early protection against sudden death by n-3 polyunsaturated fatty acids after myocardial infarction. Time-course analysis of the results of the Gruppo Italiano per lo Studio della Sopravvivenza nell'Infarto Miocardico (GISSI)-Prevenzione. *Circulation* 2002; 105: 1897-1903.

[58] Mozaffarian D, Psaty BM, Rimm EB, Lemaitre RN, Burke GL, Lyles MF, Lefkowitz D, Siscovick DS. Fish intake and risk of incident atrial fibrillation. *Circulation* 2004; 110: 368-373.

[59] Calo L, Bianconi L, Colivicchi F, Lamberti F, Loricchi L, de Ruvo E, Meo A, Pandozi C, Staibano M, Santini M. N-3 fatty acids for the prevention of atrial fibrillation after coronary artery bypass surgery. A randomized, controlled trial. *J Am Coll Cardiol.* 2005; 45: 1723-1728.

[60] Lavie CJ, Milani RV, Mehra MR, Ventura HO. Omega-3 polyunsaturated fatty acids and cardiovascular disease. *J Am Coll Cardiol* 2009; 54: 585-594.

[61] Anand RG, Alkadri M, Lavie CJ, Milani RV. The role of fish oil in arrhythmia prevention. *J Cardiopulm Rehabil* 2008; 28:92-98.

[62] Raitt MH, Connor WE, Morris C, Kron J, Halperin B, Chugh SS, McClelland J, Cook J, MacMurdy K, Swenson R, Connor SL, Gerhard G, Kraemer DF, Oseran D, Marchant C, Calhoun D, Shnider R, McAnulty J. Fish oil supplementation and risk of ventricular tachycardia and ventricular fibrillation in patients with implantable defibrillators: a randomized controlled trial. *JAMA* 2005; 293: 2884-2891.

[63] Brouwer IA, Zock PL, Camm AJ, Bocker D, Hauer RN, Wever EF, Dullemeijer C, Ronden JE, Katan MB, Lubinski A, Buschler H, Schouten EG, SOFA Study Group. Effect of fish oil on ventricular tachyarrhythmia and death in patients with implantable cardioverter defibrillators: the Study on Omega-3 Fatty Acids and Ventricular Arrhythmia (SOFA) randomized trial. *JAMA* 2006; 295: 2613-2619.

[64] Leon H, Shibata MC, Sivakumaran S, Dorgan M, Chatterley T, Tsuyuki RT. Effect of fish oil on arrhythmias and mortality: systematic review. *BMJ* 2008; 337: a2931.

[65] Macchia A, Levantesi G, Franzosi MG, Geraci E, Maggioni AP, Marfisi R, Nicolosi GL, Schweiger C, Tavazzi L, Tognoni G, Valagussa F, Marchioli R, GISSI-Prevenzione Investigators. Left ventricular systolic dysfunction, total mortality, and sudden death in patients with myocardial infarction treated with n-3 polyunsaturated fatty acids. *Eur J Heart Fail* 2005; 7: 904-909.

[66] Kowey PR, Reiffel JA, Ellenbogen KA, Naccarelli GV, Pratt CM. Efficacy and safety of prescription omega-3 fatty acids for the prevention of recurrent symptomatic atrial fibrillation: a randomized controlled trial. *JAMA* 2010; 304: 2363-2372.

[67] Assmann G, Schulte H. Relation of high-density lipoprotein cholesterol and triglycerides to incidence of atherosclerotic coronary artery disease (the PROCAM experience). *Am J Cardiol* 1992; 70: 733-737.

[68] Jeppesen J, Hein HO, Suadicani P, Gyntelberg F. Triglyceride concentration and ischemic heart disease: an eight-year follow-up in the Copenhagen Male Study. *Circulation* 1998; 97: 1029-1036.

[69] Eberly LE, Stamler J, Neaton JD, the Multiple Risk Factor Intervention Trial Research Group. Relation of triglyceride levels, fasting and nonfasting, to fatal and nonfatal coronary heart disease. *Arch Intern Med* 2003; 163: 1077-1083.

[70] Freiberg JJ, Tybjaerg-Hansen A, Jensen JS, Nordestgaard BG. Nonfasting triglycerides and risk of ischemic stroke in the general population. *JAMA* 2008; 300: 2142-2152.

[71] Faergeman O, Holme I, Fayyad R, Bhatia S, Grundy SM, Kastelein JJ, LaRosa JC, Larsen ML, Lindahl C, Olsson AG, Tikkanen MJ, Waters DD, Pedersen TR, Steering Committees of IDEAL and TNT Trials. Plasma triglycerides and cardiovascular events in the Treating to New Targets and Incremental Decrease in End-Points through Aggressive Lipid Lowering trials of statins in patients with coronary artery disease. *Am J Cardiol* 2009; 104: 459-463.

[72] Sarwar N, Danesh J, Eiriksdottir G, Sigurdsson G, Wareham N, Bingham S, Boekholdt M, Khaw KT, Gudnason V. Triglycerides and the risk of coronary heart disease: 10,158 incident cases among 262,525 participants in 29 Western prospective studies. *Circulation* 2007; 115: 450-458.

[73] Triglyceride Coronary Disease Genetics Consortium and Emerging Risk Factors Collaboration. Triglyceride-mediated pathways and coronary disease: collaborative analysis of 101 studies. *Lancet* 2010; 375: 1634-1639.

[74] Executive Summary of The Third Report of The National Cholesterol Education Program (NCEP) Expert Panel on Detection, Evaluation, And Treatment of High Blood Cholesterol In Adults (Adult Treatment Panel III). *JAMA* 2001; 285: 2486-2497.

[75] Miller M, Stone NJ, Ballantyne C, Bittner V, Criqui MH, Ginsberg HN, Goldberg AC, Howard WJ, Jacobson MS, Kris-Etherton PM, Lennie TA, Levi M, Mazzone T, Pennathur S, American Heart Association Clinical Lipidology, Thrombosis, and Prevention Committee of the Council on Nutrition, Physical Activity, and Metabolism, Council on Arteriosclerosis, Thrombosis and Vascular Biology, Council on Cardiovascular Nursing, Council on the Kidney in Cardiovascular Disease. Triglycerides and cardiovascular disease: a scientific statement from the American Heart Association. *Circulation published online Apr 18, 2011.*

[76] Grundy SM, Cleeman JI, Merz NB, Brewer B, Clark LT, Hunninghake DB, Pasternak RC, Smith SC, Stone NJ for the Coordinating Committee of the National Cholesterol Education Program. Implications of recent clinical trials for the National Cholesterol Education Program Adult Treatment Panel III guidelines. *Circulation* 2004; 110: 227-239.

[77] Brunzell JD, Davidson M, Furberg CD, Goldberg RB, Howard B, Stein JH, Witztum JL. Lipoprotein management in patients with cardiometabolic risk: consensus statement from the American Diabetes Association and the American College of Cardiology Foundation. *Diabetes Care* 2008; 31: 811-822.

[78] Christian JB, Bourgeois N, Snipes R, Lowe KA. Prevalence of severe (500 to 2,000 mg/dL) hypertriglyceridemia in United States adults. *Am J Cardiol* 2011; 107: 891-897.

[79] Karalis DG, Subramanya RD, Hessen SE, Liu L, Victor MF. Achieving optimal lipid goals in patients with coronary artery disease. *Am J Cardiol* 2011; 107: 886-890.

[80] Harris WS. N-3 fatty acids and serum lipoproteins: human studies. *Am J Clin Nutr* 1997; 65(suppl): 1645S-1654S.

[81] Bays H. Clinical overview of Omacor: a concentrated formulation of omega-3 polyunsaturated fatty acids. *Am J Cardiol* 2006;98(suppl): 71i-76i.

[82] Harris WS, Ginsberg HN, Arunakul N, Shacter NS, Windsor SL, Adams H, Berglund L, Osmundsen K. Safety and efficacy of Omacor in severe hypertriglyceridemia. *J Cardiovasc Risk* 1997; 4: 385-391.

[83] Van Dam M, Stalenhoef AH, Wittekoek J, Trip J, Prins MH, Kastelein JJ. Efficacy of concentrated n-3 fatty acids in hypertriglyceridemia. A comparison with gemfibrozil. *Clin Drug Invest* 2001; 21: 175-178.

[84] Minnema MC, Wittekoek ME, Schoonenboom N, Kastelein JJ, Hack CE, ten Cate H. Activation of the contact system of coagulation does not contribute to the hemostatic imbalance in hypertriglcyeridemia. *Arterioscler Thromb Vasc Biol* 1999; 19: 2548-2553.

[85] Stalenhoef AF, de Graaf J, Wittekoek ME, Bredie SJ, Demacker PN, Kastelein JJ. The effect of concentrated n-3 fatty acids versus gemfibrozil on plasma lipoproteins, low density lipoprotein heterogeneity and oxidizability in patients wit hypertriglyceridemia. *Atherosclerosis* 2000; 153: 129-138.

[86] Gerber JG, Kitch DW, Fichtenbaum CJ, Zackin RA, Charles S, Hogg E, Acosta EP, Connick E, Wohl D, Kojik EM, Benson CA, Aberg JA, for the AIDS Clinical Trial Group A5186 Team. *J Acquir Immune Defic Syndr* 2008; 47: 459-466.

[87] Durrington PN, Bhatnagar D, Mackness MI, Morgan J, Julier K, Khan MA, France M. An omega-3 polyunsaturated fatty acid concentrate administered for one year decreased triglycerides in simvastatin treated patients with coronary heart disease and persistant hypertriglyceridemia. *Heart* 2001; 85: 544-548.

[88] Bays HE, Maki KC, McKenney J, Snipes R, Meadowcroft A, Schroyer R, Doyle RT, Stein E. Long-term up to 24-month efficacy and safety of concomitant prescription omega-3 fatty acid ethyl esters and simvastatin in hypertriglyceridemic patients. *Curr Med Res Opin* 2010; 26: 907-915.

[89] Roth EM, Bays HE, Forker AD, Maki KC, Carter R, Doyle RT, Stein EA. Prescription omega-3 fatty acids as an adjunct to fenofibrate therapy in hypertriglyceridemic subjects. *J Cardiovasc Pharmacol* 2009; 54: 196-203.

[90] 90. Isley WL, Miles JM, Harris WS. Pilot study of combined therapy with omega-3 fatty acids and niacin in atherogenic dyslipidemia. J Clin Lipidol 2007; 1: 211-217.

[91] Morris MC, Sacks F, Rosner B. Does fish oil lower blood pressure? A meta-analysis of controlled trials. *Circulation* 1993; 88: 523-533.

[92] 92. Appel LJ, Miller ER, Seidler AJ, Whelton PK. Does supplementation of diet with "fish oil" reduce blood pressure? A meta-analysis of controlled clinical trial. *Arch Intern Med* 1993; 153: 1429-1428.

[93] Geleijnse JM, Giltay EJ, Grobbee DE, Donders AR, Kok FJ. Blood pressure response to fish oil supplementation: metaregression analysis of randomized trials. *J Hypertens* 2002; 20: 1493-1499.

[94] Yamagishi K, Iso H, Date C, Fukui M, Wakai K, Kikuchi S, Inaba Y, Tanabe N, Tamakoshi A, for the JACC Study Group. Fish, ω-3 polyunsaturated fatty acids, and mortality from cardiovascular diseases in a nationwide community-based cohort of Japanese: The JACC (Japan Collaborative Cohort Study for Evaluation of Cancer Risk) study. *J Am Coll Cardiol* 2008; 52: 988-996.

[95] Nodari S, Triggiani M, Campia U, Manerba A, Milesi G, Cesana BM, Gheorghiade M, Cas LD. Effects of n-3 polyunsaturated fatty acids on left ventricular function and functional capacity in patients with dilated cardiomyopathy. *J Am Coll Cardiol* 2011; 57: 870-879.

[96] Blackburn EH. Switching and signaling at the telomere. *Cell* 2001; 106: 661-673.

[97] Blackburn EH. Structure and function of telomeres. *Nature* 1991; 350: 569-573.

[98] Cawthon RM, Smith KR, O'Brien E, Sivatchenko A, Kerber RA. Association between telomere length in blood and mortality in people aged 60 years and older. *Lancet* 2003; 361: 393-395.

[99] Farzaneh-Far R, Cawthon RM, Na B, Browner WS, Schiller NB, Whooley MA. Prognostic value of leukocyte telomere length in patients with stable coronary artery disease: data from the Heart and Soul Study. *Arterioscler Thromb Vasc Biol* 2008; 28: 1379-1384.

[100] Farzaneh-Far R, Lin J, Epel ES, Harris WS, Blackburn EH, Whooley MA. Association of marine omega-3 fatty acid levels with telomeric aging in patients with coronary heart disease. *JAMA* 2010; 303: 250-257.

[101] Lawson LD, Hughes BG, Absorption of eicosapentaenoic acid and docosahexaenoic acid from fish oil triacylglycerols or fish oil ethyl esters coingested with a high fat meal. *Biochem Biophys Res Commu* 1988; 156: 960-963.

[102] Dyerberg J, Madsen P, Moller JM, Aardestrup I, Schmidt EB. Bioavailability of marine n-3 fatty acid formulations. *Prostaglandins Leukotrienes Essent* 2010; 83: 137-141.

[103] Luley C, Weiland H, Grunwald J. Bioavailability of omega-3 fatty acids: ethylester preparations are as suitable as triglyceride preparations. *Akt Ernahr Med* 1990; 15: 123-125.

[104] Harris WS, Zucker ML, Dujovne CA. Omega-3 fatty acids in hypertriglyceridemic patients: triglcyerides vs. ethyl esters. *Am J Clin Nutr* 1988; 48: 992-997.

[105] 105. Bays H. *AMR101: a pure-EPA omega-3 fatty acid lowers triglycerides in patients with very high triglycerides without raising LDL-C: the MARINE study.* Presented at the National Lipid Association 2011 Annual Scientific Sessions.

[106] The ANCHOR study. Available at *http://investor.aramincorp.com/releases.cfm.*

[107] Bays HE. Safety considerations with omega-3 fatty acid therapy. *Am J Cardiol* 2007; 99(suppl): 35C-43C.

[108] Hansen JB, Lyngmo V, Svensson B, Nordoy A. Inhibition of exercise-induced shortening of bleeding time by fish oil in familial hypercholesterolemia (type IIa). *Arterioscler Thromb Vasc Biol* 1993; 13: 98-104.

[109] Harris WS. Expert opinion: omega-3 fatty acids and bleeding-cause for concern? *Am J Cardiol* 2007; 99(suppl): 44C-46C.

[110] Eritsland J, Arnesen H, Gronseth K, Fjeld NB, Abdelnoor M. Effect of dietary supplementation with n-3 fatty acids on coronary artery bypass graft patency. *Am J Cardiol* 1996; 77: 31-36.

[111] Leaf A, Jorgenson MB, Jacobs AK, Cote G, Schoenfield DA, Scheer J, Weiner BH, Slack JD, Kellet MA, Raizner AE, Webner PC, Mahrer PR, Rossouw JE. Do fish oil prevent restenosis after coronary angioplasty? *Circulation* 1994; 90: 2248-2257.

[112] Bender NK, Kraynak MA, Chiquette E, Linn WD, Clark GM, Bussey HI. Effects of marine fish oils on the anticoagulation status of patients receiving chronic warfarin therapy. *J Thromb Thrombolysis* 1998; 5: 257-258

[113] Watson PD, Joy PS, Nkonde C, Hessen SE, Karalis DG. Comparison of bleeding complications with omega-3 fatty acids + aspirin + clopidogrel – versus – aspirin + clopidogrel in patients with cardiovascular disease. *Am J Cardiol* 2009; 104: 1052-1054.

[114] Mozaffarian D, Rimm EB. Fish intake, contaminants, and human health: evaluating the risk and benefits. *JAMA* 2006; 296: 1885-1899.

[115] Berquin IM, Edwards IJ, Chen YQ. Multi-targeted therapy of cancer by omega-3 fatty acids. *Cancer Letters* 2008; 269: 363-377.

[116] Kimura Y, Kono S, Toyomura K, Nagano J, Mizoue T, Moore MA, Mibu R, Tanaka M, Kakeji Y, Maehara Y, Okamura T, Ikejiri K, Futami K, Yasunami Y, Maekawa T, Takenaka K, Ichimiya H, Imaizumi N. Meat, fish, and fat intake in relation to subsite-specific risk of colorectal cancer: the Fukuoka Colorectal Cancer Study. *Cancer Sci* 2007; 98: 590-597.

[117] Theodoraou E, McNeill G, Cetnarskyj R, Farrington SM, Tenesa A, Barnetson R, Porteous M, Dunlop M, Campbell H. Dietary fatty acids and colorectal cancer: a case control study. *Am J Epidemiiol* 2007; 166: 181-195.

[118] Chavarro JE, Stampfer MJ, Li H, Campos H, Kurth T, Ma J. A prospective study of polyunsaturated fatty acid levels in blood and prostate cancer risk. *Cancer Epidemiol Biomarkers Prev* 2007; 16: 1364-1370.

[119] Ritch CR, Wan RL, Stephens LB, Taxy JB, Huo D, Gong EM, Zagaja GP, Brendler CB. Dietary fatty acids correlate with prostate cancer biopsy grade and volume in Jamaican men. *J Urol* 2007; 177: 97-101.

[120] Brasky TM, Till C, White E, Neuhouser ML, Song X, Goodman P, Thompson IM, King IB, Albanes D, Kristal AR. Serum phospholipid fatty acids and prostate cancer risk: results from the Prostate Cancer Prevention Trial. *Am J Epidemiol* (2011) first published online April 24, 2011 doi:10.1093/aje/kwr027.

In: Fish Oil: Production, Consumption and Health Benefits
Editors: Matthias Van Dijk and Jürgen Vitek
ISBN: 978-1-61470-963-3

Chapter III

Polyunsaturated Fatty Acids and Their Dietary Implications during Pregnancy

Emilio Herrera** and Encarnación Amusquivar
Faculties of Pharmacy and Medicine, University CEU San Pablo, Madrid, Spain

Abstract

Although animals can modify fatty acyl chains by introducing more than one double bond, certain limitations exist. Chain elongation alternates with desaturation, which together with peroxisomal retro-conversion reactions allow the synthesis of long-chain polyunsaturated fatty acids (LCPUFA) from linoleic acid (18:2ω6) and α-linolenic acid (18:3ω3), the only nutritionally essential fatty acids (EFA). Arachinonic acid and other C_{20} LCPUFA give rise to eicosanoids (prostaglandins, thromboxanes, leukotrienes and lipoxins), which are signaling molecules classified as local hormones. Polyunsaturated fatty acids (PUFA) are also biological regulators, and many of their effects relate to their abilities to regulate gene expression and downstream events. These effects are cell-specific and involve members of the super-family of nuclear receptors that function as transcription factors. PUFA are susceptible to autooxidation by a process that is especially complex in the cell membrane, where it increases the consumption of vitamin E – a chain-breaking antioxidant that prevents the propagation of free radical reactions. Other antioxidant defenses exist, in the form of certain enzymes (e.g., superoxide dismutases, catalase, gluthatione peroxidase and other peroxidases) and of compounds that protect against the oxidation process or repair the damage caused. Normal fetal development requires both EFA and LCPUFA, and the nutritional status of the mother during gestation has been related to fetal growth. Supplementing diets with oils rich in LCPUFA during the last trimester of gestation has been advised; however, in excess, they may cause competitive inhibition of the Δ^6 and Δ^5 desaturases that control the conversion of EFA into LCPUFA by the ω-3 and ω-6 pathways, thus inhibiting the synthesis of certain LCPUFA that could be essential for fetal growth. Maternal dietary LCPUFA are taken up by adipose tissue during early pregnancy, where they are stored temporarily,

* Corresponding author: Prof. Emilio Herrera, Universidad San Pablo-CEU, Ctra. Boadilla del Monte km 5,300, E-28668 Boadilla (Madrid), Spain, Telephone: +34 913727730, FAX: +34 913510496, e.mail: eherrera@ceu.es

before being released during late pregnancy to become available to the fetus in the last stages of its development. In maternal plasma most LCPUFA circulate in their esterified form in different lipoproteins, and around parturition they are diverted to mammary gland where – through the induction of lipoprotein lipase – they are used for milk synthesis and thus become available to the newborn. Efforts have been made to determine whether supplements with LCPUFA during different perinatal stages can improve the short- or long-term developmental outcome, but no definitive conclusion has been attained, and additional studies are required.

Keywords: Polyunsaturated fatty acids, Oxidative stress, Eicosanoids, Gene expression, Antioxidants, Pregnancy, Offspring, Dietary fatty acids, LCPUFA supplements.

Introduction

Human diets contain two main essential fatty acids (EFA), α-linolenic acid (18:3ω-3)[1] and linoleic acid (18:2ω-6), which can be elongated and desaturated in human tissues to the more highly unsaturated members of their respective long chain polyunsaturated fatty acid (LCPUFA) families (ω-3 and ω-6), principally docosahexaenoic acid (DHA, 22:6ω-3) and arachidonic acid (AA, 20:4ω-6). LCPUFA are known to play a major role in fetal development and pregnancy outcome [1,2]. DHA is essential for brain development and visual function [3,4], whereas AA is the precursor of prostaglandins and leukotrienes and is essential for neonatal growth [5,6]. For these reasons, diets have been supplemented with either specific LCPUFA or certain oils, mainly fish-oils rich in ω-3 LCPUFA, during pregnancy and lactation, to provide higher concentrations of these fatty acids to newborn infants. This practice is still controversial [7-9], since high intakes of polyunsaturated fatty acids (PUFA) may also carry a risk of adverse effects [10,11]. Excessive intake of PUFA increases lipid peroxidation and reduces antioxidant capacity [12,13], increasing susceptibility to oxidative damage [14,15]. We have shown that feeding a diet containing moderate amounts of fish oil during pregnancy and lactation in the rat decreases both α-tocopherol and AA concentrations in the pups and greatly delays postnatal development [13].

In the light of these observations, the metabolism of PUFAs, their susceptibility to peroxidation and their implications for the offspring during pregnancy and lactation are reviewed here. The intention is to present a comprehensive overview of the subject, rather than to attempt an exhaustive and detailed review of the individual parts of the subject, which in any case have been published elsewhere [3,16-24].

[1] Fatty acids are named by the number of carbon atoms in the chain (first number), the number of double bonds (the second number following the colon), and the position of the last double bond relative to the methyl end of the carbon chain (the ω carbon atom, which it is sometimes named n).

The Metabolism of PUFA – An Overview

Desaturase and Elongase Systems

Although animal tissues can modify fatty acyl chains by introducing more than one double bond, there are certain limitations [25-28]. i) The first double bond introduced is normally in the Δ^9-position[2]. ii) In animals, the second and subsequent double bonds are always inserted between an existing double bond and the carboxyl end of the acyl chain, never on the methyl side of an existing double bond; in plants, however, double bonds can be introduced between the existing double bond and the terminal methyl group as well. Since the "ω-families" of unsaturated fatty acids are defined by the number of carbons between the methyl end of the molecule and the nearest double bound, and animals are unable to alter that designation because they can only insert new double bonds at the carboxyl end of the chain, the ω-families present are determined entirely by dietary intake. iii) The introduction of conjugated double bonds is extremely rare in most organisms, and certainly so in higher animals; most pairs of double bonds are separated by a methylene group (CH_2 group). iv) All bonds introduced by the oxidative action of desaturases are *cis* geometric isomers. Thus, as shown in figure 1, animals insert double bonds at positions Δ^4, Δ^5, Δ^6 and Δ^9, but in plants they can be inserted at positions Δ^9, Δ^{12} and Δ^{15}. Microscopic algae, like *diatoms,* and photosynthetic protest like *Euglena* are, however, able to desaturate on either side of an existing bond, and this appears also to be so in insects [29], yielding double bonds in positions Δ^5, Δ^6, Δ^9, Δ^{12} and Δ^{15}.

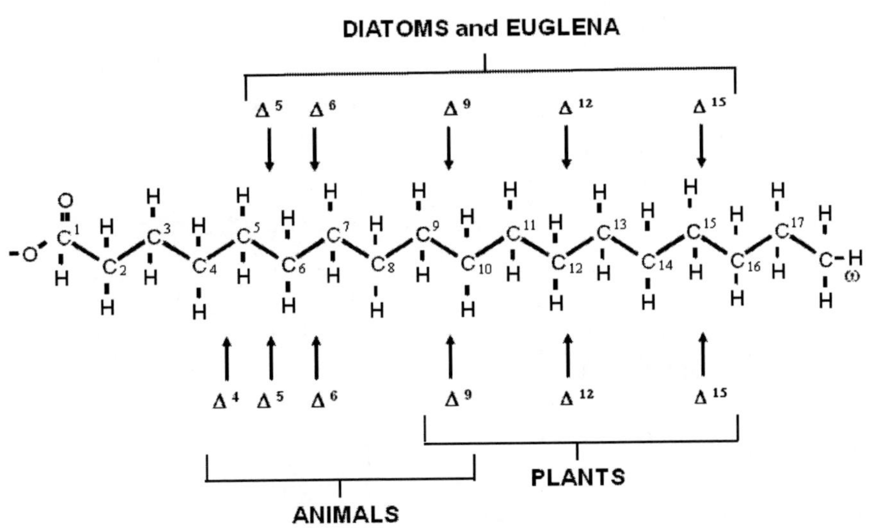

Figure 1. Positions of enzymatic fatty acyl chain desaturation in animals, plants, diatoms and Euglena. Carbon atoms are numbered from the carboxyl carbon (carbon 1); double bonds are indicated by the Δ, with the superscript indicating the first carbon number of the two affected carbons, and the terminal methyl carbon is known as the ω-carbon atom.

---

[2] Δ corresponds to the position of the double bond relative to the carboxylic carbon (# 1).

Fatty acyl chain desaturation is carried out by a desaturase system present in endoplasmic reticulum, of which the best studied is Δ^9 desaturase [27], although its mechanism of action is not yet completely understood. The system is an oxygenase type of enzyme that has been isolated from liver, mammary gland, brain, testes and adipose tissue. It acts on acyl-CoA substrates (mainly of 14 to 18 carbons), formed from non-esterified fatty acid by the action of acyl-CoA synthetase using ATP, Mg^{2+} and CoASH. The desaturase system is an electron transport system that has an absolute requirement for molecular oxygen, which acts as an electron acceptor for two pairs of hydrogen atoms, one pair from NADH and the other from the fatty acyl-CoA. It consists of three major proteins: NADH:cytocrome b_5 reductase (a flavoprotein), cytochrome b_5 (a heme-containing protein) and a terminal desaturase component, which is sensitive to cyanide inhibition and contains one non-heme iron per molecule.

As well as desaturation, most organisms, and certainly animals, also elongate fatty acids by adding 2 carbon units at a time. Mitochondrial elongation systems exist, but there is greater activity in the endoplasmic reticulum (microsomes). The microsomes contain at least two different elongation systems, one for saturated and another for unsaturated fatty acids [27,30]. These systems use malonyl-CoA plus fatty acyl-CoA (of 10 carbons or more) as substrates and four enzymes: 3-ketoacyl synthase, 3-ketoacyl reductase, 3-hydroxy acyl dehydrase and 2-trans-enoyl-CoA reductase.

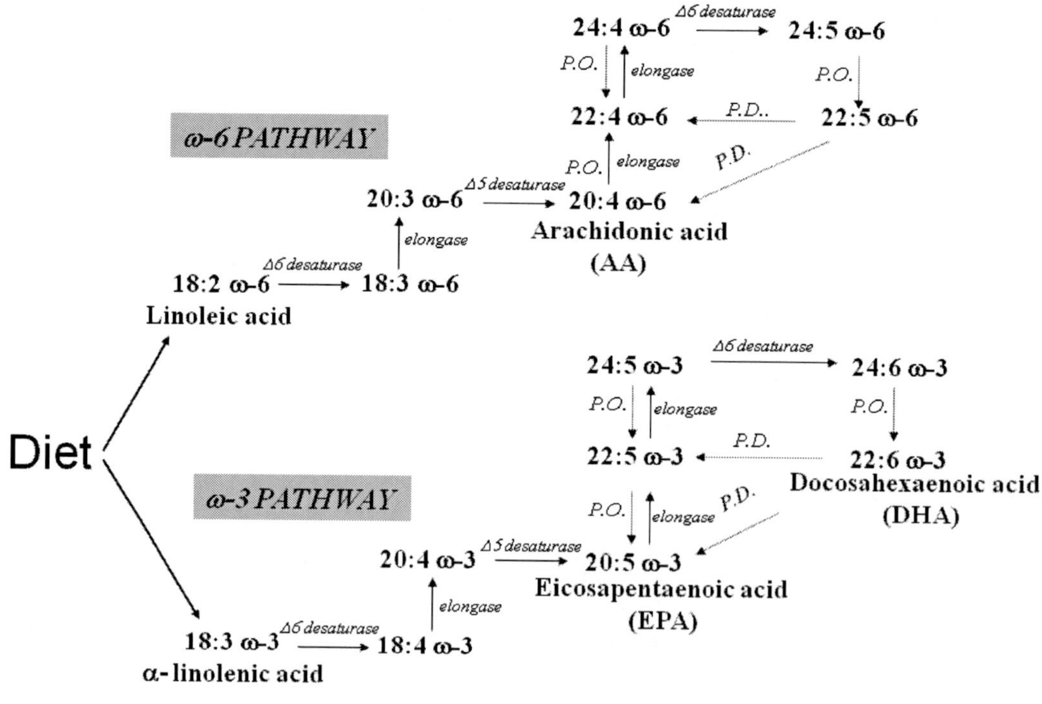

Figure 2. Major pathways of the biosynthesis of ω-6 and ω-3 long chain polyunsaturated fatty acids from their respective essential fatty acid precursor by desaturation and elongation, including the peroxisomal retroconversion reactions. Note the alternating sequence of desaturation in the horizontal direction and chain elongation in the vertical direction of the solid arrows; the partial degradation reactions taking place in peroxisomes (peroxisomal degradation, P.D.) are indicated by the dotted arrows.

In mammals, chain elongation usually alternates with desaturation to bring about the synthesis of the LCPUFA (figure 2). Thus, 18-carbon unsaturated fatty acids precursors of the ω-6- and ω-3-PUFA families are converted to corresponding highly unsaturated and elongated fatty acyl-CoAs via 24-carbon intermediates. This pathway requires the activities of Δ^6- and Δ^5-desaturases, enzymes that have been cloned [31,32]. The desaturation and elongation reactions are followed by a peroxisomal β-oxidation retro-conversion reaction, which forms the final 22-carbon products [28,33-35] (figure 2). Thanks to these series of reactions, the only fatty acids known to be nutritionally essential are linoleic acid (18:2ω6) and α-linolenic acid (18:3ω3), which are the substrates for the ω-6 and ω-3 pathways respectively (figure 2). In case of the ω-6 pathway, AA (20:4ω6) is synthesized, and is the substrate for eicosanoid synthesis (prostanoids, leukotrienes and lipoxins), as well as for fatty acids of longer chain. AA used for eicosanoid synthesis (see below) has been shown to be esterified in the phospholipids of specific cell membranes [36], from which it has to be liberated at the time of cell activation. Since there is very little AA in the diet normally, and because most of the dietary fatty acid of the ω-6 family is linoleate, an intact pathway between linoleate and arachidonate is essential for the production of eicosanoids [37]. In case of the ω-3 pathway, eicosapentaenoic (EPA, 20:5ω3) and DHA (22:6ω3) are synthesized, which together with AA play an important role as components of brain phospholipids.

The processes of desaturation and elongation are modulated by diet (31), hormones [31,38,39] and age [40-42]. They are lower in young rat's liver than in adults, but higher in the brain of young rats than in adults.

Eicosanoids Formed from C_{20} Polyunsaturated Fatty Acids

AA and some other 20 carbon polyunsaturated fatty acids give rise to eicosanoids, which are physiologically and pharmacologically active compounds known as prostaglandins (PG), thromboxanes (TX), leukotrienes (LT) and lipoxins (LX). They are signaling molecules, which are considered to be local hormones and which function through G-protein-linked receptors to elicit their biochemical effects.

Eicosanoids can be derived from 3 different sources, i) by biosynthesis from the EFA, linoleic or α-linolenic acid, ii) directly from, for example, AA and EPA in the diet, or iii) from fatty acids stored in membrane phospholipids. AA is usually present in the 2-position of phospholipids in the plasma membrane, being released by the action of phospholipase A_2 to become the substrate for the synthesis of prostanoids (PG_2 and TX_2 series) by the cycloxygenase pathway or the LT_4 and LX_4 series by the lipoxygenase pathway, with the two pathways competing for the substrate (figure 3). The ω-6 eicosanoids are generally pro-inflammatory, whereas the ω-3 family is much less so [43]. Eicosanoids of the 2-series (ω-6) promote inflammation, platelet aggregation and activate immune response, whereas prostanoids of the 3-series (ω-3) tend to ameliorate these effects [44,45]. The ω-6/ω-3 ratio in membrane phospholipids modulates the balance between prostanoids of the 2- and 3-series derived from AA and EPA, respectively. Prostanoids from series-3 are weaker agonists than the corresponding compounds of the 2-series or, in some cases, antagonists.

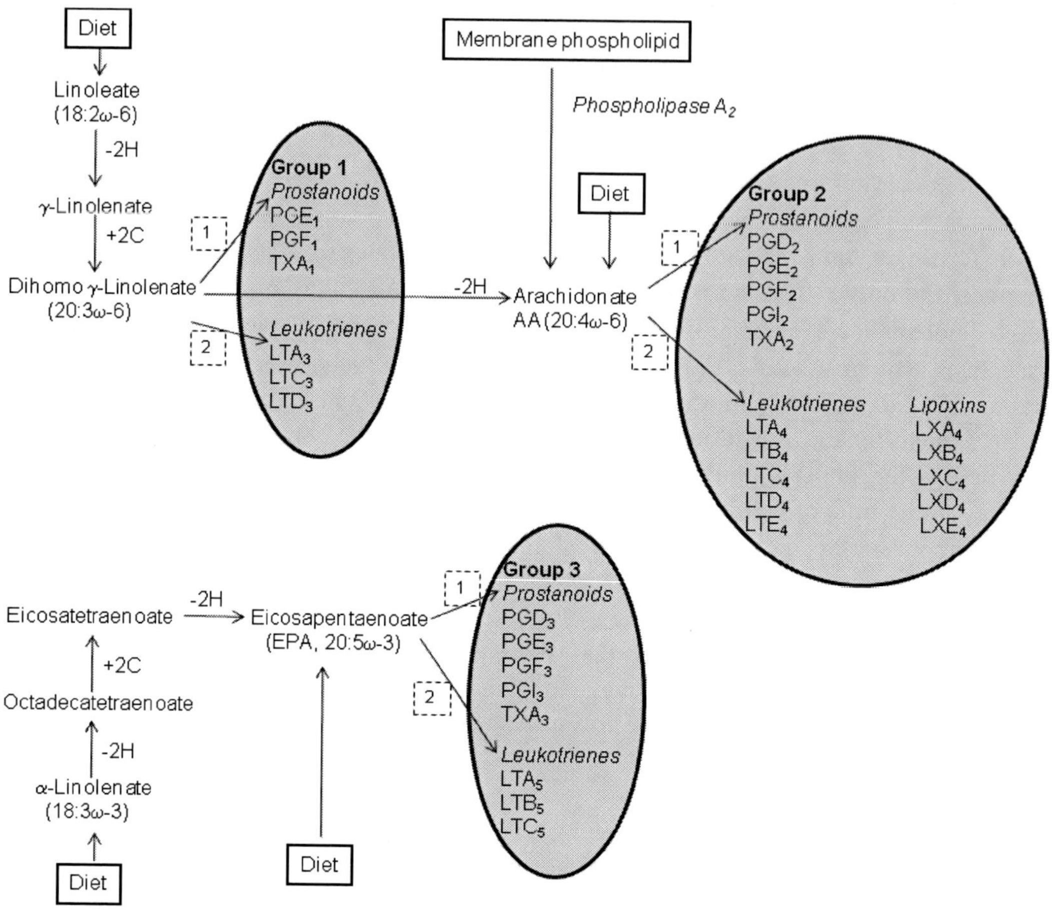

Figure 3. Schematic pathway of the biosynthesis of three groups of eicosanoids from dietary essential fatty acids (e.g. linoleate and α-linolenate), eicosapentaenoate or arachidonate, or membrane phospholipids in case of arachidonate. PG, prostaglandin; PGI, prostacyclin; TX, thromboxane; LT, leukotriene; LX, lipoxin.

Both EPA and DHA also give rise to resolvins and related compounds, like protectins, through pathways involving cyclooxygenase and lipoxygenase enzymes [46]. These mediators have been demonstrated to have potent anti-inflammatory and immunoregulatory actions at very low concentrations.

Thus LCPUFA, through the action of the cyclooxygenase or lipoxygenase pathways, form a considerable number of compounds that play key roles in modulating inflammation, cytokine release, immune response, platelet aggregation, vascular reactivity, thrombosis, and allergic phenomena including anaphalaxis.

Role of Fatty Acids Controlling Gene Expression

Fatty acids have increasingly been recognized as major biological regulators. Many of the effects of fatty acids, both in cell biology and in human health and disease, relate to their abilities to regulate gene expression and subsequent downstream events, ω-3 PUFA being especially potent in this respect [24,47-49]. The mechanism for the regulation of gene expression by fatty acids involves members of the superfamily of nuclear receptors that function as transcription factors, like the peroxisome proliferator-activated receptor (PPAR) family, the liver nuclear receptor (LXR), hepatic nuclear factor-4α (HNF-4α), sterol regulatory element-binding protein (SREBP) and NF-κB. These transcription factors are responsible for the expression of other key proteins that are pertinent to inflammation, lipid metabolism and energy utilization.

The effects of fatty acids on gene expression are cell-specific and depend on fatty acid structure and metabolism. The mechanism of action involves the fatty acid acting as a ligand for nuclear receptors, thus promoting their dimerization, either with an identical receptor (homodimer) or with a different nuclear receptor (heterodimer). The binding of the fatty acid may also facilitate the interaction of the dimer with co-activator or co-repressor proteins that determine the activity of the protein complex. The interaction of PUFA with the SREBP or with PPAR may serve as examples of their pluripotent effects on gene expression:

i. *PUFA and SREBP*. Three SREBP have been identified: SREBP1a and SREBP1c, which mainly regulate genes of fatty acid metabolism, and SREBP2, which regulates genes involved in cholesterol metabolism. Regulation of SREBP is carried out post-transcriptionally. Its inactive precursor is located in the endoplasmic reticulum (ER), linked to the SREBP cleavage-activating protein (SCAP), and the complex is anchored by another ER-resident membrane protein, Insig [50]. When the concentration of sterols is low in the cell, Insig dissociate from the SREBP/SCAP complex, which translocates to the Golgi via vesicular transport [50]. Once in the Golgi, SREBP dissociates from SCAP and undergoes a two-step proteolytic cleavage. The newly generated amino-terminal fragment of SREBP, which is the transcriptionally active end of the molecule, is released to the cytoplasm and travels to the nucleus, where it binds to sterol regulatory elements (SRE) in the promoter region of a substantial number of genes involved in lipid metabolism. Both cholesterol and oxysterols are known to regulate this pathway by feedback inhibition [51]. The LCPUFA (EPA, DHA and AA) have been shown to decrease the concentration of the transcriptionally active amino-terminal fragment of SREBP [52,53], and this inhibitory capacity on SREBP processing is greater than that shown by shorter chain PUFA, monounsaturated fatty acids or saturated fatty acids, which have practically no effect on SREBP processing [52].
ii. *PUFA, peroxisome proliferator-activated receptors (PPARs) and other transcription factors*. PPARs are members of the nuclear receptor family of ligand-activated transcription factors, and consist of three isoforms, PPARα, PPARβ/δ and PPARγ that have distinct, but interrelated, functions. These transcription factors have a ligand domain where they are activated by the binding of an agonist. Activated PPAR form a heterodimer with retinoid-X receptor (RXR) and binds a peroxisome proliferator response element in the promoter of target genes [54,55]. The PUFA, as well as their CoenzymeA derivatives, the oxidative derivatives of ω-3 PUFA, their eicosanoid products and AA metabolites (eicosanoids), but not saturated fatty acids, have been reported to bind PPARs (at least to PPARα and PPARγ) [49,56-59] and

consequently to induce physiological responses such as increasing β-oxidation of fatty acids and adipogenesis, although the effect varies according to cell type.

Substantial "cross-talk" seems to exists between PPARs, expression of SREBPs and liver X receptor (LXR) [58,60-62]. It has been shown, using cultured rat hepatocytes, that ω-3 PUFAs suppress insulin-induced SREBP1c transcription via reduced trans-activation of LXRα [60]. Further investigation is needed to determine the molecular mechanisms of this effect, as well as to determine whether such relationships are also present *in vivo*. Nevertheless, there are studies in suckling rats showing that oral treatment with Intralipid, which is rich in EFA, induces the expression of hepatic PPARα and of its target genes, like acyl-CoA oxidase and lipoprotein lipase; the effect disappears under hyperinsulinemic conditions [63-65]. This fatty acid-induced effect was not detected in adult rats, where the PPARα gene seems to be less sensitive to nutritional changes than in neonates [64]. Although the current evidence indicates that these interactions exist and are active *in vivo* during development, it appears that the overall effect is complex. The characteristics of how each PUFA can affect transcriptional processes and their potency differ, and we are still far from understanding the detailed mechanisms of how and when specific PUFAs control the expression of genes affecting lipid homeostasis.

Susceptibility of Polyunsaturated Fatty Acids to Oxidative Stress

Unlike saturated and monounsaturated fatty acids (MFA), PUFA are highly susceptible to autoxidation [66,67]. Although highly purified polyunsaturated fatty acids *in vitro* have been shown to be stable for long periods of time even in the presence of oxygen [68], autoxidation occurs readily *in vivo* and the initial stages are critical for the process. The process is autocatalytic and is summarized in figure 4. A resonance hybrid is formed (PUFA•, alkyl radical) from a PUFA (e.g., linoleic acid: 18:2ω3) either by the action of a free radical (R•), which may be formed by the presence of traces of peroxides or transition metals, by ultraviolet or ionizing radiation, by oxygen singlet formed photochemically [69] or by several other factors (figure 4a). The hybrid is already a free radical that may propagate the process by reacting with oxygen to form peroxyl radicals (PUFA-OO•), which can then initiate more peroxidation by abstracting a hydrogen atom from another molecule of substrate, converting the peroxy radicals to hydroperoxides (PUFA-OOH) (figure 4b). These latter compounds decompose under certain conditions by homolysis, giving radicals (PUFA-O•, alkoxy radical and •OH, hydroxyl radical) that may initiate a new peroxidation chain. The process may be accelerated by the presence of metal-catalyzing reactions, in which certain transition metal ions (e.g. of copper or iron or as part of metalloproteins) convert hydroperoxides (PUFA-OOH) to alkoxy radicals (PUFA-O•) and hydroxyl ion [19,70,71].

$$\text{PUFA-OOH} + M^{n+} \rightarrow \text{PUFA-O}^{\bullet} + OH^{-} + M^{(n+1)+}$$

(M = transition metal ion)

The termination of the process may occur by the coupling of two hybrid radicals, forming a product that is not a free radical (figure 4c).

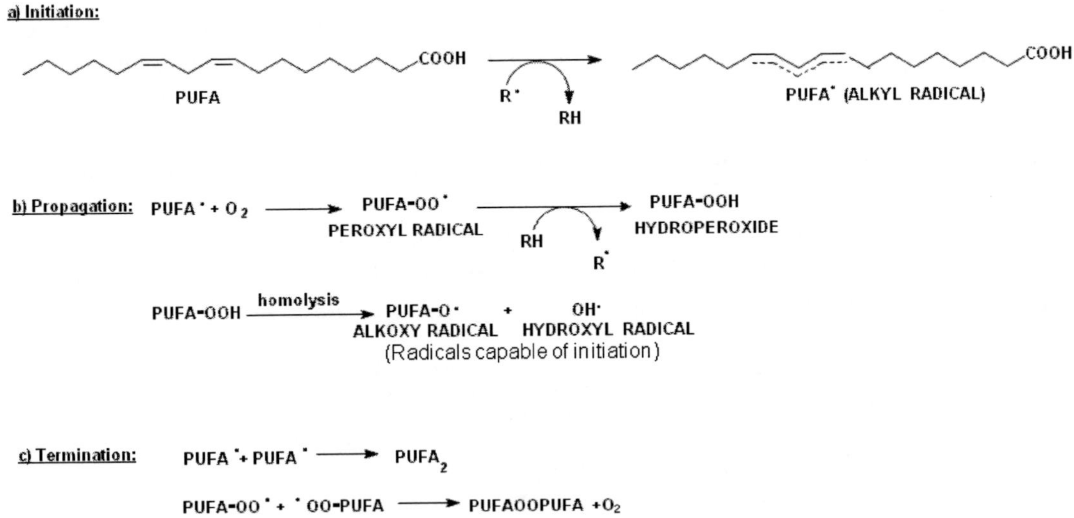

Figure 4.- Initiation, propagation and termination reactions in the autoxidation of a polyunsaturated fatty acid (PUFA) (e.g. linoleic acid, 18:2 ω-6). $PUFA^{\bullet}$ = alkyl radical; $PUFAOO^{\bullet}$ = peroxyl radical; PUFAOOH = hydroperoxide; $PUFAO^{\bullet}$ = alkoxy radical; $OH^{\bullet}$ = hydroxyl radical; $R^{\bullet}$ = free radical; RH = any hydrogen donor.

An interesting feature of the polyunsaturated fatty acid peroxidation reaction chains is that a single initiating event could convert a large number of polyunsaturated fatty acids to hydroperoxides [72]. The number of polyunsaturated fatty acids oxidized per initiated radical (R• or even PUFA-OO•, in figure 4) depends on several factors, particularly the rate of chain termination and the presence of phenolic antioxidants (AOH, e.g. vitamin E), that may scavenge the radical.

$$\text{PUFA-OO}^{\bullet} + \text{AOH} \rightarrow \text{PUFA-OOH} + \text{AO}^{\bullet}$$

In the cell membrane this process may be even more complex [73-75], and cells have the ability to mediate lipid oxidation processes. The formation not only of hydroperoxides but also lipid peroxide degradation products (e.g. endoperoxides and malondialdehyde) may disturb the structure of the membrane [76-78]. Furthermore, although PUFA in phospholipids may be more resistant to peroxidation than in its non-esterified form, when compared in purified preparations [79], phospholipid-PUFAs in the surface of cell membranes seem to be an ideal target for peroxidation, as has been shown *in vivo* [80], and by the fact that polyunsaturated oil intake decreases the concentration of vitamin E in animal tissues [12,13,81].

Antioxidant Defenses

Other powerful oxidants are also produced during the course of normal metabolism. These include reactive oxygen species, such as the superoxide anion radical ($O^{\bullet\bullet}$), hydrogen peroxide (H_2O_2), hydroxyl radical ($OH^{\bullet}$), and reactive nitrogen species. They are reactive molecules that can directly modify proteins, nucleic acids, lipids, and other molecules that can bring about a number of effects including mutations, strand breaks, tissue damage, aldehyde formation, oxidation of low density lipoproteins (LDL), and alterations in enzyme activities and signal transduction pathways. These effects may contribute to pathological conditions such as cardiovascular diseases, cancer, diabetes, aging or abnormalities in the nervous system [82-86].

The organism is able to compensate for the continuous production of these highly reactive molecules and their effects thanks to a number of antioxidant enzymes or compounds that protect against the oxidation process or repair the damage caused [87,88].

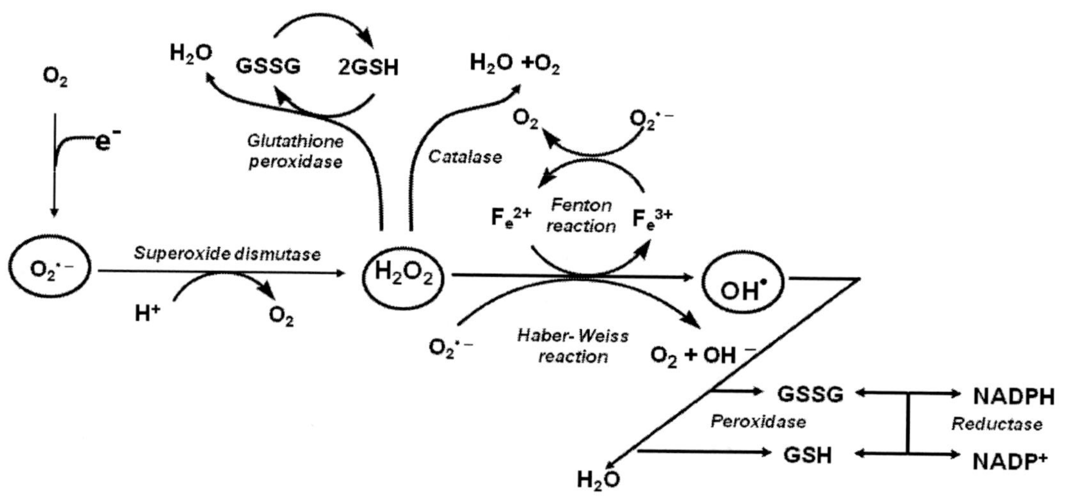

Figure 5.- Metabolism of toxic oxygen metabolites formed in one-electron reduction of molecular oxygen, as an example of the coordinated function of antioxidant enzymes. $O_2^{\bullet -}$ = superoxide anion; $OH^{\bullet}$ = hydroxyl free radical; GSH = (reduced) glutathione; GSSG = oxidized glutathione; H_2O_2 = hydrogen peroxide.

The antioxidant enzymes involved in removing reactive oxygen species are the superoxide dismutases [89], catalase [90], glutathione peroxidase [91] and other peroxidases [92]. In many cases, the action of these antioxidant enzymes is coordinated with the production of the reactive species (figure 5). Thus, in the metabolism of toxic oxygen metabolites, the reduction of molecular oxygen to form superoxide anion free radicals ($O^{\bullet -}$) may be followed rapidly by the action of superoxide dismutase, causing its conversion into hydrogen peroxide (H_2O_2), and this, by means of the Fenton and Haber-Weiss reactions, is transformed into hydroxyl free radical ($OH^{\bullet}$). The hydrogen peroxide can be destroyed by reacting with glutathione in the peroxidase reaction, or it can be converted to oxygen and water in a reaction mediated by catalase, and the hydroxyl free radical can be destroyed by reacting with glutathione.

The body has a wide range of antioxidant compounds, present at relatively low concentrations, that protect against excessive radical generation and the consequences thereof [93]. Some of them are located intracellularly where they scavenge aberrant free radical species. Other antioxidants are located extracellularly, mainly in plasma, where they intercept propagating radical reactions by removing delocalized metal ions or by sequestering the ions in forms that do not allow the stimulation of free-radical reactions. The major plasma antioxidant compounds include serum albumin, urate, ascorbate, α-tocopherol, γ-tocopherol, β-carotene, α-carotene, ubiquinol, bilirubin, reduced gluthatione and iron-transfer proteins (transferrin, ceruloplasmin, haptoglobin, hemopexin), which are present in a very wide range of concentrations [94,95].

α-Tocopherol is considered the main lipid-soluble antioxidant in the body [96], although it has been also shown to have pro-oxidant activity [97-99]. Despite its ability to decrease lipid peroxidation, studies in animal models and in clinical trials do not yet support a definitive recommendation for its therapeutic use in humans [100,101]. Pregnancy, especially with pre-eclampsia or diabetic pregnancy, is associated with high levels of lipid peroxides in serum [102-107], accompanied during normal pregnancies by higher maternal levels of vitamin E [107,108].

Dietary Fatty Acids uuring Pregnancy and Lactation

Normal fetal development needs the availability not only of EFA but also of their long chain polyunsaturated fatty acid (LCPUFA) derivatives to support the synthesis of structural lipids [109-112]. Both term and preterm infants seem to be able to form AA (20:4ω-6) and DHA (22:6ω-3) from their respective EFA precursors linoleic acid (18:2ω-6) and α-linolenic acid (18:3ω-3) (figure 2) [113-117]. The degree to which the fetus, however, is capable of fatty acid desaturation and elongation is not clear. Although fetal baboons have been shown to synthesize effectively both AA (20:4, ω-6) and DHA (22:6, ω-3) from their respective EFA precursors [118,119], in the human fetus LCPUFA synthesis seems to be negligible [120]. The endogenous synthesis of AA by newborn infants during the first week of life seems to contribute very little to the plasma AA pool [116], the limiting factor being a low Δ^5-desaturase activity.

During gestation, a reduced intake of EFA has been correlated with reduced neonatal growth [121], and, in untreated healthy women, concentrations of LCPUFA in maternal plasma consistently correlate with those in the fetus or newborn [111,122-125]. After supplementation of the maternal diet with fish-oil during pregnancy, increases in DHA levels have been found in both mothers and newborns [126,127]. These findings, which showed the important role of dietary fatty acids during pregnancy in controlling the supply of LCPUFA to the fetus and newborn, have been used to justify advice that maternal diets be supplemented with oils rich in LCPUFA during the last trimester of pregnancy [126-128].

However, specific fatty acids can cause competitive inhibition of the Δ^6- and Δ^5-desaturases that control the conversion of EFA into LCPUFA in both the ω-3 and ω-6 pathways (figure 2). An excess of one acid may inhibit the synthesis of other particular LCPUFAs that could be essential for fetal growth [7]. For example, excessive intake of safflower, sunflower or corn oils (vegetable oils rich in linoleic acid (18:2ω-6)) may inhibit Δ^6-desaturase thereby reducing the synthesis of DHA (22:6ω-3) from its parent EFA precursor, α-linolenic acid (18:3ω-3). An excess of linoleic acid has been also shown to decrease the formation of AA (20:4ω-6) [2,42,129-131]. Furthermore, when fish oil was consumed, low plasma AA levels were found [7,13], the effect being caused by the abundance in fish oil of both EPA (20:5ω-3) and DHA (22:6ω-3), which are known to inhibit the Δ^6 desaturase activity specifically [132,133], although Δ^5 and Δ^9 desaturase activities were both decreased in rats fed with diet high in fish oil [134].

The inhibitory effects of an excess of certain dietary fatty acids on LCPUFA synthetic pathways may acquire major relevance during the perinatal period, where plasma AA concentration has been correlated to body weight in preterm infants [135,136]; adverse effects of low blood concentrations of AA on growth during infancy have also been reported [137-139].

An excess of dietary LCPUFAs may also increase lipid peroxidation [140-142], reducing the antioxidant capacity [12,13] and increasing susceptibility to oxidative damage [143,144]. Increased quantities of reactive oxygen species and increased lipid peroxidation resulting in fetal damage, as well as its reversion by vitamin E treatment, have been shown experimentally to take place in diabetic pregnancy [145-151]. However, it is not yet clear whether oxidative stress plays any role in the development of complications in diabetic patients [152], and it has been shown that treating diabetic children with high doses of antioxidative agents, including vitamin E, has no effect on the preservation of beta-cell function or on metabolic balance [153]. Some studies have suggested a potential for vitamin E to be useful in the prevention of mutagenic effects caused by genotoxic free radicals, but others report no effects [18].

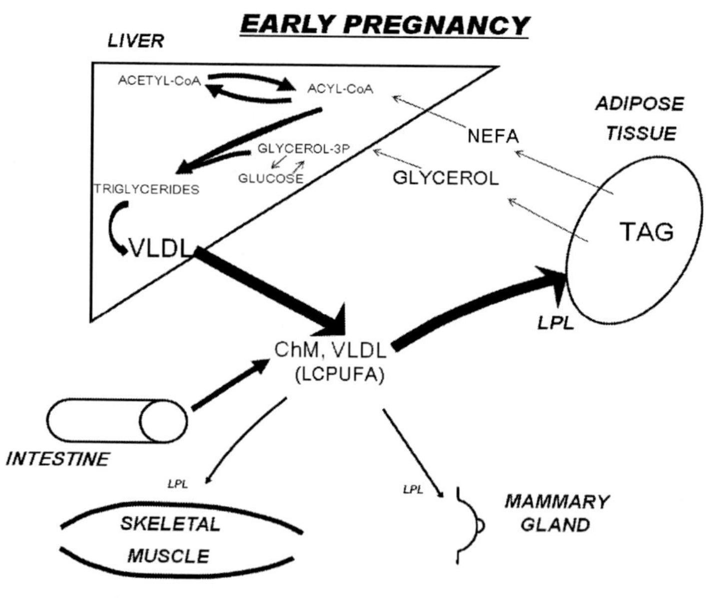

Figure 6a.-. Schematic view of main lipid metabolic adaptations taking place at two different stages of gestation. a) during early pregnancy showing the enhanced production of chylomicrons (ChM) by intestine, carrying dietary derived LCPUFA as result of maternal hyperphagia. Maternal hyperinsulinemia and slightly increased adipose tissue lipoprotein lipase (LPL) activity allow the hydrolysis of circulating triacylglycerols in chylomicrons and liver-derived very low density lipoproteins (VLDL) and the uptake of their products by adipose tissue, where LCPUFA are re-esterified for the synthesis of triacylglycerols (TAG) that become a store of those fatty acids. NEFA, non-esterified fatty acids.

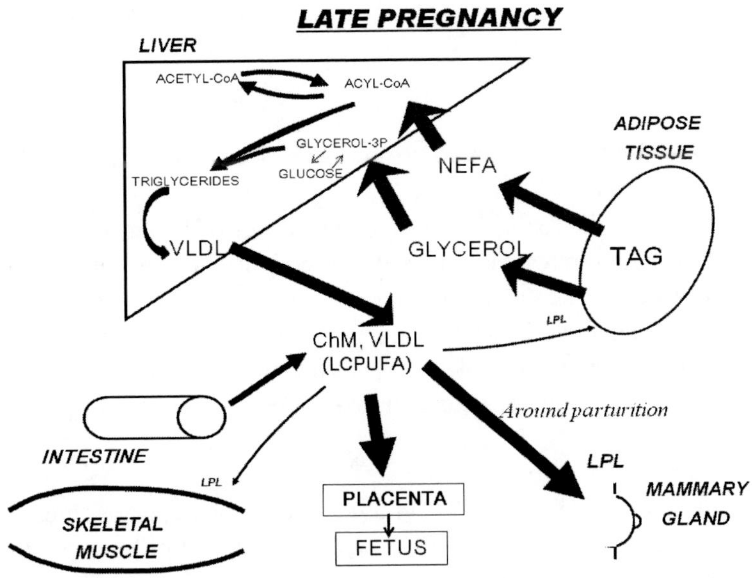

Figure 6b.- During late pregnancy a decline in adipose tissue LPL activity occurs and its lipolytic activity increases. The products, in the form of NEFA[237] (including LCPUFA accumulated at earlier stages of gestation) and glycerol, mainly travel to the liver where, among other metabolic fates, they are used for the synthesis of TAG, which are released to the circulation as components of VLDL, a process which is very active in late pregnancy. Plasma VLDL and chylomicrons arrive at the placenta, which has the appropriate biochemical machinery to take up these lipoproteins and release the LCUFA that they carry into the fetal circulation. Also, close to parturition, an induction of LPL occurs in mammary gland, causing a considerable uptake of lipids from the lipoproteins in the maternal circulation by this organ, which uses the LCPUFA it takes up for milk synthesis.

Experimental diabetic embryopathy has also been associated with an AA deficiency state [154]. Transfer and lipid distribution of AA have been shown to be altered in placentas from diabetic pregnancies [155,156]. Neonates from women with gestational diabetes do indeed have reduced levels of AA and DHA [157], but the change seems to be caused mainly by altered handling or metabolism of LCPUFA by the fetus rather than by impaired placental transfer [158].

The negative effect on offspring of high dietary fish oil intake during pregnancy could be result from either the reported decrease in AA levels [159,160], or by more rapid deplection of α-tocopherol due to the high LCPUFA content. In contrast, dietary olive oil protects the ω-3 PUFA series [161], does not affect AA concentrations [162-164], and is much more resistant to lipid peroxidation [141,165,166]. Therefore, a comparative study on these variables in rats fed a diet supplemented with moderate proportions (10%) of either fish oil or olive oil as the only non-vitamin lipid during pregnancy and lactation was carried out [13]. A decrease in both AA and α-tocopherol concentrations as well as delayed postnatal development were found in the offspring of rats given the fish oil-rich diet, and supplement experiments showed that low AA rather than α-tocopherol was responsible for the delayed postnatal development [13].

In conclusion, since on one hand, the safety of high intakes of LCPUFA during pregnancy is still unclear, and on the other hand, the risks and benefits of supplementing diets with vitamin E are not yet clearly determined, additional research is clearly needed before recommendations to increase LCPUFA intake or undertake vitamin E treatment in pregnancy can be made.

Maternal Adipose Tissue as a Storage Organ for Dietary LCPUFA

An average weight gain for a full-term pregnancy is 12.5 kg, of which approximately 3.35 kg corresponds to fat depots, and most of the remainder corresponds to the weight of the conceptus (i.e., the fetus, placenta and amniotic fluid) [167]. Thus, an increase in the size of the maternal fat depot is a characteristic feature of normal pregnancy, occurs in both women and experimental animals and takes place during the first two-thirds of gestation [168-170]. As well as being an efficient energy store, it is an effective reserve of polyunsaturated fatty acids.

Maternal insulin plays a critical role in her fat deposition. In early pregnancy, the secretion of insulin is increased [171,172] and the responsiveness of adipose tissue to insulin has been also found to increase [173]. Both changes contribute to the maternal fat accumulation that takes place. Maternal hyperphagia, which is normally present from early gestation [174], must also contribute to the increased fat depots. Moreover, studies in the rat have shown that maternal hyperinsulinemia and unchanged, or even enhanced, adipose tissue insulin responsiveness seems to be responsible for the increase in adipose tissue lipoprotein lipase (LPL) activity that takes place at this stage [169,175] . This enzyme, present in the endothelium of extra-hepatic tissues, hydrolyzes triacylglycerols circulating in plasma in the form of triacylglycerol-rich lipoproteins [176] and the hydrolytic products, fatty acids and glycerol, are taken up by the subjacent tissue [177]. Consequently, changes in adipose tissue LPL together with maternal hyperphagia may facilitate the uptake of lipids and could contribute to the fat accumulation that occurs during early pregnancy.

It is thought that the uptake of dietary derived LCPUFA by adipose tissue during early pregnancy plays a key role in their temporary storage allowing a timed release during late pregnancy. LCPUFA, thus released, become available to the fetus during the last stage of pregnancy and to the newborn via lactation. In fact, the composition of fatty acids in the diet determines their composition in adipose tissue in humans [178] and in adult rats [179], and a linear correlation between dietary fatty acids and maternal adipose tissue has also been found in the pregnant rat [180]. Those fatty acids taken up by adipose tissue are released during late pregnancy. Fat uptake by adipose tissue decreases in late pregnancy due to a lower LPL activity [181-183] and lipolytic activity is increased [184-186], causing a net breakdown of fat depots. Thus, during the final phase of pregnancy, when the foetus is growing at its maximum rate [181], maternal fat stores are mobilized, the change probably being the result of the insulin resistant condition that develops at this stage [187]. The products of adipose tissue lipolysis, nonesterified fatty acids (NEFA) and glycerol, are released into the circulation. Since the placental transfer of these products is quantitatively low [188], their main fate is maternal liver [189], where they are in part re-esterified to synthesize triacylglycerols that are released into the bloodstream as components of the very low density lipoproteins (VLDL). Indeed, most of the LCPUFA in maternal circulation are in their esterified form in plasma lipoproteins and not as NEFA [190-192].

During the last trimester of pregnancy, there is a high fetal demand for fatty acids as they are critical for normal neural and vascular development. The fetus is able to synthesize saturated and monounsaturated fatty acids but depends entirely on placental transport for its supply of the essential fatty acids linoleic acid and □-linolenic acid. As triacylglycerols are transported in the bloodstream as lipoproteins they must be hydrolyzed to release NEFA before they can be transferred across the placenta. It has been suggested that LPL is the most important hydrolase in the initial step for placental transfer of triacylglycerol-derived fatty acids, but a placenta-specific hydrolase and phospholipase A2, and receptors for very low, low and high density lipoproteins as well as scavenger receptors have been detected in the placenta [193]. Several FA transfer proteins have been identified in the placenta: FABPs, FAT/CD36, and FATPs have been implicated in the bidirectional transport of FA between the mother and the fetus [194], while others, like FAPBPpm, seem to play a role in the sequestration of certain FAs from the maternal side to the placenta [195]. Once in the placenta, FA are guided to various intracellular sites for esterification, beta-oxidation, and prostaglandin production or are transported directly to the fetal circulation. Also, EFA could be converted into their long chain derivatives, although this conversion is much lower than in other maternal tissues like liver [196].

It has been estimated that the fetus needs approximately 50 mg /kg /day of ω-3 and 400 mg /kg /day of ω-6 PUFA [197] and specifically DHA fetal accretion amounts to about 30-45 mg per day in the last trimester of gestation [198]. The brain is the organ that most of all incorporates LCPUFA for its development. DHA and AA are the major LCPUFA components in membranes of the brain and retina [199]. During gestation and infancy, exogenous LCPUFA supply can affect neural function by modulating membrane FA composition. LCPUFA are supplied to the infant through the placenta during pregnancy and in milk after birth; the rate of conversion of EFA into LCPUFA in the fetus and the neonate is low, and is insufficient on its own to support optimal growth and development if supply of LCPUFA from other sources declines [200,201]. During intrauterine life, the supply of both EFA and LCPUFA to the fetus depends on their concentration in maternal circulation as well as on their placental transfer. In fact, LCPUFA proportions in fetal circulation have been significantly correlated with their proportions in maternal plasma at the end of gestation [180]. Several studies have been carried out to demonstrate how the profile of fatty acids in the fetus or the neonate can be modified by manipulating the fatty acid profile of the mother during pregnancy [198,202-204].

In suckled newborns the availability of fatty acids depends on their profile in milk, which is influenced by those ingested by the lactating mother [205]. Milk fatty acid composition derives from two sources: i) biosynthesis of fatty acids and their subsequent esterification within the mammary gland and ii) the uptake of lipids from the plasma by the mammary gland. The influence of dietary fatty acids on milk fatty acid composition is well-recognized in humans [206-208] and has been associated with the fatty acid composition in maternal adipose tissue [209,210]. Fatty acids in milk come mostly from those carried in esterified form in maternal lipoproteins, which are taken up by the action of mammary gland LPL activity [211]. Maternal hypertriacylglyceridemia rapidly ceases around parturition [212], coinciding with a rapid increase in the mammary gland LPL activity and mRNA expression, whereas LPL activity in adipose tissue remains low, as determined in rats [213,214]. These combined changes facilitate an enhanced uptake of circulating triacygylcerols by the mammary gland, instead of their being stored in the adipose tissue. The mechanism, which regulates some of these changes in the mother, seems to be the hormonal changes occurring around parturition. The decline in plasma progesterone concentration and the subsequent release of prolactin, which occurs during the last 2 days of gestation, together with an enhanced responsiveness to insulin by mammary gland, seem to be the main factors responsible for the induction of mammary LPL expression and activity around parturition [215-219]. Several studies have demonstrated the uptake of the diet-derived LCPUFA by the mammary gland and their presence in the milk both in humans and in rats [203,208,220-224].

In view of the foregoing, we hypothesized that diet-derived LCPUFA during early pregnancy are stored in adipose tissue and released into the circulation in late pregnancy to become available to the fetus or even around parturition to be taken up by the mammary gland and become available to the newborn during suckling. Due to the similarities in the fatty acid metabolism in human and pigs [225], we determined the effect of feeding pregnant sows with either a fish oil or an olive oil supplemented diet during different stages of pregnancy [226]. When the fish oil supplemented diet was given during the first half of gestation, an increase in the □-3 PUFA, specifically in the proportion of DHA present, was found in maternal plasma at the end of the dietary period but also at day 7 of lactation in comparison with the olive group, even though the dietary treatment had stopped more than 2 months before. Furthermore, when the fatty acid profile of the lipids in colostrum and milk was analyzed, the proportion of DHA was significantly higher in the fish oil group. Finally, the proportion of DHA in the plasma from suckled piglets in the fish oil group remained higher than in the other group at day 3 of lactation [226]. The results obtained when the fish oil supplemented diet was given during the first part of gestation were even more striking that when the sow received the diet during the second stage of pregnancy. These findings indicate an important role of maternal adipose tissue during the first half of gestation as a store of dietary LCPUFA, especially DHA, which are mobilized around parturition and early lactation to be used for milk synthesis, making them available to the newborn during suckling [226].

All these findings together follow the same trend and suggest the following scheme: during pregnancy, dietary LCPUFA are taken up by adipose tissue, the action being especially effective during early pregnancy. Enhanced lypolytic activity of adipose tissue in late pregnancy releases these fatty acids into the bloodstream and, after being taken up by the liver and converted into triacyglycerols, they return to the circulation as components of VLDL, becoming an important source of LCPUFA for the fetus; around parturition they are diverted to mammary gland for milk synthesis, becoming available to the newborn during suckling.

Consequences in the Offspring of Fish Oil Supplements during the Perinatal Stages

As mentioned above, both DHA and AA are important for development of the central nervous system. During the last trimester of pregnancy and the first postnatal months there is a growth spurt in the human brain, with a large increase in the cerebral content of AA and DHA [109,227]. Since the capacity for elongation and desaturation of EFA is inadequate in the fetus and the newborn, the maternal LCPUFA status during pregnancy and lactation is critical to enable their proper availability to the fetus [228,229] and to newborn infants [230,231]. Although numerous randomized controlled trials have been undertaken to determine whether supplements with LCPUFA during different perinatal stages improves the developmental outcome, no definitive conclusion has been arrived [232,233]. However, comments on some specific aspects can be made.

In one intervention trial, carried out in a poor area of Bangladesh, the effects of fish oil supplements (4 g/day), from 25 weeks of gestation until term, were investigated [234]. At birth, no differences in length, head circumference or ponderal index between the fish oil and the soy-oil control groups were observed. Moreover, at 10 months, no difference was found between the groups in terms of weight and length or in any of the psychomotor developmental or behavioural outcomes. Another intervention study was also carried out in a low-income area (Cuernavaca, Mexico), where the effect of only DHA (400 mg/day) versus placebo from mid-pregnancy until birth was determined. Again no differences in weight, length or head circumference at birth were found [235].

There have also been a few studies on fish oil supplementation, applied just during pregnancy, carried out in better nourished areas. In one, it was reported that children in the fish-oil supplementation group (2.2 g DHA and 1.1 g EPA/day, from 20 weeks of gestation until delivery) attained higher scores for hand-eye coordination than those in the placebo group, whereas growth measurements were similar in the two groups at 30 months [236]. In another study, from 24 weeks of pregnancy until delivery, women received DHA-supplementation (300 mg/day), and at 9 months children showed improved problem solving [237]. In these two trials the sample size was relatively small, and it is difficult to exclude random error. In a more recent and larger trial, women received DHA-rich fish oil capsules (800 mg DHA/day) from less than 21 weeks of gestation until delivery. In children at 18 months of age no significant benefit to mean cognitive and language scores was found in those born from fish-oil supplemented women when compared to those from mothers receiving matched vegetable oil capsules without DHA [238].

Whereas DHA and AA are absent in most infant formulae, they are present in breast milk, although their concentrations are variable, depending on the mother's diet [239,240]. In any case, it is now well-established that breastfeeding is associated with a better neurological, cognitive and behavioural outcome than formula feeding [241-244]. It is however not clear to what extent the composition of human milk explains the difference in neurological development. The finding that prolongation of the duration of breastfeeding was associated with better cognitive scores at six years [245] suggests that the composition of human milk plays a positive role in the association between breastfeeding and outcome. One of the differences that may contribute to the differences between human milk and commercial formulae is the presence of LCPUFA in the former [246]. However, interpreting studies on the effect of supplementing of formula with LCPUFA is not straightforward and depends on the outcome studied and on the age at which the outcome was studied. Thus, a review of papers on the subject shows that supplementation of formula with LCPUFA is associated with a beneficial effect on short-term neuro-developmental outcome (i.e., until the age of four months) [247]. However, when the motor, visual and cognitive outcome of the LCPUFA-supplemented formula are the assessed, outcomes measured between 6 and 24 months of age usually reveal no differences between supplemented and non-supplemented groups [248,249]. The consumption by healthy term infants of formula containing LCPUFA for the first 2 months after birth has been shown not to alter neurological function at school age (i.e., 9 years old) [244].

Thus, no long-term beneficial effects of LCPUFA supplementation in term infants have been demonstrated. However, the human brain takes more than 20 years before attaining its adult configuration; the available information on the effects of LCPUFA supplementation on neuro-development beyond the school age is quite limited. It may happen that the effects of LCPUFA supplementation emerge at early postnatal stages to re-emerge at later ages, when more complex neural functions are expressed. A biphasic response in the comparison between breast-fed and formula-fed infants has been described in the Netherlands, where at three months the breastfed infants show a better neurological status than the formula-fed infants [250], the difference disappearing at 18 months [251] to re-emerge at 3.5 years [252]. The need for more studies to confirm and characterize this biphasic response is obvious.

Conclusion

Normal fetal development needs both EFA and LCPUFA, which must be obtained from its mother by the placental transfer. During early pregnancy, when fetal size is still small, dietary derived fatty acids are accumulated in maternal adipose tissue. However, during late pregnancy when fetal growth rate is higher, maternal adipose tissue switches to a catabolic condition and lipolytically released LCPUFA are mainly carried as their esterified form in plasma lipoproteins and become available to be transferred through the placenta. The enhanced adipose tissue lipolysis is maintained around parturition, and circulating LCPUFA are diverted to mammary gland for milk synthesis thanks to the induction of the expression and activity of mammary gland lipoprotein lipase. As a result, the LCPUFA become available to the newborn during suckling. The importance of both DHA and AA for development of central nervous system and growth has motivated the use of supplements of LCPFA during different perinatal stages. Several intervention trials of LCPUFA supplementation have been carried out, but the short- and long-term responses in the offspring have been very variable and no clear beneficial effects were demonstrated; although a biphasic response has been proposed further studies are needed.

Acknowledgments

This study has been carried out with the financial support of the Spanish Ministry of Science and Innovation (SAF2008-04518) and Universidad San Pablo CEU (USP-BSCH-05/08, USP-PC09-12). The authors wish to thank Milagros Morante for her excellent technical assistance and pp-science-editing.com for editing and linguistic revision of the manuscript.

References

[1] Al, Mdm; Van Houwelingen, Ac; Hornstra, G . Long-Chain Polyunsaturated Fatty Acids, Pregnancy, And Pregnancy Outcome. *American Journal Of Clinical Nutrition* 2000, *71*, 285s-291s.

[2] Innis, Sm . Essential Fatty Acids In Growth And Development. *Progress In Lipid Research* 1991, *30*, 39-103.

[3] Lauritzen, L; Hansen, Hs; Jorgensen, Mh; Michaelsen, Kf . The Essentiality Of Long Chain *N*-3 Fatty Acids In Relation To Development And Function Of The Brain And Retina. *Progress In Lipid Research* 2001, *40*, 1-94.

[4] Innis, Sm . Dietary (N-3) Fatty Acids And Brain Development. *Journal Of Nutrition* 2007, *137*, 855-859.

[5] Carlson, Se; Cook, Rj; Werkman, Sh; Tolley, Ea . First Year Growth Of Preterm Infants Fed Standard Compared To Marine Oil N-3 Supplemented Formula. *Lipids* 1992, *27*, 901-907.

[6] Carlson, Se . Arachidonic Acid Status Of Human Infants: Influence Of Gestational Age At Birth And Diets With Very Long Chain N-3 And N-6 Fatty Acids. *Journal Of Nutrition* 1996, *126 Suppl.*, 1092s-1098s.

[7] Uauy-Dagach, R; Mena, P . Nutritional Role Of Omega-3 Fatty Acids During The Perinatal Period. *Clin.Perinatol.* 1995, *22*, 157-175.

[8] Hamosh, M . Long-Chain Polyunsaturated Fatty Acids: Who Needs Them? *Biochem.Soc.Trans.* 1998, *26*, 96-103.

[9] Jensen, Cl . Effects Of N-3 Fatty Acids During Pregnancy And Lactation. *American Journal Of Clinical Nutrition* 2006, *83 (Suppl)*, 1452s-1457s.

[10] Eritsland, J . Safety Considerations Of Polyunsaturated Fatty Acids. *American Journal Of Clinical Nutrition* 2000, *71*, 197s-201s.

[11] Olafsdottir, As; Skuladottir, Gv; Thorsdottir, I; Hauksson, A; Thorgeirsdottir, H; Steingrimsdottir, L . Relationship Between High Consumption Of Marine Fatty Acids In Early Pregnancy And Hypertensive Disorders In Pregnancy. *Br.J.Obstet.Gynaec.* 2006, *113*, 301-309.

[12] Cho, S-H; Choi, Y . Lipid Peroxidation And Antioxidant Status Is Affected By Different Vitamin E Levels When Feeding Fish Oil. *Lipids* 1994, *29*, 47-52.

[13] Amusquivar, E; Rupérez, Fj; Barbas, C; Herrera, E . Low Arachidonic Acid Rather Than A-Tocopherol Is Responsible For The Delayed Postnatal Development In Offspring Of Rats Fed Fish Oil Instead Of Olive Oil During Pregnancy And Lactation. *Journal Of Nutrition* 2000, *130*, 2855-2865.

[14] Mazière, C; Meignotte, A; Dantin, F; Conte, Ma; Maziére, Jc . Oxidized Ldl Induces An Oxidative Stress And Activates The Tumor Suppressor P53 In Mrc5 Human Fibroblasts. *Biochemical And Biophysical Research Communications* 2000, *276*, 718-723.

[15] Bougnoux, P . N-3 Polyunsaturated Fatty Acids And Cancer. *Curr.Opin.Nutr.Metab.Care* 1999, *2*, 121-126.

[16] Herrera, E; Barbas, C . Vitamin E: Action, Metabolism And Perspectives. *J.Physiol.Biochem.* 2001, *57*, 43-56.

[17] Woollett, La . The Origins And Roles Of Cholesterol And Fatty Acids In The Fetus. *Current Opinion In Lipidology* 2001, *12*, 305-312.

[18] Claycombe, Kj; Meydani, Sn . Vitamin E And Genome Stability. *Mutation Research: Fundamental And Molecular Mechanisms Of Mutagenesis* 2001, *475*, 37-44.

[19] Mashima, R; Witting, Pk; Stocker, R . Oxidants And Antioxidants In Atherosclerosis. *Current Opinion In Lipidology* 2001, *12*, 411-418.

[20] Herrera, E; Ortega-Senovilla, H . Maternal Lipid Metabolism During Normal Pregnancy And Its Implications To Fetal Development. *Clin.Lipidol.* 2010, *5*, 899-911.

[21] Herrera, E.; Ortega, H. Hyperlipidemia And Vitamin E Metabolism In Pregnancy, In *Antioxidants: New Research*, Panglossi, H. V., Editor; Nova Science Publishers, Inc.: 2006; Chapter 5, Pp. 111-130.

[22] Koletzko, B; Lien, E; Agotini, C; Böles, H; Campoy, C; Cetin, I; Decsi, T; Dudenhausen, Jw; Dupont, C; Forsyth, S; Hoesli, I; Holzgreve, W; Lapillonne, A; Putet, G; Secher, Nj; Symonds, M; Szajewska, H; Willatts, P; Uauy, R . The Roles Of Long-Chain Polyunsaturted Fatty Acids In Pregnancy, Lactation And Infancy: Review Of Current Knowledge And Consensus Recommendatios. *J.Perinat.Med.* 2008, *36*, 5-14.

[23] Muhlhausler, Bs; Gibson, Ra; Makrides, M . Effect Of Long-Chain Polyunsaturated Fatty Acid Supplementation During Pregnancy Or Lactation On Infant And Child Body Composition: A Systematic Review. *Am.J.Clin.Nutr.* 2010, *92*, 857-863.

[24] Sampath, H; Ntambi, Jm . Polyunsaturted Fatty Acid Regulation Of Genes Of Lipid Metabolism. *Annual Review Of Nutrition* 2005, *25*, 317-340.

[25] Holloway, Pw; Peluffo, R; Wakil, Sj . On The Biosynthesis Of Dienoic Fatty Acid By Animal Tissues. *Biochem.Biophys.Res.Commun.* 1963, *12*, 300-304.

[26] Brenner, Rr . The Oxidative Desaturation Of Unsaturated Fatty Acids In Animals. *Molecular And Cellular Biochemistry* 1974, *3*, 41-52.

[27] Cook, H. W. Fatty Acid Desaturation And Chain Elongation In Eucaryotes, In *Biochemistry Of Lipids, Lipoproteins And Membranes*, Vance, D. E.; Vance, J., Editors; Elsevier: Amsterdam, The Netherlands, 1991; Vol. 20, Pp. 141-169.

[28] Sprecher, H . Metabolism Of Highly Unsaturated *N*-3 And *N*-6 Fatty Acids. *Biochimica Et Biophysica Acta: Molecular And Cell Biology Of Lipids* 2000, *1486*, 219-231.

[29] De Renobales, M; Cripps, C; Stanley-Samuelson, Dw; Jurenka, Ra; Blomquist, Gj . Biosynthesis Of Linoleic Acid In Insects. *Trends In Biochemical Sciences* 1987, *12*, 364-366.

[30] Seubert, W; Podack, Er . Mechanisms And Physiological Roles Of Fatty Acid Elongation In Microsomes And Mitochondria. *Molecular And Cellular Biochemistry* 1973, *1*, 29-40.

[31] Cho, Hp; Nakamura, Mt; Clarke, Sd . Cloning, Expression, And Nutritional Regulation Of The Mammalian D-6 Desaturase. *Journal Of Biological Chemistry* 1999, *274*, 471-477.

[32] Aki, T; Shimada, Y; Inagaki, K; Higashimoto, H; Kawammoto, S; Shigeta, S; Ono, K; Suzuki, O . Molecular Cloning And Functional Characterization Of Rat Delta-6 Fatty Acid Desaturase. *Biochemical And Biophysical Research Communications* 1999, *255*, 575-579.

[33] Moore, Sa; Hurt, E; Yoder, E; Sprecher, H; Spector, Aa . Docosahexaenoic Acid Synthesis In Human Skin Fibroblasts Involves Peroxisomal Retroconversion Of Tetracosahexaenoic Acid. *Journal Of Lipid Research* 1995, *36*, 2433-2443.

[34] Sprecher, H; Luthria, D; Mohammed, Bs; Baykousheva, Sp . Reevaluation Of The Pathway For The Biosynthesis Of Polyunsaturated Fatty Acids. *Journal Of Lipid Research* 1995, *36*, 2471-2477.

[35] Voss, A; Reinhart, M; Sankarappa, S; Sprecher, H . The Metabolism Of 7,10,13,16,19-Docosapentaenoic Acid To 4,7,10,16,19-Docosahexaenoic Acid In Rat Liver Is Independent Of A 4-Desaturase. *Journal Of Biological Chemistry* 1991, *266*, 19995-20000.

[36] Capriotti, Am; Furth, Ee; Arrasmith, Me; Laposata, M . Arachidonate Released Upon Agonist Stimulation Preferentially Originates From Arachidonate Most Recently Incorporated Into Nuclear Membrane Phospholipids. *Journal Of Biological Chemistry* 1988, *263*, 10029-10034.

[37] Laposata, M . Fatty Acids: Biochemistry To Clinical Significance. *Am.J.Clin.Pathol.* 1995, *104*, 172-179.

[38] Brenner, Rr . Endocrine Control Of Fatty Acid Desaturation. *Biochemical Society Transactions* 1990, *18*, 773-775.

[39] Jeffcoat, R . The Biosynthesis Of Unsaturated Fatty Acids And Its Control In Mammalian Liver. *Essays Biochem.* 1979, *15*, 1-36.

[40] Cook, Hw; Spence, Mw . Formation Of Monoenoic Fatty Acids By Desaturation In Rat Brain Homogenate. Effect Of Age, Fasting And Refeeding And Comparisons With Liver Enzyme. *Journal Of Biological Chemistry* 1973, *248*, 1793-1796.

[41] Cook, Hw . In Vitro Formation Of Polyunsaturated Fatty Acids By Desaturation In Rat Brain: Some Properties Of The Enzymes. *Journal Of Neurochemistry* 1978, *30*, 1327-1334.

[42] Sprecher, H . Biochemistry Of Essential Fatty Acids. *Progress In Lipid Research* 1981, *20.*, 13-22.

[43] Calder, Pc . Omega-3 Fatty Acids And Inflammatory Processes. *Nutrients* 2010, *2*, 355-374.

[44] Whelan, J . Antagonistic Effects Of Dietary Arachidonic Acid And N-3 Polyunsaturated Fatty Acids. *Journal Of Nutrition* 1996, *126*, 1086s-1091s.

[45] Calder, Pc . N-3 Polyunsaturated Fatty Acids And Cytokine Production In Health And Disease. *Annals Of Nutrition And Metabolism* 1997, *41*, 203-234.

[46] Serhan, Cn; Chiang, N; Van Dyke, Te . Resolving Inflammation: Dual Anti-Inflammatory And Pro-Resolution Lipid Mediators. *Nature Rev.Immunol.* 2008, *8*, 349-361.

[47] Clarke, Sd . Polyunsaturated Fatty Acid Regulation Of Gene Transcription: A Molecular Mechanism To Improve The Metabolic Syndrome. *Journal Of Nutrition* 2002, *132*, 1129-1132.

[48] Jump, Db . Dietary Polyunsaturated Fatty Acids And Regulation Of Gene Transcription. *Current Opinion In Lipidology* 2002, *13*, 155-164.

[49] Deckelbaum, Rj; Worgall, Ts; Seo, T . N-3 Fatty Acids And Gene Expression. *American Journal Of Clinical Nutrition* 2006, *83*, 1520s-1525s.

[50] Yang, T; Espenshade, Pj; Wright, Me; Yabe, D; Gong, Y; Aeberson, R; D'agostino, Rb; Goldstein, Jl; Brown, Ms . Crucial Step In Cholesterol Homeostasis: Sterols Promote Binding Of Scap To Nsig-1, A Membrane Protein That Facilitates Retention Of Srebps In Er. *Cell* 2002, *110*, 489-500.

[51] Adams, Cm; Reitz, J; De Brabander, Jk; Feramisco, Jd; Li, L; Brown, Ms; Goldstein, Jl . Cholesterol And 25-Hydroxycholesterol Inhibit Activation Of Srebps By Different Mechanisms, Both Involving Scap And Insigs. *Journal Of Biological Chemistry* 2004, *279*, 52772-52780.

[52] Worgall, Ts; Sturley, Sl; Seo, T; Osborne, Tf; Deckelbaum, Rj . Polyunsaturated Fatty Acids Decrease Expression Of Promoters With Sterol Regulatory Elements By Decreasing Levels Of Mature Sterol Regulatory Element-Binding Protein. *Journal Of Biological Chemistry* 1998, *273*, 25537-25540.

[53] Hannah, Vc; Ou, Jf; Luong, A; Goldstein, Jl; Brown, Ms . Unsaturated Fatty Acids Down-Regulate Srebp Isoforms 1a And 1c By Two Mechanisms In Hek-293 Cells. *Journal Of Biological Chemistry* 2001, *276*, 4365-4372.

[54] González, M. C.; Panadero, M. I.; Herrera, E.; Bocos, C. Ppara As Target For Pharmacological And Nutritional Agents Affecting Lipid Metabolism, In *New Emerging Pharmacological Targets In Metabolic Diseases*, Vázquez-Carrera, M., Editor; Transworld Research Network: Kerala, 2007; Pp. 1-48.

[55] Panadero, Mi; González, Mc; Herrera, E; Bocos, C . Factors Modulating Fibrates Response: Therapeutic Implications And Alternative Strategies. *Endocr., Metab.& Immun.Disorders-Drug Targets* 2009, *9*, 219-236.

[56] Bell-Parikh, Lc; Ide, T; Lawson, Ja; Mcnamara, P; Reilly, M; Fitzgerald, Ga . Biosynthesis Of 15-Deoxy-Delta12,14-Pgj2 And The Ligation Of Ppargamma. *Journal Of Clinical Investigation* 2003, *112*, 945-955.

[57] Ide, T; Egan, K; Bell-Parikh, Lc; Fitzgerald, Ga . Activation Of Nuclear Receptors By Prostaglandins. *Thromb.Res.* 2003, *110*, 311-315.

[58] Mishra, A; Chaudhary, A; Sethi, S . Oxidized N-3 Fatty Acids Inhibit Nf-Kappab Activation Via A Pparalpha-Dependent Patway. *Arteriosclerosis, Thrombosis, And Vascular Biology* 2004, *24*, 1621-1627.

[59] Hostetler, Ha; Petrescu, Ad; Kier, Ab; Schoeder, F . Peroxisome Proliferator Activated Receptor Alpha Interacts With High Affinity And Is Conformationally Responsive To Endogenous Ligands. *J.Biol.Chem* 2005, *280*, 18667-18682.

[60] Howell Iii, G; Deng, X; Yellaturu, C; Park, Ea; Wilcox, Hg; Raghow, R; Elam, Mb . N-3 Polyunsaturated Fatty Acids Suppress Insulin-Induced Srebp-1c Transcription Via Reduced Trans-Activating Capacity Of Lxra. *Biochim.Biophys.Acta* 2009, *1791*, 1190-1196.

[61] Ide, T; Shimano, H; Yoshikawa, T; Yahagi, N; Amemiya-Kudo, M; Matsuzaka, T; Nakakuki, M; Yatoh, S; Iizuka, Y; Tomita, S; Ohashi, K; Takahashi, A; Sone, H; Gotoda, T; Osuga, J; Ishibashi, S; Yamada, N . Cross-Talk Between Peroxisome Proliferator-Activated Receptor (Ppar) A And Liver X Receptor (Lxr) In Nutritional Regulation Of Fatty Acid Metabolism. Ii. Lxrs Suppress Lipid Degradation Gene Promoters Through Inhibition Of Ppar Signaling. *Molecular Endocrinology* 2003, *17*, 1255-1267.

[62] Yoshikawa, T; Ide, T; Shimano, H; Yahagi, N; Amemiya-Kudo, M; Matsuzaka, T; Yatoh, S; Kitamine, T; Okazaki, H; Tamura, Y; Sekiya, M; Takahashi, A; Hasty, Ah; Sato, R; Sone, H; Osuga, J; Ishibashi, S; Yamada, N . Cross-Talk Between Peroxisome Proliferator-Activated Receptor (Ppar) A And Liver X Receptor (Lxr) In Nutritional Regulation Of Fatty Acid Metabolism. I. Ppars Supress Sterol Regulatory Element Binding Protein-1c Promoter Through Inhibition Of Lxr Signaling. *Molecular Endocrinology* 2003, *17*, 1240-1254.

[63] Panadero, M; Vidal, H; Herrera, E; Bocos, C . Nutritionally Induced Changes In The Peroxisome Proliferator-Activated Receptor-A Gene Expression In Liver Of Suckling Rats Are Dependent On Insulinaemia. *Archives Of Biochemistry And Biophysics* 2001, *394*, 182-188.

[64] Panadero, M; Herrera, E; Bocos, C . Different Sensitivity Of Ppar-A Gene Expression To Nutritional Changes In Liver Of Suckling And Adult Rats. *Life Sciences* 2005, *76*, 1061-1072.

[65] Panadero, M; Bocos, C; Herrera, E . Relationship Between Lipoprotein Lipase And Peroxisome Proliferator-Activated Receptor-A Expression In Rat Liver During Development. *J.Physiol.Biochem.* 2006, *62*, 189-198.

[66] Cho, S-Y; Miyashita, K; Miyazawa, T; Fujimoto, K; Kaneda, T . Autoxidation Of Ethyl Eicosapentaenoate And Docosahexaenoate. *Journal Of The American Oil Chemists' Society* 1987, *64*, 876-879.

[67] Mead, J. F.; Alfin-Slater, R. B.; Howton, D. R.; Popják, G. The Amphipathic Lipids, In *Lipids: Chemistry, Biochemistry And Nutrition*, Plenum Press: New York, 1986; Pp. 369-404.

[68] Privett, Os; Blank, Ml . The Initial Stages Of Autoxidation. *Journal Of The American Oil Chemists' Society* 1962, *39*, 465-469.

[69] Rawls, Hr; Van Santen, Pj . A Possible Role For Singlet Oxygen In The Initiation Of Fatty Acid Autoxidation. *Journal Of The American Oil Chemists' Society* 1970, *47*, 121-125.

[70] Marnett, Lj; Wilcox, Al . The Chemistry Of Lipid Alkoxyl Radicals And Their Role In Metal-Amplified Lipid Peroxidation. *Biochem.Soc.Symp.* 1995, *61*, 65-72.

[71] Pryor, Wa . Free Radicals And Their Importance In Biochemical Systems. *Fed.Proc.* 1973, *32*, 1862-1869.

[72] Esterbauer, H. The Chemistry Of Oxidation Of Lipoproteins, In *Oxidative Stress, Lipoproteins And Cardiovascular Dysfunction*, Rice-Evans, C.; Bruckdorfer, K. R., Editors; Portland Press: London, 1995; Chapter 3, Pp. 55-79.

[73] Barber, Aa; Bernheim, F . Lipid Peroxidation: Its Measurement, Occurrence And Significance In Animal Tissues. *Advanc.Gerontol.Res.* 1967, *2*, 355-403.

[74] Fong, Kl; Mccay, P; Poyer, Jl; Keele, Bb; Misra, H . Evidence That Lipid Peroxidation Of Lysosomal Membranes Is Initiated By Hydroxyl Free Radicals Produced During Flavin Enzyme Activity. *Journal Of Biological Chemistry* 1973, *248*, 7792-7797.

[75] Pryor, Wa; Stanley, Jp; Blair, F . Autoxidation Of Polyunsaturated Fatty Acids: Ii. A Suggested Mechanism For The Formation Of Tba-Reactive Materials From Prostaglandin-Like Endoperoxides. *Lipids* 1976, *11*, 370-379.

[76] Kowaltowski, Aj; Castilho, Rf; Vercesi, Ae . Mitochondrial Permeability Transition And Oxidative Stress. *Febs Letters* 2001, *495*, 12-15.

[77] Logani, Mk; Davies, Re . Lipid Oxidation: Biologic Effects And Antioxidants-A Review. *Lipids* 1980, *15*, 485-495.

[78] Tappel, Al . Lipid Peroxidation Damage To Cell Components. *Fed.Proc.* 1973, *32*, 1870-1874.

[79] Song, Jh; Inoue, Y; Miyazawa, T . Oxidative Stability Of Docosahexaenoic Acid-Containing Oils In The Form Of Phospholipids, Triacylglycerols, And Ethyl Esters. *Biosci.Biotechnol.Biochem.* 1997, *61*, 2085-2088.

[80] Song, Jh; Fujimoto, K; Miyazawa, T . Polyunsaturated (N-3) Fatty Acids Susceptible To Peroxidation Are Increased In Plasma And Tissue Lipids Of Rats Fed Docosahexaenoic Acid-Containing Oils. *Journal Of Nutrition* 2000, *130*, 3028-3033.

[81] Leibowitz, Be; Hu, M-L; Tappel, Al . Lipid Peroxidation In Rat Tissue Slices: Effect Of Dietary Vitamin E, Corn Oil-Lard And Menhaden Oil. *Lipids* 1990, *25*, 125-129.

[82] Halliwell, B . Antioxidants And Human Disease: A General Introduction. *Nutr.Rev.* 1997, *55*, S44-S49.

[83] Keyse, S. M. *Stress Response: Methods And Protocols;* Humana Press: Totowa,Nj, 2000; Vol. 99.

[84] Ogino, T.; Packer, L.; Traber, M. C. Oxidant Stress And Host Oxidant Defense Mechanisms, In *Nutritional Oncology*, Heber, D.; Blackburn, G. L.; Go, V. L. W., Editors; Academic Press: San Diego, Ca, 1999; Pp. 253-275.

[85] Haffner, Sm . Clinical Relevance Of The Oxidative Stress Concept. *Metabolism: Clinical And Experimental* 2000, *49*, 30-34.

[86] Morgan, Mj; Liu, Z . Crosstalk Of Reactive Oxygen Species And Nf-Kb Signaling. *Cell Res.* 2011, *21*, 103-115.

[87] Scandalios, J. G. *Oxidative Stress And The Molecular Biology Of Antioxidant Defenses;* Plainview,Ny, 1997.

[88] Özben, T. *Free Radicals, Oxidative Stress, And Antioxidants: Pathological Significance;* Plenum Press: New York, 1998.

[89] Fridovich, I . The Biology Of Oxygen Radicals. *Science* 1978, *201*, 875-880.

[90] Ogura, Y; Yamazaki, I . Steady-State Kinetics Of The Catalase Reaction In The Presence Of Cyanide. *J.Biochem.* 1983, *94*, 403-408.

[91] Cohen, G; Hochstein, P . Glutathione Peroxidase: The Major Pathway Of Peroxide Detoxication In Erytrocytes. *Biochemistry* 1963, *2*, 1420-1428.

[92] Bhabak, Kp; Mugesh, G . Functional Mimics Of Glutathione Peroxidase: Bioinpired Synthetic Antioxidants. *Acc.Chem.Res.* 2010, *43*, 1408-1419.

[93] Halliwell, B . How To Characterize A Biological Antioxidant. *Free Rad.Res.Comm.* 1990, *9*, 1-32.

[94] Rice-Evans, C. Free Radicals And Antioxidants In Normal And Pathological Processes, In *Oxidative Stress, Lipoproteins And Cardiovascular Dysfunction*, Rice-Evans, C.; Bruckdorfer, K. R., Editors; Portland Press: London, 1995; Chapter 1, Pp. 1-32.

[95] Tulipani, S; Romandini, S; Busco, F; Bompadre, S; Mezzetti, B; Battino, M . Ascorbate, Not Urate, Modulates The Plasma Antioxidant Capacity After Strawberry Intake. *Food Chemistr.* 2009, *117*, 181-188.

[96] Packer, L; Weber, Su; Rimbach, G . Molecular Aspects Of A-Tocotrienol Antioxidant Action And Cell Signalling. *Journal Of Nutrition* 2001, *131*, 369s-373s.

[97] Thomas, Sr; Stocker, R . Molecular Action Of Vitamin E In Lipoprotein Oxidation: Implications For Atherosclerosis. *Free Radical Biology And Medicine* 2000, *28*, 1795-1805.

[98] Stocker, R . The Ambivalence Of Vitamin E In Atherogenesis. *Trends In Biochemical Sciences* 1999, *24*, 219-223.

[99] Kontush, A; Finckh, B; Karten, B; Kohlschütter, A; Beisiegel, U . Antioxidant And Prooxidant Activity Of A-Tocopherol In Human Plasma And Low Density Lipoprotein. *Journal Of Lipid Research* 1996, *37*, 1436-1448.

[100] Steinberg, D . Is There A Potential Therapeutic Role For Vitamin E Or Other Antioxidants In Atherosclerosis? *Current Opinion In Lipidology* 2000, *11*, 603-607.

[101] Jialal, I; Traber, M; Devaraj, S . Is There A Vitamin E Paradox? *Current Opinion In Lipidology* 2001, *12*, 49-53.

[102] Uotila, Jt; Tuimala, Rj; Aarnio, Tm; Pyykkö, Ka; Ahotupa, Mo . Findings On Lipid Peroxidation And Antioxidant Function In Hypertensive Complications Of Pregnancy. *Br.J.Obstet.Gynaecol.* 1993, *100*, 270-276.

[103] Carone, D; Loverro, G; Greco, P; Capuano, F; Selvaggi, L . Lipid Peroxidation Products And Antioxidant Enzymes In Red Blood Cells During Normal And Diabetic Pregnancy. *European Journal Of Obstetrics, Gynecology And Reproductive Biology* 1993, *51*, 103-109.

[104] Morris, Jm; Gopaul, Nk; Endresen, Mjr; Knight, M; Linton, Ea; Dhir, S; Änggård, Ee; Redman, Cwg . Circulating Markers Of Oxidative Stress Are Raised In Normal Pregnancy And Pre-Eclampsia. *British Journal Of Obstetrics And Gynaecology* 1998, *105*, 1195-1199.

[105] Uotila, Jt; Tuimala, R; Aarnio, T; Pyykko.K.; Ahotupa, M . Lipid Peroxidation Products, Selenium-Dependent Glutathione Peroxidase And Vitamin E In Normal Pregnancy. *European Journal Of Obstetrics, Gynecology And Reproductive Biology* 1991, *42*, 95-100.

[106] Wang, Yp; Walsh, Sw; Guo, Jd; Zhang, Jy . Maternal Levels Of Prostacyclin, Thromboxane, Vitamin E, And Lipid Peroxides Throughout Normal Pregnancy. *American Journal Of Obstetrics And Gynecology* 1991, *165*, 1690-1694.

[107] De Vriese, Sr; Dhont, M; Christophe, Ab . Oxidative Stability Of Low Density Lipoproteins And Vitamin E Levels Increase In Maternal Blood During Normal Pregnancy. *Lipids* 2001, *36*, 361-366.

[108] Oostenbrug, Gs; Mensink, Rp; Al, Mdm; Van Houwelingen, Ac; Hornstra, G . Maternal And Neonatal Plasma Antioxidant Levels In Normal Pregnancy, And The Relationship With Fatty Acid Unsaturation. *British Journal Of Nutrition* 1998, *80*, 67-73.

[109] Clandinin, Mt; Chappell, Je; Leong, S; Heim, T; Swyer, Pr; Chance, Gw . Intrauterine Fatty Acid Accretion Rates In Human Brain: Implications For Fatty Acid Requirements. *Early Human Development* 1980, *4*, 121-129.

[110] Foreman-Van Drongelen, Mmhp; Van Houwelingen, Ac; Kester, Adm; Hasaart, Thm; Blanco, Ce; Hornstra, G . Long-Chain Polyunsaturated Fatty Acids In Preterm Infants: Status At Birth And Its Influence On Postnatal Levels. *Journal Of Pediatrics* 1995, *126*, 611-618.

[111] Leaf, Aa; Leightfield, Mj; Casteloe, Kl; Crawford, Ma . Long-Chain Polyunsaturated Fatty Acids And Fetal Growth. *Early Human Development* 1992, *30*, 183-191.

[112] Neuringer, M; Connor, We . Omega-3 Fatty Acids In The Brain And Retina: Evidence Of Their Essentiality. *Nutrition Reviews* 1986, *44*, 285-294.

[113] Demmelmair, H;, Ru; Behrendt, E; Sauerwald, T; Koletzko, B . Estimation Of Arachidonic Acid Synthesis In Full Term Neonates Using Natural Variation Of ^{13}c-Abundance. *J.Pediatr.Gastroent.Nutr.* 1995, *21*, 31-36.

[114] Salem, N, Jr.; Wegher, B; Mena, P; Uauy, R . Arachidonic And Docosahexaenoic Acids Are Biosynthesized From Their 18-Carbon Precursors In Human Infants. *Proceedings Of The National Academy Of Sciences Of The United States Of America* 1996, *93*, 49-54.

[115] Carnielli, Vp; Wattimena, Dh; Luijendijk, Iht; Boerlage, A; Degenhart, Hj; Sauer, Pjj . The Very Low Birth Weight Premature Infant Is Capable Of Synthesizing Arachidonic And Docosahexaenoic Acid From Linoleic And Linolenic Acid. *Pediatric Research* 1996, *40*, 169-174.

[116] Szitanyi, P; Koletzko, B; Mydlilova, A; Demmelmair, H . Metabolism Of ^{13}c-Labeled Linoleic Acid In Newborn Infants During The First Week Of Life. *Pediatric Research* 1999, *45*, 669-673.

[117] Uauy, R; Mena, P; Wegher, B; Nieto, S; Salem, N, Jr. Long Chain Polyunsaturated Fatty Acid Formation In Neonates: Effect Of Gestational Age And Intrauterine Growth. *Pediatric Research* 2000, *47*, 127-135.

[118] Su, Hm; Corso, Tn; Nathanielsz, Pw; Brenna, Jt . Linoleic Acid Kinetics And Conversion To Arachidonic Acid In The Pregnant And Fetal Baboon. *Journal Of Lipid Research* 1999, *40*, 1304-1311.

[119] Su, Hm; Huang, Mc; Saad, Nmr; Nathanielsz, Pw; Brenna, Jt . Fetal Baboons Convert 18:3n-3 To 22:6n-3 In Vivo: A Stable Isotope Tracer Study. *Journal Of Lipid Research* 2001, *42*, 581-586.

[120] Haggarty, P . Effect Of Placental Function On Fatty Acid Requirements During Pregnancy. *European Journal Of Clinical Nutrition* 2004, *58*, 1559-1570.

[121] Jumpsen, J.; Van Aerde, J.; Clandinin, M. T. Fetal Lipid Requirements: Implications In Fetal Growth Retardation, In *Placental Function And Fetal Nutrition*, Battaglia, F. C., Editor; Nesttec Ltd., Vevey/Lippincott-Raven Publ.: Philadelphia, 1997; Vol. 9, Pp. 157-165.

[122] Al, Mdm; Hornstra, G; Van Der Schouw, Yt; Bulstra-Ramakers, Mtew; Huisjes, Hj . Biochemical Efa Status Of Mothers And Their Neonates After Normal Pregnancy. *Early Human Development* 1990, *24*, 239-248.

[123] Matorras, R; Perteagudo, L; Sanjurjo, P; Ruiz, Ji . Intake Of Long Chain ω3 Polyunsaturated Fatty Acids During Pregnancy And The Influence Of Levels In The Mother On Newborn Levels. *European Journal Of Obstetrics, Gynecology And Reproductive Biology* 1999, *83*, 179-184.

[124] Crastes De Paulet, P.; Sarda, P.; Boulot, P.; Crastes De Paulet, A. Fatty Acids Blood Composition In Foetal And Maternal Plasma, In *Essential Fatty Acids And Infant Nutrition*, Ghisolfi, J.; Putet, G., Editors; John Libbey Eurotext: Paris, 1992; Chapter 7, Pp. 65-77.

[125] Herrera, E; Amusquivar, E . Lipid Metabolism In The Fetus And The Newborn. *Diabetes Metab.Res.Rev.* 2000, *16*, 202-210.

[126] Connor, We; Lowensohn, R; Hatcher, L . Increased Docosahexaenoic Acid Levels In Human Newborn Infants By Administration Of Sardines And Fish Oil During Pregnancy. *Lipids* 1996, *31*, S183-S187.

[127] Van Houwelingen, Ac; Sorensen, Jd; Hornstra, G; Simonis, Mmg; Boris, J; Olsen, Sf; Secher, Nj . Essential Fatty Acid Status In Neonates After Fish-Oil Supplementation During Late Pregnancy. *British Journal Of Nutrition* 1995, *74*, 723-731.

[128] Warstdt, K; Furuhjelm, C; Duchén, K; Falth-Magnusson, K; Fageras, M . The Effects Of Omega-3 Fatty Acid Supplementation In Pregnancy On Maternal Eicosanoid, Cytokine, And Chemokine Secretion. *Pediatric Res.* 2009, *66*, 212-217.

[129] Brenner, Rr; Peluffo, Ro . Regulation Of Unsaturated Fatty Acid Biosynthesis. *Biochim.Biophys.Acta* 1969, *176*, 471-479.

[130] Simopoulos, Ap . W-3 Fatty Acids In Health And Disease And In Growth And Development. *American Journal Of Clinical Nutrition* 1991, *54*, 438-463.

[131] Willis, A. L. Essential Fatty Acids, Prostaglandins And Related Eicosanoids, In *Present Knowledge In Nutrition*, Olson, R. E., Editor; The Nutrition Foundation: Washington,D.C., 1984; Pp. 90-113.

[132] Raz, A; Kamin-Belsky, N; Przedecki, F; Obukowicz, Mg . Fish Oil Inhibits Delta 6 Desaturase Activity In Vivo: Utility In A Dietary Paradigm To Obtain Mice Deplected Of Arachidonic Acid. *J.Nutr.Biochem.* 1997, *8*, 558-565.

[133] Garg, Ml; Thomson, Abr; Clandinin, Mt . Interactions Of Saturated, N-6 And N-3 Polyunsaturated Fatty Acids To Modulate Arachidonic Acid Metabolism. *Journal Of Lipid Research* 1990, *31*, 271-277.

[134] Christiansen, En; Lund, Js; Rortveit, T; Rustan, Ac . Effect Of Dietary N-3 And N-6 Fatty Acids On Fatty Acid Desaturation In Rat Liver. *Biochim.Biophys.Acta* 1991, *1082*, 57-62.

[135] Leaf, Aa; Leighfield, Mj; Costeloe, Kl; Crawford, Ma . Factors Affecting Long-Chain Polyunsaturated Fatty Acid Composition Of Plasma Choline Phosphoglycerides In Preterm Infants. *J.Pediatr.Gastroent.Nutr.* 1992, *14*, 300-308.

[136] Woltil, Ha; Van Beusekom, Cm; Schaafsma, A; Muskiet, Faj; Okken, A . Long-Chain Polyunsaturated Fatty Acid Status And Early Growth Of Low Birth Weight Infants. *European Journal Of Pediatrics* 1998, *157*, 146-152.

[137] Carlson, Se; Cooke, Rj; Rhodes, Pg; Peeples, Jm; Werkman, Sh; Tolley, Ea . Long-Term Feeding Of Formulas High In Linolenic Acid And Marine Oil To Very Low Birth Weight Infants: Phospholipid Fatty Acids. *Pediatr.Res.* 1991, *30*, 404-412.

[138] Carlson, Se; Werkman, Sh; Pepples, Jm . Arachidonic Acid Status Correlates With First Year Growth In Preterm Infants. *Proceedings Of The National Academy Of Sciences Of The United States Of America* 1993, *90*, 1073-1077.

[139] Koletzko, B; Braun, M . Arachidonic Acid And Early Human Growth: Is There A Relation? *Annals Of Nutrition And Metabolism* 1991, *35*, 128-131.

[140] Esterbauer, H . Cytotoxicity And Genotoxicity Of Lipid-Oxidation Products. *American Journal Of Clinical Nutrition* 1993, *57 Suppl.*, 779s-786s.

[141] Berry, Em; Eisenberg, S; Haratz, D; Friedlander, Y; Norman, Y; Kaufman, Na; Stein, Y . Effects Of Diets Rich In Monounsaturated Fatty Acids On Plasma Lipoproteins - The Jerusalen Nutrition Study: High Mufas Vs High Pufas. *American Journal Of Clinical Nutrition* 1991, *53*, 899-907.

[142] Halliwell, B; Chirico, S . Lipid Peroxidation: Its Mechanism, Measurement, And Significance. *American Journal Of Clinical Nutrition* 1993, *57 Suppl.*, 715s-725s.

[143] Mazière, C; Dantin, F; Conte, Ma; Degonville, J; Ali, D; Dubois, F; Mazière, Jc . Polyunsaturated Fatty Acid Enrichment Enhances Endothelial Cell-Induced Low-Density-Lipoprotein Peroxidation. *Biochemical Journal* 1998, *336*, 57-62.

[144] Haegele, Ad; Briggs, Sp; Thompson, Hj . Antioxidant Status And Dietary Lipid Unsaturation Modulate Oxidative Dna Damage. *Free Radical Biology And Medicine* 1994, *16*, 111-115.

[145] Viana, M; Herrera, E; Bonet, B . Teratogenic Effects Of Diabetes Mellitus In The Rat. Prevention By Vitamin E. *Diabetologia* 1996, *39*, 1041-1046.

[146] Simán, Cm; Eriksson, Uj . Vitamin E Decreases The Occurrence Of Malformations In The Offspring Of Diabetic Rats. *Diabetes* 1997, *46*, 1054-1061.

[147] Reece, Ea; Wu, Yk . Prevention Of Diabetic Embryopathy In Offspring Of Diabetic Rats With Use Of A Cocktail Of Deficient Substrates And An Antioxidant. *American Journal Of Obstetrics And Gynecology* 1997, *176*, 790-797.

[148] Wentzel, P; Welsh, N; Eriksson, Uj . Developmental Damage, Increased Lipid Peroxidation, Diminished Cyclooxygenase-2 Gene Expression, And Lower Pge2 Levels In Rat Embryos Exposed To A Diabetic Environment. *Diabetes* 1999, *48*, 813-820.

[149] Viana, M; Aruoma, Oi; Herrera, E; Bonet, B . Oxidative Damage In Pregnant Diabetic Rats And Their Embryos. *Free Radicals Biology And Medicine* 2000, *29*, 1115-1121.

[150] Cederberg, J; Eriksson, Uj . Increased Rate Of Lipid Peroxidation And Protein Carbonylation In Experimental Diabetic Pregnancy. *Diabetologia* 2001, *44*, 766-774.

[151] Eriksson, Uj; Borg, Lah . Protection By Free Oxygen Radical Scavenging Enzymes Against Glucose-Induced Embryonic Malformations In Vitro. *Diabetologia* 1991, *34*, 325-331.

[152] Jain, Sk . Should High-Dose Vitamin E Supplementation Be Recommended To Diabetic Patients. *Diabetes Care* 1999, *22*, 1242-1244.

[153] Ludvigsson, J; Samuelsson, U; Johansson, C; Stenhammar, L . Treatment With Antioxidants At Onset Of Type 1 Diabetes In Chilcren: A Randomized, Double-Blind Placebo-Controlled Study. *Diabetes Metab.Res.Rev.* 2001, *17*, 131-136.

[154] Reece, Ea; Wu, Yk; Wiznitzer, A; Homko, C; Yao, J; Borenstein, M; Sloskey, G . Dietary Polyunsaturated Fatty Acid Prevents Malformations In Offspring Of Diabetic Rats. *American Journal Of Obstetrics And Gynecology* 1996, *175*, 818-823.

[155] Kuhn, Dc; Crawford, Ma; Stuart, Mj; Botti, Jj; Demers, Lm . Alterations In Transfer And Lipid Distribution Of Arachidonic Acid In Placentas Of Diabetic Pregnancies. *Diabetes* 1990, *39*, 914-918.

[156] Bitsanis, D; Ghebremeskel, K; Moodley, T; Crawford, Ma; Djahanbakhch, O . Gestational Diabetes Mellitus Enhances Arachidonic And Docosahexaenoic Acids In Placental Phospholipids. *Lipids* 2006, *41*, 341-346.

[157] Thomas, B; Ghebremeskel, K; Lowy, C; Offley-Shore, B; Crawford, Ma . Plasma Fatty Acids Of Neonates Born To Mothers With And Without Gestational Diabetes. *Prostaglandins, Leukotrienes And Essential Fatty Acids* 2005, *72*, 335-341.

[158] Ortega-Senovilla, H; Alvino, G; Taricco, E; Cetin, I; Herrera, E . Gestational Diabetes Mellitus Upsets The Proportion Of Fatty Acids In Umbilical Arterial But Not Venous Plasma. *Diabetes Care* 2009, *32*, 120-122.

[159] Bourre, Jm; Bonneil, M; Dumont, O; Piciotti, M; Calaf, R; Portugal, H; Nalbone, G; Lafont, H . Effect Of Increasing Amounts Of Dietary Fish Oil On Brain And Liver Fatty Acid Composition. *Biochim.Biophys.Acta* 1990, *1043*, 149-152.

[160] Bourre, Jm; Bonneil, M; Dumont, O; Nalbone, G; Lafont, H . High Dietary Fish Oil Alters The Brain Polyunsaturated Fatty Acid Composition. *Biochim.Biophys.Acta* 1988, *960*, 458-461.

[161] Navarro, Md; Periago, Jl; Pita, Ml; Hortelano, P . The N-3 Polyunsaturated Fatty Acid Levels In Rat Tissue Lipids Increase In Response To Dietary Olive Oil Relative To Sunflower Oil. *Lipids* 1994, *29*, 845-849.

[162] Girón, Md; Mataix, Fj; Faus, Mj; Suárez, Md . Effect Of Long-Term Feeding Olive And Sunflower Oils On Fatty Acid Composition And Desaturation Activities Of Liver Microsomes. *Biochem.Internat.* 1989, *19*, 645-656.

[163] Periago, Jl; Suarez, Md; Pita, Ml . Effect Of Dietary Olive Oil, Corn Oil And Medium-Chain Triglycerides On The Lipid Composition Of Rat Red Blood Cell Membranes. *Journal Of Nutrition* 1990, *120*, 986-994.

[164] Rao, Cv; Zang, E; Reddy, B . Effect Of High Fat Corn Oil, Olive Oil And Fish Oil On Phospholipid Fatty Acid Composition In Male F344 Rats. *Lipids* 1993, *28*, 441-447.

[165] Scaccini, C; Nardini, M; D'aquino, M; Gentili, V; Di Felice, M; Tomassi, G . Effect Of Dietary Oils On Lipid Peroxidation And On Antioxidant Parameters Of Rat Plasma And Lipoprotein Fractions. *Journal Of Lipid Research* 1992, *33*, 627-633.

[166] Öztezcan, S; Toker, G; Uysal, M . The Susceptibility Of Plasma To Lipid Peroxidation In Rats Fed On Diets Supplemented With Olive Oil And Sunflower Seed Oil. *Biochem.Arch.* 1996, *12*, 13-18.

[167] Hytten, F. E.; Leitch, I. The Gross Composition Of The Components Of Weight Gain, In *The Physiology Of Human Pregnancy*, 2 Ed.; Hytten, F. E.; Leitch, I., Editors; Blackwell: Oxford, 1971; Chapter 12, Pp. 370-387.

[168] Hytten, F. E.; Leitch, I. The Physiology Of Human Pregnancy., Oxford Ed.; Blackwell Scientific: 1971.

[169] Knopp, Rh; Boroush, Ma; O'sullivan, Jb . Lipid Metabolism In Pregnancy. Ii. Postheparin Lipolytic Acitivity And Hypertriglyceridemia In The Pregnant Rat. *Metabolism* 1975, *24*, 481-493.

[170] López-Luna P.; Maier, I; Herrera, E . Carcass Ans Tissue Fat Content In The Pregnant Rat. *Biol Neonate* 1991, *60*, 29-38.

[171] Muñoz, C; López-Luna P.; Herrera, E . Glucose And Insulin Tolerance Tests In The Rat In Different Days Of Gestation. *Biol Neonate* 1995, *68*, 282-291.

[172] Sorenson, Rl; Brelje, Tc . Adaptation Of Islets Of Langerhans To Pregnancy: B-Cell Growth, Enhanced Insulin Secretion And The Role Of Lactogenic Hormones. *Horm Metab Res* 1997, *29*, 301-307.

[173] Ramos, P; Crespo-Solans, Md; Del Campo, S; Cacho, J; Herrera, E . Fat Accumulation In The Rat During Early Pregnancy Is Modulated By Enhanced Insulin Responsiveness. *Am J Physiol Endocrinol Metab* 2003, *285*, E318-E328.

[174] Murphy, Sp; Abrams, Bf . Changes In Energy Intakes During Pregnancy And Lactation In A National Sample Of Us Women. *Am J Public Health* 1993, *83*, 1161-1163.

[175] Herrera, E.; Lasunción, M. A.; Martín, A.; Zorzano, A. Carbohydrate-Lipid Interactions In Pregnancy, In *Perinatal Biochemistry*, Herrera, E.; Knopp, R. H., Editors; Crc Press: Boca Raton, 1992; Pp. 1-18.

[176] Braun, Jea; Severson, Dl . Regulation Of Synthesis, Processing And Translocation Of Lipoprotein Lipase. *Biochem J* 1992, *287*, 337-347.

[177] Lasunción, Ma; Herrera, E . Changes With Starvation In The Rat Of The Lipoprotein Lipase Activity And Hydrolysis Of Triacylglycerols From Triacylglycerol-Rich Lipoproteins In Adipose Tissue Preparations. *Biochem J* 1983, *210*, 639-643.

[178] Leaf, Da; Connor, We; Barstad, L; Sexton, G . Incorporation Of Dietary N-3 Fatty Acids Into The Fatty Acids Of Human Adipose Tissue And Plasma Lipid Classes. *Am J Clin Nutr* 1995, *62*, 68-73.

[179] Weber, N; Klein, E; Mukherjee, Kd . The Composition Of The Major Molecular Species Of Adipose Tissue Triacylglycerols Of Rats Reflects Those Of Dietary Rapeseed, Olive And Sunflower Oils. *J Nutr* 2002, *132*, 726-732.

[180] Amusquivar, E; Herrera, E . Influence Of Changes In Dietary Fatty Acids During Pregnancy On Placental And Fetal Fatty Acid Profile In The Rat. *Biol Neonate* 2003, *83*, 136-145.

[181] Herrera, E; Lasunción, Ma; Gómez-Coronado, D; Aranda, P; López-Luna P.; Maier, I . Role Of Lipoprotein Lipase Activity On Lipoprotein Metabolism And The Fate Of Circulating Triglycerides In Pregnancy. *Am J Obstet Gynecol* 1988, *158*, 1575-1583.

[182] Hamosh, M; Clary, Rt; Chernick, Ss; Scow, Ro . Lipoprotein Lipase Activity Of Adipose And Mammary Tissue And Plasma Triglyceride In Pregnant And Lactating Rats. *Biochim Biophys Acta* 1970, *210*, 473-482.

[183] Alvarez, Jj; Montelongo, A; Iglesias, A; Lasunción, Ma; Herrera, E . Longitudinal Study On Lipoprotein Profile, High Density Lipoprotein Subclass, And Postheparin Lipases During Gestation In Women. *Journal Of Lipid Research* 1996, *37*, 299-308.

[184] Knopp, Rh; Herrera, E; Freinkel, N . Carbohydrate Metabolism In Pregnancy.Viii. Metabolism Of Adipose Tissue Isolated From Fed And Fasted Pregnant Rats During Late Gestation. *Journal Of Clinical Investigation* 1970, *49*, 1438-1446.

[185] Williams, C; Coltart, Tm . Adipose Tissue Metabolism In Pregnancy: The Lipolytic Effect Of Human Placental Lactogen. *Br.J.Obstet.Gynaecol.* 1978, *85*, 43-46.

[186] Coltart, Tm; Williams, C . Effect Of Insulin On Adipose Tissue Lipolysis In Human Pregnancy. *Br.J.Obstet.Gynaecol.* 1976, *83*, 241-244.

[187] Ramos, P; Herrera, E . Reversion Of Insulin Resistance In The Rat During Late Pregnancy By 72-H Glucose Infusion. *Am J Physiol Endocrinol Metab* 1995, *269*, E858-E863.

[188] Herrera, E.; Lasunción, M. A. Maternal-Fetal Transfer Of Lipid Metabolites, In *Fetal And Neonatal Physiology*, 3 Ed.; Polin, R. A.; Fox, W. W.; Abman, S. H., Editors; Saunders: Philadelphia, 2004; Pp. 375-388.

[189] Mampel, T; Villarroya, F; Herrera, E . Hepatectomy-Nephrectomy Effects In The Pregnant Rat And Fetus. *Bichem Biophys Res Commu* 1985, *131*, 1219-1225.

[190] Herrera, E; Ortega-Senovilla, H . Maternal Lipid Metabolism During Normal Pregnancy And Its Implications To Fetal Development. *Clin Lipidol* 2010, *5*, 899-911.

[191] Amusquivar, E; Herrera, E . Influencia De Los Ácidos Grasos De La Dieta En Su Distribución Entre Las Lipoproteínas Circulantes Y En Su Asequibilidad Al Feto En La Rata Preñada. *Clin Invest Arterioscl* 2003, *15*, 91-98.

[192] Herrera, E . Lipid Metabolism In Pregnancy And Its Consequences In The Fetus And Newborn. *Endocrine* 2002, *19*, 43-55.

[193] Herrera, E; Ortega-Senovilla, M . Meternal Lipid Metabolism During Normal Pregnancy And Its Implications To Fetal Development. *Clin.Lipidol.* 2010, *5*, 899-911.

[194] Cetin, I; Alvino, G; Cardellicchio, M . Long Chain Fatty Acids And Idetary Fats In Fetal Nutrition. *J Physiol* 2009, *587.14*, 3441-3451.

[195] nsaturated Fatty Acids In The Human Placenta. *Am J Clin Nutr* 2000, *71 (Suppl)*, 315s-322s.

[196] Crawford, Ma . Placental Delivery Of Arachidonic And Docosahexaenoic Acids: Implications For The Lipid Nutrition Of Preterm Infants. *Am J Clin Nutr* 2000, *71 (Suppl)*, 275-284.

[197] Clandinin, Mt; Chapell, Je; Leong, S; Heim, T; Swyer, Pr; Chance, Gw . Intrauterine Fatty Acid Accretion Rates In Human Brain: Implications For Fatty Acid Requirements. *Early Hum Dev* 1980, *120*, 121-130.

[198] Koletzko, B; Cetin, I; Brenna, Jt . Dietary Fat Intakes For Pregnant And Lactating Women. *Br J Nutr* 2007, *98*, 873-877.

[199] Clandinin, Mt; Jumpsen, J; Suh, M . Relationship Between Fatty Acid Accretion, Membrane Composition And Biologic Functions. *J Pediatr* 1994, *125*, S25-S32.

[200] Demmelmair, H; Schenk, U; Behrendt, E; Sauerwald, T; Koletzko, B . Estimation Of Arachidonic Acid Synthesis In Full Term Neonates Using Natural Variation Of ^{13}c Content. *Journal Of Pediatric Gastroenterology And Nutrition* 1995, *21*, 31-36.

[201] Aerde, J. E.; Wilke, M. S.; Feldman, M.; Clandinin, M. T. Accretion Of Lipid In The Fetus And Newborn, In *Fetal And Neonatal Physiology*, 3 Ed.; Polin, R. A.; Fox, W. W.; Abman, S. H., Editors; W.B.Saunders Co.: Philadelphia, 2004; Pp. 388-404.

[202] Sanjurjo, P; Matorras, R; Perteagudo, L . Influence Of Fatty Fish Intake During Pregnancy In The Polyunsaturated Fatty Acids Of Erythrocyte Phospholipids In The Mother At Labor And Newborn Infant. *Acta Obstet Gynecol Scand* 1995, *74*, 594-598.

[203] Rooke, Ja; Shanks, M; Edwards, Sa . Effect Of Offering Maize, Linseed Or Tuna Oils Throughout Pregnancy And Lactation On Sow And Piglet Tissue Composition And Piglet Performance. *Animal Science* 2000, *71*, 289-299.

[204] Fleith, M; Clandinin, Mt . Dietary Pufa For Preterm And Term Infants: Review Of Clinical Studies. *Clinical Reviews In Food Science And Nutrition* 2005, *45*, 205-229.

[205] Arbuckle, Ld; Innis, Sm . Docosahexaenoic Acid Is Transferred Through Maternal Diet To Milk And To Tissues Of Natural Milk-Fed Piglets. *J Nutr* 1993, *123*, 1668-1675.

[206] Hachey, Dl; Thomas, Mr; Emken, Ea; Garza, C; Brown-Booth, L; Adlof, Ro; Klein, Pd . Human Lactation: Maternal Transfer Of Dietary Triglycerides Labeled With Stable Isotopes. *J.Lipid Res.* 1987, *28*, 1185-1192.

[207] Scopesi, F; Ciangherotti, S; Lantieri, Pb; Risso, D; Bertini, I; Campone, F; Pedrotti, A; Bonacci, W; Serra, G . Maternal Dietary Pufas Intake And Human Milk Content Relationships During The First Month Of Lactation. *Clin.Nutr.* 2001, *20*, 393-397.

[208] Chappell, Je; Clandinin, Mt; Kearney-Volpe, C . Trans Fatty Acids In Human Milk Lipids: Influence Of Maternal Diet And Weight Loss. *Am J Clin Nutr* 1985, *42*, 49-56.

[209] Martin, Jc; Bougnoux, P; Fignon, A; Theret, V; Antoine, Jm; Lamisse, F; Couet, C . Dependence Of Human Milk Essential Fatty Acids On Adipose Stores During Lactation. *Am.J.Clin.Nutr.* 1993, *58*, 653-659.

[210] Martin, Jc; Niyongabo, T; Moreau, L; Antoine, Jm; Lanson, M; Berger, C; Lamisse, F; Bougnoux, P; Couet, C . Essential Fatty Acid Composition Of Human Colostrum Triglycerides: Its Relationship With Adipose Tissue Composition. *Am.J.Clin.Nutr.* 1991, *54*, 829-835.

[211] Fielding, Ba; Frayn, K . Lipoprotein Lipase And The Disposition Of Dietary Fatty Acids. *British Journal Of Nutrition* 1998, *80*, 495-502.

[212] Alvarez, Jj; Montelongo, A; Iglesias, A; Lasunción, Ma; Herrera, E . Longitudinal Study On Lipoprotein Profile, High Density Lipoprotein Subclas, And Postheparin Lipases During Gestation In Women. *J Lipid Res* 1996, *37*, 299-308.

[213] Ramírez, I; Llobera, M; Herrera, E . Circulating Triacylglicerols, Lipoproteins, And Tissue Lipoprotein Lipase Activities In Rat Mothers And Offspring During The Perinatal Period: Effect Of Postmaturity. *Metabolism* 1983, *32*, 333-341.

[214] ulation Of Lipoprotein Lipase Messenger Ribonucleic Acid And Activity In Mammary Gland. *Endocrinology* 1999, *140*, 1089-1093.

[215] Ramirez, I; Llobera, M; Herrera, E . Circulating Triacylglycerols, Lipoproteins, And Tissue Lipoprotein Lipase Activities In Rat Mothers And Offspring During The Perinatal Period: Effect Of Postmaturity. *Metabolism* 1983, *32*, 333-341.

[216] Carrascosa, Jm; Ramos, P; Molero, Jc; Herrera, E . Changes In The Kinase Activity Of The Insulin Receptor Account For An Increased Insulin Sensitivity Of Mammary Gland In Late Pregnancy. *Endocrinology* 1998, *139*, 520-526.

[217] Martín-Hidalgo, A.; Ramos, P.; Blanco, L.; Herrera, E. Regulation Of Rat Mammary Gland Activity And Mrna By Insulin During Pregnancy And Lactation. Easd Study Group "Control Of Metabolism And Insulin Action" (Aachen) .Abstract, 1995.

[218] Ramos, P; Herrera, E . Comparative Responsiveness To Prolonged Hyperinsulinemia Between Adipose-Tissue And Mammary-Gland Lipoprotein Lipase Activities In Pregnant Rats. *Early Pregnancy: Biol.And Med.* 1996, *2*, 29-35.

[219] Ramos, P; Martín-Hidalgo, A; Herrera, E . Insulin-Induced Up-Regulation Of Lipoprotein Lipase Messenger Ribonucleic Acid And Activity In Mammary Gland. *Endocrinology* 1999, *140*, 1089-1093.

[220] Hachey, Dl; Thomas, Mr; Emken, Ea; Garza, C; Brown-Booth, L; Adlof, Ro; Klein, Pd . Human Lactation: Maternal Transfer Of Dietary Triglycerides Labeled With Stable Isotopes. *J.Lipid Res.* 1987, *28*, 1185-1192.

[221] Argilés, J; Herrera, E . Appearance Of Circulating And Tissue ^{14}c-Lipids After Oral ^{14}c-Tripalmitate Administration In The Late Pregnant Rat. *Metabolism* 1989, *32*, 333-341.

[222] Rooke, Ja; Sinclair, Ag; Edwards, Sa . Feeding Tuna Oil To The Sow At Different Times During Pregnancy Has Different Effects On Piglet Long-Chain Polyunsaturated Fatty Acid Composition At Birth And Subsequent Growth. *British Journal Of Nutrition* 2001, *86*, 21-30.

[223] Fritsche, Kl; Huang, Sc; Cassity, Na . Enrichment Of Omega-3 Fatty Acids In Suckling Pigs By Maternal Dietary Fish Oil Supplementation. *J.Anim Sci.* 1993, *71*, 1841-1847.

[224] Scopesi, F; Ciangherotti, S; Lantieri, Pb; Risso, D; Bertini, I; Campone, F; Pedrotti, A; Bonacci, W; Serra, G . Maternal Dietary Pufas Intake And Human Milk Content Relationships During The First Month Of Lactation. *Clin.Nutr.* 2001, *20*, 393-397.

[225] Innis, Sm . The Colostrum-Deprived Piglet As A Model For Study Of Infant Lipid Nutrition. *J Nutr* 1993, *123*, 386-390.

[226] Amusquivar, E; Laws, J; Clarke, L; Herrera, E . Fatty Acid Composition Of The Maternal Diet During The First Or The Second Half Of Gestation Influences The Fatty Acid Composition Of Sows' Milk And Plasma, And Plasma Of Their Piglets. *Lipids* 2010, *45*, 409-418.

[227] Crawford, Ma; Hassan, Ag; Williams, G; Whitehouse, Wl . Essential Fatty Acids And Fetal Brain Growth. *Lancet* 1976, *I*, 452-453.

[228] Al, Md; Hornstra, G; Van Der Schouw, Yt; Bulstra-Ramakers, Mt; Hisjes, Hj . Biochemical Efa Status Of Mothers And Their Neonates Afte Normal Pregnancy. *Early Human Development* 1990, *24*, 239-248.

[229] Herrera, E; Ortega, H; Alvino, G; Giovannini, N; Cetin, I . Relationship Between Plasma Fatty Acid Profile And Antioxidant Vitamins During Normal Pregnancy. *Eur.J.Clin.Nutr.* 2004, *58*, 1231-1238.

[230] Farquharson, J; Cockburn, F; Patrick, Wa; Jamieson, Ec; Logan, Rw . Infant Cerebral Cortex Phospholipid Fatty-Acid Composition And Diet. *Lancet* 1992, *340*, 810-813.

[231] Makrides, M; Neumann, Ma; Byard, Rw; Simmer, K; Gibson, Ra . Fatty Acid Composition Of Brain, Retina, And Erytrocytes In Breast- And Formula-Fed Infants. *American Journal Of Clinical Nutrition* 1994, *60*, 189-194.

[232] Meldrum, Sj; Smith, Ma; Prescott, Sl; Hird, K; Simmer, K . Achieving Definitive Results In Long-Chain Polyunsaturated Fatty Acid Supplementation Trials Of Term Infants: Factors For Consideration. *Nutrition Reviews* 2011, *69*, 205-214.

[233] Makrides, M; Collins, Ct; Gibson, Ra . Impact Of Fatty Acid Status On Growth And Neurobehavioural Development In Humans. *Maternal And Child Nutrition* 2011, *7 (Suppl. 2)*, 80-88.

[234] Tofail, F; Kabir, I; Hamadani, Jd; Chowdhury, F; Yesmin, S; Mehreen, F; Huda, Sn . Supplementation Of Fish-Oil And Soy-Oil During Pregnancy And Psycomotor Development Of Infants. *J.Health, Population And Nutr.* 2006, *24*, 48-56.

[235] Ramakrishnan, U; Stein, Ad; Parra-Cabrera, S; Wang, M; Imhoff-Kunsch, B; Juarez-Marquez, S; Rivera, J; Martorell, R . Effects Of Docosahexaenoic Acid Supplementation During Pregnancy On Estational Age And Size At Birth: Randomized, Double Bind, Placebo-Controlled Trial In Mexico. *Food And Nutrition Bull.* 2010, *31*, S108-S116.

[236] Dunstan, Ja; Simmer, K; Dixon, G; Prescott, Sl . Cognitive Assessment Of Children At Age 2(1/2) Years After Maternal Fish Oil Supplementation In Pregnancy: A Randomised Controlled Trial. *Arch.Dis.Child Fetal Neonatal Ed* 2008, *93*, F45-F50.

[237] Judge, Mp; Harel, O; Lammi-Keefe, Cj . Maternal Consumption Of A Docosahexaenoic Acid-Containing Functional Food During Pregnancy: Benefit For Infant Performance On Problem-Solving But Not On Recognition Memory Tasks At Age 9 Mo. *American Journal Of Clinical Nutrition* 2007, *85*, 1572-1577.

[238] Makrides, M; G; I; B; S; O; N; ; R; .; A; .Mcphee, Aj; Yelland, L; Quinlivan, J; Ryan, P . Effcet Of Dha Supplementation During Pregnancy On Maternal Depression And Neurodevelopment Of Young Children: A Rabdomized Controlled Trial. *Journal Of The American Medical Association* 2010, *304*, 1675-1683.

[239] Innis, Sm; Kuhnlein, Hv . Long-Chain N-3 Fatty Acids In Breast Milk Of Inuit Women Consuming Traditional Foods. *Early Human Development* 1988, *18*, 185-189.

[240] Helland, Ib; Saarem, K; Saugstad, Od; Drevon, Ca . Fatty Acid Composition In Maternal Milk And Plasma During Supplementation With Cod Liver Oil. *Eur.J.Clin.Nutr.* 1998, *52*, 839-845.

[241] Lanting, Ci; Fidler, V; Huisman, M; Touwen, Bc; Boersma, Bc . Neurological Differences Between 9-Year Old Children Fed Breast-Milk Or Formula-Milk As Babies. *Lancet* 1994, *344*, 1319-1322.

[242] Anderson, Jw; Johnstone, Bm; Remley, Dt . Breast-Feeding And Co.Nitive Development: A Meta-Analysis. *J.Clin.Nutr.* 1999, *70*, 525-535.

[243] ulvez, J; Ribas-Fitó, N; Forns, M; Garcia-Esteban, R; Torrent, M; Sunyer, J . Attention Behaviour And Hyperactivity At Age 4 And Duration Of Breast-Feeding. *Acta Paediatr.* 2007, *96*, 842-847.

[244] ong, Cd; Kikkert, Hk; Fidler, V; Hadders-Algra, M . The Groningen Lcpufa Study: No Effect Of Postnatal Long-Chain Polyunsaturated Fatty Acids In Healthy Term Infants On Neurological Condition At 9 Years. *British Journal Of Nutrition* 2010, *104*, 566-572.

[245] Kramer, Ms; Aboud, F; Mironova, E; Vanilovich, I; Platt, Rw; Matush, L; Igumnov, S; Fombonne, E; Bogdanovich, N; Ducruet, T; Collet, Jp; Chalmers, B; Hodnett, E; Davidovsky, S; Skugarevsky, O; Trofimovich, O; Kozlova, L; Shapiro, S . Promotion Of Breastfeeding Intervention Trial (Probit) Study Group. Breastfeeding And Child

Cognitive Development: New Evidence From A Large Randomized Trial. *Arch.Gen.Psychiatry* 2008, *65*, 578-584.

[246] Brenna, Jt; Varamini, Bi; Jensen, Rg; Diersen-Schade, Da; Boettcher, Ja; Arterbum, Lm . Docosahexaenoic And Arachidonic Acid Concentration In Human Breast Milk Worldwibe. *American Journal Of Clinical Nutrition* 2007, *85*, 1457-1464.

[247] Hadders-Algra, M . Effect Of Long-Chain Polyunsaturated Fatty Acid Supplementation On Neurodevelopmental Outcome In Full-Term Infants. *Nutrients* 2010, *2*, 790-804.

[248] Simmer, K.; Patole, S. K.; Rao, S. C. The Cochrane Database Of Systematic Reviews. *Longchain Polyunsaturated Fatty Acid Supplementation In Infants Born At Term.* 2008.

[249] Simmer, K.; Schulzke, S. M.; Patole, S. K. *The Cochrane Database Of Systematic Reviews. Longchain Polyunsaturated Fatty Acid Supplementation In Preterm Infants.* 2008.

[250] Bouwstra, H; Dijck-Brouwer, Daj; Wildeman, Jal; Tjoonk, Hm; Van Der Heide, Jc; Boersma, Er; Muskiet, Faj; Hadders-Algra, M . Long-Chain Polyunsaturated Fatty Acids Have A Positive Effect On The Quality Of General Movements Of Healthy Term Infants. *American Journal Of Clinical Nutrition* 2003, *78*, 313-318.

[251] Bouwstra, H; Dijck-Brouwer, Daj; Boehm, G; Boersma, Er; Muskiet, Faj; Hadders-Algra, M . Long-Chain Polyunsaturated Fatty Acids And Neurological Developmental Outcome At 18 Months In Healthy Term Infants. *Acta Paediatrica* 2005, *94*, 26-32.

[252] Lanting, Ci; Patandin, S; Weisglas-Kuperus, N; Touwen, Bc; Boersma, Er . Breastfeeding And Neurological Outcome At 42 Months. *Acta Paediatr.* 1998, *87*, 1224-1229.

In: Fish Oil: Production, Consumption and Health Benefits
Editors: Matthias Van Dijk and Jürgen Vitek
ISBN: 978-1-61470-963-3

Chapter IV

Beneficial Effects of a Fish Oil Diet for the Correction of the Fatty Acid Pattern of Intestinal, Liver, Red Blood Cells, Brain and Adipose Tissue Lipids in Rats Deprived of Long-Chain Polyunsaturated Ω3 Fatty Acids

Willy J. Malaisse and Yvon A. Carpentier
Laboratories of Experimental Hormonology and Surgery,
Université Libre de Bruxelles, Brussels, Belgium

Abstract

The initial aim of the present chapter was to assess the suitability of a fish oil diet to correct the metabolic and hormonal defects otherwise encountered in rats deprived of a dietary supply of long-chain polyunsaturated ω3 fatty acids. For such a purpose, 8 groups of 4 rats each were first exposed from the 8th week after birth and for the ensuing 3 months to either a soya oil or sunflower oil diet and then examined at the end of this 3 months initial period or after a further period of one, two or 8 weeks exposure to a fish oil diet. The fatty acid profile of jejunum, caecum, liver, red blood cells and brain phospholipids, as well as liver triglycerides and visceral adipose tissue lipids, was analyzed. Changes in food intake, body weight and the HOMA index for insulin resistance were also monitored. The results document the efficiency of this procedure for the correction of both the ω3 deficiency and insulin resistance, without any undesirable increase in liver steatosis, visceral obesity, food intake or body weight. Emphasis is also placed on the dual regulation of the lipid fatty acid profile as attributable to either a direct link with the fatty acid content of the diet or the transfer of information from one organ to another.

Introduction

The bolus intravenous injection of a novel medium-chain triglyceride:fish oil emulsion was recently proposed as a suitable tool to increase within 60 min the long-chain polyunsaturated ω3 fatty acid content of cell phospholipids [1]. The optimal procedure for the dietary correction of the metabolic and hormonal disturbances found in situations of ω3-depletion, in terms of the total lipid content and source of ω3 fatty acids in the diet, as well as the time course for the enrichment of tissue lipids in these ω3 fatty acids requires, however, further attention [2]. In such a perspective, the present report deals mainly with the effects of a diet containing 5% (w/w) fish oil diet, as assessed in rats first exposed for 3 months to an ω3-deficient sunflower oil (also 5%) diet.

Materials and Methods

Eight groups of 4 fed female rats each were examined in the present study. Four groups consisted of control animals exposed from the age of 8 weeks after birth to a diet containing 5% (w/w) soya oil diet and examined either at the end of this initial 3 months period or one, two and 8 weeks later whilst being exposed to a 5% (w/w) fish oil diet. The other 4 groups of rats were first exposed during the initial 3 months period to a diet containing 5% (w/w) sunflower oil diet (ω3D rats) and examined either at the end of this 3 months initial period or after further exposure for one, two or eight weeks to the fish oil diet. Four further control animals were maintained on the soya oil for 8 weeks after the initial period, whilst six further ω3D rats were maintained after the initial period and for the ensuing 8 weeks to the sunflower oil. In the present report, the findings recorded in these two additional groups of rats are restricted to the measurements of food intake and body weight.

The rats were eventually sacrificed after CO2 inhalation. The methods used for collection of intestinal mucosa at the jejunal and caecal level [3], liver [4], red blood cell [5], brain [6] and both visceral and parametrial adipose tissue [7] sampling, lipid extraction [8], separation by thin-layer chromatography [9] and determination of lipid fatty acid pattern by gas-liquid chromatography [10], food intake measurements [11], and plasma D-glucose [12] and insulin [13] determinations were previously described in the cited references.

All results are presented as mean values (± SEM) together with the number of individual observations (n) or degree of freedom (df). Except if otherwise mentioned, all tabulated values refer to four individual determinations. In the case of RBC, however, the measurements listed for rats examined 1 or 2 weeks after the switch in diet refer to single measurements made in pooled material from four rats. The statistical significance of differences between mean values was assessed by use of Student's *t*-test.

Results

1. Fatty Acid Profile of Intestinal Phospholipids

1.1. Long-Chain Polyunsaturated Ω3 Fatty Acids

At the end of the 3 months initial period, the relative weight content of most long-chain polyunsaturated ω3 fatty acids (C18:3ω3, C22:5ω3 and C22:6ω3) in jejunal phospholipids was higher ($p < 0.01$ or less) in control animals than in ω3D rats (Table 1). No C20:5ω3 was detected, however, whether in control animals or ω3D rats. In both the control animals and ω3D rats examined one week after the switch to the fish oil diet, no C18:3ω3 was anymore detected in jejunal phospholipids, whilst the relative weight content of the other three long-chain polyunsaturated ω3 fatty acids was considerably increased ($p < 0.002$ or less). No significant difference between control animal and ω3D rats was anymore observed one week after the switch in diet. Pooling together the results recorded in control animals and ω3D rats, the enrichment of C20:5ω3, C22:5ω3 and C22:6ω3 in the jejunal phospholipids, resulting from the switch in diet and expressed as an increment in relative weight content, averaged respectively 53.8 ± 3.7‰, 11.0 ± 1.1‰ and 89.1 ± 8.0‰. There was a tight ($r = + 0.9969$) and significant ($p = 0.05$) correlation between the latter three mean values and the relative weight content of the corresponding ω3 fatty acids in the fish oil diet, i.e. 7.1, 1.3 and 13.4% in the case of C20:5ω3, C22:5ω3 and C22:6ω3, respectively.

Table 1. Relative weight content (‰) of long-chain polyunsaturated ω3 fatty acids in jejunal and caecal phospholipids

Rats	C18:3ω3	C20:5ω3	C22:5ω3	C22:6ω3
Jejunum				
Control before	7.10±1.46	0.00±0.00	4.18±0.39	39.51±2.00
after (1wk)	0.00±0.00	61.59±4.84	13.04±1.14	113.50±12.39
ω3D before	0.00±0.00	0.00±0.00	0.00±0.00	14.86±1.62
after (1wk)	0.00±0.00	46.04±4.07	13.22±1.34	119.08±6.43
Caecum				
Control before	1.46±1.46	2.76±1.60	2.74±2.74	49.94±6.83
after (1wk)	0.00±0.00	16.34±9.43	11.85±6.91	114.32±6.36
ω3D before	0.00±0.00	0.00±0.00	0.00± 0.00	5.49±5.49
after (1wk)	0.00±0.00	16.70±5.58	19.22±1.55	86.38±9.97

At the end of the 3 months initial period, only the relative weight content of C22:6ω3 in caecal phospholipids was significantly lower ($p < 0.004$) in ω3D rats than in control animals. Such was no more the case ($p < 0.06$) one week after the switch in diet. Except in the case of C18:3ω3, which remained below the limit of detection in the caecum phospholipids, all other long-chain polyunsaturated ω3 fatty acids (C20:5ω3, C22:5ω3 and C22:6ω3) yielded higher mean relative weight content after than before the switch in diet, whether in control animals or ω3D rats (Table 1). Pooling together the results recorded in control animals and ω3D rats, the enrichment of C20:5ω3, C22:5ω3 and C22:6ω3 in the caecal phospholipids, as attributable to the switch in diet, averaged respectively (expressed as an increment in relative weight content) 15.1 ± 5.3‰, 14.2 ± 3.9‰ and 72.6 ± 7.4‰. Only the first of these three mean values differed significantly ($p < 0.001$) from the corresponding value found at the jejunal level.

1.2. Long-Chain Polyunsaturated Ω6 Fatty Acids

Before the switch in diet, higher mean values for the C20:2ω6 ($p < 0.02$), C22:4ω6 ($p < 0.09$) and C22:5ω6 ($p < 0.003$) relative weight content of jejunal phospholipids were found in the ω3D rats than in the control animals (Table 2). Such was no more the case one week after the switch in diet. In the ω3D rats, the C20:2ω6 ($p < 0.007$) and C22:5ω6 ($p < 0.004$) content of jejunal phospholipids were indeed significantly lower after then before the switch in diet. A dramatic decrease of the C18:2ω6 relative weight content of jejunal phospholipid ($p < 0.001$) was also observed after the switch in diet, whether in control animals or ω3D rats. This coincided with the much lower content of C18:2ω6 in the fish oil diet (2.0%) than in either the soya oil diet (56.5%) or sunflower oil diet (65.6%).

At the caecal level, the sole significant difference between control animals and ω3D rats examined before the switch in diet consisted in the higher content ($p < 0.001$) of C22:5ω6 in the phospholipids of the latter rats as compared to former animals. Except in the case of C20:3ω6 in the ω3D rats, the mean values for all ω6 fatty acids were lower after then before the switch in diet, whether in control animals or ω3D rats. Such differences achieved statistical significance ($p < 0.04$ or less) in both control animals and ω3D rats in the case of C18:2ω6, C20:4ω6 and C22:4ω6, as well as in the case of C22:5ω6 in ω3D rats ($p < 0.001$).

Table 2. Relative weight content (‰) of long-chain polyunsaturated ω6 fatty acids in jejunal and caecal phospholipids

Rats	C18:2ω6	C20:2ω6	C20:3ω6	C20:4ω6	C22:4ω6	C22:5ω6
Jejunum						
Control before	314.40±19.28	1.16±0.68	5.71±0.45	175.68±21.41	4.24±0.60	0.00±0.00
after (1wk)	136.94±11.78	1.10±0.64	6.57±0.11	147.45±17.69	2.90±1.21	0.00±0.00
ω3D before	316.85±16.43	4.61±0.71	6.31±0.75	173.77±8.19	7.94±1.66	16.80 ±3.09
after (1wk)	122.96±1.23	0.64±0.64	6.80±0.12	154.07±8.37	4.75±0.51	1.37±0.80
Caecum						
Control before	192.02±12.80	3.40±1.96	16.50±0.36	164.85±12.04	16.69±5.70	2.13±1.32
after (1wk)	90.00±28.59	0.00±0.00	0.00±0.00	82.60±15.23	0.00±0.00	0.00±0.00
ω3D before	189.76±8.28	0.00±0.00	7.42±4.34	200.00±13.13	29.56±3.28	26.47±1.36
after (1wk)	142.22±9.97	0.00±0.00	9.44±3.15	156.93±8.18	14.52±1.36	2.61±1.97

1.3. Saturated Fatty Acids

Before the switch in diet, no significant difference in the relative weight content of saturated fatty acids (C14:0, C16:0, C18:0, C20:0, C22:0 and C24:0) in jejunal phospholipids was observed between control animals and ω3D rats (Table 3). Such was also the case after the switch in diet. Both the C14:0 ($p < 0.001$) and C16:0 ($p < 0.025$ or less) content of jejunal phospholipids were higher after then before the switch in diet, whether in control animals or ω3D rats. This coincided with the higher C14:0 content (2.0%) and C16:0 content (13.2%) of the fish oil diet as compared to soya oil or sunflower oil diet. As a matter of fact, when the overall mean values for the enrichment of jejunal phospholipids in C14:0 (5.26 ± 0.55‰) and C16:0 (34.05 ± 7.18‰) attributable to the switch in diet were divided by the just mentioned relative content of these fatty acids in the fish oil diet, virtually identical quotients ($p > 0.49$) were reached for C14:0 (2.63 ± 0.28) and C16:0 (2.58 ± 0.54).

Likewise, at the caecal level, no significant difference in the content of saturated fatty acids were observed between control animals and ω3D rats examined before the switch in diet. The sole significant difference ($p < 0.025$) between the mean results recorded either before or after the switch in diet consisted in a higher value of C14:0 in the caecal phospholipids of control animals after the switch in diet.

Table 3. Relative weight content (‰) of saturated fatty acids in jejunum and caecum phospholipids

Rats	C14:0	C16:0	C18:0	C20:0	C22:0	C24:0
Jejunum						
Control before	0.00±0.00	167.22±3.42	198.25±9.42	7.00±0.79	7.58±0.53	6.25±0.51
after (1wk)	5.35±0.89	198.25±7.42	193.87±2.56	8.53±2.30	7.51±1.80	4.00±1.92
ω3D before	0.78±0.45	164.31±10.29	204.77±5.02	9.32±3.02	10.83±2.73	9.24±2.38
after (1wk)	5.95±0.57	201.38±6.90	192.11±2.76	10.28±1.40	8.16±1.01	6.92±0.80
Caecum						
Control before	7.79±3.03	247.74±15.67	123.27±10.61	15.05±3.28	18.09±5.06	18.20±7.70
after (1wk)	29.14±6.44	321.53±40.38	140.13±11.33	33.79±7.44	31.04±6.38	34.68±8.73
ω3D before	9.01±0.69	242.60±10.81	129.05±4.07	11.83±2.12	12.85±1.75	9.61±1.39
after (1wk)	6.47±2.17	243.79±12.27	129.27±5.02	14.91±1.95	13.40±1.63	6.97±2.60

1.4. Monodesaturated Fatty Acids

The relative weight content of the four monodesaturated fatty acids listed in Table 4 (C16:1ω7, C18:1ω9, C20:1ω9 and C22:1ω9) failed to differ significantly ($p > 0.06$ or more) in the jejunal phospholipids of control animals and ω3D rats examined before the switch in diet. Such was also the case one week after the switch in diet ($p > 0.3$ or more). The difference between the results recorded before and after the switch in diet averaged, in the case of C16:1ω7 and C20:1ω9, 11.0 ± 1.0‰ and 17.9 ± 1.3‰ (pooled data collected in both control animals and ω3D rats), these enrichments being commensurate with the C16:1ω7 content (7.7%) and C20:1ω9 content (13.0%) of the fish oil diet. In the case of the two other monodesaturated fatty acids (C18:1ω9 and C22:1ω9), a significant increase ($p < 0.02$) was only observed for the C18:1ω9 content of jejunal phospholipids in the ω3D rats.

Likewise, at the caecal level, no significant difference ($p > 0.15$ or more) in the relative weight content of monodesaturated fatty acids was observed between control animals and ω3D rats examined before the switch in diet. Once again, such was also the case ($p > 0.07$ or more) after the switch in diet. Moreover, no significant difference was detected, at the caecal level, when comparing the relative weight content of each monodesaturated fatty acids before and after the switch in diet, whether in control animals or ω3D rats.

Table 4. Relative weight content (‰) of monodesaturated fatty acids in jejunum and caecum phospholipids

Rats	C16:1ω7	C18:1ω9	C20:1ω9	C22:1ω9
Control before	3.70±0.70	58.03±2.03	0.00±0.00	0.00±0.00
after (1wk)	13.47±1.43	68.53±5.33	17.26±1.91	0.00±0.00
ω3D before	2.50±0.92	64.77±2.11	0.43±0.43	0.00±0.00
after (1wk)	14.69±0.75	72.81±0.54	18.91±1.81	1.06±1.06
Caecum				
Control before	5.54±3.34	120.28±1.42	0.00±0.00	0.00±0.00
after (1wk)	3.40±3.40	89.34±15.62	0.00±0.00	0.00±0.00
ω3D before	12.18±2.09	118.44±4.76	1.01±0.1	0.00±0.00
after (1wk)	11.49±3.96	125.77±5.55	1.36±1.36	0.00±0.00

2. Fatty Acid Profile of Liver Phospholipids

2.1. Long-Chain Polyunsaturated Ω3 Fatty Acids

Sizeable amounts of C18:3ω3 were found in the liver phospholipids of all control animals, except 8 weeks after the switch from the soya oil diet to the fish oil diet. In the ω3D rats, however, such was the case only in four out of 16 samples, null values being again recorded in all ω3D rats examined 8 weeks after the switch from the sunflower oil diet to the fish oil diet. Pooling all available measurements made at the end of the 3 months initial period and one or two weeks thereafter, the overall mean value for C18:3ω3 averaged 1.94 ± 0.17‰ (n = 12) in the control animals, as distinct ($p < 0.001$) from only 0.49 ± 0.21‰ (n = 12) in the ω3D rats (Table 5).

The mean relative weight content of C20:5ω3 in liver phospholipids was always lower ($p < 0.02$ or less) in ω3D rats than in control animals, whether before or at any time after the switch in diet. In both the control animals and ω3D rats, it underwent a progressive increase after the switch in diet. Even after two weeks exposure to the fish oil diet, the increment in the C20:5ω3 content of liver phospholipids above the mean corresponding value found at the end of the 3 months initial period did not exceed 66.9 ± 5.6% (df = 12; $p < 0.03$) of that recorded in the same type of rats (control animals or ω3D rats) 8 weeks after the switch in diet (100.0 ± 12.8%; df = 12).

The C22:5ω3 relative weight content of liver phospholipids remained significantly lower ($p < 0.03$ or less) in ω3D rats than in control animals up to the second week after the switch in diet. In the case of C22:6ω3, however, no significant difference between control animals and ω3D rats prevailed whether 2 or 8 weeks after the switch in diet. The latter situation obviously contrasts with that described above in the case of C20:5ω3. Nevertheless, in the case of C22:6ω3, like in that of C20:5ω3, the increment recorded 2 weeks after the switch to the fish oil diet did not exceed 76.8 ± 4.9% (df = 12; $p < 0.004$) of that recorded in the same type of rats after 8 weeks exposure to the fish oil diet (100.0 ± 5.7%; df = 12).

Table 5. Relative weight content (‰) of long-chain polyunsaturated ω3 fatty acids in liver phospholipids

Rats	C18:3ω3	C20:5ω3	C22:5ω3	C22:6ω3
Control before	2.30±0.19	5.05±1.12	9.00±0.41	169.11±4.49
after (1wk)	1.56±0.35	58.18±2.63	12.90±0.68	226.13±2.19
after (2wk)	1.97±0.23	72.00±11.08	12.82±0.53	232.33±6.22
after (8wk)	0.00±0.00	105.51±5.59	17.13±0.63	260.13±8.43
ω3D before	0.35±0.35	0.00±0.00	1.56±0.80	54.52±5.32
after (1wk)	0.76±0.44	20.83±1.51	9.88±0.34	208.41±2.60
after (2wk)	0.36±0.36	36.45±1.90	10.64±0.51	228.77±6.40
after (8wk)	0.00±0.00	54.23±14.14	15.13±1.83	261.68±10.48

2.2. Long-Chain Polyunsaturated Ω6 Fatty Acids

The C22:4ω6 and C22:5ω6 relative weight contents of liver phospholipids were higher ($p < 0.02$ or less) in the ω3D rats than in the control animals examined before the switch in diet (Table 6). No significant difference between control animals and ω3D rats was observed at that time for the five other long-chain polyunsaturated ω6 fatty acids. With the outstanding exception of C20:3ω6, which displayed higher mean values after than before the switch in diet, the relative weight content of all other long-chain polyunsaturated ω6 fatty acids in liver phospholipids decreased after the switch in diet. In the case of C20:3ω6, a time-related increase of its content in liver phospholipids was observed in ω3D rats, yielding in a semi-logarithmic analysis a significant positive correlation ($r = + 0.6658$; $n = 16$; $p < 0.007$) as a function of the length of exposure to the fish oil diet; such was not the case in the control animals. The time course for the decrease in the relative weight content of the other long-chain polyunsaturated ω6 fatty acids was quite rapid. Only one week after the switch in diet, the overall mean value for the decrease in the relative weight content observed in both control animals and ω3D rats achieved statistical significance ($p < 0.007$ or less) in all cases (C18:2ω6, C20:2ω6, C18:3ω3, C20:4ω6, C22:4ω6 and C22:5ω6). A further progressive decrease after 2 to 8 weeks exposure to the fish oil was noticed in most cases. Thus, at the exclusion of C20:2ω6, which yielded the lowest mean relative weight content, at least in the

Table 6. Relative weight content (‰) of long-chain polyunsaturated ω6 fatty acids in liver phospholipids

Rats	C18:2ω6	C20:2ω6	C18:3ω6	C20:3ω6	C20:4ω6	C22:4ω6	C22:5ω6
Control before	82.51±5.16	1.59±0.18	1.72±0.25	6.05±0.63	303.65±5.77	2.87±0.16	5.27±0.48
after (1wk)	60.90±4.56	0.27±0.27	0.57±0.33	6.66±0.54	199.92±2.10	1.26±0.47	1.19±0.46
after (2wk)	57.88±8.86	0.79±0.28	0.47±0.27	8.02±1.33	182.65±11.29	1.10±0.06	1.47±0.14
after (8wk)	52.69±2.69	0.59±0.20	0.37±0.21	6.70±0.52	131.84±3.86	0.72±0.24	0.00±0.00
ω3D before	77.83±2.73	2.78±0.80	2.03±0.20	5.44±0.44	342.83±4.45	8.54±0.31	72.67±8.82
after (1wk)	60.99±7.06	1.27±0.22	0.72±0.24	6.23±0.31	271.84±2.81	2.41±0.25	4.02±0.50
after (2wk)	51.35±1.56	0.75±0.25	0.57±0.33	7.02±0.45	244.30±7.93	2.16±0.20	3.26±0.46
after (8wk)	59.22±9.21	0.90±0.05	0.65±0.23	8.56±1.30	184.79±22.41	1.17±0.06	1.50±0.24

control animals examined before the switch in diet, a highly significant negative correlation (r = - 0.3599; n = 120; p < 0.001) prevailed, in a semi-logarithmic analysis, between the length of exposure to the fish oil diet and the relative weight contents of the five remaining ω6 fatty acids (C18:2ω6, C18:3ω3, C20:4ω6, C22:4ω6 and C22:5ω6) all expressed relative to the mean value for the same fatty acid found in either control animals or ω3D rats one, two and eight weeks after the switch in diet, i.e. as derived from 12 individual values in each case.

2.3. Saturated Fatty Acids

No obvious difference between control animals and ω3D rats examined before the switch in diet and no obvious trend of changes after the switch in diet were observed in the relative weight content of C14:0 and C16:0 in liver phospholipids (Table 7). Before the switch in diet, the C20:0 content of liver phospholipids was higher (p < 0.05) in control animals than in ω3D rats, this coinciding with the higher C20:0 content of the soya oil diet (0.5%) as distinct from sunflower oil diet (0.0%). After the switch in diet, 23 out of 24 samples did not more contain any detectable amount of C20:0, this again coinciding with the low C20:0 content of the fish oil diet (0.1%). Before the switch in diet, the mean relative weight contents of C18:0, C22:0 and C24:0 were higher (p < 0.025 or less) in ω3D rats than in control animals. Such differences disappeared after the switch in diet. Thus, the mean values recorded after the switch in diet were, in the case of C18:0, virtually identical (p > 0.7) in control animals (234.08 ± 2.28‰; n = 12) and ω3D rats (235.48 ± 2.93‰; n = 12) and, in the case of C24:0, no more significantly higher (p > 0.2) in ω3D rats (4.40 ± 0.14‰; n = 12) than in control animals (4.09 ± 0.18‰; n = 12). In the case of C22:0, such values were slightly higher (p < 0.04) in control animals (1.95 ± 0.09‰; n = 12) than in ω3D rats (1.43 ± 0.20%; n = 12).

Table 7. Relative weight content (‰) of saturated fatty acids in liver phospohlipids

Rats	C14:0	C16:0	C18:0	C20:0	C22:0	C24:0
Control before	1.56±0.15	133.92±2.71	237.04±4.67	0.70±0.01	2.23±0.69	6.84±0.34
after (1wk)	2.19±0.16	152.13±3.05	231.59±3.71	0.00±0.00	2.25±0.10	3.92±0.20
after (2wk)	1.98±0.14	147.75±4.66	232.45±5.26	0.00±0.00	2.00±0.08	3.69±0.27
after (8wk)	1.82±0.05	131.57±2.63	238.19±2.67	0.00±0.00	1.59±0.03	4.67±0.29
ω3D before	1.86±0.22	144.02±5.75	273.82±1.42	0.20±0.20	4.42±0.20	9.63±0.24
after (1wk)	1.64±0.11	131.23±2.70	246.09±2.07	0.00±0.00	1.10±0.37	4.87±0.19
after (2wk)	1.78±0.07	145.39±4.52	226.22±4.66	0.00±0.00	1.47±0.49	4.15±0.29
after (8wk)	1.51±0.22	131.44±3.55	234.13±1.32	0.13±0.13	1.73±0.02	4.19±0.05

2.4. Monodesaturated Fatty Acids

No significant difference (p > 0.17) was found between control animals and ω3D rats for the C16:1ω7 content of liver phospholipids, the values recorded in the latter rats averaging 88.1 ± 6.8% (n = 16) of the mean corresponding values found at the same time in the former animals (100.0 ± 5.2%; n = 6). In both control animals and ω3D rats, the C16:1ω7 content progressively increased from 5.50 ± 0.67‰ (n = 8) before the switch in diet to 7.13 ± 0.51‰,

8.99 ± 0.62‰ and 9.82 ± 0.72‰ (n = 8 in all cases), respectively one, two and eight weeks after the switch to the fish oil diet (Table 8). Such an increase coincided with the higher C16:1ω7 relative content of the fish oil diet (7.7%), as distinct from either the soya oil diet (0.1%) or sunflower oil diet (0.1%).

Likewise, no significant difference ($p > 0.27$) was observed between control animals and ω3D rats for the C18:1ω9 content of liver phospholipids, the measurements made in the latter ω3D rats averaging 93.5 ± 4.9% (n = 16) of those recorded at the same time in control animals (100.0 ± 2.9%; n = 16). After the switch in diet, a modest but progressive and significant increase of the C18:1ω9 content was only observed in the control animals.

Whether in control animals or ω3D rats, the C20:1ω9 content of liver phospholipids was much higher after the switch in diet than at the end of the 3 months initial period. This again coincided with the higher relative content of C20:1ω9 in the fish oil diet (13.0%) as distinct from either soya oil diet (0.2%) or sunflower oil diet (0.0%).

Although a comparable difference in the C22:1ω9 relative content of the fish oil diet (13.4%) as compared to the soya oil diet (0.0%) or sunflower oil diet (0.0%), the C22:1ω9 relative weight content of liver phospholipids decreased, in both control animals and ω3D rats, after the switch in diet, eventually reaching null values. In other words, the C22:1ω9/C20:1ω9 paired ratio decreased from 2.65 ± 0.47 (in two control animals) and infinite values (in all other six rats) before the switch in diet to 1.20 ± 0.16 (n = 8), 0.76 ± 0.17 (n = 8) and 0.00 ± 0.00 (n = 8) one, two and eight weeks thereafter.

Whether in the case of C20:1ω9 or C22:1ω9, the mean values recorded at each time point in the ω3D rats never differed significantly from those found in the control animals.

Table 8. Relative weight content (‰) of monodesaturated fatty acids in liver phospholipids

Rats	C16:1ω7	C18:1ω9	C20:1ω9	C22:1ω9
Control before	5.16 ± 1.06	23.91 ± 2.57	0.33 ± 0.19	2.04 ± 0.24
after (1 wk)	8.32 ± 0.40	27.43 ± 1.26	1.70 ± 0.07	2.12 ± 0.42
after (2 wk)	9.31 ± 0.89	30.02 ± 0.70	1.85 ± 0.36	0.90 ± 0.35
after (8 wk)	11.23 ± 0.38	33.32 ± 1.56	1.92 ± 0.12	0.00 ± 0.00
ω3D before	5.83 ± 0.96	27.04 ± 2.78	0.00 ± 0.00	2.92 ± 0.63
after (1 wk)	5.94 ± 0.31	22.39 ± 1.09	1.61 ± 0.08	1.79 ± 0.19
after (2 wk)	8.67 ± 0.98	26.48 ± 1.94	1.68 ± 0.08	1.78 ± 0.34
after (8 wk)	8.42 ± 0.99	30.37 ± 3.32	1.72 ± 0.20	0.00 ± 0.00

2.5. Comparison of Intestinal And Liver Data

In the case of the four long-chain polyunsaturated ω3 fatty acids, there was a highly significant positive correlation ($r = + 0.8975$; $n = 16$; $p < 0.001$) between the mean values for the relative weight content of a given fatty acid in jejunal and liver phospholipids in the rats examined before the switch in diet and one week thereafter, with only two (out of sixteen) negative xy products. More importantly, however, even when the individual measurements recorded in each group of 4 rats were expressed relative to the mean value found for the same variable in the same group of rats, in order to rule out any group effect, there remained a significant correlation between these normalized values for jejunal and hepatic data. More precisely, such a comparison was restricted to the data relative to the C22:5ω3 and C22:6ω3 content of phospholipids since, in this case, only these measurements concerning the C22:5ω3 content of phospholipids in the ω3D rats examined before the switch in diet were not taken into account because of the null values recorded at the jejunal level. Under these analytical conditions, a significant positive correlation ($r = + 0.4932$; $n = 28$; $p < 0.009$) indeed prevailed between the individual normalized values for the relative weight content of C22:5ω3 and C22:6ω3 in jejunal and hepatic phospholipids.

In the case of the seven long-chain polyunsaturated ω6 fatty acids, there was also a highly significant positive correlation ($r = + 0.6395$; $n = 28$; $p < 0.001$) between the mean values for the relative weight content of a given fatty acid in jejunal and liver phospholipids in the rats examined before the switch in diet and one week thereafter, with only one (out of 28) negative xy product. Moreover and once again, a significant positive correlation ($r = + 0.3794$; $n = 32$; $p < 0.04$) was also observed between selected normalized values (see above) for the relative weight content of long-chain polyunsaturated ω6 fatty acids in jejunal and liver phospholipids. In this case, the just mentioned correlation concerned both C18:2ω6 and C20:4ω6, selected as the two most abundant ω6 fatty acids in both jejunal and liver phospholipids.

In the case of both saturated and monodesaturated fatty acids, significant positive correlations were also observed between the normalized values for the relative weight content of a given fatty acid in jejunal and liver phospholipids. For instance, in the case of C14:0 and C16:1ω7, respectively, the correlation coefficient between normalized values ($n = 16$ in both cases) amounted to + 0.6400 ($p < 0.009$) and + 0.6066 ($p < 0.02$).

Taken as a whole, these findings are compatible with a tight alignment, at the individual level and independently of any group effect, of the relative abundance of selected fatty acids in jejunal and liver phospholipids. In this respect, it should be emphasized that the dispersion of the normalized values was often quite modest. To cite only one example, the variation coefficient (i.e. the SD/mean ratio) of the normalized values relative to the C20:4ω6 weight content of liver phospholipids did not exceed 6.0% in the 16 rats (control animals and ω3D rats) examined before the switch in diet and one week thereafter.

3. Fatty Acid Profile or RBC Phospholipids

3.1. Long-Chain Polyunsaturated Ω3 Fatty Acids

Before the switch in diet, the C18:3ω3 relative weight content of RBC phospholipids was higher ($p < 0.005$) in the control animals than in the ω3D rats. Whilst, in the control animals, the C18:3ω3 relative weight content of RBC phospholipids was lower ($p < 0.02$) after 8 weeks exposure to the fish oil diet than before such a switch, the mean value recorded in the ω3D rats after the switch in diet (1.64 ± 0.05‰; $n = 6$) was higher ($p < 0.01$) than that recorded in the ω3D rats examined at the end of the 3 months initial period (Table 9). This coincided with the fact that the C18:3ω3 relative content of the fish oil diet (1.2%) was lower than that of the soya oil diet (7.1%), but higher than that of the sunflower oil diet (0.2%).

Before the switch in diet, the C20:5ω3 and C22:6ω3 content of RBC phospholipid was again lower in ω3D rats than in control animals. It progressively increased after the switch in diet, eventually reaching in both control animals and ω3D rats much higher values than those recorded before the switch in diet. Once again, this coincided with the higher relative content of C20:5ω3 (7.1%), C22:5ω3 (1.3%) and C22:6ω3 (13.4%) in the fish oil diet, as distinct from soya oil diet and sunflower oil diet, which both did not contain any detectable amount of these three ω3 fatty acids.

Table 9. Relative weight content (‰) of long-chain polyunsaturated ω3 fatty acids in RBC phospholipids

Rats	C18:3ω3	C20:5ω3	C22:5ω3	C22:6ω3
Control before	2.11±0.14	4.33±0.57	19.11±0.63	68.11±1.39
after (1wk)	1.70 (1)	26.93 (1)	21.00 (1)	79.20 (1)
after (2wk)	1.80 (1)	37.08 (1)	21.39 (1)	84.42 (1)
after (8wk)	0.45±0.45	82.71±2.36	39.61±0.87	108.57±6.81
ω3D before	0.62±0.36	0.00±0.00	1.82±0.14	19.76±1.12
after (1wk)	1.83 (1)	15.31 (1)	6.67 (1)	50.09 (1)
after (2wk)	1.66 (1)	20.64 (1)	12.03 (1)	68.93 (1)
after (8wk)	1.59±0.04	50.10±5.59	32.97±1.16	111.56±3.75

3.2. Long-Chain Polyunsaturated Ω6 Fatty Acids

Before the switch in diet, only the C22:4ω6 and C22:5ω6 relative weight contents of RBC phospholipids were significantly higher ($p < 0.001$) in ω3D rats than in control animals (Table 10). Surprisingly, the C20:3ω6 content progressively increased after the switch in diet, whether in control animals or ω3D rats, with an overall mean value for the difference in content before the switch in diet and 8 weeks thereafter of 1.65 ± 0.59‰ ($p < 0.02$). In the case of C18:2ω6, C20:4ω6, C22:4ω6 and C22:5ω6, a progressive decrease in relative weight content was always observed after the switch in diet, whether in control animals or ω3D rats. This coincided with the much lower content of the precursor C18:2ω6 fatty acid in the fish oil diet (2.0%) than in either the soya oil diet (56.5%) or sunflower roil diet (65.6%).

Table 10. Relative weight content (‰) of long-chain polyunsaturated ω6 fatty acids in RBC phospholipids

Rats	C18:2ω6	C18:3ω6	C20:2ω6	C20:3ω6	C20:4ω6	C22:4ω6	C22:5ω6
Control before	80.09±4.08	0.17±0.17	0.00±0.00	4.44±0.20	330.00±6.00	13.35±0.79	5.48±0.31
after (1wk)	52.29 (1)	0.00 (1)	0.00 (1)	4.35 (1)	291.24 (1)	11.68	3.90 (1)
after (2wk)	55.05 (1)	0.00 (1)	0.00 (1)	5.20 (1)	266.00 (1)	10.19	3.77 (1)
after (8wk)	45.65±2.80	0.00±0.00	0.00±0.00	6.32±1.01	201.44±3.35	0.00±0.00	0.00±0.00
ω3D before	78.13±0.51	0.22±0.22	0.00±0.00	3.69±0.22	341.09±10.40	25.21±0.43	31.37±3.66
after (1wk)	52.78 (1)	0.00 (1)	1.29 (1)	3.93 (1)	328.63 (1)	19.63 (1)	17.30 (1)
after (2wk)	51.02 (1)	0.00 (1)	0.00 (1)	4.52 (1)	314.25 (1)	16.73 (1)	14.51 (1)
after (8wk)	46.99±2.53	0.00±0.00	0.00±0.00	5.11±0.60	243.28±8.96	3.38±0.08	1.89±0.19

3.3. Saturated Fatty Acids

A sizeable amount of C12:0 (0.40‰) was only detected in one out of 20 samples.

The C10:0 relative weight content of RBC phospholipids averaged 0.19 ± 0.13‰ (n = 8) before the switch in diet. Thereafter, it increased ($p < 0.001$) to 0.95 ± 0.11‰ (n = 12), without any significant difference between the various groups of rats. Only one minor difference was encountered when comparing the data collected before the switch in diet in control animals and ω3D rats (Table 11). Thus, the C18:0 content was slightly higher ($p < 0.04$) in ω3D rats than in control animals. Likewise, significant changes after the switch in diet were only observed in a few instances. For instance, the C14:0 content was, in both control animals and ω3D rats, higher ($p < 0.001$) after the switch in diet (2.19 ± 0.08‰; n = 12) than before such a switch (1.43 ± 0.04‰; n = 8). In the control animals, the C16:0 content was also higher ($p < 0.002$) after the switch in diet (229.76 ± 1.90‰; n = 12) than before such a switch (212.94 ± 3.33‰; n = 4). Last, in the control animals and ω3D rats, the C20:0 content decreased ($p < 0.001$) from a mean value of 1.19 ± 0.04‰ (n = 8) before the switch in diet to 0.91 ± 0.04‰ (n = 8) eight weeks thereafter.

Table 11. Relative weight content (‰) of saturated fatty acids in RBC phospholipids

Rats	C14:0	C16:0	C18:0	C20:0	C22:0	C24:0
Control before	1.56±0.04	212.94±3.33	179.33±2.25	1.15±0.04	6.38±0.26	15.03±0.77
after (1wk)	2.12 (1)	230.03 (1)	185.28 (1)	1.28 (1)	7.20 (1)	16.32 (1)
after (2wk)	2.07 (1)	227.16 (1)	192.22 (1)	1.18 (1)	6.97 (1)	18.16 (1)
after (8wk)	2.42±0.07	230.34±2.89	184.66±2.82	0.85±0.02	5.14±0.16	15.77±1.06
ω3D before	1.50±0.06	219.93±8.24	189.75±3.12	1.23±0.08	6.52±0.33	13.46±0.52
after (1wk)	2.18 (1)	219.92 (1)	193.41 (1)	1.13 (1)	7.17 (1)	15.18 (1)
after (2wk)	1.75 (1)	217.48 (1)	185.11 (1)	1.06 (1)	7.27 (1)	19.44 (1)
after (8wk)	2.11±0.16	226.37±3.98	180.76±1.27	0.97±0.07	5.74±0.34	15.24±0.92

Table 12. Relative weight content of monodesaturated fatty acids in RBC phospholipids

Rats	C16:1ω7	C18:1ω9	C20:1ω9	C22:1ω9
Control before	2.80±0.28	53.99±2.36	0.00±0.00	0.00±0.00
after (1wk)	4.22 (1)	55.44 (1)	1.81 (1)	0.00 (1)
after (2wk)	4.87 (1)	58.88 (1)	2.32 (1)	0.00 (1)
after (8wk)	0.50±0.17	69.97±2.29	3.87±0.12	0.00±0.00
ω3Dbefore	2.58±0.41	52.91±2.47	0.00±0.00	8.14±0.20
after (1wk)	0.00 (1)	52.29 (1)	1.69 (1)	7.26 (1)
after (2wk)	4.16 (1)	55.06 (1)	2.29 (1)	0.00 (1)
after (8wk)	0.00±0.00	65.91±0.87	3.63±0.27	1.01±0.24

3.4. Monodesaturated Fatty Acids

The most obvious difference between control animals and ω3D rats examined before the switch in diet consisted in the higher C22:1ω9 content of RBC phospholipids ($p < 0.001$) in the latter rats than in the former animals. After the switch in diet, progressive increases in the C18:1ω9 and C20:1ω9 of RBC phospholipids were observed in both control animals and ω3D rats. The high initial content of C22:1ω9 in the latter ω3D rats eventually reached close-to-null values after the switch in diet (Table 12).

3.5. Comparison of Liver and RBC Data

The comparison of the relative weight content of long-chain polyunsaturated ω3 fatty acids in liver and RBC phospholipids revealed three sets of findings suggesting a transfer of information from the liver to the RBC.

First, in both control animals and ω3D rats, the enrichment of phospholipids in C20:5ω3, C22:5ω3 and C22:6ω3 progressed more slowly in RBC than in liver. Thus relative to the mean increment recorded 8 weeks after the switch in diet in the same type of rats (control animals or ω3D rats), that observed after only one week exposure to the fish oil diet averaged 24.1 ± 3.9% ($n = 6$) in RBC as distinct ($p < 0.001$) from 55.9 ± 5.2% ($n = 6$) in the liver. Likewise, after two weeks exposure to the fish oil diet, such increments averaged 36.8 ± 5.8% ($n = 6$) in RBC as distinct ($p < 0.004$) from 66.9 ± 4.8% ($n = 6$) in the liver.

A second argument to suggest a delayed alignment of RBC to liver data resulted for the paired comparison in each rat of the normalized value for the relative weight content of each ω3 fatty acid in liver and RBC phospholipids (Table 13). Such normalized values are taken as the individual value found in each rat relative to the mean value recorded in the same group of four rats, in order to rule out any group effect. Whether in the case of C20:5ω3, C22:5ω3 or C22:6ω3 highly significant correlations ($p < 0.001$ in all cases) were found between the liver and RBC normalized values collected in the control animals and ω3D rats examined before the switch in diet and 8 weeks therefore, with 16 sets of data for each ω3 fatty acid. As indicated in Table 13, the few negative xy products related to 12 out of 48 individual comparisons, in which the individual deviation (Δ) from the 100% reference value did not exceed 4.4 ± 0.9% ($n = 24$) as distinct ($p < 0.02$) from a mean deviation of 17.3 ± 3.0% ($n = 64$) in the case of the 32 positive xy products.

Table 13. Comparison of the normalized values for ω3 fatty acids in liver and RBC phospholipids

Variable	C20:5ω3	C22:5ω3	C22:6ω3
Correlation coefficient	+ 0.9640	+ 0.8371	+ 0.7713
p value	< 0.001	< 0.001	< 0.001
Liver variation coefficient (%)	30.99	47.52	10.15
RBC variation coefficient (%)	15.70	8.57	8.35
Negative xy (n)	2/16	6/16	4/16
Negative Δ (10^{-2})	0.95±0.23 (4)	5.94±1.46 (12)	3.88±0.95 (8)
Positive Δ (10^{-2})	23.22±4.39 (20)	21.86±8.06 (20)	8.46±1.13 (24)
ΔRBC/Δliver (%)	49.75±6.44 (10)	32.95±7.68 (10)	127.43±17.50 (12)

A further argument emerged from the finding that the coefficient of variation was always higher for the normalized liver data than for the normalized RBC data. Such a difference was most modest with C22:6ω3, in which case the paired ratio between the RBC/liver Δ yielded, in the comparisons with a positive xy product, a mean value (1.27 ± 0.18; n = 12) not significantly different from unity ($p > 0.15$). In the case of C20:5ω3 and C22:6ω3 however, the same ratio between the RBC/liver Δ averaged, respectively, 0.50 ± 0.06 (n = 10) and 0.33 ± 0.08 (n = 10), these two mean values being both significantly different from unity ($p < 0.001$). The latter finding clearly indicates that, at least in the case of C20:5ω3 and C22:6ω3, the dispersion of individual values within the same group of rats represents in RBC an attenuated and, hence, likely consequential picture of that prevailing in liver.

It should be underlined that a comparable situation prevailed when only those data collected in the control animals and ω3D rats examined at the end of the 3 months initial period, hence under presumably steady-state conditions, were taken into account. For instance, in the comparison concerning the normalized values for the relative weight content of long-chain polyunsaturated ω3 fatty acids in liver and RBC, significant positive correlations were recorded in the case of C20:5ω3 (r = + 0.9816; n = 8; $p < 0.001$), C22:5ω3 (r = + 0.8790; n = 8; $p < 0.001$) and C22:6ω3 (r = + 0.8879; n = 8; $p < 0.005$). Moreover, the variation coefficients were always lower for the BC data than for the liver data, averaging in the first case 12.2 ± 2.8% (n = 3), i.e. a value representing no more than 45.4 ± 14.3% (n = 3; $p < 0.07$) of that recorded for the same ω3 fatty acids in the liver (36.6 ± 16.1%; n = 3). Such a difference became highly significant, with a RBC/liver ratio for the variation coefficient averaging 59.7 ± 0.1% (n = 2; $p < 0.001$) when considering only the C20:5ω3 and C22:6ω3 data.

Comparable observations were made in the case of selected long-chain polyunsaturated ω6 fatty acids. Indeed, in the case of several long-chain polyunsaturated ω6 fatty acids, the alignment of RBC to liver phospholipids was also obviously delayed. In this respect, the salient exception concerned the precursor C18:2ω6 fatty acid. In this case, the decrement recorded one to two weeks after the switch in diet, when expressed relative to the decrement recorded for the same fatty acid in the same type of rats (control animals or ω3D rats) indeed failed to differ significantly ($p > 0.3$) in RBC (80.3 ± 3.0%; n = 4) and liver (97.0 ± 15.5%; n = 4). Pooling all available data collected in the case of C18:2ω6, C20:4ω6, C22:4ω6 and C22:5ω6 the decrement in the relative weight content of a given fatty acid, as judged from the mean values recorded at each time point and as expressed relative to the decrement found in the same type of rats (control animals or ω3D rats) 8 weeks after the switch in diet averaged, in the liver phospholipids, 75.0 ± 5.8% (n = 8) and 87.0 ± 8.8% (n = 8), respectively, one and two days after the switch in diet. With the already mentioned exception of C18:2ω6, much lower percentages were recorded in the RBC than in the liver. Thus, in the case of C20:4ω6, C22:4ω6 and C22:5ω6, the decrements recorded one to two days after the switch in diet (always expressed relative to those found eight weeks after the switch in diet) only represented in RBC 41.9 ± 4.3% (n = 12; $p < 0.001$) of the corresponding value found under the same experimental conditions in liver phospholipids.

Moreover, there were also highly significant positive correlations between the normalized values for either C20:4ω6 (r = + 0.7139; n = 16; $p < 0.004$) or C22:5ω6 (r = + 0.8689; n = 12; $p < 0.001$) in the liver and RBC phospholipids of the control animals and ω3D rats examined before the switch in diet or 8 weeks thereafter. In the case of C22:5ω6, the data collected in the control animals 8 weeks after the switch in diet were not taken into account, however, since null values were recorded in the RBC phospholipids of these four control animals. When the results collected in the case of C22:4ω6 (at the exclusion of the same four control rats examined 8 weeks after the switch in diet and again displaying null values in their RBC phospholipids) were pooled together with those obtained for C20:4ω6 and C22:5ω6, a highly significant positive correlation ($r = + 0.7703$; $n = 40$; $p < 0.001$) was again documented between the normalized values in liver and RBC phospholipids.

Last, as already noticed in the case of the long-chain polyunsaturated ω3 fatty acids, the variation coefficients for the normalized values were always higher in the liver than in the RBC, the difference between liver and RBC being most obvious in the case of C20:4ω6 and C22:5ω6 and averaging, in these two instances, 6.93 ± 0.39% ($n = 2$; $p < 0.05$), with overall mean values for the three ω6 fatty acid under consideration of 14.32 ± 4.41% ($n = 3$) in liver and 9.14 ± 3.33% ($n = 3$) in RBC and a mean paired RBC/liver ratio of 63.7 ± 11.1% ($n = 3$).

Selected findings based on the measurements of the relative weight content of saturated and monodesaturated fatty acids in liver and RBC phospholipids provided further support to the concepts here under consideration. First, when comparing the time course for the enrichment of C20:1ω9 in liver and RBC phospholipids, the increment reached one and two day after the switch in diet averaged, in the RBC phospholipids, respectively 46.7 ± 0.1% and 61.4 ± 1.7% ($n = 2$ in both cases) of that reached in the same type of rats (control animals or ω3D rats) 8 weeks after the switch in diet as distinct ($p < 0.01$ or less) from corresponding values of 89.9 ± 3.7% and 96.6 ± 1.0% ($n = 2$ in both cases) in the liver. In other words, the increments (Δ) reached in RBC phospholipids compared to those reached at the same time and in the same type of rats in liver phospholipids and all expressed relative to the corresponding increment recorded 8 weeks after the switch in diet yielded a mean RBC/liver Δ ratio averaging 57.8 ± 3.5% ($n = 4$; $p < 0.002$). Second, significant positive correlations were found between the individual normalized values for the relative weight content of some saturated or monodesaturated fatty acids in liver and RBC phospholipids. For instance, the data relative to the C14:0 content of liver and RBC phospholipids recorded before the switch in diet and 8 weeks thereafter in either control animals or ω3D rats indeed yielded, for the relevant normalized values, a significant positive correlation ($r = + 0.5860$; $n = 16$; $p < 0.03$). Likewise, the data relative to the C16:1ω7 content of liver and RBC phospholipid recorded before the switch in diet in both control animals and ω3D rats again yielded a significant positive correlation between normalized values ($r = + 0.9059$; $n = 8$; $p < 0.003$). Moreover, in these two instances, the variation coefficient for the normalized values was higher in liver than in RBC, with a paired difference of 10.2 ± 0.3% ($n = 2$; $p < 0.025$). At this point, it should be underlined that the comparison between the data relative to the C16:1ω7 relative weight content of liver and RBC phospholipids was restricted to the measurements made before the switch in diet, because of the high prevalence (5 out of 8 measurements) of null values in RBC phospholipids eight weeks after the switch in diet. Hence, the tight individual coupling between liver and RBC phospholipid fatty acid profile was also operative under close to steady-state conditions, such as those presumably prevailing after 3 months exposure to a given diet. As a matter of fact, the latter view was supported by the analysis of the C20:5ω3, C22:5ω3 and C22:6ω3 relative weight content of liver and RBC phospholipids in the control animals and ω3D rats examined at the end of the 3 months initial period and, hence, before any switch in diet (see above).

4. Fatty Acid Profile of Brain Phospholipids

4.1. Long-Chain Polyunsaturated Ω3 Fatty Acids

Table 14. Relative weight content (‰) of long-chain polyunsaturated ω3 fatty acids in brain phospholipids

Rats	C18:3ω3	C20:5ω3	C22:5ω3	C22:6ω3
Control before	0.00±0.00	0.00±0.00	2.29±0.04	235.93±6.60
after (1wk)	0.00±0.00	0.22±0.22	3.01±0.07	227.20±6.88
after (8wk)	0.00±0.00	2.35±0.36	6.23±0.48	233.37±3.72
ω3Dbefore	0.00±0.00	0.00±0.00	0.00±0.00	186.65±5.01
after (1wk)	0.00±0.00	0.00±0.00	2.13±0.16	201.84±3.23
after (8wk)	0.00±0.00	0.53±0.31	4.39±0.12	231.88±5.91

No C18:3ω3 was detected in any of the 24 samples of brain phospholipids (Table 14). A sizeable amount of C20:5ω3 was only detected in one out of 8 samples obtained one week after the switch in diet, i.e. in a control animal and, in 6 out of 8 samples obtained 8 weeks after the switch in diet, i.e. in all four control animals and two ω3D rats. The C22:5ω3 and C22:6ω3 relative weight content of brain phospholipids was lower ($p < 0.002$ or less) in the ω3D rats than in the control animals examined before the switch in diet. After the switch in diet, the C22:5ω3 content of brain phospholipids increased in both control animals and ω3D rats, but remained lower ($p < 0.001$) in the latter rats than in the former animals, averaging in the ω3D rats 70.6 ± 2.6% (n = 8) of the mean values recorded at the same time after the switch in diet in the control animals (100.0 ± 3.7%; n = 8). Last, the C22:6ω3 relative weight content of brain phospholipids progressively increased after the switch in diet in the ω3D rats ($p < 0.002$), eventually reaching after 8 weeks exposure to the fish oil diet a mean value virtually identical to that recorded at the same time in control animals (Table 14).

4.2. Long-Chain Polyunsaturated Ω6 Fatty Acids

Before the switch in diet, only the relative weight content of C22:5ω6 differed significantly ($p < 0.001$) in control animals and ω3D rats (Table 15). After the switch in diet, the mean C20:3ω6 content of brain phospholipids was higher than that recorded before such a switch. Such an increase only achieved statistical significance ($p < 0.05$) in the control animals, the measurements made after the switch in diet averaging 120.6 ± 5.9% (n = 8) of the mean corresponding value found before such a switch. All five other ω6 fatty acids displayed a progressive decrease after the switch in diet. In the case of C18:2ω6, C20:2ω6, C20:4ω6 and C22:4ω6, the measurements collected one and eight weeks after the switch in diet, expressed relative to those recorded for the same ω6 fatty acid in the same type of rats (control animals or ω3D rats) before the switch in diet averaged 94.4 ± 1.8% (n = 32) and 79.3 ± 2.2% (n = 32), respectively, as compared to a reference value of 100.0 ± 2.1% (n = 32). Thus, a significant decrease ($p < 0.05$) was already observed after one week exposure to the fish oil diet, followed by a further decrease ($p < 0.001$) after eight weeks exposure to the same diet. Lower mean percentages were recorded in the control animals in the case of C22:5ω6, i.e. 76.6 ± 5.8% (n = 4; p < 0.05) and 62.2 ± 9.9% (n = 4; p < 0.025), one and eight weeks after the switch in diet, as compared to a reference value of 100.0 ± 7.4% (n = 4). The former two percentages were indeed lower (p < 0.02 or less) than those mentioned above for the four other ω6 fatty acids. Last, an even more pronounced relative decrease was observed in the case of C22:5ω6 in the ω3D rats, i.e. 61.0 ± 5.2% (n = 4) and 15.3 ± 1.4% (n = 4), one and eight weeks after the switch in diet, as compared to a reference value of 100.0 ± 6.4% (n = 4). The relative magnitude of the decrease in the C22:5ω6 content of brain phospholipids was thus indeed more pronounced (p < 0.005) in the ω3D rats than in the control animals examined after eight weeks exposure to the fish oil diet.

Table 15. Relative weight content (‰) of long-chain polyunsaturated ω6 fatty acids in brain phospholipids

Rats	C18:2ω6	C20:2ω6	C20:3ω6	C20:4ω6	C22:4ω6	C22:5ω6
Control before	7.16±0.39	1.31±0.06	2.48±0.09	131.66±6.04	26.85±1.70	3.12±0.23
after (1wk)	6.51±0.61	1.35±0.10	2.90±0.26	120.43±4.65	25.93±0.90	2.39±0.18
after (8wk)	4.55±0.18	1.16±0.08	3.08±0.16	111.14±7.33	22.68±1.02	1.94±0.31
ω3D before	6.27±0.58	1.34±0.14	2.07±0.21	137.94±7.23	30.21±1.63	22.94±1.46
after (1wk)	5.62±0.21	1.32±0.06	3.18±0.86	124.50±4.60	28.74±1.51	13.99±1.19
after (8wk)	5.17±0.18	1.20±0.03	2.54±0.15	104.93±6.62	19.81±1.75	3.52±0.33

4.3. Saturated Fatty Acids

The sole consistent difference in the relative weight content of saturated fatty acids concerned the rapid increase in the C20:0, C22:0 and C24:0 relative content of brain phospholipids observed after the switch in diet (Table 16). In the control animals, the values recorded after the switch in diet averaged 149.2 ± 7.8% (n = 24; p < 0.001) of the mean corresponding values found before such a switch (100.0 ± 3.4%; n = 12). In the ω3D rats, however, the mean value recorded after the switch in diet (109.9 ± 4.7%; n = 24) was no more significantly different (p > 0.28) from that found before the switch to the fish oil diet (100.0 ± 8.9%; n = 12). Such changes represented a mirror image of those found in either liver or RBC phospholipids.

Table 16. Relative weight content (‰) if saturated fatty acids in brain phospholipids

Rats	C14:0	C16:0	C18:0	C20:0	C22:0	C24:0
Control before	1.03±0.06	228.96±6.45	184.97±2.01	3.06±0.14	2.90±0.18	6.90±0.58
after (1wk)	0.94±0.03	200.38±7.24	189.93±1.32	4.24±0.51	4.68±0.82	10.85±1.43
after (8wk)	0.92±0.04	202.12±6.41	187.77±1.22	4.40±0.47	4.55±0.68	9.51±1.24
ω3D before	1.11±0.07	232.34±6.19	188.85±2.19	3.44±0.38	3.54±0.80	8.65±1.62
after (1wk)	1.08±0.09	215.94±5.10	191.13±1.47	4.04±0.33	4.26±0.43	10.27±1.12
after (8wk)	1.27±0.09	239.91±11.56	175.22±1.73	3.71±0.35	3.62±0.43	8.02±1.07

4.4. Monodesaturated Fatty Acids

Table 17. Relative weight content (‰) of monodesaturated fatty acids in brain phospholipids

Rats	C16:1ω7	C18:1ω9	C20:1ω9	C22:1ω9
Control before	3.20±0.16	149.78±3.34	8.39±1.01	0.00±0.00
after (1wk)	3.47±0.04	180.94±11.22	13.69±2.56	0.91±0.91
after (8wk)	3.81±0.07	183.93±10.54	13.88±2.67	2.67±0.57
ω3D before	3.05 ±0.24	161.33±13.22	9.70±2.38	0.58±0.58
after (1wk)	3.36±0.16	176.11±9.41	11.41±1.49	1.06±0.65
after (8wk)	4.13±0.09	177.74±8.12	10.82±1.64	1.57±0.53

Before the switch in diet, no significant difference between control animals and ω3D rats was observed in terms of the relative weight content of monodesaturated fatty acids (C16:1ω7, C18:1ω9, C20:1ω9 and C22:1ω9) in brain phospholipids (Table 17). The mean values recorded after the switch in diet were always higher than those found before such a switch. Such a difference, expressed in terms of the relative weight content (‰) of brain phospholipids was often more pronounced in the control animals than in the ω3D rats. Thus, in the case of C18:1ω9, C20:1ω9 and C22:1ω9, the increments recorded in the ω3D rats after 8 weeks exposure to the fish oil diet only represented 35.2 ± 24.0% ($p < 0.05$) of those recorded for the same monodesaturated fatty acid in the control animals (100.0 ± 25.0%). Nevertheless, when pooling together the results recorded in the control animals and ω3D rats, the increase in the relative weight content observed 8 weeks after the switch in diet above the values measured before such a switch achieved statistical significance in the case of C16:1ω7 ($p < 0.001$), C18:1ω9 ($p < 0.025$) and C22:1ω9 ($p < 0.005$). Only the increase in the C20:1ω9 content of brain phospholipids failed to achieve statistical significance ($p > 0.10$).

4.5. Comparison of Liver and Brain Data

In the seven rats displaying a sizeable amount of C20:5ω3 in brain phospholipids, a positive correlation ($r = + 0.7466$; $n = 7$; $p < 0.06$) prevailed between the relative weight content of this ω3 fatty acid in liver and brain phospholipids. The correlation line between these two variables yielded a positive intercept with the abscissa (39.40‰), suggesting a kind of threshold phenomenon for the accumulation of C20:5ω3 in brain phospholipids as a function of the C20:5ω3 relative weight content of liver phospholipids.

As illustrated in Fig. 1, highly significant positive correlations were found between the liver and brain relative content of either C22:5ω3 ($r = + 0.9040$; $n = 24$; $p < 0.001$) or C22:6ω3 ($r = + 0.6765$; $n = 24$; $p < 0.001$). The pattern of such relationships differed, however, with these two ω3 fatty acids. Indeed, whilst the C22:5ω3 data follow a pattern close to a rule of proportionality, the C22:6ω3 relationship displayed an obvious intercept with the ordinates, suggesting that a regulatory process operative in the brain favoured the maintenance of a close-to-normal C22:6ω3 content in brain phospholipids at the expense of null values for all other three long-chain polyunsaturated ω3 fatty acids (C18:3ω3, C20:5ω3 and C22:5ω3), as already documented by the data listed in Table 14. No significant correlation was found, however, between the normalized values for the C22:5ω3 (r = + 0.0247; n = 24) or C22:6ω3 (r = 0.0000; n = 24) relative weight content of liver and brain phospholipids.

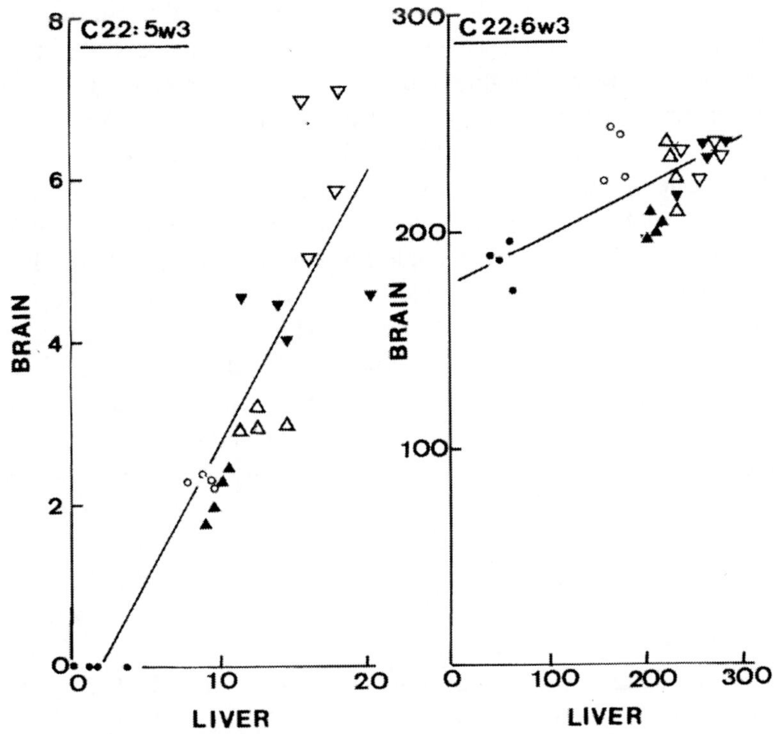

Figure 1. Relationship between the relative weight content (‰) of C22:5ω3 (left panel) and C22:6ω3 (right panel) in brain *versus* liver phospholipids in control animals (open symbols) and ω3D rats (closed symbols) examined before the switch to the fish oil diet (circles) and either one week (triangles pointing upwards) or eight week (triangles pointing downwards) thereafter. The oblique lines correspond to the regression lines.

The time course for the enrichment of brain phospholipids in long-chain polyunsaturated ω3 fatty acids was delayed relative to that observed in liver phospholipids. Thus, in the brain, even if ignoring the data relative to the C22:6ω3 content of brain phospholipids in the control animals, which failed to display any increase above the initial value recorded at the end of the 3 months initial period, the mean increment above the latter initial value reached after one week exposure to the fish oil diet, as expressed relative to the corresponding mean increment observed after 8 weeks exposure to the fish oil diet, did not exceed 21.5 ± 8.7% (n = 5), as distinct ($p < 0.007$) from 56.3 ± 1.5% (n = 6) in the liver. The brain/liver ratio for the increments found one week after the switch in diet and expressed as just indicated averaged 35.1 ± 13.4% (n = 5; $p < 0.009$ *versus* unity) with each fatty acid in each type of rats (control animals or ω3D rats). Moreover, the values recorded in the brain did not differ significantly ($p > 0.56$ or more) from those prevailing in RBC, i.e. 24.1 ± 3.9% (n = 6) for the week-1/week-8 incremental ratio and 44.5 ± 8.8% (n = 6) for the paired RBC/liver ratio between corresponding relative increments.

In the case of the five long-chain polyunsaturated ω6 fatty acids undergoing a progressive decrease of their relative weight content in brain phospholipids (C18:2ω6, C20:2ω6, C20:4ω6, C22:4ω6 and C22:5ω6), there was an obvious delay in the alignment of the brain data on the liver data. Thus, for these five ω6 fatty acids, the decrement observed one week after the switch in diet above the mean corresponding value found for the same fatty acid and in the same type of rats (control animals or ω3D rats), when expressed relative to the corresponding decrement recorded eight weeks after the switch in diet, averaged 31.1 ± 8.6% (n = 10) in brain, as compared ($p < 0.001$) to 81.3 ± 7.3% (n = 10) in liver. The values relative to such a fractional decrement represented in the brain 45.3 ± 11.5% (n = 10; $p < 0.002$) of the corresponding value found for the same ω6 fatty acid in the same type of rats.

The correlation between the normalized values for the relative weight content of C20:4ω6, C22:4ω6 and C22:5ω6 in liver and brain phospholipids barely reached significance in the case of C20:4ω6 (r = + 0.4090; n = 24; $p < 0.05$), whilst failing to do so in the case of C22:4ω6 (r = - 0.1445; n = 24) or C22:5ω6 (r = + 0.0355; n = 24), yielding a mean value for the correlation coefficients not exceeding + 0.1000 ± 0.1630 (n = 3). When pooling together these three sets of comparisons, the correlation coefficient was as low as – 0.0012 (n = 72). In other words, the obvious positive correlations found between the liver and brain values for the relative weight content of C20:4ω6 (r = + 0.7144; n = 24; $p < 0.001$), C22:4ω6 (r = + 0.5488; n = 24; $p < 0.008$) and C22:5ω6 (r = + 0.8566; n = 24; $p < 0.001$) reflected largely a group effect, whilst often failing to achieve statistical significance at the individual level within each group of rats, as assessed by the analysis of the corresponding normalized values.

It should not be ignored, however, that, in the analysis of the results obtained either separately for each of these three ω6 fatty acids or for the pooled data, the variation coefficient for the normalized values was always lower in brain than in liver, with a mean brain/liver ratio averaging (geometric mean) 49.7 ± 13.3% (n = 4; $p < 0.04$). Incidentally, such was also the case with the absolute values for the relative weight content of the concerned ω6 fatty acids, with a mean brain/liver ratio for the variation coefficients averaging 36.9 ± 10.2% (n = 3; $p < 0.03$).

The data concerning the relative weight content of saturated fatty acids provided another indication of the occasional dissociation between liver and brain data. First, as already mentioned, the changes in the C20:0, C22:0 and C24:0 content of brain phospholipids after the switch in diet represented a mirror image of those found in the liver phospholipids. Second, no significant correlation was found between the normalized values of the C14:0 (r = + 0.0491; n = 24), C16:0 (r = - 0.0197; n = 24) or C18:0 (r = + 0.0518; n = 24) relative weight content in liver and brain phospholipids.

At the exception of C22:1ω9, which displayed opposite changes in response to the switch in diet in liver and brain, a highly significant positive mean correlation (0.4804 ± 0.0840; n = 72; $p < 0.001$) prevailed between the relative weight content of C16:1ω7, C18:1ω9 and C20:1ω9 in liver and brain phospholipids. Even the normalized values for the C16:1ω7 and C18:1ω9 relative weight content of liver and brain phospholipids yielded an overall significant positive correlation (r = + 0.4573 ± 0.1305; $p < 0.03$ or less). Moreover, the variation coefficient for such normalized values only represented, in brain, 52.8 ± 16.0% (n = 2) of that found in liver. No delayed alignment, however, of the brain phospholipid content in monodesaturated fatty acids on that of the liver phospholipid content in the same fatty acid was observed. In the liver, the increments recorded one week after the switch in diet, expressed relative to those found for the same monodesaturated fatty acid in the same type of rats (control animals or ω3D rats) did not exceed 61.6 ± 11.9% (n = 5), even after exclusion of three values yielding a negligible (n = 1) or negative (n = 2) increment after one week exposure to the fish oil diet. In the brain, such relative increments averaged 61.9 ± 11.2% (n = 7), even after exclusion of one day-1/day-8 incremental ratio exceeding unity (152.7%). Thus, in this analytical procedure, the day-1/day-8 incremental ratio for monodesaturated fatty acids was virtually identical ($p > 0.98$) in liver and brain phospholipids.

5. Fatty Acid Profile of Liver Triglycerides

The total fatty acid content of liver triglycerides was not significantly higher ($p > 0.89$) in ω3D rats (12.55 ± 1.19 mg/g wet wt.; n = 16) than in control animals (12.32 ± 1.35 mg/g wet wt.; n = 15).

5.1. Long-Chain Polyunsaturated Ω3 Fatty Acids

A sizeable amount of C18:4ω3 was only detected in two out of 32 samples, such being the case in two control animals. Before the switch in diet, the C18:3ω3, C20:5ω3, C22:5ω3 and C22:6ω3 relative weight content of liver triglycerides was always higher ($p < 0.02$ or less) in control animals than in ω3D rats. In the control animals, the C18:3ω3 relative weight content of liver triglycerides failed to differ significantly ($p > 0.43$) before the switch in diet (12.82 ± 2.96‰; n = 4) and thereafter (10.40 ± 1.44‰; n = 12). In all other instances, however, a pronounced increase of the long-chain polyunsaturated ω3 fatty acids relative weight content of liver triglycerides was observed after the switch in diet (Table 18). For instance, in the ω3D rats, the C18:3ω3 content of liver triglycerides increased ($p < 0.005$) from 1.81 ± 0.69‰ (n = 4) before the switch in diet to 4.54 ± 0.41‰ (n = 12) thereafter. Nevertheless, the latter value remained significantly lower ($p < 0.001$) than that recorded, also after the switch in diet, in the control animals. Such was not the case for C20:5ω3, C22:5ω3 and C22:6ω3, which reached, after the switch in diet, much higher values than those recorded in the control animals at the end of the initial 3 months period, such high values failing to differ significantly in control animals and ω3D rats ($p > 0.27$ or more).

Table 18. Relative weight content (‰) of long-chain polyunsaturated ω3 fatty acids in liver triglycerides

Rats	C18:3ω3	C20:5ω3	C22:5ω3	C22:6ω3
Control before	12.82±2.96	2.01±0.27	3.41±0.56	7.04±1.08
after (1wk)	8.51±1.42	12.17±3.59	10.52±3.37	28.85±7.51
after (2wk)	12.92±3.78	19.22±6.86	14.05±4.80	41.30±12.84
after (8wk)	9.76±1.73	20.94±5.62	14.58±4.39	43.14±10.10
ω3Dbefore	1.81±0.69	0.00±0.00	0.00±0.00	0.48±0.48
after (1wk)	5.26±0.39	12.74±2.33	12.72±2.01	38.49±6.01
after (2wk)	5.03±0.79	10.56±2.24	9.20±1.86	27.71±5.58
after (8wk)	3.32±0.54	17.02±2.86	15.45±2.24	50.65±7.79

5.2. Long-Chain Polyunsaturated Ω6 Fatty Acids

Before the switch in diet, no significant difference in the relative weight content of C18:2ω6, C18:3ω6, C20:2ω6, C20:3ω6 and C20:4ω6 in liver triglycerides was observed between control animals and ω3D rats, the measurements collected in the latter rats averaging 119.9 ± 14.3% ($n = 20$; $p > 0.2$) of the mean corresponding values found in the former control animals (100.0 ± 4.5%; $n = 20$). The C22:4ω6 ($p < 0.05$) and C22:5ω6 ($p < 0.005$) relative weight content of liver triglycerides were higher, however, in ω3D rats than in control animals, both examined before the switch in diet (Table 19). Thereafter, however, the relative weight content of all long-chain polyunsaturated ω6 fatty acids decreased, whether in control animals or ω3D rats, from a mean initial reference value of 100.0 ± 6.1% ($n = 56$) to 61.8 ± 15.6 % ($n = 56$; $p < 0.025$) after one week exposure to the fish oil diet, with a further decrease ($p < 0.04$) to 27.0 ± 3.8% ($n = 56$) after two weeks exposure to the fish oil diet. No further significant decrease ($p > 0.84$) in these overall mean values was observed after eight weeks exposure to the fish oil diet, at which time the results averaged 28.1 ± 4.2% ($n = 56$) of the mean corresponding initial values.

Table 19. Relative weight content (‰) of long-chain polyunsaturated ω6 fatty acids in liver triglycerides

Rats	C18:2ω6	C18:3ω6	C20:2ω6	C20:3ω6	C20:4ω6	C22:4ω6	C22:5ω6
Control before	235.21±34.54	5.35±0.38	1.78±0.09	1.65±0.22	20.14±2.57	2.61±0.63	0.73±0.45
after (1wk)	115.58±21.23	0.99±0.58	0.30±0.30	0.13±0.13	9.88±2.73	0.27±0.27	2.29±1.34
after (2wk)	99.94±35.53	0.32±0.32	0.53±0.30	0.18±0.18	11.08±2.75	1.26±0.61	0.00±0.00
after (8wk)	68.36±11.48	0.44±0.25	0.48±0.28	0.00±0.00	5.50±1.40	1.85±0.47	0.00±0.00
ω3D before	237.23±42.90	6.17±0.88	1.75±0.65	1.92±0.83	33.93±6.30	6.15±1.30	4.62±0.78
after (1wk)	170.71±32.64	2.04±0.71	0.83±0.48	1.81±0.62	20.85±3.16	3.64±0.48	1.48±0.65
after (2wk)	110.49±13.13	1.49±0.50	0.34±0.34	0.32±0.32	14.81±1.63	2.14±0.26	0.00±0.00
after (8wk)	97.39±26.02	0.85±0.53	0.86±0.50	0.95±0.55	10.84±2.23	2.45±0.36	0.25±0.25

5.3. Saturated Fatty Acids

The mean C12:0 relative weight content of liver triglycerides was lower ($p < 0.07$) in ω3D rats (0.22 ± 0.10‰; $n = 16$) than in control animals (0.63 ± 0.19‰; $n = 16$). Despite comparable values ($p > 0.85$) for the relative weight content of C14:0 in the liver triglycerides of control animals and ω3D rats examined before the switch in diet (Table 20), the higher values recorded thereafter yielded a mean value in the control animals (18.67 ± 0.86‰; $n = 12$) which exceeded ($p < 0.05$) that recorded in the ω3D rats (15.62 ± 1.10‰; $n = 12$). The two latter mean values were significantly higher ($p < 0.03$ or less) than the overall mean value recorded before the switch in diet (11.73 ± 1.06‰; $n = 8$). A possible explanation for these findings could be that, after the switch in diet, the food intake becomes lower in ω3D rats than in control animals. The measurements of the C16:0 relative weight content of liver triglycerides provided an information closely comparable to that just described in the case of C14:0. First, the mean relative weight content of C16:0 did not differ significantly ($p > 0.55$) in the control animals and ω3D rats examined before the switch in diet, with an overall mean value of 299.73 ± 12.14‰ (n = 8). Second, higher values were recorded after the switch in diet, whether in control animals ($p < 0.009$) or ω3D rats ($p < 0.05$). Third, the mean value reached after the switch in diet was lower, albeit not significantly so ($p > 0.25$) in ω3D rats (344.91 ± 14.58‰; n = 12) than in control animals (370.37 ± 17.38‰; n = 12). As a matter of fact, the difference between the mean values recorded after and before the switch in diet amounted to 37.34‰ and 78.46‰ in the ω3D rats and control animals, respectively, yielding a ω3D/control ratio of 47.6%. A comparable analysis of the data recorded with C14:0 yielded differences of 3.70‰ and 7.13‰ in ω3D rats and control animals and a ω3D/control ratio of 51.9%, virtually identical to that found with C16:0.

In the control animals, the C18:0 relative weight content of liver triglycerides was also higher ($p < 0.05$) after the switch in diet (28.52 ± 1.60‰; n = 12) than therefore (21.83 ± 2.40‰; n = 4). The former value was not significant different ($p > 0.76$) from that recorded in the ω3D rats before the switch in diet and identical to that reached in the ω3D rats after the switch in diet (28.52 ± 1.76‰; n = 12).

A sizeable amount of C20:0 was only detected in three control animals examined before the switch in diet (n = 2) or one week thereafter (n = 1). The C22:0 content of liver triglycerides averaged 0.30 ± 0.17‰ (n = 16) and 0.81 ± 0.30‰ (n = 16) in control animals and ω3D rats, such mean values failing to differ significantly from one another ($p > 0.15$). No C24:0 was detected in any of the 32 samples of liver triglycerides.

Table 20. Relative weight content (‰) of saturated fatty acids in liver triglycerides

Rats	C12:0	C14:0	C16:0	C18:0	C20:0	C22:0	C24:0
Control before	0.77±0.26	11.54±1.47	291.91±14.36	21.83±2.40	0.41±0.23	0.00±0.00	0.00±0.00
after (1wk)	0.71±0.51	19.60±1.33	381.39±32.13	27.30±2.42	0.10±0.10	0.02±0.02	0.00±0.00
after (2wk)	0.53±0.31	17.65±2.16	356.25±40.25	29.51±3.82	0.00±0.00	1.19±0.47	0.00±0.00
after (8wk)	0.51±0.30	18.76±0.98	373.47±23.68	28.76±2.59	0.00±0.00	0.00±0.00	0.00±0.00
ω3D before	0.21±0.21	11.92±1.75	307.56±20.99	29.56±3.48	0.00±0.00	0.66±0.38	0.00±0.00
after (1wk)	0.00±0.00	14.45±2.34	332.65±36.55	28.22±3.74	0.00±0.00	0.00±0.00	0.00±0.00
after (2wk)	0.00±0.00	16.26±0.76	344.18±10.58	25.07±1.41	0.00±0.00	2.57±0.39	0.00±0.00
after (8wk)	0.68±0.24	16.16±2.55	357.82±28.07	32.27±3.09	0.00±0.00	0.00±0.00	0.00±0.00

5.4. Monodesaturated Fatty Acids

The mean relative weight content of C18:1ω9 in the liver triglycerides did not differ significantly from one another in the eight groups of rats listed in Table 21.

The data concerning the C16:1ω7 and C20:1ω9 content of liver triglycerides provided comparable information. First, in the case of these two monodesaturated fatty acids, the relative weight content of liver triglycerides was somewhat lower, albeit not significantly so ($p > 0.48$ or more), in the ω3D rats than in the control animals examined before the switch in diet. Second, the mean values recorded after the switch in diet were always higher than those recorded before the switch in diet, whether in control animals or ω3D rats. Such increases averaged 20.65 ± 6.94‰ (df = 28; $p < 0.007$) and 4.04 ± 0.54‰ (df = 28; $p < 0.001$) in the case of C16:1ω7 and C20:1ω9 respectively. Last, in both cases, the mean values reached after the switch in diet were lower, albeit not significantly so, in the ω3D rats than in the control animals, averaging in the former rats 91.1 ± 4.8% ($n = 24$; $p > 0.22$) of the mean corresponding values recorded in the control animals (100.0 ± 5.3%; $n = 24$).

A sizeable amount of C22:1ω9 was only detected in two control animals examined 8 weeks after the switch in diet.

Taken as a whole, the findings collected in the liver triglycerides again suggest a double regulatory process. Thus, on one hand, the increase in the content of the long-chain polyunsaturated ω3 fatty acids, C14:0, C16:0, C16:1ω7 and C20:1ω9 recorded after the switch in diet, as well as the decrease in the C18:2ω6 content of liver triglycerides after the switch in diet, could be attributed mainly to the higher content of C20:5ω3, C22:5ω3, C22:6ω3, C14:0, C16:0, C16:1ω7 and C20:1ω9 and lower content of C18:2ω6 in the fish oil diet than in either the soya oil diet or sunflower oil diet. On the other hand, the decrease in the liver triglyceride content of C18:3ω3, C20:2ω6, C20:3ω6, C22:4ω6 and C22:5ω6 observed after the switch in diet can only be attributed to secondary regulatory processes, since the relative abundance of these long-chain polyunsaturated ω6 fatty acids in the fish oil diet is not lower than that found in either the soya oil or sunflower oil diet.

Table 21. Relative weight content (‰) of monodesaturated fatty acids in liver triglycerides

Rats	C16:1ω7	C18:1ω9	C20:1ω9	C22:1ω9
Control before	54.15±9.90	325.12±16.65	1.29±0.14	0.00±0.00
after (1wk)	69.78±4.64	306.35±4.59	5.03±0.82	0.00±0.00
after (2wk)	73.15±10.49	315.60±10.53	5.21±0.90	0.00±0.00
after (8wk)	82.88±3.18	323.76±12.69	6.15±1.08	0.57±0.34
ω3D before	45.40±6.55	309.22±20.00	1.27±0.49	0.00±0.00
after (1wk)	45.55±7.84	302.73±7.92	5.67±0.37	0.00±0.00
after (2wk)	84.27±7.70	340.76±17.51	4.72±0.68	0.00±0.00
after (8wk)	67.18±3.67	325.32±8.67	5.17±0.58	0.00±0.00

6. Fatty Acid Profile of Adipose Tissue Lipids

The wet weight of visceral adipose tissue collected along the intestinal tract did not differ significantly in control animals (11.01 ± 1.50 g; $n = 16$) and ω3D rats (11.74 ± 1.05 g; $n = 16$). Such was also the case when comparing the wet weight of parametrial adipose tissue in control animals (17.93 ± 2.09 g; $n = 16$) and ω3D rats (18.09 ± 1.82 g; $n = 16$).

The total fatty acid content of visceral adipose tissue lipids was slightly higher ($p < 0.04$) in ω3D rats (1.21 ± 0.02 mg/mg wet wt.; $n = 8$) than in control animals (1.14 ± 0.02 mg/mg wet wt.; $n = 8$).

6.1. Long-Chain Polyunsaturated Ω3 Fatty Acids

The C18:3ω3 relative weight content of visceral adipose tissue lipids decreased ($p < 0.003$) in the control animals from 20.36 ± 0.83‰ to 11.48 ± 1.51‰ ($n = 4$ in both cases) after 8 weeks exposure to the fish oil diet (Table 22). On the contrary, it increased ($p < 0.001$) from a null value to 3.15 ± 0.46‰ ($n = 4$) over the same period in the ω3D rats. These findings coincide with the hierarchy for the relative weight content of C18:3ω3 in the soya oil diet (7.1%), fish oil diet (1.2%) and sunflower oil diet (0.2%).

No C20:5ω3 was detected in the adipose tissue lipids before the switch in diet, whether in control animals or ω3D rats, whilst sizeable amounts of this ω3 fatty acid were always found 8 weeks after the switch in diet.

The C22:5ω3 content of adipose tissue lipids was higher ($p < 0.002$) in control animals than ω3D rats examined before the switch in diet. It increased after exposure to the fish oil diet to values largely exceeding those found before such a switch. This was also the case for the C22:6ω3 content of adipose tissue lipid. In the case of C20:5ω3, C22:5ω3 and C22:6ω3, the mean measurements made after the switch in diet were always lower in the ω3D rats than in the control animals, averaging in the former ω3D rats 80.7 ± 7.1% ($n = 12$; $p < 0.05$) of the mean corresponding values found in the control animals (100.0 ± 5.5%; $n = 12$).

Table 22. Relative weight content (‰) of long-chain polyunsaturated ω3 fatty acids in visceral adipose tissue lipids

Rats	C18:3ω3	C20:5ω3	C22:5ω3	C22:6ω3
Control before	20.36±0.83	0.00±0.00	1.10±0.19	0.00±0.00
after (8wk)	11.48±1.51	4.66±0.53	5.82±0.52	17.12±1.93
ω3D before	0.00±0.00	0.00±0.00	0.00±0.00	0.00±0.00
after (8wk)	3.15±0.46	3.33±0.62	4.86±0.71	14.92±2.33

6.2. Long-Chain Polyunsaturated Ω6 Fatty Acids

No C18:3ω6 was detected in the 16 samples of adipose tissue lipids. The C20:2ω6 content of such lipids was comparable in the four groups of rats listed in Table 23. Except in the case of C20:3ω6, the mean values recorded before the switch in diet were higher in ω3D rats than in control animals. Such a difference, however, only achieved statistical significance ($p < 0.001$) in the case of C22:5ω6.

As already observed in the liver triglycerides, the C18:2ω6, C20:4ω6 and C22:4ω6 content of adipose tissue lipids decreased after the switch in diet, in both control animals and ω3D rats. In relative terms, i.e. relative to the mean value recorded in the same type of rats (control animals or ω3D rats) before the switch indiet, such a decrease averaged 35.1 ± 5.10% ($df = 14$; $p < 0.001$) in the case of C18:2ω6, 28.4 ± 11.6% ($df = 14$; $p < 0.03$) in the case of C20:4ω6, and 18.8 ± 12.5% ($df = 14$; $p > 0.1$) in the case of C22:4ω6. As judged from the just mentioned relative values recorded 8 weeks after the switch in diet, the extent of the decrease in the C18:2ω6, C20:4ω6 and C22:4ω6 content of adipose tissue lipids only represented, in the ω3D rats, 65.9 ± 13.7% ($n = 12$; $p < 0.05$) of the mean corresponding value found in ω3D rats (100.0 ± 7.8%; $n = 12$).

In sharp contrast to the liver triglyceride data, the relative weight content of C20:3ω6 in adipose tissue lipids increased ($p < 0.001$) after the switch in diet in both control animals and ω3D rats, this coinciding with the presence of a modest but sizeable amount of this fatty acid in the fish oil diet, as distinct from soya oil or sunflower oil diet.

Incidentally, in the ω3D rats, the paired ratio between the relative weight content of C22:5ω6 in RBC phospholipids/adipose tissue lipid averaged 22.86 ± 3.61 ($n = 4$) before the switch in diet, as distinct ($p < 0.002$) from 1.92 ± 0.22 ($n = 4$) 8 weeks thereafter. In the light of prior proposals to estimate adipocyte lipolysis [14, 15], the present finding would be compatible with the view that, in the ω3D rats, the correction of ω3 fatty acid deficiency coincides with a decrease in adipocyte lipolysis, itself coinciding with a decrease of insulin resistance.

Table 23. Relative weight content (‰) of long-chain polyunsaturated ω6 fatty acids in visceral adipose tissue lipids

Rats	C18:2ω6	C20:2ω6	C20:3ω6	C20:4ω6	C22:4ω6	C22:5ω6
Control before	303.07±13.00	2.52±0.06	0.00±0.00	6.72±1.13	1.28±0.29	0.00±0.00
after (8wk)	194.65±7.82	2.61±0.07	0.75±0.07	4.11±0.41	0.97±0.06	0.00±0.00
ω3D before	324.61±23.71	2.67±0.10	0.00±0.00	8.21±0.93	2.09±0.25	1.45±0.22
after (8wk)	212.81±20.44	2.82±0.05	1.15±0.08	6.73±0.86	1.81±0.12	1.00±0.10

6.3. Saturated and Monodesaturated Fatty Acids

At the exception of C12:0 and C18:0, the relative content of with in the fish oil diet does not exceed that found in either the soya oil or sunflower oil diet, all other saturated (C14:0, C16:0) and monodesaturated (C16:1ω7, C18:1ω9 and C20:1ω9) fatty acids yielded higher mean values for their relative weight content in adipose tissue lipids after than before the switch in diet, whether in control animals or ω3D rats (Table 24). Except in the case of C18:1ω9, the relative weight content of these fatty acids (C14:0, C16:0, C16:1ω7 and C20:1ω9) is also higher in the fish oil diet than in the soya oil or sunflower oil diet. Expressed in terms of relative weight content, the increments attributable to the exposure to the fish oil diet, averaged ($df = 12$ in all cases) 4.49 ± 1.03‰ ($p < 0.001$) for C14:0, 24.91 ± 8.81‰ ($p < 0.02$) for C16:0, 12.77 ± 4.52‰ ($p < 0.02$) for C16:1ω7, 34.99 ± 11.89‰ ($p < 0.02$) for C18:1ω9, and 12.26 ± 1.89‰ ($p < 0.001$) for C20:1ω9.

Table 24. Relative weight content (‰) of saturated and monodesaturated fatty acids in visceral adipose tissue lipids

Rats	C12:0	C14:0	C16:0	C16:1ω7	C18:0	C18:1ω9	C20:1ω9
Control before	0.72±0.09	9.57±0.93	253.51±5.71	39.95±3.73	30.07±1.20	328.06±7.87	1.83±0.11
after (8wk)	0.84±0.04	15.23±0.97	280.68±8.91	50.45±1.39	34.80±0.78	357.54±6.73	17.36±2.56
ω3D before	0.77±0.07	10.57±1.13	253.17±11.65	38.03±7.35	34.09±1.78	321.17±9.81	1.75±0.16
after (8wk)	0.76±0.07	13.89±1.02	275.81±9.32	53.06±4.12	30.63±3.11	361.67±19.98	10.74±2.30

7. Food Intake and Body Weight

As was also the case before the switch in diet, the food intake over the last 8 weeks of the present experiments was higher ($p < 0.002$) in the ω3D rats maintained on the sunflower oil diet than in the control animals maintained on the soya oil diet, the measurements collected in the former ω3D rats averaged 112.1 ± 2.5% of the corresponding values recorded at the same time in the latter control animals (100.0 ± 1.6%).

Likewise over the 8 weeks following the switch in diet, the food intake by the ω3D rats exposed to the fish oil diet averaged 107.3 ± 1.5% ($p < 0.004$) of the corresponding values recorded in the control animals also exposed to the fish oil diet (100.0 ± 1.8%). In the control animals eventually exposed to the fish oil diet, the food intake only represented 91.6 ± 2.0% ($p < 0.005$) of that recorded at the same time in control animals maintained on the soya oil diet (100.0 ± 1.6%). Also in the ω3D rats eventually exposed to the fish oil diet, the food intake did not exceed 93.7 ± 1.6% ($p < 0.005$) of that recorded in the ω3D rats switched from the sunflower oil diet to the soya oil diet (100.0 ± 1.5%).

These findings were in good agreement with those concerning the relative gain in body weight over the last 7 weeks of the present experiments. Thus, over this period, the relative gain in body weight was higher ($p < 0.008$) in the ω3D rats maintained on the sunflower oil diet (+ 24.7 ± 1.3%) than in the control animals maintained on the soya oil diet (+ 13.3 ± 1.4%). The relative gain in body weight was lower in the control animals eventually exposed to the fish oil diet than in the control animals maintained on the soya oil diet, as well as in the ω3D rats switched to the fish oil diet than in the ω3D rats maintained on the sunflower oil diet, the values recorded in the rats switched to the fish oil diet representing 91.4 ± 1.7% ($p < 0.002$) of the mean corresponding values found in the same type of rats (control animals or ω3D rats) maintained on their initial diet (100.0 ± 0.8%).

8. Insulin Resistance

The HOMA index for insulin resistance, i.e. the product of plasma insulin times plasma D-glucose concentration, was measured in both control animals and ω3D rats before the switch in diet and one, two or eight weeks thereafter, with 3 individual determinations at each time point and in each type of rats. Before the switch in diet, such an index was higher ($p < 0.04$) in ω3D rats than in control animals.

After only one week exposure to the fish oil diet, the paired ratio between the HOMA index in ω3D/control rats (logarithmic values) was significantly lower ($p < 0.004$) than that recorded before the switch in diet. A further decrease ($p < 0.002$) was observed when comparing the values found one week after the switch in diet and those collected two to eight weeks after such a switch. There was indeed a significant negative correlation ($r = -0.5925$; $n = 12$; $p < 0.05$) between the logarithmic values of the ω3D/control paired ratio and the length of exposure to the fish oil diet. As a matter of fact, the overall mean value for such a ratio during exposure to the fish oil diet was no more significantly different from unity (118.0 ± 21.8%; $n = 9$; $p > 0.43$).

Conclusion

The present experimental design prevents any undesirable aggravation of liver steatosis and visceral obesity, as well as increase in food intake, otherwise resulting from an increase in the lipid content of the diet from 5 to 10% [4, 11, 16]. The finding that exposure of the rats to the fish oil diet both decreased food intake and minimized the gain in body weight may represent another favourable attribute of the present design in the perspective of preventing or correcting, if so required, excess of body weight.

The exposure of the ω3D rats to the fish oil diet also allowed the repletion of long-chain polyunsaturated ω3 fatty acids in the intestinal tract, liver, red blood cells and brain phospholipids.

The changes in the fatty acid pattern of tissue lipids were not always merely and directly attributable to the respective content of each diet in a given fatty acid, as documented by the accumulation of selected long-chain polyunsaturated ω6 fatty acids in the phospholipids of ω3D rats and the correction of this anomaly after the switch to the fish oil diet.

The present findings also support the view that a transfer of information takes place between the liver and either RBC or brain, as documented for instance by the delayed alignment of the fatty acid pattern in the latter two sites on that prevailing at the hepatic level. This is not meant to deny the operation of distinct regulatory processes in distinct organs (e.g. brain *versus* liver) in the fine adjustment of the relative weight content of selected fatty acids in cell phospholipids, as suggested in the present study, for instance, by the comparison between the fatty acid pattern of long-chain polyunsaturated ω3 fatty acids in liver and brain phospholipids.

Last, the present findings further evidence the fact that changes in the dietary supply of ω3 fatty acids may also affect the relative content of tissue lipids in selected saturated and monodesaturated fatty acids.

Further investigations are required to extend to human subjects the possible beneficial effects of a fish oil diet on the various parameters considered in this chapter.

Acknowledgment

We are grateful to C. Demesmaeker for secretarial help.

References

[1] Carpentier, YA; Hacquebard, M; Portois, L; Dupont, IE; Deckelbaum, RJ; Malaisse WJ. Rapid cellular enrichment of eicosapentaenoate after a single intravenous injection of a novel medium-chain triacylglycerol:fish oil emulsion in humans. *American Journal of Clinical Nutrition*, 2010, 91, 875-882.

[2] Malaisse, WJ; Hacquebard, M; Zhang, Y; Bulur, N; Sener, A; Carpentier, YA. The metabolic syndrome of ω3-depleted rats. X. Comprenhensive view. *The Open Physiology Journal*, 2011, 4, 1-10.

[3] Hacquebard, M; Portois, L; Malaisse, WJ; Carpentier, YA. The metabolic syndrome of ω3-depleted rats. IV. Intestinal phospholipid ω3 fatty acids. *International Journal of Molecular Medicine,* 2009, 24, 859-865.

[4] Malaisse, WJ; Bulur, N; Zhang, Y; Hacquebard, M; Portois, L; Sener, A; Carpentier, YA. The metabolic syndrome of ω3-depleted rats. I. Liver data. *International Journal of Molecular Medicine,* 2009, 24, 111-123.

[5] Carpentier, YA; Zhang, J; Hacquebard, M; Malaisse, WJ. The metabolic syndrome of ω3-depleted rats: dietary changes in lipid fatty acid pattern without changes in total lipid content. V. Red blood cell phospholipids. *Metabolic and Functional Research on Diabetes*, 2011, 4 (suppl 1), 28-32.

[6] Portois, L; Hacquebard, M; Malaisse, WJ; Carpentier, YA. The metabolic syndrome of ω3-depleted rats. III. Brain phospholipids. *International Journal of Molecular Medicine,* 2009, 24, 269-278.

[7] Portois, L; Delporte, C; Malaisse, WJ; Carpentier, YA. Fatty acid pattern of epiploic and parametric lipids in second generation rats depleted in long-chain polyunsaturated ω3 fatty acids. *Trends Cell Molecular Biology*, 2007, 2, 55-68.

[8] Folch, J; Lees, M; Sloane-Stanley, GH. A simple method for the isolation and purification of total lipids from animal tissues. *Journal of Biological Chemistry*, 1957, 226, 497-509.

[9] Dahlan, W; Richelle, M; Kulapongse, S; Rössle, C; Deckelbaum, RJ; Carpentier, YA. Effects of essential fatty acid contents of lipid emulsions on erythrocyte polyunsaturated fatty acid composition in patients on long-term parenteral nutrition. *Clinical Nutrition*, 1992, 11, 262-268.

[10] Lepage, G; Roy, CC. Direct transesterification of all classes of lipids in a one step reaction. *Journal of Lipid Research*, 1986, 48, 2463-2470.

[11] Zhang, Y; Bulur, N; Louchami, K; Hacquebard, M; Larondelle, Y; Carpentier, YA; Sener, A; Malaisse, WJ. The metabolic syndrome of ω3-depleted rats. IX. Food intake. *The Open Physiology Journal*, 2010, 3, 10-15.

[12] Lowry, OH; Passonneau, JV. A flexible system of enzymatic analysis. Academic Press. New York; 1972; 174.

[13] Leclercq-Meyer, V; Marchand, J; Woussen-Colle, MC; Girois, M-H; Malaisse, WJ. Multiple effects of leucine on glucagon, insulin and somatostatin secretion from the perfused rat pancreas. *Endocrinology*, 1985, 116, 1168-1174.

[14] Malaisse, WJ; Sener, A; Carpentier, YA. Plasma phospholipid-mediated transfer of docesahexaenoic acid from liver to brain phospholipids in Type 1 and Type 2 diabetic rats. *Molecualr Medicine Reports*, 2010, 3, 977-981.

[15] Zhang, J; Hacquebard, M; Malaisse, WJ; Carpentier, YA. The metabolic syndrome of ω3-depleted rats. XII. Adipose tissue lipids. *Metabolic and Functional Research on Diabetes,* 2011, 4 (suppl 1), 67-71.

[16] Sener, A; Zhang, Y; Bulur, N; Louchami, K; Malaisse, WJ; Carpentier, YA. The metabolic syndrome of ω3-depleted rats. II. Body weight, adipose tissue mass and glycemic homeostasis. *International Journal of Molecular Medicine*, 2009, 24, 125-129.

In: Fish Oil: Production, Consumption and Health Benefits
Editors: Matthias Van Dijk and Jürgen Vitek
ISBN: 978-1-61470-963-3

Chapter V

Beneficial Effects of Fish Oil and its Applications in Human Health

K.Dhanapal*[*], *A. Devivaraprasad Reddy and G. Vidya Sagar Reddy
Department of Fish Processing Technology, College of Fishery Science,
Sri Venkateswara Veterinary University, Muthukur, India

Abstract

Omega–3 and Omega–6 Fatty Acids are predominant in fish oils compared to other animal oils. Omega–3 polyunsaturated fatty acids (PUFA) such as Docosahexaenoic acid (DHA) and Eicosapentaenoic acid (EPA) have attracted considerable interest in both nutraceutical and pharmaceutical fields. The major beneficial role of omega – 3 fatty acids is to reduce the risk of coronary heart disease and help in brain, neural and retinal developments. Consumption of diet containing PUFA reduces blood pressure, plasma triglycerides and cholesterol levels, thereby increasing the blood coagulation time, which are responsible for maintenance of normal blood flow by preventing platelets from sticking to each other. PUFA not only alleviates blood vessel disorders and inflammatory diseases, but also controls immune functions resulting in alleviation of autoimmune diseases such as arthritis and certain types of dermatitis. Human diet deficient in DHA and EPA can cause several disorders such as restrictive growth, abnormality of skin and hair, damage of reproductive system and abnormal composition of serum and tissue fatty acids. Fish oil rich in PUFA, is also associated with decreased risk of Dementia and Alzheimer's disease. Increased levels of DHA in brain are believed to reduce ageing.

This chapter describes the beneficial effects of consumption of fish oil containing PUFA in protecting human health; besides addressing certain individual diseases.

* Corresponding author. Tel.: +91-0861 2377596, Fax: +91-0861 2377886, E-mail address: kdhanpal@yahoo.com (K. Dhanapal)

1. Introduction

The Greek physician Hippocrates, the father of medicine in the 4th century, advised "Let food be your medicine and medicine be your food" started attracting increasing attention by the modern world. Historically, the importance of diet in maintenance of health is been known from time immemorial in some parts of the world. In Asia, the concept is rooted in a tradition, known as Ayurveda, "The Science of Life", which had its origin some 5000 years ago. The science of life recognized the importance of a balanced diet (Venugopal 2009).

Unsaturated fatty acids consist of monounsaturates and polyunsaturates. There are two classes of PUFAs, omega-3 (n-3) and omega-6 (n-6). The distinction between omega-3 and omega-6 fatty acids is based on the location of the first double bond, counting from the methyl end of the fatty acid molecule. Monounsaturates are represented by oleic acid, which can be synthesized by all mammals including humans. Its double bond is between the 9th and 10th carbon atoms. Omega-3 and omega-6 fatty acids are also known as essential fatty acids (EFAs) because humans like all we mammals cannot make them and must obtain them in their diet. Omega-6 fatty acids are represented by linoleic acid (LA) and omega-3 fatty acids by alpha-linolenic acid (ALA). Fish oils are rich sources of n-3 fatty acids (FAs), especially eicosapentaenoic acid (EPA; C20:5) and docosahexaenoic acid (DHA; C22:6).

Lipids play a major role in human nutrition and health while accounting for about 40% of the total calories in most of the industrialized countries. Fish oils, especially of marine origin are unique compared to other lipids. Fish oils or lipids (mainly marine lipids) have been considered as an available source of omega – 3 fatty acids especially DHA & EPA. Several studies have demonstrated beneficial effects of omega-3/omega-6 consumption for the prevention or treatment of various diseases. However, in most cases a number of studies have shown no beneficial effect of omega-3/omega-6 consumption on disease risk or progression. Although, some discrepancy may occur due to differences in the experimental design and methods used in different studies, it is becoming increasingly more apparent that the genetic make-up and physiological wellbeing of individuals in the study population also has a strong influence on study outcome.

Better understanding of the mechanism of action of omega-3/omega-6 in biological systems will aid in determining the type of individual most likely to benefit from omega-3/omega-6. In this chapter, several new studies on determining the mechanism of action of omega-3/omega-6 have been focussed.

2. Coronary Heart Disease (CHD)/ Cardio Vascular Disease (CVD)

Death from CHD – i.e, documented or suspected fatal myocardial infection and sudden death – i.e, a sudden pulseless condition of presumed cardiac etiology – are clinically defined entities often sharing the final common pathway of ventricular arrhythmia, often ischemia – induced ventricular fibrillation (Mozaffarian and Rimm 2006).

Much of the interest in a marine diet and fish oil comes from the pioneering study of Greenland Eskimos by Dyerberg et al. (1978) more than 30 years ago. They found that even though Eskimos had a diet rich in fat, they had a very low rate of ischemic heart disease (Harris 2004a). Their findings spawned numerous research studies and has resulted in recommendations from major public health organisations for increased intake of omega-3 PUFA (fish, seal, salmon, whale meat & fish oil) for reducing the risk of myocardial interact and researchers have proposed the mechanism associated with this effect was the reduction of thrombosis risk (Harris 2004a; Nunes et al., 2011). Since then, the effects of the omega-3 fatty acids in alleviating the clinical symptoms of cardiovascular heart disease have been well examined.

Many years of epidemiological research have shown that populations consuming diets high in saturated fatty acids show relatively high levels of serum cholesterol and carry a high prevalence of coronary heart disease (Caggiula and Mustad 1997). Based on the evidence of various studies conducted, it is generally accepted that high levels of serum cholesterol, particularly LDL, promote the development of atherosclerosis or coronary heart disease. Mensink and Katan (1990) suggested that *trans* fats increased low density lipoprotein (LDL) and decreased the beneficial high density lipoprotein (HDL) resulting in a less desirable LDL/HDL ratio. Invariably, it was established that *trans* fatty acids (TFA) could be worse than the saturated fatty acids. The concept has become widely accepted that lowering LDL cholesterol by any means will reduce the risk of coronary heart disease. It has been estimated that dietary TFAs from partially hydrogenated oils may be responsible for 30,000–100,000 premature coronary deaths per year in the United States (Dhaka et al., 2011).

The omega 3 index is the percentage of total red blood cell fatty acids, which is composed of eicosapentaenoic acid (EPA) and docohexaneoic acid (DHA), the primary long chain omega 3 fatty acids found in fish. This measure has been found to correlate with myocardial omega 3 fatty acid levels (Harris et al. 2004b), and individuals in the highest quartile of omega 3 fatty acid blood level have 81% to 90% lower risks of sudden cardiac deaths (SCD) as compared to those in the lowest quartile in healthy populations (Siscovick et al., 1995). In addition, dietary intake of long-chain omega 3 fatty acids from fish has been inversely associated with SCD risk in four observational studies among primarily healthy populations, (Albert et al., 1998; Mozaffarian et al., 2005) and a supplement of omega3 fatty acids lowered SCD risk in a randomized trial among post–myocardial infarction (MI) patients. Based upon these data, it has been proposed that low levels of the omega-3 fatty acid index might identify those at higher risk for SCD (von Schacky and Harris 2007). In addition, if the observed associations are causal, then raising an individual's omega3 fatty acid level by increasing dietary or supplement intake of omega3 fatty acids might lower their risk of SCD.

Further, epidemiological studies suggested that individuals at risk of CHD/CVD are benefited from the consumption of plant and marine derived omega – 3 PUFA may be present in a large proportion of the population and might be a factor in CHD (de Deckere et al., 1998).

Across different studies, compared with little or no intake, modest consumption (250 – 500 mg/day of EPA & DHA) lowers relative risk by 25% or more. The various mechanisms by which EPA & DHA prevent / modify cardio vascular diseases have been the subject of a thorough research over 3 decades. Clinical & Nutritional researchers continue to demonstrate the benefits of omega – 3 long chain PUFA'S. These studies conclusively showed that diets rich in fish and fish oils are associated with a reduced risk of coronary heart disease (He 2009).

Marine oils which are rich in EPA & DHA, has several biological functions in the body system. EPA & DHA lower elevated triglyceride levels, afford protection to the cardiovascular system, have anti – inflammatory and immune – modulating properties and are beneficial for the skeletal muscles and gastro intestinal systems. Solid compelling evidence that two long chain omega – 3 fatty acids – eicosapentaenoic acid (EPA) and docosahexaenoic acid (DHA) help in preventing coronary heart disease (He 2009).

Currently, data from one large randomized trial, the GISSI-Prevenzione trial, suggest that these agents may prevent SCD after recent myocardial infarction (Marchioli et al., 2002), prompting the American Heart Association and other international agencies to recommend omega3 fatty acid intakes of 1g of the EPA and DHA in these patients. The enthusiasm for such an apparently simple, low-cost, and low-risk intervention has been high; prompting the American Heart Association to recommend that all adults eat fatty fish at least 2 times per week and those patients with coronary heart disease consume approximately 1 g/day of EPA and DHA through diet or supplements (Kris-Etherton et al., 2002 and 2003).

There are also planned or ongoing trials in patients with diabetes and/or other cardiac risk factors but currently no trials in healthy populations. Although the actions of omega 3 fatty acids may not be so simple, the potential public health impact of preventing SCD with this relatively low-cost intervention, even if only in certain subgroups of patients, is quite large. Therefore, the benefits and risks of omega-3 fatty acids require and deserve to be adequately tested in randomized trials.

3. Thrombosis

It is recognised that up to 85% of cases of vascular access failure may be due to thrombosis caused by myointimal hyperplasia (proliferation of the cells lining the blood vessel), particularly in prosthetic grafts. Thrombosis is a major complication of coronary atherosclerosis that can lead to myocardial infarction. The omega-3 fatty acids from fish oil have powerful antithrombotic action. EPA inhibits the synthesis of thromboxane A2 from arachidonic acid in platelets. This prostaglandin causes platelet aggregation and vasoconstriction. As a result, fish oil ingestion by human increases the bleeding time and decreases the stickiness of the platelets for aggregation to glass beads. In addition, the administration of fish oil enhances the production of prostacyclin, a prostaglandin that produces vasodilation and less sticky platelets. The Schmitz trial (Schmitz et al., 2002) examined the effects of fish oil versus placebo on graft thrombosis. Two out of 12 participants taking fish oil developed a thrombosis compared with nine out of 12 who received placebo. The studies conducted by several scientists favored consumption of fish oil for prevention of thrombosis (Osborn et al., 2008).

4. Brain Development, Function, Disease and Mental Health

Numerous studies over the past 40 years have evaluated the impact of nutrition in early life on central nervous system development. Omega-3 long chain polyunsaturated fatty acids (LCPUFAs) have an important role in brain development and function. Although it is known that the brain contains large amounts of omega-3 LCPUFAs, how the LCPUFAs present in the brain influence brain function is less clear. The effects of Omega-3 deficiency on the nervous system suggest that omega-3 fatty acids may be key to its adequate development and functioning. This notion is further supported by the high concentrations of Omega-3 long chain PUFA (Omega – 3 LCPUFAs) such as DHA in the cerebral cortex and retina, a brain derived neuronal network specialized for photo – signal transduction and processing. Indeed, the dry weight of the human brain is predominantly lipid, with 22% of the cerebral cortex and 24% of white matter consisting of phospholipids (Uauy and Dangour 2006).

Nutrition Effects on the Brain

The cell itself needs proper nutrition to carry on its function just like any other cell in the body.

1. The myelin sheath covers the axon of the cell like insulation covering electrical wires. It speeds transmission of electrical signals along the axons, the "wires" of the brain. Deficiencies of nutrients that compose myelin, such as essential fatty acids, delay nerve impulse transmission.
2. The neurotransmitters, such as serotonin, dopamine, and norepinephrine, carry messages from one cell to the other and affect mood as well as thoughts and actions.
3. Some of the nutrients in the food we eat become part of the neurotransmitters that help us think. Neurotransmitters are probably the biological explanation for the food-mood connection.

The brain uses carbohydrates for energy and omega-3 fatty acids for forming its cell structure. The nervous system relies on neurotransmitters to communicate messages within the brain. Such as those that regulate mood, hunger, and sleep. DHA is the primary structural component of brain tissue, so a deficiency of DHA in the diet could lead to a deficiency in brain function. In fact, research is recognizing the possibility that DHA has a crucial influence on neurotransmitters in the brain, helping brain cells better communicate with each other. Omega -3 fatty acids are essential to the optimum performance of the brain. Lack of Omega - 3 fats in the diet can lead to depression, poor memory, low IQ, learning disabilities, and dyslexia.

Certain foods when consumed directly affect the performance of the brain. It has been proved that by eating the right food, we can boost our IQ, improve our mood, be more emotionally stable, sharpen our memory and keep mind young. If we give our brain the right nutrients, we will be able to think quicker, have a better memory, be better coordinated and balanced and have improved concentration (Vora and Deshpande 2010). Omega-3 fatty acids, found mainly in fish oils, are said to be beneficial in conditions from Alzheimer disease to Zellweger syndrome.

a.) Multiple Sclerosis

Neurons are responsible for relaying signals from the brain to other parts of the body. The axon of a neuron is surrounded by a sheath known as myelin. Myelin is composed of 80% lipids and 20% proteins and is important for signal transduction. Degradation of the myelin sheath (demyelination) is a major factor causing the symptoms of multiple sclerosis.

Multiple sclerosis (MS) is an inflammatory and demyelinating disease of the central nervous system. MS is the most important non-traumatic cause of neurological disability in young adults, especially women, typically striking between 20 and 40 years of age. Although MS etiology and pathogenesis remain poorly understood, it is widely accepted that the disease has an immune-mediated basis and occurs in genetically susceptible individuals. Despite limited advances in treatments, there is still no cure. Management is largely directed to relieving symptoms, which arise variably in the course of the disease. Because available conventional therapies are only partially effective and may produce side effects, people with MS widely use treatments proposed by complementary and alternative medicine (CAM). Studies in several countries, including the United States, Canada, Netherlands, Germany and Australia, showed that about a half to three quarters of people with MS use some form of CAMs in conjunction with conventional medicine (Bowling and Stewart 2003; Farinotti et al., 2007).

Several epidemiological studies have considered various nutritional factors in relation to MS, as summarised by Lauer (1997) and dietary interventions appear to have the potential to favourably influence the prognosis of MS. Several pathophysiological mechanisms were proposed as a rational basis for the therapeutic use of PUFAs for MS including immunomodulatory and anti-inflammatory actions, effects on microcirculation and erythrocyte aggregation, antioxidant action, and also effects related to their role as constituents of the myelin membrane (Das 2003; Swank and Goodwin 2003; Schwarz and Leweling 2005; Farinotti et al., 2007).

Scientists in Italy investigated the effect of EPA and DHA on the expression of several myelin proteins. A single dose of EPA or DHA was injected directly into the cerebral cortex of two-day old rats. Rats were euthanised three days later and the levels of RNA for specific myelin proteins were measured in three areas of the brain, the cortex, cerebellum and medulla. Both EPA and DHA increased expression of RNA for myelin proteins but EPA had a stronger effect than DHA (Salvati et al., 2008). Although much more research is required, to raise the possibility that EPA or DHA treatment may aid in preventing demyelination or in the repair of a damaged myelin sheath.

b.) Alzheimer's Disease

Congruent with the graying demographic trend in many developed countries, it is projected that there will be an exponential rise in the prevalence of age-associated diseases like dementia. Based on demographic projections, it has been estimated that the number of cases of Alzheimer's disease (AD) in developed countries has risen to around 40% between 1990 and 2010 (Lim et al., 2006). Alzheimer's disease is characterised by the formation of plaques within brain tissue. These plaques are made from the protein β-amyloid which is believed to be toxic to neurons. Neuron destruction is believed to be the primary cause of the symptoms of Alzheimer's disease. LR11 is a brain protein which prevents the formation of these plaques. In late-onset Alzheimer's patients, LR11 is present in very low amounts. Investigators have found that treatment of cultured rat and human neuronal cells results in increased LR11 levels. Similarly feeding mice and rats with DHA has also been shown to increase LR11 in the animals' brain (Ma et al., 2007). The US NIH is currently carrying out a clinical study to investigate the effect of DHA supplementation on LR11 protein levels in patients with established Alzheimer's Disease.

Another group of researchers found feeding DHA to rats or gerbils resulted in increased levels of phosphatides and pre-synaptic and post-synaptic proteins in brain cells as well as increased number of dendritic spines and post-synaptic neurons (Cansev et al., 2008). "Synapse" is the sending of a signal from one neuron to another. Phosphatides are important components of the membranes at which synapse occurs and pre- and post-synaptic proteins are involved in the sending and receipt of the signal between neurons. Dendritic spines are formed once synapse has occurred and may be important for memory. Alzheimer's patients have smaller and fewer synapses, reduced levels of membrane phosphatides and reduced levels of synaptic proteins. It is possible that DHA treatment may aid in combating synaptic loss associated with Alzheimer's and other neurodegenerative diseases as well as neural damage which occur as a result of stroke or trauma.

However, in a study with transgenic mouse model of Alzheimer's disease, consumption of a high fish oil diet (4% menhaden oil) for 5½-7 months had no effect on cognitive function (Arendash et al., 2007). Although there is promising data to suggest a role for omega-3 LCPUFAs in combating the neurodegeneration associated with Alzheimer's and other similar diseases, due to the complexity of the disease process as well as limitations associated with the use of model systems to study the disease, there is still much work to be done to determine which LCPUFAs are effective, if effective at what dose and at what extent.

c.) Epilepsy

Detrimental changes in the integrity of the brain cell membranes as well as in the ability of brain cells to utilise energy may occur in diseases such as epilepsy. In a recent pilot study, epileptic patients were supplemented with either placebo or high doses of EPA and DHA (1g EPA and 0.8g DHA per day) for 12 weeks. Using ^{31}Phosphous neurospectroscopy, the composition of phosphorylated compounds in the patients' brains was determined. The relative amount of the different types of phosphorylated compounds in brain tissue provides information on the biochemical activity occurring within the brain (Kruger and Poulsen 2008).

Significant effects of EPA/DHA supplementation were observed on the levels of two phosphorylated compounds: PDE (phosphodiesters), γ-NTP (gamma nucleotide triphosphate) as well as in the amount of BBC (broadband component) resonance. PDE is an index of membrane phospholipids catabolism. Levels of PDE were found to be significantly lower in patients receiving the EPA/DHA supplement than in patients receiving the placebo suggesting the n-3 LCPUFAs may protect phospholipids membranes from degradation. BBC is an indicator of the level of phospholipids incorporated within membranes of brain cells. The level of BBC was significantly higher in LCPUFA- treated patients compared to placebo-controls suggesting LCPUFAs may increase the incorporation of phospholipids within cell membranes. Finally, levels of γ-NTP were significantly higher in EPA/DHA supplemented patients than controls indicating improved brain energy metabolism in supplemented patients (Puri et al., 2007). Although this was a very small study involving just seven patients (3 receiving EPA/DHA supplementation and 4 receiving placebo), that significant differences between treated and untreated patients were observed in three of the parameters measured suggests EPA/DHA treatment has a major effect on these parameters. How EPA and DHA increase brain phospholipid incorporation, decrease phospholipid degradation and improve brain energy metabolism and the consequences of this for epilepsy sufferers will no doubt be a focus for further research.

d.) Depression

Although many studies have been reported on the effect of n-3 LCPUFA intake on depression, there remains a lack of consensus as to the efficacy of LCPUFAs as potential means of reducing the severity or preventing the onset of depression. Supplementation of EPA & DHA (1.5g/day) for 3 months in the diet of 190 patients suffering with mild to moderate depression had no effect on mood or congnitive function (Rogers et al., 2008). However, in another study, 60 patients with major depressive disorder, treatment with 1g of EPA per day for 8 weeks resulted in significant improvement in the severity of depression. Combined treatment with EPA (1g/day) and fluoxetine, a pharmaceutical anti- depressant, had greater therapeutic effects in alleviating depressive symptoms than either treatment alone (Jazayeri et al., 2008).

e.) Cognitive Function

For some time it has been suggested that increased n-3 LCPUFA intake may aid in reducing age-related cognitive decline. Although some studies have demonstrated a beneficial effect of n-3 LCPUFA intake on cognitive ability, others have not. This is the case with many fields of nutritional research. One reason for the apparent conflict in results obtained from studies is that certain nutrients may have certain effects in some individuals like those with a certain genetic profile or with a certain disease but have a different effect in other individuals. There is some evidence that n-3 LCPUFAs are more beneficial in reducing cognitive decline in hypertensive patients than in normotensive individuals. In a large-scale epidemiological study in 10,000 US men and women with hypertension, a positive association between n-3 LCPUFA intake and reduced risk of 6-year cognitive decline in verbal fluency was reported (Beydoun et al., 2008).

5. Lung Disease

The typical human lung has between 30 and 100 m^2 of exposed surface area. Because the function of the lung is gas exchange, the type of protection available to the skin is not feasible for this organ. Not surprisingly, inflammation is common in the lung. What is surprising is that in response to this inflammatory activity, fibrosis is rare. This contrasts with most other tissues in the body. Clearly, the lung has evolved mechanisms to protect itself; however, the evolutionary need for such mechanisms to function beyond child-rearing age is not clear. In any case, the human lung evolved during a period when the total intake of fatty acids and the distribution of types of dietary fatty acids were considerably different from those of today. This raises the question of whether the current mix and amount of fatty acid intake has consequences for the lung in health and disease (Schwartz 2000).

a. Asthma in Children

Two studies from Australia reported that dietary fish intake is protective against asthma prevalence in children. These studies are notable in that they did not depend solely on questionnaire data, but also included an assessment of airway responsiveness. Peat et al. (1992) found that children who ate fish more than once per week had lower rates of airway hyperresponsiveness than children who ate fish less often. Hodge et al. (1996) reported that consumption of fresh fish, and particularly oily fish, was protective against wheeze and asthma.

b. Asthma in Adults

Schwartz (2000) reported a dose-dependent decrease in risk of chronic obstructive pulmonary disease with increasing intake of n-3 fatty acids. In a reanalysis stimulated by the paper of Sharp et al. (1995), they also found an interaction with pack-years of smoking (number of packs of cigarettes smoked per day times the number of years smoked). The risk of an additional 10 pack years declined in a dose-dependent manner with increasing intake of n-3 fatty acids. Schwartz and Weiss (1990) reported that dietary fish intake was protective against frequent wheeze apart from colds. Troisi et al. (1995) examined the incidence of asthma in the Nurses' Health Study and found no significant association with dietary fish intake.

The evidence for bronchitis is considerably stronger. The importance of neutrophil activity in this disease is unchallenged, and the epidemiologic data are much more consistent. There is still the possibility that dietary fish intake is merely a marker of good diet, but given the changes seen in intermediate markers of disease, a moderately good case exists for a role of dietary fish intake. In this regard it is interesting to note that wild game contains only 4% fat, compared with almost 25% fat in corn-fed beef. Hence, in prehistoric times, dietary intake of saturated animal fat was much lower than it is today. Dietary intake of linoleic acid would also have been quite low before the development of agriculture. Hence, it is likely that our species evolved during a time when fatty acids from fish were a larger constituent of total fatty acid intake than is true today.

6. Obesity

Obesity has led to alarming increase in the incidence of many chronic diseases, including type 2 diabetes and cardiovascular disease (CVD). Since the over nutrition leads to obesity, manipulation of dietary nutrient content is a logical means of alleviating this problem. Adipose tissue (AT) plays an important role in regulating lipid homeostasis by storing excess energy in the form of Triglyceride (TG). The lipid storage function of AT is critical in buffering the daily influx of dietary fatty acids entering the circulation. Further, AT controls the plasma levels of free fatty acids (FFAs) by suppressing the release of non-esterified fatty acids into the circulation. Impairment of AT storage function, as seen in obesity and lipodystrophic conditions, is associated with increased lipolysis. This results in excessive release of FFAs into the circulation, which leads to ectopic lipid deposition, thereby contributing to the development of insulin resistance (IR). It has been well established that AT not only is an inert storage organ but also secretes many bioactive substances called adipokines. Adiponectin and leptin are two important adipokines secreted by AT that have an undeniable influence in modulating glucose and lipid metabolism via their autocrine and paracrine effects. In addition to the above mentioned adipokines, AT in obesity releases several inflammatory mediators, such as monocyte chemoattractant protein-1, interleukin-6 (IL-6) and tumor necrosis factor α (TNFα). Mounting evidence suggests that macrophages accumulate in AT in obesity and secrete these inflammatory mediators, thereby activating inflammatory pathways in obese AT (Weisberg et al., 2003). It is now widely accepted that AT inflammation modulates the storage and/or secretory functions of AT. Because of its crucial role in energy homeostasis, AT is now considered to be a potential target for therapeutic agents and dietary factors that are known to improve features of metabolic syndrome (Puglisi et al., 2011).

One mechanism by which dietary fish oil may exert its favorable effects in AT is by incorporation of n–3 fatty acids eicosapentaenoic acid (EPA) and docosahexaenoic acid (DHA) into lipid fractions of the adipocytes. Luo et al. (1996) demonstrated that feeding Sprague– Dawley rats with a fish oil diet for 6 weeks increased the incorporation of n–3 fatty acids into the membrane phospholipid fraction of adipocytes. This was associated with increased insulin sensitivity in the adipocytes, as insulin-stimulated glucose uptake was positively correlated with the degree of unsaturation of membrane phospholipid fatty acids (Puglisi et al., 2011). Fickova et al. (1998) also demonstrated the incorporation of n–3 fatty acids into adipocyte membrane phospholipids after feeding of male Wistar rats with a fish oil diet for only 1 week. This was associated with significantly lower concentrations of serum TG, cholesterol and insulin. Fish oil feeding has also been shown to increase incorporation of n–3 fatty acids into the TG fraction of AT in rats (Puglisi et al., 2011). Several other human studies have shown that intake of dietary omega–3 fatty acids results in accumulation of these lipids in AT (Krebs et al., 2006). Thus, dietary fish oils clearly make their way into the membrane phospholipids and TG lipid droplets of adipocytes, where they have the potential to modulate signaling events, thereby altering the metabolic activity of AT (Puglisi et al., 2011).

7. Diabetes Mellitus

The prevalence of Type – II (non-insulin-dependent) diabetes mellitus is increasing rapidly in the United States and the worldwide. Prevalence of diabetes in adults throughout the world is estimated to reach 5.4% and the number of adults with diabetes is expected to reach 300 million worldwide in the year 2025. The toll on diabetes on health and the economy is enormous and will continue to rise. Because there is no cure for diabetes, primary prevention through diet and lifestyle modification is of paramount importance (Hu et al., 2001). Diabetes mellitus is a metabolic disorder caused by an absolute or relative lack of insulin. The metabolic abnormalities include hyperglycemia, hypertriglyceridemia, and other lipoprotein disorders.

Type 2 diabetes is a multigenic, multifactorial disorder. Several environmental factors contribute to insulin resistance. The importance of genetic predisposition and its interaction with diet and exercise in the development of type 2 diabetes has been known since the time of Hippocrates, but progress in the genetics of type 2 diabetes has been slow until recently. The observation that fatty acids can regulate gene expression in adipose cells introduces a link between the composition of diets and the hyperplastic and hypertrophic responses of white adipose tissue. The characterization of fatty acid–responsive genes may also produce some clues about the development of an insulin-resistant state and cell hypertrophy. Type 2 diabetes is characterized by hyperglycemia in the presence of insulin resistance, hypertriglyceridemia, and the development of vascular complications. Men and women with type 2 diabetes have 3-fold and 5-fold higher cardiovascular mortality, respectively, than the non-diabetic population, and this higher risk is also carried by nondiabetic first-degree relatives of type 2 diabetes subjects. Clustering of atherogenic (e.g., dyslipidemia, hypertension) and thrombotic (e.g., plasminogen activator inhibitor 1, factor VII, and fibrinogen) risk factors in association with insulin resistance may explain the higher risk. EPA and DHA decrease plasminogen activator inhibitor 1, factor VII, and serum fibrinogen concentrations (Simopoulos 1999).

Borkman et al. (1993) showed that hyperinsulinemia and insulin resistance are inversely associated with the amount of 20- and 22-carbon fatty acids in the phospholipids of muscle cell membrane in patients with coronary heart disease and in normal volunteers. Such decreases in 20- and 22-carbon fatty acid concentrations could occur as a result of 1) low dietary intake of 20- and 22-carbon fatty acids (current Western diets are characterized by low amounts of EPA and DHA relative to LA and Arachidonic acid); 2) high dietary intake of trans fatty acids, which interfere with the desaturation and elongation of LA and ALA and thus lower Arachidonic acid (AA), EPA, and DHA concentrations; 3) genetic defects of D6 and D5 desaturase; 4) genetic defects that interfere with the transport or binding of 20- and 22-carbon fatty acids, such as in intestinal fatty acid–binding protein; 5) high dietary intake of LA, leads to decreased production of AA and interferes with the desaturation and elongation of ALA to EPA and DHA; or 6) increased catabolism of AA, which reduces the number of available 20- and 22-carbon atoms.

An increase in 20- and 22-carbon PUFAs, ie, AA, EPA, and DHA, leads to increase in membrane fluidity, the number of insulin receptors, and insulin action. In humans, the ratio of n–6 to saturated fatty acids in serum phospholipids correlates with insulin sensitivity. *Trans* Fatty acids are incorporated into cell membrane phospholipids, resulting in decreased fluidity of membranes and binding of insulin to its receptor, leading to impaired insulin action, insulin resistance, and hyperinsulinemia. In animal experiments, isomeric *trans* fatty acids increased LA and lowered AA concentrations in tissue phospholipids, indicating inhibition of D6 desaturase.

8. Tumour

Chance et al. (1996) compared metabolic changes between two lipid emulsions (Intralipid versus fish oil) in tumor-bearing rats. Although tumor growth, skeletal muscle atrophy, and gut hypoplasia were not reduced in the tumor-bearing group maintained on fish oil–based

TPN, immunosuppression in the Intralipid-based TPN group, as measured by the mitogen response of cultured splenocytes, was significantly improved in the rats maintained on fish oil–based TPN. Mendez et al. (1992) demonstrated that the lipid source in a TPN solution can influence tumor and host protein metabolism, and a structured lipid composed of MCT and fish oil seems to improve protein metabolism in host tissue without stimulating tumor growth. Ling et al. (1991) compared the effects of a structured lipid composed of fish oil and MCT on tumor and host metabolism with conventional fat emulsion in tumor-bearing rats and found that fish oil/MCT feeding decrease tumor protein synthesis and inhibit tumor growth (Chen and Yeh 2003).

9. Immune System

Feeding EPA and DHA has been shown to modulate specific functions of innate and acquired immunity. In general, feeding high levels (>10% of total fat) of n-3 PUFA (compared with diets high in n-6 PUFA) to healthy animals or human subjects results in suppression of the ability of lymphocytes to respond to mitogen stimulation, NK cell activity, and delayed-type hypersensitivity (DTH) reactions (Calder 1998). Suppression of these functions has been demonstrated in studies supplementing as little as 180 mg EPA + DHA/day or up to 6 g DHA/day (Kelley et al., 1999) to the diet of humans or by feeding animals from 1% w/w purified EPA or DHA (Hosack-Fowler et al., 1993) up to 20% w/w fish oil (approximately 3.5% w/w EPA+DHA). Feeding long-chain n-3 PUFA was shown to significantly decrease the production of interleukin (IL)-1, IL-6, and TNF-α by peripheral blood mononuclear cells in humans and by peritoneal macrophages in animals after mitogen stimulation. However, there is some discrepancy with respect to TNF- α production in animals, because many studies have shown to increase TNF- α production after stimulation when EPA/DHA were fed. Conversely, a number of studies have shown that feeding more moderate amounts of n-3 PUFA (i.e., fed at <10% of fat to animals and <1 g EPA+DHA/day to humans) is not immunosuppressive, and can even enhance immune functions such as lymphocyte proliferation/activation, NK cell activity, macrophage activation, and IL-1, IL-2, and TNF- α production after mitogen stimulation. Adding a small amount of DHA [and arachidonic acid (AA)] to infant formula alters the maturation (expression of the CD45RO+ antigen on CD4+ cells) of T cells in preterm infants to be more similar to that of infants fed human milk. These contradictory observations of the effect of omega-3 fatty acids on immune function in healthy humans and animals may be a result of the overall content of polyunsaturated fat in the diet and found that n-3 PUFA reduce splenocyte proliferation in healthy rats when fed in a high polyunsaturated fat diet, but not when fed in a diet with a low polyunsaturated fat level, which is more representative of the diet consumed by most North Americans (Field et al., 2002).

10. Cancer

One third of human cancers might be associated with dietary habits and lifestyle and the amount and type of dietary fat consumed are of particular importance (Reddy et al., 1985;

Bartsch et al., 1999). Studies in humans and experimental animals have indicated that the protective effect of fish oils which are rich in n-3 polyunsaturated fatty acids such as EPA and DHA; the mechanism of protection is thought to be mainly related to their interference with biosynthesis of two-series of prostaglandins from arachidonic acid (Rao et al., 2001). Other fatty acids may also have antitumorigenic properties.

Several studies have shown the effect of omega 3 PUFA against cancer. Prostate cancer is one of the most common types of cancer particularly in Western countries. An inverse relationship has been noted between blood levels of EPA and DHA and the risk of prostate cancer and adenocarcinoma. Scientists at the Paterson Institute for Cancer Research, in U.K. found that the fatty acids found in salmon, mackerel, and fresh tuna can help prevent the spread of prostate cancer to other parts of the body, which was attributed to omega 3 fatty acids. In addition, EPA and DHA have also been reported to act positively against cancer effects such as cachexia (abnormal weight loss) or survival rate in end-stage cancer (Venugopal 2009). In a systematic review about the effect of omega-3 PUFA on cancer risks, MacLean et al. (2006), observed a delay in the onset of some cancer types (viz., breast, lung, colorectal and prostate) with the intake of fatty acids. In the case of aero-digestive, bladder, lymphoma, ovarian, pancreatic, and stomach cancer, no correlation was observed between omega 3 PUFA intake and the cancer incidence. Chapkin et al. (2007) showed that omega 3 PUFA suppressed the mediating inflammatory Th 1 cells that are linked to the occurrence of colon cancer. A research team at the St. George's Hospital in South London, found that the consumption of the fish oil capsules rich in omega 3 fatty acids restored the cell protection to normal levels in bowel cancer patients.

Nutrition at the time of surgery is known to influence surgical outcome. Takeuchi et al. (2007) sought to determine whether intake of fish oil had beneficial effects on recovery from surgery in cancer patients. Following esophagectomy, patients are fed an enteral diet through a tube directly into the jejunum (jejunostomy). Fourty patients who underwent surgery for esophageal cancer were studied. Twenty patients served as controls and received a normal enteral diet post-surgery (Group A). Six other patients received the normal enteral diet supplemented with arginine, omega-3 fatty acids and RNA, all substrates believed to have immune-enhancing effects, after surgery (Group B). Another 14 patients also received the arginine, omega-3 and RNA-supplemented enteral diet but were fed this diet both before and after surgery (Group C). The incidence of incisional wound infection and the duration of post-surgery systemic inflammation were significantly lower in patients in Group C compared to patients in Group A suggesting beneficial effects of arginine, omega-3 fats and/or RNA on surgery outcome.

Dysfunctional interactions between tumour cells and normal healthy cells of the body result in a range of pathologies including fatigue, weakness, cachexia, anorexia, early satiety and chronic nausea. Collectively these pathologies are known as SIMS (systemic immune-metabolic syndrome). Reducing or eliminating SIMS is not only important for maintaining the quality of life of cancer patients but may also aid in improving the prognosis of cancer outcome. SIMS may be a side effect of the chronic systemic inflammation associated with cancer. As n-3 LCPUFAs are known to have anti-inflammatory activity, a group of researchers investigated whether inclusion of n- 3 LCPUFAs in the diet of cancer patients alleviated some of the symptoms of SIMS. Twenty-two patients with advanced stage lung cancer and SIMS were supplemented with either fish oil capsules (2g per day) alone or fish oil capsules (2g per day) with the cyclooxygenase-2 (cox-2) inhibitor celecoxib (200mg) for 6 weeks. Compared to baseline, appetite was significantly improved, fatigue significantly reduced and circulating levels of the inflammatory marker C-reactive protein (CRP) were significantly reduced in all patients receiving the fish oil supplement. Body weight and muscle strength were significantly improved in patients receiving fish oil + celecoxib compared to baseline and were significantly higher than in patients receiving fish oil supplementation alone (Cerchietti et al. 2007). This study also demonstrates that fish oil improves symptoms of SIMS possibly by reducing inflammation. Specific inhibition of cox-2, the cyclooxygenase responsible for synthesis of pro-inflammatory eicosanoids from n-6 LCPUFAs, in conjunction with fish oil supplementation further reduces symptoms of SIMS in cancer patients. In spite of these reports, recent analysis of a large body of literature spanning numerous cohorts from many countries with different demographic patterns, apprehension has been raised on significant association between omega 3 fatty acids and cancer incidence.

11. Bone

Inflammation is characterized symptomatically by pain, redness, and swelling; disordered or excessive inflammation also entails loss of function (James et al., 2000). Osteoarthritis is an inflammatory disease of the joints. The pain and loss of joint mobility known as arthritis is largely as a result of destruction of cartilage within the joint. Matrix metalloproteinases (MMPs) are enzymes responsible for the degradation of the cartilage tissue matrix. Normally MMPs remove fatigued or damaged cartilage as a part of the self-repair process which occurs in all tissues. Increased expression or activity of MMPs or loss of the normal inhibitors of MMPs results in an inappropriate increase in tissue breakdown. Beneficial effects of n-3 LCPUFAs in reducing the symptoms associated with osteoarthritis have previously been reported in some clinical studies. Hansen et al. (2008) explained the mechanism by which n-3 LCPUFAs reduces osteoarthritis. This study revealed that different LCPUFAs have different effects in bone. Bone is continually broken down and replaced. Usually in adults bone resorption is completely balanced by bone formation and net bone mass remains unchanged. However, menopause leads to conditions which favour bone resorption over formation. Bone mass can be preserved post-menopause either by inhibiting bone resorption or by promoting bone formation. The effect of LCPUFAs on osteoclast activity (the cells responsible for bone resorption) and osteoclastogenesis have recently been investigated.

One of the signalling pathways responsible for promoting osteoclastogenesis is the RANKL pathway. This pathway involves three proteins: two receptors (RANK and OPG) and a ligand (RANKL). RANK is present on the outer membrane of osteoclast precursors. When it binds to RANKL which is mainly present on the outer membrane of mature osteoblasts (the cells responsible for bone formation), maturation of the osteoclast precursors are initiated to form into fully-functional osteoclasts. OPG is secreted by osteoblasts and will also bind to RANK. Binding of RANK to OPG however does not trigger osteoclast maturation and henceis known as a decoy receptor. Osteoclastogenesis can be inhibited by reducing synthesis of RANKL and/or by increasing synthesis of OPG. Inflammatory eicosanoids such as prostaglandin E2 (PGE2) synthesised from n-6 LCPUFAs promote RANKL expression and therefore promote osteoclastogenesis. The effects of DHA and EPA on the expression of

RANKL and OPG in the MC3T3-E1/4 osteoblast cell line were recently studied. EPA and DHA were equally effective in inhibiting the PGE2-induced increase in RANKL expression in MC3T3-E1/4 cells. Neither had any effect on OPG secretion or on RANKL expression in cells not treated with PGE2 (Poulsen et al. 2008). Results of this study suggest that EPA and DHA may have a role in inhibiting the increase in bone resorption which occurs under inflammatory conditions (Kruger and Poulsen 2008).

Once RANKL binds to RANK a signalling cascade is initiated which ultimately leads to osteoclastogenesis. Influencing RANKL expression, EPA and DHA also appear to influence factors downstream in this signalling cascade. In RAW 264.7 cells (a cell line capable of differentiating into mature osteoclasts), DHA and to a lesser extent EPA, were found to reduce the number of mature osteoclasts formed after treatment of RAW cells with RANKL (Rahman et al. 2008). Results of the above studies suggest that DHA may be more effective than EPA in maintaining bone mass post-ovariectomy due at least in part to its ability to inhibit RANKL-mediated osteoclastogenesis. Whether DHA is also effective in helping to minimise bone loss in post-menopausal women remains to be investigated (Kruger and Poulsen 2008).

12. Other Benefits

Fish – derived PUFA, particularly DHA are beneficial in infant nutrition and development. Omega – 3 fatty acids are reported to associate with the brain development and important for the vision and the functions of reproductive systems (pregnancy and infancy). More persistent benefits of DHA supplementation on visual acuity, mental development and age-relatated declines in neural function is key to preserving the autonomy and well-being of older people (Uauy and Dangour 2006; Narayan et al., 2006). It was also reported that the combination of fish oil and fish protein hydrolysate in the diet profoundly reduced the plasma cholesterol level mainly due to lowering of high-density lipo protein (HDLP) cholesterol. HDLP has been beneficial to control high blood pressure. A decrease of diastolic pressure by 3 mm Hg and systolic pressure by 6 mm Hg by regular consumption of EPA and DHA has been reported in a population based intervention trial (Venugopal 2009). The positive effect of EPA in schizophrenia treatment was demonstrated when it was added to usual antipsychotic agent. The other studies show a positive role in risk in reduction of postpartum depression, bipolar disorder, humor fluctuations and kidney transplantations (Nunes et al., 2011).

13. Conclusions

Seafood is an important source of nutrients, which are fundamental for a balanced diet. The dietary recommendations for long-chain omega 3 PUFA are a still a matter of debate. Recommendations vary depending on desired disease prevention. Daily ranges for EPA and DHA begin from 180 (for healthy adults) to 500 mg (to decrease the prevalence of heart disease) to 1000 mg (to decrease the prevalence of mental illness). Various levels of consumption of fatty fish or fish oil have been recommended by different agencies to derive health benefits. The consumption of two fish meals a week or atleast a mean level of 500 mg of EPA+DHA per day are actually strongly recommended by several health authorities. In the case of secondary prevention, a double dose of 1g per day is advised. The American Heart Association recommends healthy individuals to consume 2-3 oz serving of fatty fish per week and that the persons diagnosed with CHD/CVD consume 1g each of the fatty acid per day. The World Health Organisation recommends consumption of 1-2 servings of fish, containing 200-500 mg of EPA and DHA, per week. The challenge for nutritionists now is to integrate existing scientific knowledge and further advance applied research on effective ways to attain and maintain brain function throughout the life. So, the recognized beneficial effects of omega-3 & omega-6 enriched fatty acids make fish as food item especially recommended for human health and well-being.

References

Albert, C.M., Hennekens, C.H., O'Donnell, C.J., Ajani, U.A., Carey, V.J., Willet, W.C., Ruskin, J.N, and Manson, J.E. 1998. Fish consumption and risk of sudden cardiac death. *JAMA* 279, 23-28.

Arendash, G. W., Jensen, M. T., Salem, N., Hussein, N., Cracchiolo, J., Dickson, A., Leighty, R, and Potter, H. 2007. A diet high in omega-3 fatty acids does not improve or protect cognitive performance in alzheimer's transgenic mice. *Neurosci.* 149(2), 286-302.

Bartsch, H., Nair, J, and Owen, R.W. 1999. Dietary polyunsaturated fatty acids and cancers of the breast and colorectum: emerging evidence for their role as risk modifiers. *Carcinogenesis* 20, 2209–2218.

Beydoun, M. A., Kaufman, J. S., Sloane, P. D., Heiss, G, and Ibrahim, J. 2008. N-3 fatty acids, hypertension and risk of cognitive decline among older adults in the atherosclerosis risk in communities (aric) study. *Public Health Nut.* 11(1), 17-29.

Borkman, M., Storlien, L.H., Pan, D.A., Jenkins, A.B., Chisholm, D.J. and Campbell, L.V. 1993. The relation between insulin sensitivity and the fattyacid composition of skeletal-muscle phospholipids. *N. Engl. J. Med.* 328, 238–244.

Bowling, A.C, and Stewart, T.M. 2003. Current Complementary and Alternative Therapies for Multiple Sclerosis. *Curr. Treat. options in Neurol.* 5,55–68.

Caggiula, A.W, and Mustad, V.A. 1997. Effects of dietary fat and fatty acids on coronary artery disease risk and total and lipoprotein cholesterol concentrations: epidemiologic studies. *Am. J. Clin. Nutr.* 65,1597S–1610S.

Calder, P. C. 1998. Dietary fatty acids and the immune system. *Nutr. Rev.* 56, S70–S83.

Cansev, M., Wurtman, R., Sakamoto, J, and Ulus, I. 2008. Oral administration of circulating precursors for membrane phosphatides can promote the synthesis of new brain synapses. *Alzheimers and Dementia* 4(1), S153-S168.

Cerchietti, L., Navigante, A, and Castro, M. 2007. Effects of eicosapentaenoic and docosahexaenoic n-3 fatty acids from fish oil and preferntial cox-2 inhibition on systemic syndromes in patients with advanced lung cancer. *Nut.Cancer Int. J.* 59(1), 14-20.

Chance, W.T., Ogle, C.K., Thomas, I., Zhou, L., Zhang, X., Basanta, M, and Fischer, E. 1996. Immunostimulation following fish oil-based parenteral nutrition in tumor-bearing rats. *Nutr. Cancer* 26(3), 303-312.

Chapkin, R.S., Davidson, L.A., Ly, L., Weeks, B.R., Lupton, J.R, and McMurray, D.N. 2007. Immunomodulatory effects of (n-3) fatty acids: putative link to inflammation and colon cancer. *J. Nut.* 137, 200S-204S.

Chen, W.J, and Yeh, S.L. 2003. Effects of fish oil in parenteral nutrition. *Nut.* 19, 275–279.

Das UN. 2003. Is there a role for saturated and long-chain fatty acids in multiple sclerosis?. *Nut.*19,163–166.

de Deckere, E., Korver, O., Verschuren, and Katan, M.B. 1998. Health aspects of fish and n-3 polyunsaturated fatty acids from plant and marine origin. *Eur. J. Cli. Nut.* 52, 749-753.

Dhaka, V., Gulia, N., Ahlawat, K. S. and Khatkar, B. S. 2011. Trans fats—sources, health risks and alternative approach - A review. *J. Food Sci. Technol.* In Press (Publsihed in Online: 28 January, 2011; DOI 10.1007/s13197-011-0269-4).

Dyerberg, J., Bang, H.O., Stoffersen, E., Moncada, S. and Vane, J. 1978. Eicosapentaenoic acid and prevention of thrombosis and atherosclerosis?. *Lancet* 2, 117-119.

Farinotti, M., Simi, S., Di Pietrantonj, C., McDowell, N., Brait, L., Lupo, D, and Filippini, G. 2007. Dietary interventions for multiple sclerosis. *Cochrane Database Sys.Rev.*, Issue 1. Art. No.: CD004192. DOI: 10.1002/14651858.CD004192.pub2.

Fickova, M, Hubert, P, Cremel, G, and Leray, C. 1998. Dietary (n–3) and (n–6) polyunsaturated fatty acids rapidly modify fatty acid composition and insulin effects in rat adipocytes. *J. Nutr.*128, 512–519.

Field, C.J., Johnson, I.R, and Schley, P.D. 2002. Nutrients and their role in host resistance to infection. *J. Leukocyte Biol.* 71, 16-32.

Hansen, R. A., Harris, M. A., Pluhar, G. E., Motta, T., Brevard, S., Ogilvie, G. K., Fettman, M. J, and Allen, K. G. D. 2008. Fish oil decreases matrix metalloproteinases in knee synovia of dogs with inflammatory joint disease. *J. Nut. Biochem.* 19(2), 101-108.

Harris, W.S. 2004a. Fish oil supplementation: Evidence for health benefits. *Cleveland Clinic J. Med.* 71, 208 – 221.

Harris, W.S., Sands, S.A., Windsor, S.L., Ali, H.A., Stevens, T.L., Magalski, A., Porter, C.B. and Borkon, A.M. 2004b. Omega-3 fatty acids in cardiac biopsies from heart transplantation patients: correlation with erythrocytes and response to supplementation. *Circulation,* 110, 1645-1649.

He, K. 2009. Fish, Long-Chain Omega-3 Polyunsaturated Fatty Acids and Prevention of Cardiovascular Disease—Eat Fish or Take Fish Oil Supplement?. *Progress Cardiovasc. Dis.* 52, 95–114.

Hodge, L., Salome, C.M., Peat, J.K., Haby, M.M.m Xuan, W, and Woolcock, A.J. 1996. Consumption of oily fish and childhood asthma risk. *Med. J. Aust.* 164, 137–140.

Hosack-Fowler, K., Chapkin, R. S, and McMurray, D. N. 1993. Effects of purified dietary n-3 ethyl esters on murine T lymphocyte function. *J. Immunol.* 151, 5186–5197.

Hu, F.B., van Dam, R.M. and Liu, S. 2001. Diet and risk of type II diabetes: the role of types of fat and carbohydrates. *Diabetologia* 44, 805-817.

James, M. J., Gibson, R. A. and Cleland, L. G. 2000. Dietary polyunsaturated fatty acids and inflammatory mediator Production. *Am. J. Clin. Nutr.* 71(suppl):343S–348S.

Jazayeri, S., Tehrani-Doost, M., Keshavarz, S., Hosseini, M., Djazayery, A., Amini, H., Jalali, M, and Peet, M. (2008). Comparison of therapeutic effects of eicosapentaenoic acid (epa), fluoxetine, separately and in combination, in major depressive disorder. *Australian & New Zealand J. Psychiatry* 42(3): 192-198.

Kelley, D. S., Taylor, P. C., Nelson, G. J., Schmidt, P. C., Ferretti, A., Erickson, K. L., Yu, R., Chandra, R. K, and Mackey, B. E. 1999. Docosahexaenoic acid ingestion inhibits natural killer cell activity and production of inflammatory mediators in young healthy men. *Lipids* 34, 317–324.

Krebs, J.D, Browning, L.M., McLean, N.K., Rothwell, J.L., Mishra, G.D., Moore, C.S, and Jebb, S.A. 2006. Additive benefits of long-chain n–3 polyunsaturated fatty acids and weight-loss in the management of cardiovascular disease risk in overweight hyperinsulinaemic women. *Int. J. Obes. (Lond.),* 30, 1535–1544.

Kris-Etherton, P.M., Harris, W.S, and Appel, L.J. 2002. Fish consumption, fish oil, omega-3 fatty acids, and cardiovascular disease. *Circulation* 106, 2747-57.

Kris-Etherton, P.M., Harris, W.S, and Appel, L.J. 2003. Omega-3 fatty acids and cardiovascular disease: new recommendations from the American Heart Association. *Arterioscler. Thromb. Vasc. Biol.* 23, 151-2.

Kruger, M. and Poulsen, R. 2008. Health benefits of salmon and omega 3 oil supplementation. Confidential report to New Zealand King Salmon. Institute of Food, Nutrition & Human Health, Massey University. 19pp.

Lauer, K. 1997. Diet and multiple sclerosis. *Neurol.* 49 (Suppl 2), S55–S61.

Lim, W.S., Gammack, J.K., Van Niekerk, J.K, and Dangour, A. 2006. Omega 3 fatty acid for the prevention of dementia. *Cochrane Database Sys. Rev.* Issue 1. Art. No.: CD005379. DOI: 10.1002/14651858.CD005379.pub2.

Ling, P.R., Istfan, N.W., Lopes, S.M., Babayan, V.K., Blackburn, G.L, and Bistrain, B.R. 1991. Structured lipid made from fish oil and medium-chain triglycerides alters tumor and host metabolism in Yoshidasarcoma- bearing rats. *Am. J. Clin. Nutr.* 53, 1177-1184.

Luo, J., Rizkalla, S.W., Boillot, J., Alamowitch, C., Chaib, H., Bruzzo, F., Desplanque, N., Dalix, A.M., Durand, G, and Slama, G. 1996. Dietary (n–3) polyunsaturated fatty acids improve adipocyte insulin action and glucose metabolism in insulin-resistant rats: relation to membrane fatty acids. *J. Nutr.* 126, 1951–8.

Ma, Q. L., Teter, B., Ubeda, O. J., Morihara, T., Dhoot, D., Nyby, M. D., Tuck, M. L., Frautschy, S. A, and Cole, G. M. 2007. Omega-3 fatty acid docosahexaenoic acid increases sorla/lr11, a sorting protein with reduced expression in sporadic alzheimer's disease (ad): Relevance to ad prevention. *J. Neurosci.* 27(52), 14299-14307.

Marchioli, R., Barzi, F., Bomba, E., Chieffo, C., Di Gregorio, D., Di Mascio, R., Franzosi, M.G., Geraci, E., Levantesi, G., Maggioni, P., Mantini, L., Marfisi, R.M., Mastrogiuseppe, G., Mininni, N., Nicolosi, G. L., Santini, M., Schweiger, C., Tavazzi, L., Tognoni, G., Tucci, C, and Valagussa, F. 2002. Early protection against sudden death by n-3 polyunsaturated fatty acids after myocardial infarction: time-course analysis of the results of the Gruppo Italiano per lo Studio della Sopravvivenza nell'Infarto Miocardico (GISSI)-Prevenzione. *Circulation* 105, 1897-1903.

MacLean, CH., Newberry, SJ., Mojica, WA., Khanna, P., Issa, A.M., Suttorp, M.J., Lim, Y., Traina, S.B., Hilton, L., Garland, R, and Morton, S.C. 2006. Effects of omega-3 fatty acids on cancer risk. *JAMA* 295, 403-415

Mendez, B., Ling, P.R., Istfan, N.W., Babayan, V.K, and Bistrian, B.R. 1992. Effects of different lipid sources in total parenteral nutrition on whole body protein kinetics and tumor growth. *JPEN* 16, 545-551

Mensink, R.P, and Katan, M.B. 1990. Effect of dietary trans fatty acids on high-density and low density lipoprotein cholesterol levels in healthy subjects. *N. Engl. J. Med.* 323, 439–445

Mozaffarian, D., Ascherio, A., Hu, F.B., Stanfer, M.J., Willett, W.C., Siscovick, D.S. and Rimm, E.B. 2005. Interplay between different polyunsaturated fatty acids and risk of coronary heart disease in men. *Circulation* 111, 157-64.

Mozaffarian, D. and Rimm, E. 2006. Fish intake, contaminants and human health: evaluating the risk and the benefits. *JAMA* 296, 1885-1899.

Narayan, B., Miyashita, K, and Hosakawa, M. 2006. Physiological effects of eicosapentaenoic acid (EPA) and docosahexaenoic acid (DHA)-A Review. *Food Rev. Int.* 22,291–307.

Nunes, M.L., Bandarra, N.M. and Batista, I. 2011. Health benefits associated with seafood consumption. In: Handbook of seafood quality, safety and health applications, Alasalvar, C., Shahidi, F., Miyashita, K. and Wanasundara, U. (Eds.), Blackwell Publishing Ltd.United Kingdom, 542pp.

Osborn, G., Escofet, X, and Da Silva, A. 2008. Medical adjuvant treatment to increase patency of arteriovenous fistulae and grafts. *Cochrane Database Sys. Rev.* Issue 4: 1-28. Art. No.: CD002786. DOI: 10.1002/14651858.CD002786.pub2.

Peat, J.K., Saolme, C.M, and Woolcock, A.J. 1992. Factors associated with bronchial hyperresponsiveness in Australian adults and children. *Eur. Respir. J.* 5, 921–9.

Poulsen, R. C., Wolber, F. M., Moughan, P. J., and Kruger, M. C. 2008. Long chain polyunsaturated fatty acids alter membrane-bound rank-l expression and osteoprotegerin secretion by mc3t3-el osteoblast-like cells. *Prostaglandins & Other Lipid Mediators* 85(1-2), 42-48.

Puglisi, M.J., Hasty, A.H. and Saraswathi, V. 2011. The role of adipose tissue in mediating the beneficial effects of dietary fish oil. *J. Nut. Biochem.* 22, 101–108.

Puri, B. K., Koepp, M. J., Holmes, J., Hamilton, G, and Yuen, A. W. C. 2007. A 31-phosphorus neurospectroscopy study of [omega]-3 long-chain polyunsaturated fatty acid intervention with eicosapentaenoic acid and docosahexaenoic acid in patients with chronic refractory epilepsy. *Prostaglandins, Leukotrienes and Essential Fatty Acids* 77(2): 105-107.

Rahman, M. A., Bhattacharya, A, and Fernandes, G. 2008. Docosahexaenoic acid is more potent inhibitor of osteoclast differentiation in raw 264.7 cells than eicosapentaenoic acid. *J. Cell. Physiol.* 214(1), 201-209.

Rao, C.V., Hirose, Y., Indranie, C, and Reddy, B.S. 2001. Modulation of experimental colon tumorigenesis by types and amounts of dietary fatty acids. *Cancer Res.,* 61, 1927–1933.

Reddy, B.S., Tanaka, T, and Simi, B. 1985. Effect of different levels of dietary trans fat or corn oil on azoxymethane-induced colon carcinogenesis in F344 rats. *J. Natl. Cancer Inst.* 75, 791–798.

Rogers, P., Appleton, K., Kessler, D., Peters, T., Gunnell, D., Hayward, R., Heatherly, S., LM, C., McNaughton, S.Ness, A. (2008). No effect of n-3 long-chain polynsaturated fatty acid (epa and dha) supplementation on depressed mood and cognitive function: A randomised controlled trial. *British J. Nut.* 99(2): 421-431.

Salvati, S., Natali, F., Attorri, L., Di Benedetto, R., Leonardi, F., Di Biase, A., Feri, F., Fortuna, S., Lorenzini, P., Sanchez, M., Ricceri, L. and Vitelli, L. 2008. Eicosapentaenoic acid stimulates the expression of myelin proteins in rat brain. *J. Neurosci. Res.* 86, 776-784.

Schmitz, P.G., McCloud, L.K., Reikes, S.T., Leonard, C.L. and Gellens, M.E. 2002. Prophylaxis of Hemodialysis Graft Thrombosis with Fish Oil: Double-Blind, Randomized, Prospective Trial. *J. Am. Soc. Nephrol.* 13, 184-190.

Schwartz, J, and Weiss, S.T. 1990. Dietary factors and their relation to respiratory symptoms. *Am. J. Epidemiol.* 132, 67–76.

Schwartz, J. 2000. Role of polyunsaturated fatty acids in lung disease. *Am. J. Clin. Nutr.* 71(suppl), 393S–6S.

Schwarz, S., Leweling, H. 2005. Multiple sclerosis and nutrition. *Multiple sclerosis* 11, 24–32.

Sharp, D., Rodrigues, B.L., Shahar, E., Hwang, L.J, and Burchfiel, C.M. 1995. Fish consumption may limit the damage of smoking on the lung. *Am. J. Respir. Crit. Care Med.* 150, 983–987.

Simopoulos, A. P. 1999. Essential fatty acids in health and chronic disease. *Am. J. Clin. Nutr.* 70 (suppl), 560S–569S.

Siscovick, D.S., Raghunathan, T.E., King, I., Weinmann, S., Bovbjerg, V. E., Kushi, L., Cobb, L. A., Copass, M. K., Psaty, B. M., Lemaitre, R., Retzlaff, B. and Knopp, R. H. 1995. Dietary intake and cell membrane levels of long-chain n-3 polyunsaturated fatty acids and the risk of primary cardiac arrest. *JAMA* 274,1363-1367.

Swank, R.L, and Goodwin, J.W. 2003. How saturated fats may be a causative factor in multiple sclerosis and other diseases. *Nut.* 19(5), 478.

Takeuchi, H., Ikeuchi, S., Kawaguchi, Y., Kitagawa, Y., Isobe, Y., Kubochi, K., Kitajima, M, and Matsumota, S. 2007. Clinical significance of perioperative immunonutrition forpatients with esophageal cancer. *World J. Surgery* 31, 2160-2167.

Troisi, R.J., Willett, W.C., Weiss, S.T., Trichopoulos, D., Rosner, B, and Speizer, F.E. 1995. A prospective study of diet and adult-onset asthma. *Am. J. Respir. Crit. Care Med.* 151, 1401–1408.

Uauy, R. and Dangour, A.D. 2006. Nutrition in brain development and aging: role of essential fatty acids. *Nut. Rev.,* 64, S24-S33.

Venugopal, V. 2009. Marine products for healthcare: Functional and bioactive nutraceutical compounds from the ocean. CRC Press, Taylor & Francis Group, 527pp.

von Schacky, C, Harris, W.S. 2007. Cardiovascular benefits of omega-3 fatty acids. *Cardiovasc. Res.* 73, 310-315.

Vora, J.D., Deshpande, D.D. 2010. Food for healthy brain function. *Everyman's Sci.* Vol XLV(3), 166-168.

Weisberg, S.P., McCann, D., Desai, M., Rosenbaum, M., Leibel, R.L., Ferrante, Jr. A.W. 2003. Obesity is associated with macrophage accumulation in adipose tissue. *J. Clin. Invest.* 112, 1796–808.

In: Fish Oil: Production, Consumption and Health Benefits
Editors: Matthias Van Dijk and Jürgen Vitek
ISBN: 978-1-61470-963-3

Chaper VI

Plant-Derived Antioxidants as Potential Omega-3 PUFA Stabilizers

Priya Kathirvel and H. P. Vasantha Rupasinghe*
Department of Environmental Sciences, Nova Scotia Agricultural College,
Truro, Nova Scotia, Canada

1. Introduction

The dietary intake of omega-3 fatty acids, which are long chain polyunsaturated fatty acids (PUFA), commonly found in fish or fish oil has numerous health benefits such as the prevention of heart diseases, cancer, dementia and several neurological and psychiatric diseases. The effect of omega-3 fatty acids, especially in the form of eicosapentaenoic acid (EPA) and docosahexaenoic acid (DHA) in the prevention of primary and secondary cardiovascular diseases is well addressed [1, 2]. Their cardioprotective mechanisms extend from antiartherosclerotic [3] to antithrombotic [4, 5], antiarrhythmic [6, 7] and anti-inflammatory activity including lowering of blood pressure and triglyceride levels [8]. Moreover, omega-3 PUFA have been shown to inhibit the formation of various types of cancers [9, 10] and have also been implicated in the brain and eye development in infants and young children [11, 12].

Due to many health benefits of omega-3 fatty acids, inclusion of these essential fatty acids in the diet has been recommended. The World Health Organization (WHO) has recommended one to two servings of fatty fish per week (each serving should provide the equivalent of 200 to 500 mg of EPA+DHA) and is generally being considered as a standard reference in terms of dietary intake of omega-3 fatty acids [13]. However, various organizations worldwide have established their own recommendations for the consumption of omega-3 fatty acids for health promotion and prevention of various chronic diseases [14].

* Correspondance to: H.P. Vasantha Rupasinghe, Tree Fruit Bio-product Research Program, Department of Environmental Sciences, Nova Scotia Agricultural College, P.O. Box 550, Truro, Nova Scotia, B2N 5E3 Canada. Phone: +1 902 893 6623; E-mail: vrupasinghe@nsac.ca

Currently, the dietary recommendations for EPA and DHA are being met by the intake of omega-3 fatty acids rich fish, fish oil supplements as well as algal supplements. Unfortunately, the PUFA present in fish oil are vulnerable to oxidation which decreases the shelf life and nutritional value of the fish oil. In this chapter, we have briefly discussed about lipid oxidation in fish oil, synthetic antioxidants and plant-derived natural antioxidants.

2. Lipid Oxidation in Fish Oil

Fish oil is highly susceptible to lipid oxidation mainly due to the presence of multiple double bonds in PUFA. Lipid oxidation leads to the development of off-flavors, odors and colors which in turn decreases the nutritional value of the oil. This poses a major challenge in the production and marketing of fish oils or fish oil containing products. Oxidation of fish oil is usually accelerated by various factors including exposure to light, oxygen, prooxidants and high temperatures [15]. The process of autoxidation of polyunsaturated lipids generally involves three steps: initiation (production of lipid free radicals), propagation, and termination (production of nonradical products).

Initiation $RH \rightarrow R\bullet + H\bullet$

Propagation $R\bullet + O_2 \rightarrow ROO\bullet$

$ROO\bullet + RH \rightarrow R\bullet + ROOH$

Termination

$$\left.\begin{array}{l} R\bullet + R\bullet \\ R\bullet + ROO\bullet \\ ROO\bullet + ROO\bullet \end{array}\right\} \text{nonradical products}$$

Oxidation of PUFA leads to the formation of primary lipid oxidation products, lipid hydroperoxides. Lipid hydroperoxides are unstable at high temperatures and in the presence of transition metals decompose quickly [15]. The breakdown products of lipid hydroperoxides include aldehydes, ketones, alcohols, acids, hydrocarbons and epoxides, of which certain compounds are responsible for the rancid off-flavor of fish oils. Docosahexaenoic acid (DHA) has been estimated to be over 50 times more susceptible to oxidation than oleic acid and can be detected at very early stages of oxidation [16].

The oxidative status of oil samples is determined preferably by analysis of the peroxide value (primary oxidation products) showing the onset of oxidation and the TBA-value or para-anisidine value (secondary oxidation products), which is a marker for the volatile oxidation products [16]. Several other methods that are employed to assess the progression of lipid oxidation in fish oils include head space analysis, fourier transform infrared (FT-IR) spectroscopy and nuclear magnetic resonance (NMR) spectroscopy [16, 17, 18]. Apart from this sensory evaluation also provides valuable information on the overall acceptability of fish oils.

Oxidation products of fatty acids in fish oils have been shown to induce aging and carcinogenesis [19]. Increased thiobarbituric acid reactive substances (TBARS) values of plasma and liver microsomes in animals fed oxidized oils have been reported [20, 21]. The breakdown products of lipid oxidation, such as malonaldehyde have been reported to cause adverse health effects due to their cytotoxic and genotoxic effects [22, 23].

3. Methods to Control Lipid Oxidation in Fish Oil

Omega-3 PUFA in fish oil are oxidatively unstable, only very little oxygen is needed to initiate as well as to maintain lipid oxidation process. The quality of fish oil usually deteriorates with time and hence inclusion of fish oils in foods becomes limited. In order to delay the oxidation process and to increase the overall stability of oils, many methods including application of synthetic and natural antioxidants as well as microencapsulation are widely practised in the industry. Currently, combination of both methods is often adopted for better stability of omega-3 PUFA.

3.1. Microencapsulation

Encapsulation is currently a widely practised technology in the food industry which consists of packing solid, liquid or gaseous materials in small sealed capsules. The main advantages of encapsulation include stabilization of active components in the capsules and controlled release of components in the digestive system. Microencapsulation of fish oil has facilitated the incorporation of omega-3 PUFA in foods without the development of any undesirable flavour or odor during storage. Increased sensory acceptance, prolonged shelf-life and enhanced bioavailability and efficacy of omega-3 PUFA in fortified foods have been depicted as the positive outcomes of microencapsulation of fish oil.

Spray-drying is one among the various techniques available for the encapsulation of fish oil and involves four stages: preparation of a dispersion or emulsion; homogenization of the dispersion; atomisation of the feed emulsion and dehydration of the atomized particles [24]. The high temperatures used in spray drying during the drying process poses a problem in terms of accelerating the oxidation of oils. Production of dried microencapsulated fish oil by freezing and subsequent freeze-drying has been reported to yield product with high oxidative stability [25]. Ultrasonic atomization of the feed emulsion and freeze drying has been demonstrated as a promising alternative method for tuna oil encapsulation [26]. Other techniques such as fluidized bed coating and extrusion as well as protein and biopolymer based encapsulation (polymer gelation and coacervation with subsequent cross-linking) have been considered to be superior techniques for microencapsulation compared to spray drying [27].

Although encapsulation reduces the susceptibility of fish oil to oxidation, the possibility of oxygen permeation through the wall cannot be ruled out. Hence, further stabilization is achieved by the addition of antioxidants during the homogenization as well as the microencapsulation stages. A combination of δ-tocopherol with lecithin or citric acid esters from monoglycerides and ascorbyl palmitate has been reported to be effective in stabilizing microencapsulated fish oil [28]. A combination of lipophilic antioxidants (a combination of tocopherols rich in δ-derivative and low in α-derivative), synergestic compounds (ascorbyl palmitate) and a metal chelator (lecithin) provided protection against lipid oxidation in microencapsulated fish oils [29].

3.2. Antioxidants

Antioxidants are substances that, when present in foods at low concentrations compared with that of an oxidizable substrate, markedly delay or prevent the oxidation of the substrate [30]. Antioxidants protect the lipids against oxidation by quenching the free radicals, scavenging other reactive oxygen species (ROS), chelating metals, inactivating the lipid peroxides or by reacting with secondary lipid oxidation products that impart rancidity to fish oils [31]. Based on the mechanism of action, antioxidants are broadly classified into primary and secondary antioxidants. Primary antioxidants break the chain reaction of lipid oxidation by donating hydrogen atom and producing more stable radicals where as secondary antioxidants slow down the rate of oxidation by various mechanisms including decomposition of hydroperoxides, regeneration of primary antioxidants, binding metals and scavenging of oxygen among others. Secondary antioxidants often act synergistically with primary antioxidants and have been shown to enhance the activity of the primary antioxidants [32]. A wide variety of natural as well as synthetic compounds offer protection in retarding or inhibiting lipid oxidation processes in foods. Selecting a proper antioxidant is necessary in terms of improving the oxidative stability of fish oils or fish oil fortified foods. Factors that could influence the activity of antioxidants in foods include the chemical nature of the compounds, physical location of the antioxidants in the food system, effective concentration, stability of the compounds and interaction with other food components to name a few.

3.2.1. Synthetic Antioxidants

Synthetic antioxidants that are widely used in the industry consist of four phenolic compounds: namely, butylated hydroxyanisole (BHA), butylated hydroxytoluene (BHT), tert-butylhydro-quinone (TBHQ) and propyl gallate (PG).

BHA is a mixture of two isomers (2-*tertiary*-butyl-4-hydroxyanisole and 3-*tertiary*-butyl-4-hydroxyanisole) (Figure 1). It is a monohydroxy phenol and frequently used for the preservation of fats and oils. BHT is also a monophenolic antioxidant (Figure 1) and is used alone or in combination with BHA for better antioxidant activity [33]. Both BHA and BHT are fat soluble antioxidants. Among the two, BHA has been reported to be thermally stable compared to BHT [32]. BHA and BHT have been shown to effectively inhibit lipid oxidation in fish oil as well as other omega-3 PUFA oxidation model systems [34, 35, 36]. The level of usage of BHA/BHT mixtures in foods have been limited to 0.02% based on lipid weight [32, 37].

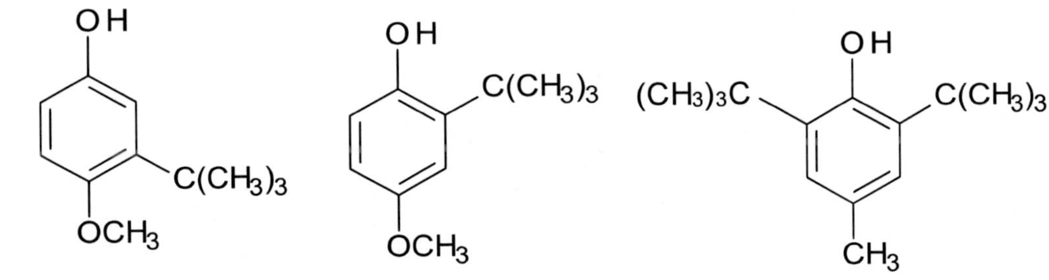

BHA (2-isomer) BHA (3-isomer) BHT

Figure 1. Chemical structures of BHA (2-isomer and 3-isomer) and BHT molecules.

tert-Butylhydroquinone (TBHQ) is another synthetic food grade antioxidant and exhibits a good stabilizing effect in unsaturated fats, particularly polyunsaturated vegetable oils, fish oils and animal fats (Figure 2). TBHQ is a diphenolic antioxidant and is considered to be a more effective antioxidant than BHA and BHT in fish oil and fish skin lipids [36, 38]. The higher efficacy of TBHQ results from the presence of two hydroxyl groups which can scavenge the free radicals formed during the oxidation process. The recommended level of usage of TBHQ in foods is 0.02% based on lipid weight.

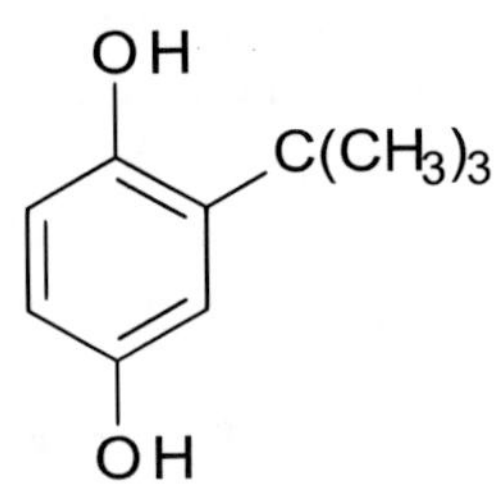

TBHQ

Figure 2. Chemical structure of TBHQ.

Propyl gallate is a food grade antioxidant slightly soluble in both water and fat and is the only gallate that is permitted in foods in the United States and Canada [32] (Figure 3). Other gallic acid esters, such as octyl and lauryl gallates are approved in several European countries as food antioxidants [32]. Propyl gallate exhibited better antioxidant activity in bulk cod liver oil compared to hydroxytyrosol and comparable activity in emulsions and frozen fish muscle [39]. Propyl gallate has been shown to be highly effective in inhibiting the formation of hydroperoxides and conjugated dienes in fish oils [40]. Propyl gallate can also act as a pro-oxidant under certain conditions due to its ability to form complexes with iron and copper and converting the metal to its active form [41, 42]. A pro-oxidant effect of propyl gallate was observed in omega-3 fatty acids enriched mayonnaise due to the activation of protein bound metal ions by the gallate [43].

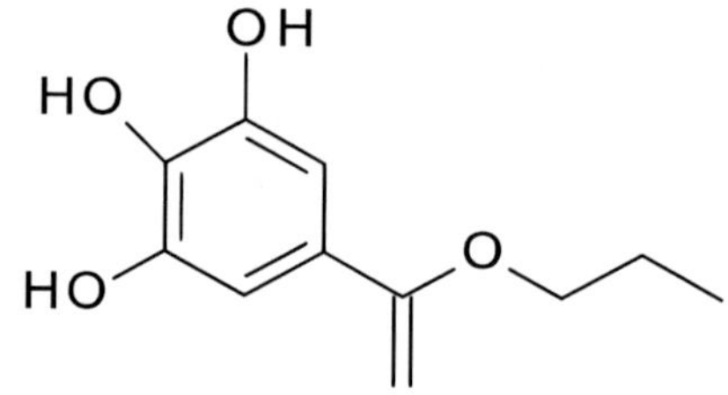

Propyl gallate

Figure 3. Chemical structure of propyl gallate.

Synthetic antioxidants have been a topic of debate due to safety concerns among the food scientists, health officials and consumers. Studies have shown that BHT could possibly induce severe tissue damage in the liver and kidney of rats [44]. High doses of BHA and BHT have been implicated in the development of tumours in the fore stomach and liver of rats [45]. In addition to this, BHA and BHT have also been reported to be cytotoxic [46, 47, 48]. Detrimental effects of BHA and BHT (at concentration of 0.75%) in the circulatory system of rats have also been observed [49]. Moreover, synthetic antioxidants like BHA, TBHQ and propyl gallate have the potential to form molecular complexes with nucleic acids and promote DNA damage [50]. Some studies indicate that low doses of BHA and BHT nowadays used in foods do not pose any cancer hazard to humans, but exert anticarcinogenic and antimutagenic properties [51, 52, 53, 54]. Similar health beneficial properties of TBHQ and propyl gallate have also been reported [52, 55]. However, growing concerns about the safety of synthetic antioxidants have led to extensive research on alternative methods such as microencapsulation as well as the use of natural sources of antioxidants in food systems.

3.2.2. Natural Antioxidants from Plant Sources

An increasingly high consumer health consciousness has led to the demand for safe and natural alternatives to synthetic antioxidants. Antioxidants of plant origin, derived from fruits, vegetables, and other plant tissues including leaves and bark have received much attention for their potential antioxidative properties. These phytochemicals are involved in normal physiological functions and have been implicated in preventing many diseases. In the past few years, extensive research has been done on the use of these phytochemicals to improve the quality and shelf life of foods as well as to provide various health benefits to the consumers.

Natural antioxidants have many advantages as well as drawbacks; advantages being its safety compared to synthetic antioxidants, health beneficial properties as well as allowing the food processors to label products with all natural ingredients; and drawbacks among several others include its low potency and high usage levels which might produce undesirable flavour or odor in the foods [32]. The two natural antioxidants that are commercially available and commonly used in foods are tocopherols and ascorbic acid. Many phenolic antioxidant rich extracts from plant sources have also been identified as natural antioxidants and tested in a variety of food model systems for their efficacy.

3.2.2.1. Tocopherols and Tocotrienols

Tocopherols and tocotrienols are distributed in the plant tissues and are commonly used as antioxidants in various foods. The chemical structure of tocopherols and tocotrienols consists of a chromanol ring with a hydroxyl group that is capable of donating hydrogen to free radicals and a long hydrophobic side chain which offers lipophilicity to the molecule (Figure 4). The tocotrienol differs from tocopherol in possessing three double bonds in the hydrophobic side chain. Both tocopherol and tocotrienols exists in four forms, alpha, beta, gamma and delta and is named based on the number and position of methyl groups in the chromanol ring.

A

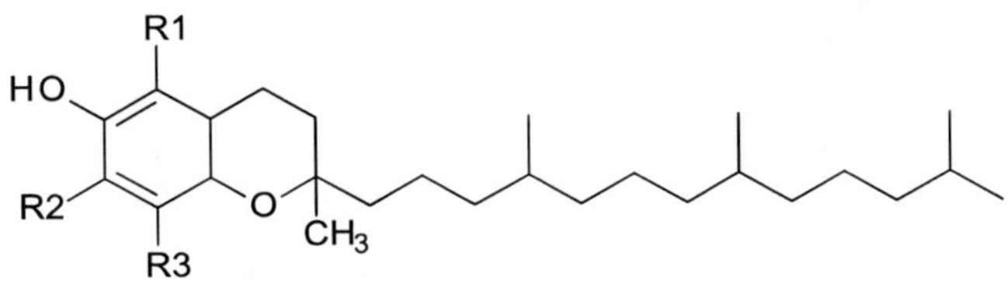

R1	R2	R3	
CH_3	CH_3	CH_3	α-tocopherol
CH_3	H	CH_3	β-tocopherol
H	CH_3	CH_3	γ-tocopherol
H	H	CH_3	δ-tocopherol

B

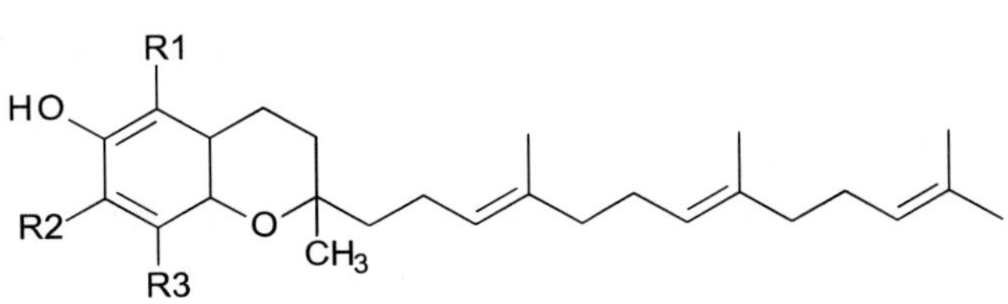

R1	R2	R3	
CH_3	CH_3	CH_3	α-tocotrienol
CH_3	H	CH_3	β-tocotrienol
H	CH_3	CH_3	γ-tocotrienol
H	H	CH_3	δ-tocotrienol

Figure 4. Chemical structures of tocopherols (A) and tocotrienols (B).

The main sources of tocopherol are vegetable oils, nuts, seeds and whole grain. Soyabean oil is considered to be the main commercial source of natural tocopherols. Mixed tocopherols range between 550 and 1000 μg/g in refined, bleached and deodorized soybean oil [56]. However, synthetic tocopherol consists of alpha, gamma and delta isomers of tocopherols. Another form of tocopherol available is tocopherol acetate. A water soluble form of tocopherol known as Trolox is also available commercially. Tocotrienols are present in rice bran oil, coconut oil, palm oil, cocoa butter, barley and wheat germ [57]. The current commercial sources of tocotrienols are rice, palm and annatto [58].

The oxidation of polyunsaturated fatty acids results in the formation of alkoxyl and peroxyl radicals which in turn can react with more lipids and propagate lipid oxidation. Tocopherols scavenge the alkoxyl and peroxyl radicals thereby stopping the chain propagation of lipid oxidation. Tocopherols thus act as chain-breaking antioxidants in food systems. Tocopherols, being lipophilic are more effective in oil-in water emulsions than in bulk oil due to its ability to orient and function at the oil-water interface or inside the oil droplets which are the major sites of lipid oxidation [59]. Different tocopherol homolog differ in their antioxidant activity based on the temperature, unsaturated substrates used, rate of oxidation and the methods used to analyze oxidation [60, 61, 62]. A mixture of α-tocopherol and ascorbic acid exhibit a strong synergistic effect which is facilitated by reduction of the tocopheroxyl radical intermediate by ascorbic acid to regenerate α-tocopherol. Apart from the redox mechanism, synergism also occurs by means of metal inactivation by ascorbic acid thereby preventing the decomposition of tocopherol by metals.

Tocopherols are regarded as safe food additives and the recommended level of usage in fats and oil varies between 200 ppm to 500 ppm in various countries. Various studies on the effect of addition of tocopherol on lipid oxidation in fish oil as well as fish oil fortified foods have been carried out. The antioxidant effect of tocopherols in fish oil systems has been reported [63, 64]. Low doses of tocopherol (<100ppm) in combination with storage at low temperature (-40 C) has been reported to be effective in terms of controlling lipid oxidation in mackerel oil [65]. α-Tocopherol was a better antioxidant than δ-tocopherol in bulk menhaden oil where as δ-tocopherol was more effective than α-tocopherol in menhaden oil in water emulsions [66]. Application of α-tocopherol in combination with synergists such as ascorbic acid and lecithin improved the oxidative stability of sardine skin lipids [67]. In fish oil enriched energy bars, γ-tocopherol reduced lipid oxidation during storage at a concentration above 440 μg/g fish oil [68]. In the same study, concentrations lower than 220 μg/g fish oil increased the formation of lipid hydroperoxides, volatile secondary oxidation products as well as the development of rancid-off flavors. In contrary, other studies have reported prooxidative effects of tocopherols at high concentrations whereas lower concentrations were found to be ineffective or antioxidative in nature [69, 70]. γ-Tocopherol alone or in combination with ascorbic acid ethylenediaminetetraacetic acid (EDTA) protected fish oil-enriched salad dressing during a storage period of six weeks [71].

3.2.2.2. Ascorbic Acid

Ascorbic acid or Vitamin C occurs in plant tissues and is used in various foods as antioxidants (Figure 5). It is water soluble and has limited applications in fats and oils. Ascorbic acid is considered a secondary antioxidant and exhibits synergestic interactions with α-tocopherol, BHT, BHA and other metal chelators in fish oil or fish oil fortified food systems [36, 67, 72]. It functions mainly by regeneration of primary antioxidants, reduction of free radicals, metal inactivation and scavenging reactive oxygen species [73, 74].

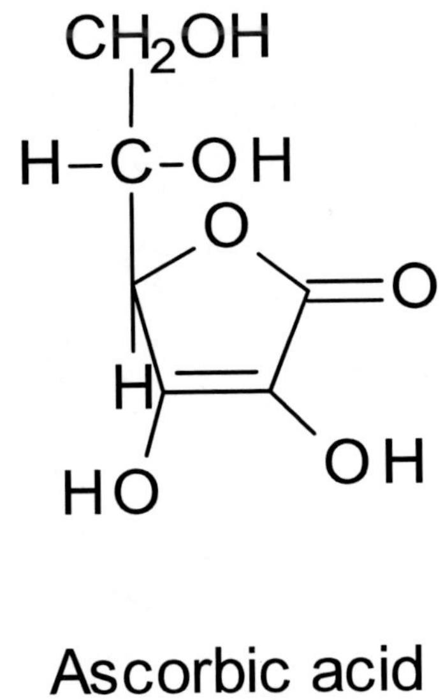

Figure 5. Chemical structure of ascorbic acid.

The lipohilic derivative of ascorbic acid, ascorbyl palmitate is also available as a food antioxidant. According to the polar paradox theory [59], ascorbic acid being polar is effective in non-polar media like bulk oils where as ascorbyl palmitate being non-polar is effective in polar systems like oil-in water emulsions. Ascorbic acid can also act as pro-oxidants under certain conditions. Reduction of Fe^{3+} to Fe^{2+} by ascorbic acid resulted in the formation of an ascorbic acid-Fe complex which reacted with lipid hydroperoxides promoting lipid oxidation and formation of rancid fishy off-flavors in fish oil-enriched mayonnaise [75]. Specific limits on the use of ascorbic acid in foods have not been recommended.

3.2.2.3. Carotenoids

Carotenoids are isoprenoid pigments that are widely distributed in plants, fruits and vegetables. They include α- and β-carotene, lycopene, lutein, canthaxanthin, astaxanthin and zeaxanthin (Figure 6). The main mechanisms by which carotenoids act as antioxidants in food systems include quenching of singlet oxygen and by trapping the free radicals [32]. However, carotenoids are highly unstable in the presence of heat, light, oxygen, pH and metals and have limited applications as food antioxidants.

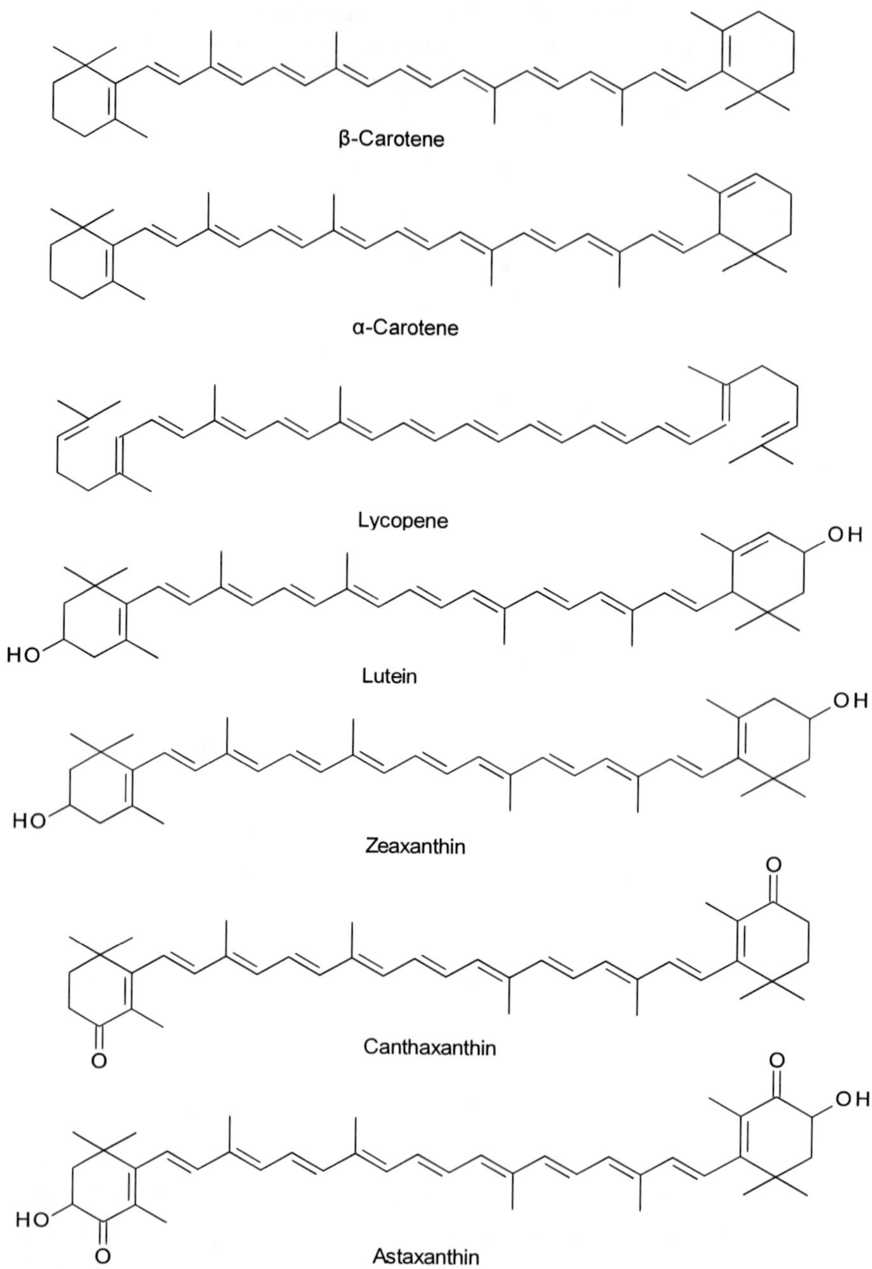

Figure 6. Structures of major carotenoids in plants.

3.2.2.4. Rosemary and Sage

Rosemary (*Rosmarinus officnalis*) belongs to the Labiatae plant family and is known for its culinary as well as medicinal uses. Rosemary extract is now commercially available as a natural antioxidant and has gained much popularity in the food industry as well as among the consumers. It is currently considered as the most commonly used natural alternative to synthetic antioxidants. Various forms of rosemary extract including water soluble and lipid soluble extracts have been formulated for delivery into food systems. Water soluble extracts are good for application in salad dressings, brines and beverages whereas oil-soluble formulation is effective in fats and oils. Rosemary extracts are produced through solvent extraction, water extraction, oil extraction or supercritical CO_2 extraction [76].

The main compounds in rosemary extract are carnosic acid, carnosol, and other phenolic diterpenes such as rosmanol, epirosmanol, isorosmanol, rosmaridiphenol, rosmadial, rosmariquinone, 6-7 dehydrocarnosic acid, and 7-ketocarnosic acid and phenolic acids such as rosmarinic acid as well as flavonoids. Some of the major rosemary antioxidant compounds are given in Figure 7. Carnosic acid is the major diterpene present in the rosemary extract where as carnosol, rosmanol and galdosol are oxidation products of carnosic acid.

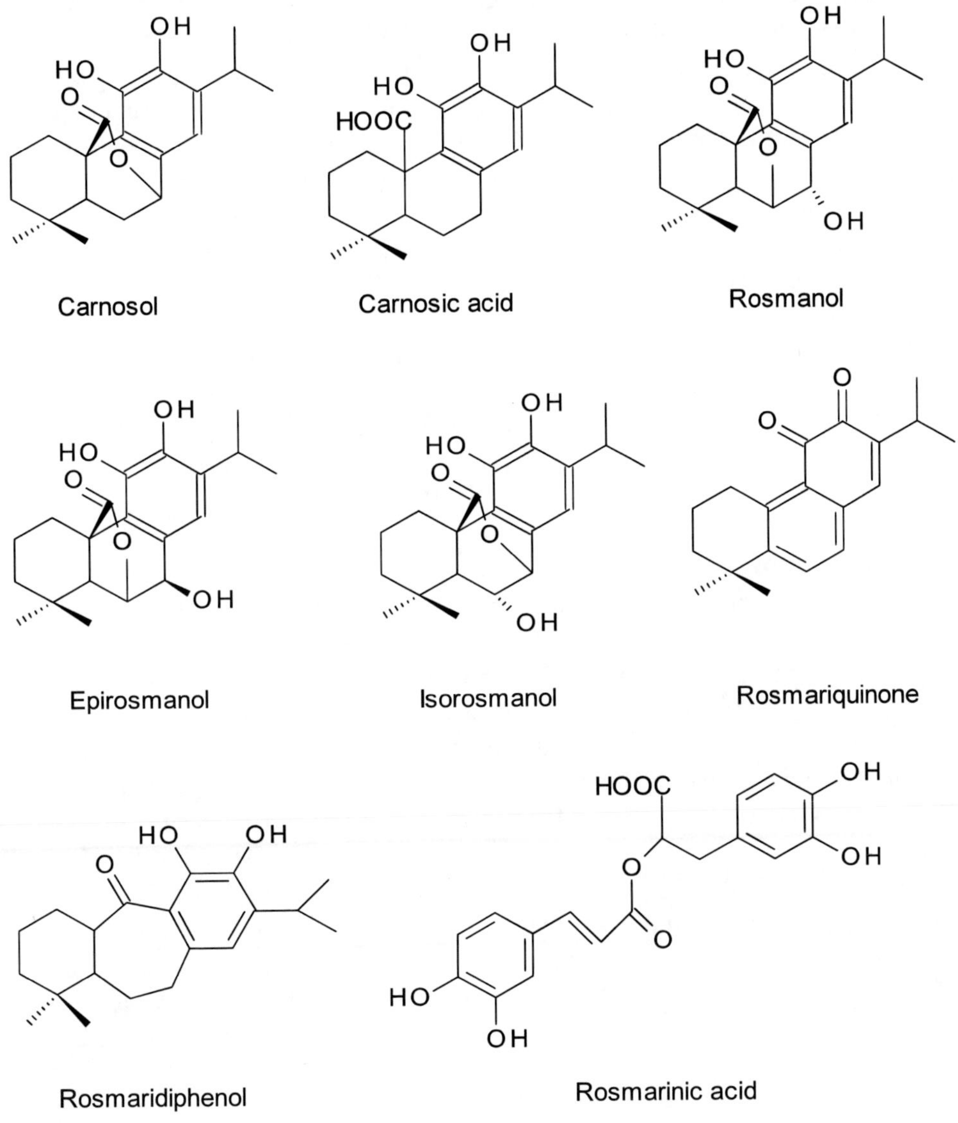

Figure 7. Structures of various compounds present in rosemary and sage.

Rosemary antioxidants have been tested in a wide variety of fats and oils and have been shown to provide oxidative stability equivalent to that provided by BHA and BHT [76, 77]. Hydrophilic rosemary antioxidants, carnosic acid and carnsol were effective in inhibiting lipid oxidation in bulk fish oil by orienting at the air-oil interface where as in oil-in water emulsions, they were not effective due to their partitioning into the aqueous phase [74]. Carnosic acid and its oxidative derivates such as carnosol and rosmanol contribute to the high antioxidant activity of rosemary extract in food systems and they function by scavenging the free radicals and chelating iron [78]. Rosemary extract increased the oxidative stability of gels prepared from fish fortified with omega-3 PUFA that underwent high pressure and thermal treatments [79]. Extracts from rosemary leaves prevented lipid oxidation in fish oil-in-water emulsions as determined by the formation of conjugated dienes, trienes and fluorescent products formed during storage [80]. A synergistic effect between fish proteins and rosemary extracts in preventing the formation of hydroperoxides have been suggested to be an important mechanism in inhibiting lipid oxidation in fish muscle emulsion [80]. Rosemary compounds have been shown to act synergistically with α-tocopherol in sardine oil at 30° C and in frozen crushed fish meat models [81]. Suggested mechanism of synergism involved regeneration of α-tocopheroxyl radical to α-tocopherol by rosemary extract through hydrogen atom donation. The use of rosemary as an antioxidant in cod or pollack liver oil systems reduced the production of primary lipid oxidation products during storage [82]. Addition of rosemary extract significantly protected the omega-3 PUFA, DHA and EPA against oxidation during heating and storage [83].

Sage (*Salvia officinalis* L) is another herb that is used commonly in foods and belongs to the same family as rosemary. The major compounds that are present in sage consist of carnosol, carnosic acid, rosmanol, rosmarinic acid and rosmadial similar to what is present in rosemary (Figure 7). Carnosic acid, carnosol and rosmarinic acid are reported to be responsible for the antioxidant activity of sage [84,85].

3.2.2.5. Flavonoids

Flavonoids are a group of naturally occurring compounds ubiquitously found in the plant kingdom. The basic structure of a flavonoid consists of a flavan nucleus (2-phenyl-benzo-γ-pyrane), with two benzene rings (A and B) combined by an oxygen containing pyran ring C (Figure 8). There are various sub classes of flavonoids depending on the saturation/substitution of the C ring including flavan-3-ols, flavonols, anthocyanidins, flavones and flavanones. Flavan-3-ols contain a C ring with methylene at position 4 (eg. catechins have an OH group at 5, 7, 3', 4' positions) where as flavonols contain a keto group at position 4 in the C ring (e.g. quercetin, myrcetin etc. with OH groups at 5, 7, 3', 4' positions and 5, 7, 3', 4', 5' positions, respectively). Flavonols usually occur in their glycosylated forms. Anthocyanidins are sugar free counter parts of anthocyanins based on the flavyllium ion, which usually exists as cation forming salts with organic acids (cyanidin with OH on 5, 7, 3', 4' and glucoside on the 3-position) and procyanidins are oligomers of flavan-3-ols.

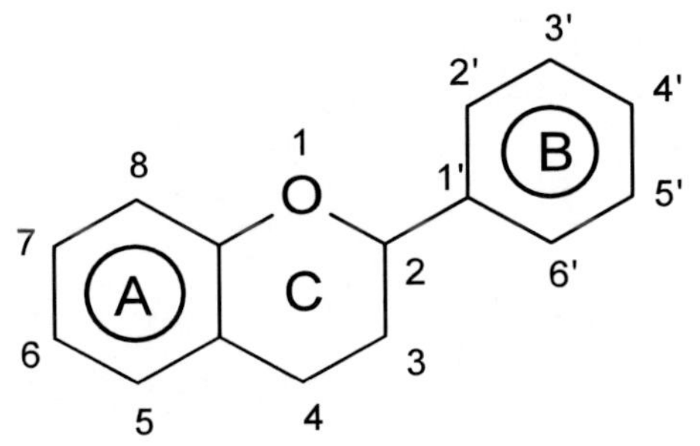

Figure 8. The basic chemical structure of flavonoids.

Flavonoids act as antioxidants mainly due to their ability to scavenge the free radicals as well as to chelate the metal ions [86, 87, 88]. The free radical scavenging activity of the flavonoids is due to the hydroxyl groups in the B-ring as well as the 2, 3 double bond in conjugation with the keto group in position 4 in the C ring. The binding sites for trace metals to flavonoids are the 3- or 5-hydroxyl and keto group in position 4 of the C ring or the hydroxyl groups in the B-ring. Some of the major flavonoids found in plants and examples are given in Table 1.

Table 1. Major flavonoids found in plants and examples.

Flavonoids	Examples
Flavan-3-ols	catechin, epicatechin, epicatechin gallate and epigallocatechin-3-gallate
Flavonols	quercetin, myrcetin, kaempferol
Anthocyanidins	delphinidin, petunidin, cyanidin, peonidin, malvidin
Isoflavonoids	genistein, diadzein, formononetin, coumestrol, glycitein
Flavones	apigenin, luteolein, chrysin
Flavanones	hesperidin, naringin, naringenin

Some of the natural extracts prepared from plant sources which are rich in flavonoids, that have received much attention in the recent years for stabilizing omega-3 PUFA are discussed below.

3.2.2.5.1. Green Tea

Green tea leaves consists of 36% of polyphenols on the dry weight basis and catechins form the most predominant group of polyphenols. Catechins are a group of flavonoids that fall under the class of flavan-3-ols. The six major catechins in green tea leaves are (+)-catechin (C), (-)-epicatechin (EC), (-)-gallocatechin (GC), (-)-epicatechin gallate (ECG), (-)-epigalocatechin (EGC) and (-)-epigalocatechin gallate (EGCG) (Figure 9). The total content of catechins in green tea has been estimated to be 420 mg/L [89]. Other important group of polyphenols present in tea is flavonols, major compounds being quercetin, myricetin and kaempferol existing mainly as glycosides [90, 91].

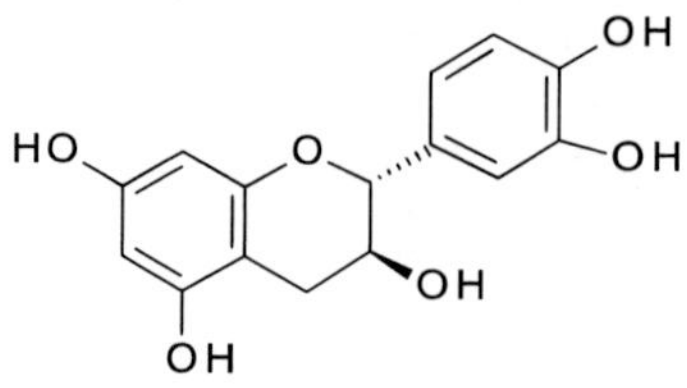

(+) - catechin [C]

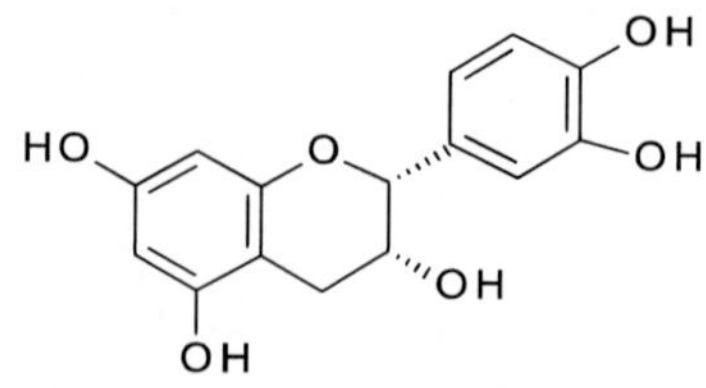

(-) - epicatechin [EC]

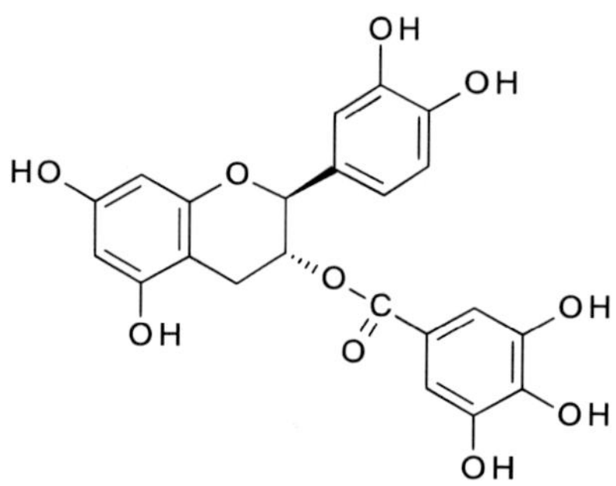

(-) - catechin gallate [GC]

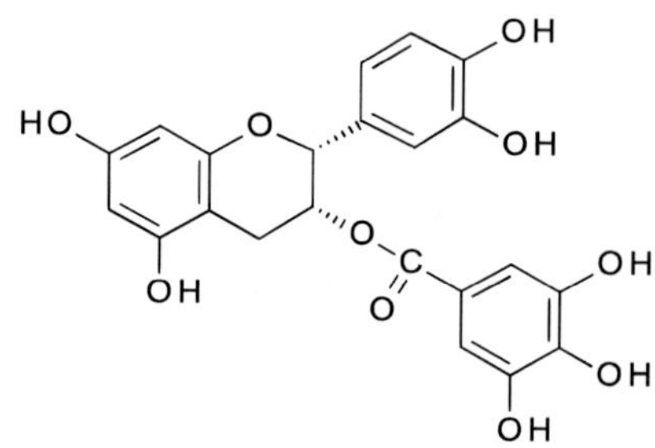

(-) - epicatechin gallate [ECG]

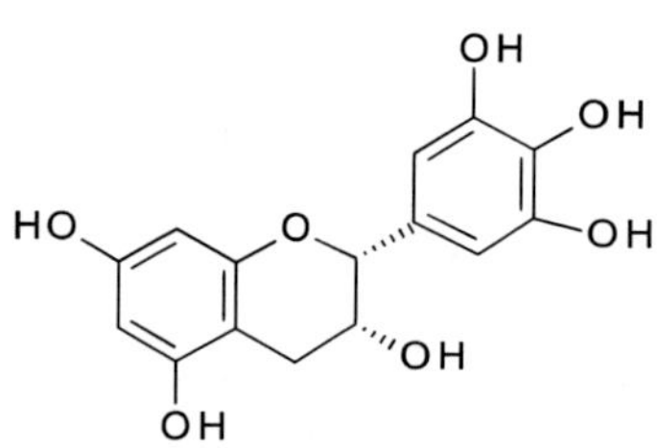

(-) - epigallocatechin [EGC]

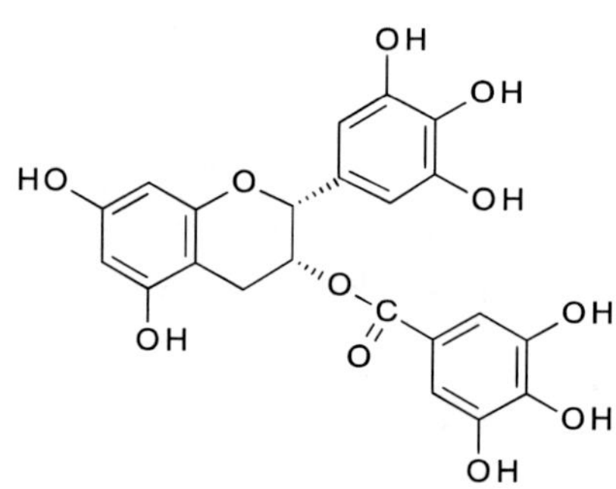

(-) - epigallocatechin gallate [EGCG]

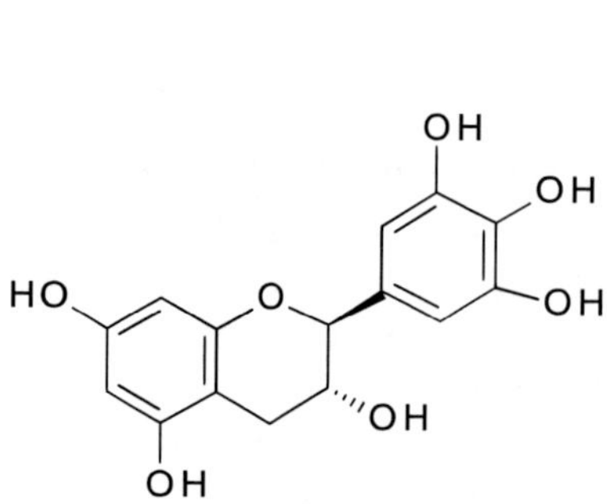

(+) - gallocatechin [GC]

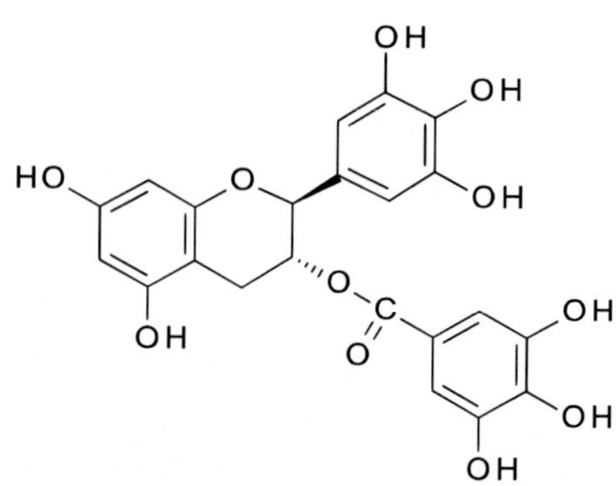

(-) - gallocatechin gallate [GCG]

Figure 9. Structures of major green tea catechins.

Green tea extracts are commercially available and are used as antioxidants in food systems. Green tea catechins enhanced the oxidative stability of fish oils in comparison with α-tocopherol, BHT, BHA and TBHQ [92]. In this study, the researchers found the activity of catechins in the following order: ECG >EGCG>EGC>EC. Catechins and other flavonoids have been shown to be efficient in scavenging oxygen radicals and chelating metals [93, 94, 95]. The possible regeneration of tocopherol by green tea catechins have also been reported [96]. A pro-oxidant effect of green tea extract was seen in marine oils due to the presence of chlorophyll in the extract where as dechlorophyllized green tea extract was effective in preventing lipid oxidation in oils [97]. Fish fillets given a dip/glazing treatment in green tea extract solutions delayed the formation of secondary lipid oxidation products during storage [98]. A better antioxidant activity of green tea extract was observed in cod liver oil and white pollack liver oil when compared to other natural antioxidants [82]. Crude tea extracts, ground green tea and individual catechins exhibited excellent antioxidant activities in fish meat system. The varied potency of tea catechins in inhibiting lipid oxidation was related to the number of hydroxyl groups in the catechin molecule which in turn changes the hydrophilicity/hydrophobicity of the catechins [99]. In a recent study, EGCG was shown to trap reactive carbonyl species, acrolein and reduce the peroxidation of seal blubber oil [100].

3.2.2.5.2. Grapes

Extensive research on the utilization of grape seeds and skins as natural sources of polyphenolic antioxidants have been carried out. The main phenolic compounds present in grape seeds are monomeric flavan-3-ols, (+)-catechin, oligomeric flavan-3-ols (proanthocyanidins), flavonols and anthocyanins (Figure 10) [101,102]. Grape skins also contain high levels of ellagic acid, myricetin, kaempferol and trans-resveratrol along with monomeric and oligomeric flavan-3-ols.

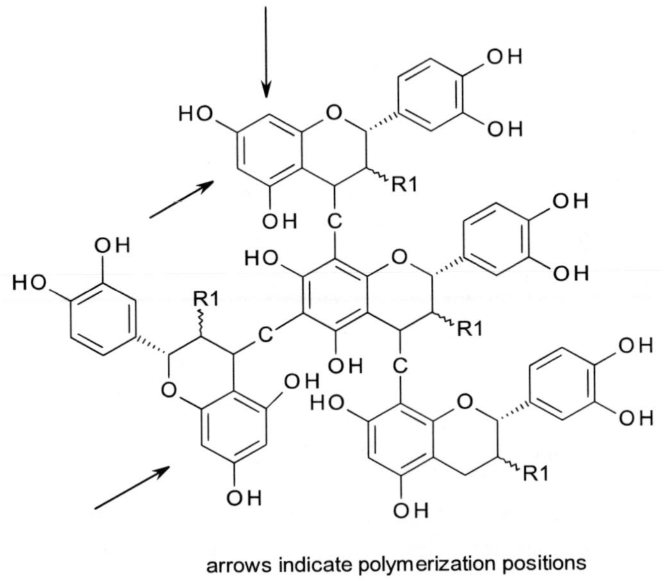

Figure 10. (continued).

Oligomeric flavan-3-ols (proanthocyanidins)

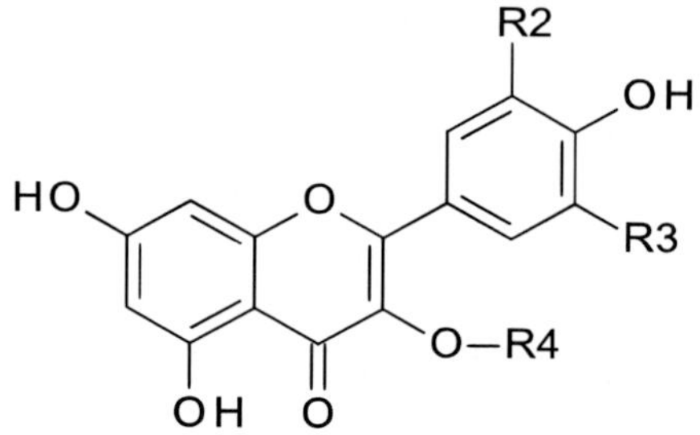

R2 = R3 = H, R4 = H: Kaempferol

R2 = OH, R3 = H, R4 = H: Quercetin

R4 = Saccharide: flavonol glycosides

Flavonols

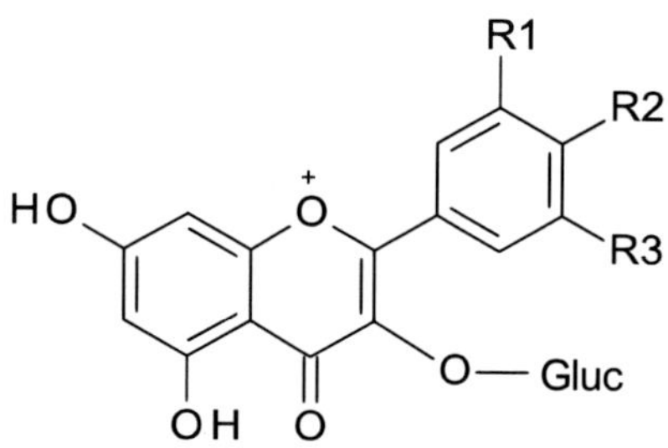

anthocyanins

	R1	R2	R3
peonidin-3-*O*-glucoside	OCH_3	OH	-
petunidin-3-*O*-glucoside	OH	OH	OCH_3
malvidin-3-*O*-glucoside	OCH_3	OH	OCH_3
cyanidin-3-*O*-glucoside	OH	OH	-
delphinindin-3-*O*-glucoside	OH	OH	OH

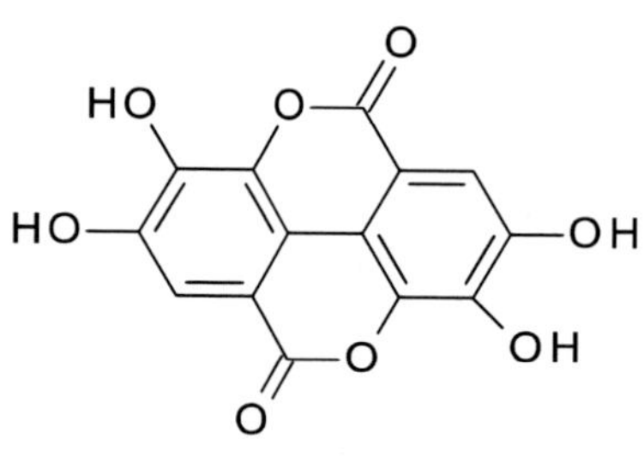

Ellagic acid

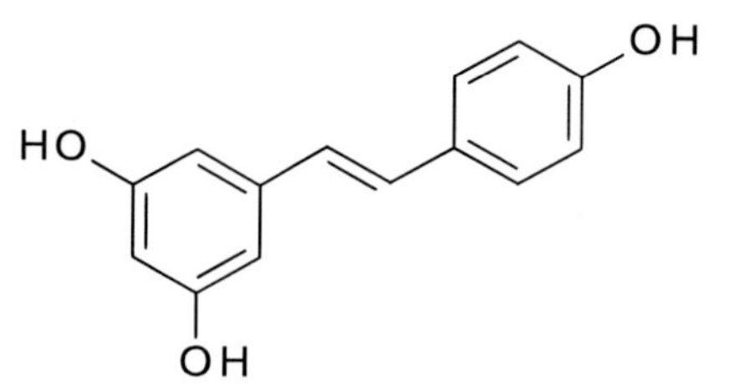

Resveratrol

Figure 10. Structures of some phenolic compounds in grapes.

The flavonoids extracted from grapes as well as its by-products differ greatly in their molecular structure as well as their antioxidant capacity [40, 101, 103, 104]. A fraction consisting of monomeric flavan-3-ols isolated from grape by-products such as skins, stems and seeds were more effective in fish oil than monomeric flavonols, whereas in fish oil emulsions, a fraction containing oligomeric flavan-3-ols with intermediate degree of polymerization and percentage galloylation as well as the crude extract were the most efficient antioxidants [40]. Grape seed extract has been shown to be an excellent food preservative for fish muscle as well as fish oil [105]. Dietary fiber concentrate obtained from white grapes prevented the oxidation of polyunsaturated fatty acids in regular as well as lipid fortified washed cod mince [106]. Resveratrol effectively inhibited the formation of conjugated diene and triene hydroperoxides in fish oil-in water emulsions during oxidation at 40° C where as lipophilization of resveratrol did not improve its antioxidant activity in emulsions [107]. This could be possibly due to the location of the lipophilized resveratrol in the interior of the oil droplet rather than at the oil-water interface.

3.2.2.5.3. Apples

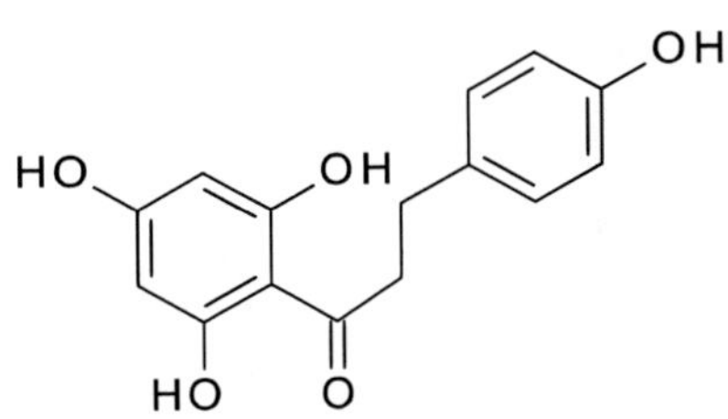

Phloretin

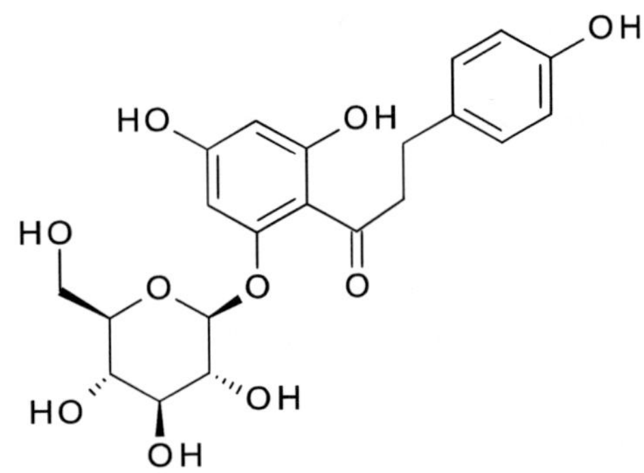

Phloridzin

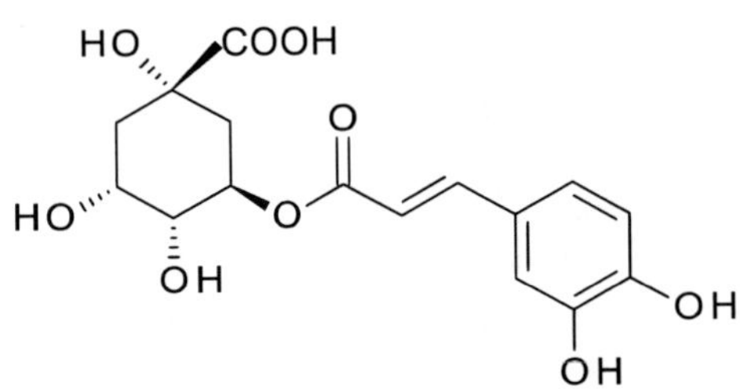

Chlorogenic acid

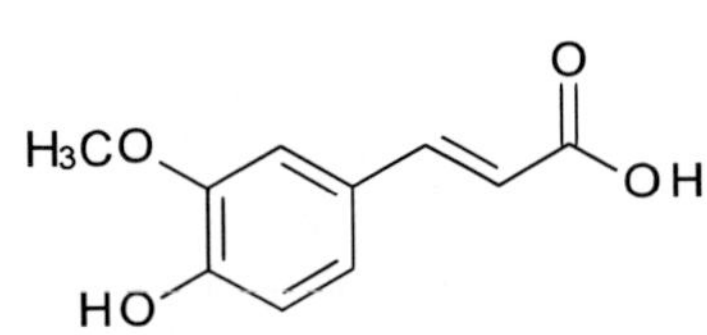

Ferulic Acid

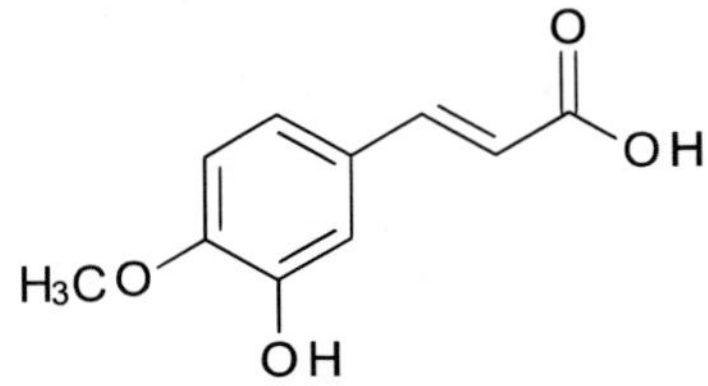

Isoferulic acid

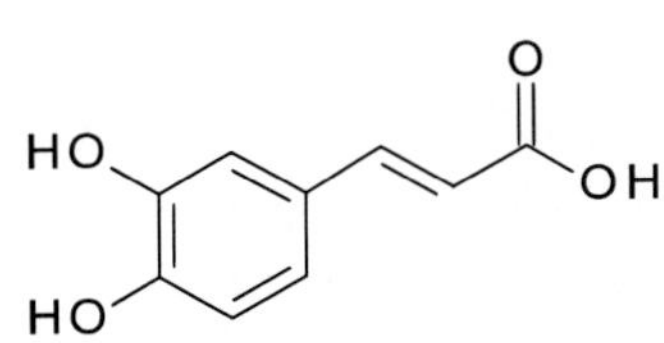

Caffeic acid

Figure 11. Structures of dihydrochalcones and some phenolic acids present in apples.

Apples are a good source of phenolic compounds and provide about 22% of the dietary phenolics in the North American and European diets [108]. The phenolic composition of apples varies with growing season, geographical location, genetic variation and growth period [109, 110]. The major polyphenolic groups in various apple varieties include anthocyanins, flavan-3-ols, flavonols, dihydrochalcones and phenolic acids (Figure 11) [111].

Flavan-3-ols exist in the form of monomers (catechin and epicatechin), oligomers and polymers (procyanidins); flavonols are associated with sugar moieties such as glucose, galactose, rhamnose, arabinose and xylose; dihydrochalcones are associated with glucose and xyloglucose.

Apple skin has 3-6 times higher flavonoid content than apple flesh and has been shown to possess powerful antioxidant activity [112, 113]. Apple skin extracts (ASE1 and ASE2) prepared from apple skin powder inhibited heat-, UV light- and peroxyl radical-induced oxidation in fish oil as well as in EPA emulsions (Table 2) [34].

Table 2. Percent inhibition of heat-, UV-light and peroxyl radical-induced lipid oxidation in bulk fish oil and oil-in water emulsion by apple skin extracts (ASE1 and ASE2), BHT and α-tocopherol determined by ferric thiocyanate test

% Inhibition								
	EPA Emulsion				Fish oil			
Antioxidant	**conc (μg/ml)**	**Heat**	**UV light**	**AAPH**	**conc (μg/ml)**	**Heat**	**UV light**	**AAPH**
ASE 1	200	53	41	54	2000	25	35	66
ASE 2	4	60	64	61	400	51	61	97
BHT	20	82	70	70	20	87	63	89
α-tocopherol	200	13	35	35	200	33	58	82

Oxidation was induced by

i) heating at 50 °C for 2 min (EPA emulsion) and 70 °C for 10 min (fish oil)

ii) exposing to UV light at room temperature for 20 min (EPA emulsion) and 60 min (fish oil)

iii) adding peroxyl radical generator, AAPH (100 μl of 100 mM) and incubating at room temperature for 40 min (EPA emulsion) and 10 μl of 100 mM and incubating at room temperature for 60 min (fish oil)

Adapted from Rupasinghe et al. (2010); ref 34.

In this study, the removal of sugars and organic acids from the crude apple skin extract (ASE1) enhanced the antioxidant properties of the extract (ASE2) in both the emulsion and bulk fish oil systems. The phenolic concentration of ASE2 was found to be 105-times higher than ASE1 and could have possibly contributed to the higher antioxidative properties of the de-sugared extract even at a lower concentration.

In another study by the same group, naturally occurring flavonols, quercetin and its various glycosides were incorporated into selected PUFA or fish oil in aqueous emulsions and bulk oil systems to evaluate their antioxidant efficacy in omega-3 fatty acid model systems [35]. Quercetin and quercetin-3-*O*-glucoside were effective antioxidants than BHT in bulk fish oil; however, the reverse was observed in PUFA and fish oil emulsion systems, which is in agreement with the polar paradox theory. The glycosylation at C-3 position of quercetin did not influence the lipid oxidation inhibition activity in PUFA emulsions. Various studies by researchers have shown quercetin to be an excellent antioxidant in marine oils rich in PUFA [114, 115, 116].

The two predominant dihydrochalcones in apples, phloretin and phloridzin have also been shown to protect PUFA from oxidation (Table 3) [117].

Table 3. Percent inhibition of peroxyl radical-induced lipid oxidation in ML, MEPA and MDHA oil-in water emulsion and heat-induced lipid oxidation in bulk fish oil by phloretin, phloridzin, BHT and α-tocopherol determined by thiobarbituric acid reactive substances (TBARS) assay

% Inhibition						
	Peroxyl radical-induced				Heat-induced	
Antioxidant	**conc(mmole/L)**	**ML**	**MEPA**	**MDHA**	**conc(mmole/L)**	**Fish oil**
Phloretin	1	100	91	74	50	31
Phloridzin	1	82	73	61	50	49
BHT	1	100	93	77	50	79
α-Tocopherol	1	11	9	8	50	90

Oxidation was induced by adding peroxyl radical generator, AAPH (100μl of 100mM) and incubating at 37° C for 24 hrs for fatty acid emulsions
and by heating at 70° C for 3 hrs for fish oil.
Adapted from Rupasinghe et al. (2010); ref 117.

Two model systems, namely peroxyl radical-induced oxidation of methyl esters of linolenic acid (ML), EPA (MEPA) and DHA (MDHA) in oil-in-water emulsion and heat-induced oxidation of fish oil were employed. Phloretin being lipophilic in nature compared to phloridzin exhibited greater antioxidant activity in terms of inhibiting the formation of thiobarbituric acid reactive substances (TBARS) in oil-in water emulsions. In bulk oil system, phloridzin was effective compared to its aglycone counterpart; however, was less effective compared to α-tocopherol and BHT.

3.2.2.5.4. Berries

Berries are rich in phenolic compounds: flavonoids, phenolic acids, lignans and polymeric tannins. Anthocyanins impart color to the berries and are found in high concentrations in many berries including bilberry, raspberry, strawberry, chokeberry, blueberry, lingonberry, and crowberry. Cloudberry, raspberry and strawberry contain ellagitannins; cowberry and cranberry are rich in flavonols and procyanidins [118].

Berry extracts have been used to protect omega-3 PUFA against oxidation. The antioxidative effects of berry phenolics in methyl linolenate fatty acid as well as methyl linolenate emulsions have been reported [118, 119]. Black raspberry seed flour extract reduced the degradation of omega-3 PUFA in menhaden oil under accelerated oxidation conditions [105].

3.2.2.5.5. Other Spices

Oregano (*Oreganum vulgare* L) and thyme (*Thymus vulgaris* L) are two spices that are valued for its antioxidant as well as antimicrobial properties. Some of the compounds isolated from oregano includes rosmarinic acid, caffeic acid, protocatechuic acid, carvacrol, thymol and some flavonoids such as apigenin, eriodictyol, dihydrokaempferol and dihydroquercetin [120, 121, 122, 123] (Figure 12). In thyme, the principal compounds are carvacol and thymol [124].

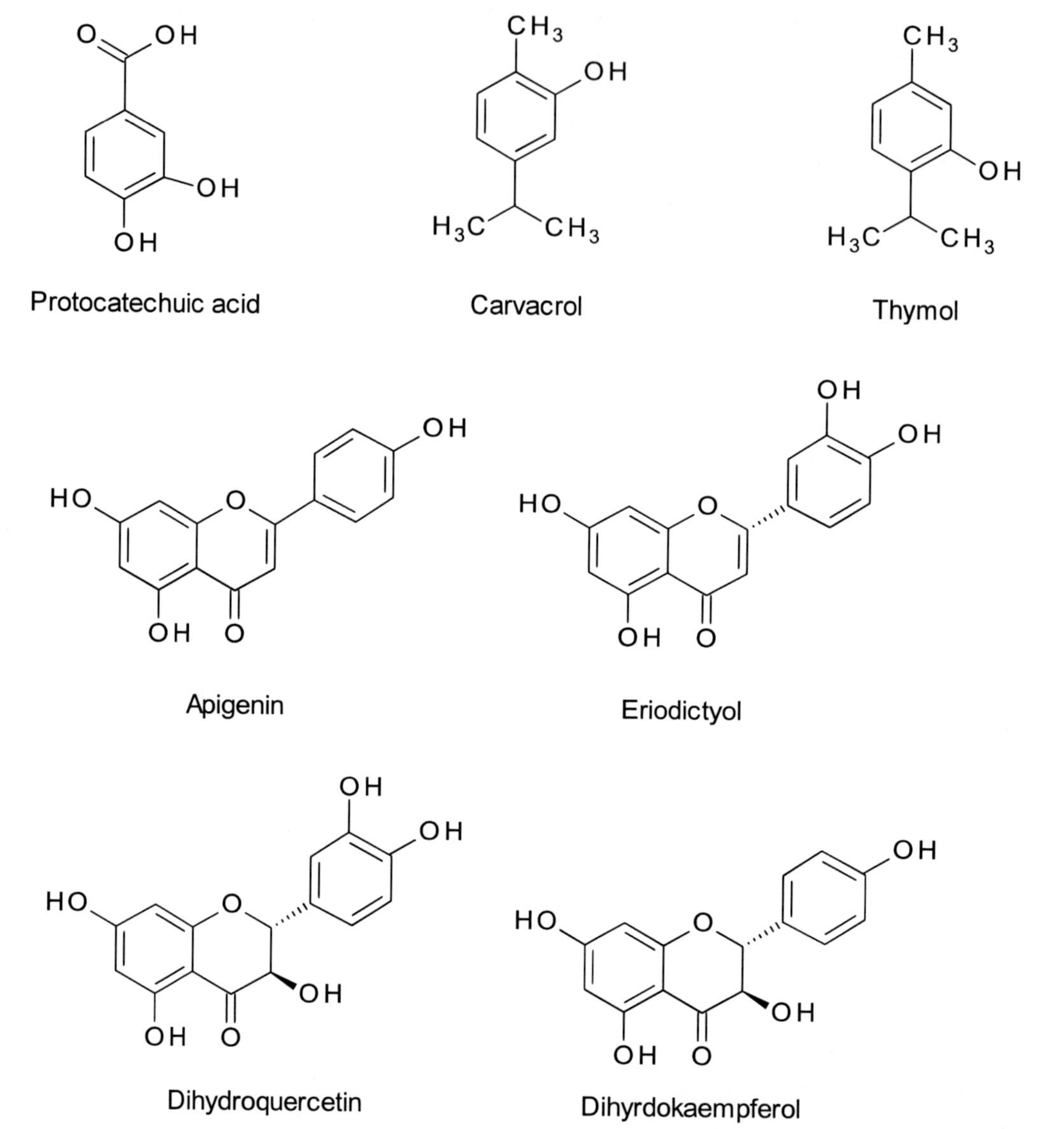

Figure 12. Structures of some compounds present in oregano and thyme.

Dry oregano powder was effective in retarding lipid oxidation in mackerel oil stored at 40 °C when added at 1% level where as a concentration dependant effect of oregano extract was observed in terms of retaining DHA and EPA in menhaden oil subjected to heating at 150 °C for 30 min [83, 125]. Oregano and thyme incorporated in fish oil-enriched tuna salads at 1% improved the oxidative stability of the salads during storage [126].

3.2.2.5.6. Soybean

Tocopherols, phenolic acids and isoflavones are some of the major compounds present in soybeans. Isoflavones represent the most predominant flavonoid group in soybean [128]. They include glucosides of genistein, diadzein and glycitein (Figure 13) [129]. The phenolic acids exist in the form of esters; Defatted soyflour extracts when added to menhaden oil at 5% reduced heat-induced oxidation of oil and retained 60% of EPA and DHA.

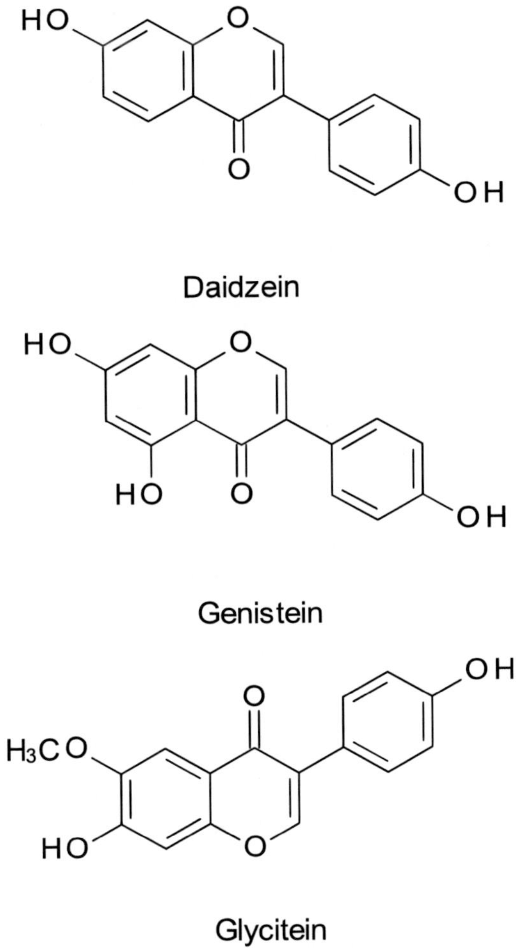

Figure 13. Structures of major isoflavone aglycones in soybean.

4. Conclusion

The use of plant-derived natural extracts serves as a potential alternative to synthetic antioxidants. A large variety of natural plant extracts have been evaluated in fish oils and in fish oil fortified foods to understand the antioxidative properties of the extracts as well as the different components in the extracts. However, the most widely used natural antioxidants in fish oils are tocopherols, ascorbic acid or its derivatives, rosemary and green tea extracts. Further research on the commercialization of other plant extracts as safe food antioxidants is highly warranted.

References

[1] Lavie, C.J., Milani, R.V., Mehra, M.R., Ventura, H.O. Omega-3 polyunsaturated fatty acids and cardiovascular diseases. *Journal of the American College of Cardiology*, 2009, 54, 585-594.

[2] Defilippis, A.P., Blaha, M.J., Jacobson, T.A. Omega-3 Fatty acids for cardiovascular disease prevention. *Current Treatment Options in Cardiovascular Medicine*, 2010, 12, 365-80.

[3] Nadine, M.Z., Paula, M. Fish oil: Getting to the heart of it. *The Journal for Nurse Practitioners*, 2007, 3,104-109.

[4] Engstrom, K., Wallin, R., Saldeen, T. Effect of low-dose aspirin in combination with stable fish oil on whole blood production of eicosanoids. *Prostaglandins Leukotrienes and Essential Fatty Acids*, 2001, 64, 291–297.

[5] Kramer, H.J., Stevens, J., Grimminger, F., Seeger, W. Fish oil fatty acids and human platelets: dose dependent decrease in dienoic and increase in trienoic thromboxane generation. *Biochemical Pharmacology*, 1996, 52, 1211–1217.

[6] Reiffel, J.A., McDonald, A. Antiarrhythmic effects of omega-3 fatty acids. *American Journal of Cardiology,* 2006, 98, 50i–60i.

[7] Leaf, A., Kang, J.X., Xiao, Y.F., Billman, G.E. Clinical prevention of sudden cardiac death by n-3 polyunsaturated fatty acids and mechanism of prevention of arrhythmias by n-3 fish oils. *Circulation*, 2003,107, 2646-2652.

[8] Davidson, M.H., Stein, E.A., Bays, H.E. Efficacy and tolerability of adding prescription omega-3 fatty acids 4 g/d to simvastatin 40 mg/d in hypertriglyceridemic patients: an 8-week, randomized, double-blind, placebo-controlled study. *Clinical Therapeutics,* 2007, 29, 1354–1367.

[9] Gleissman, H., Johnsen, J.I., Kogner, P. Omega-3 fatty acids in cancer, the protectors of good and the killers of evil? *Experimental Cell Research*, 2010, 316, 1365-73.

[10] Pauwels, E.K., Kairemo, K. Fatty acid facts, part II: role in the prevention of carcinogenesis, or, more fish on the dish? *Drug News and Perspective*, 2008, 21, 504–510.

[11] Innis, S.M. Dietary omega-3 fatty acids and the developing brain. *Brain Research*, 2008, 1237, 35-43.

[12] Hodge, W., Barnes, D., Schachter, H., Pan, Y., Lowcock, E., Zhang, L., Sampson, M., Morrison, A., Tran, K., Miguelez, M., Lewin, G. *Effects of Omega-3 Fatty Acids on Eye Health*. Evidence Report/Technology Assessment No. 117 (Prepared by University of Ottawa Evidence-based Practice Center under Contract No. 290-02-0021.) AHRQ Publication No. 05-E008-2. Rockville, MD: Agency for Healthcare Research and Quality. July 2005.

[13] *FAO/WHO Technical Report N. Diet, nutrition and the prevention of chronic diseases.* World Health Organization, Geneva, Switzerland, 2003.

[14] Kris-Etherton, P., Grieger, J.A., Etherton, T.D. Dietary reference intakes for DHA and EPA. *Prostaglandins, Leukotrienes and Essential Fatty Acids*, 2009, 81, 99-104.

[15] Choe, E., Min, D.B. Mechanisms and factors for edible oil oxidation. *Comphrehensive Reviews in Food Science and Food Safety*, 2006, 5, 169-186.

[16] Frankel, E. *Lipid oxidation. 2nd edn.* Bridgwater TA7 OYZ, U. K.: The Oily Press, 2005.

[17] Van de Voort, F.R., Ismail, A.A., Sedman, J., Dubois, J., Nicodemo, T. The determination of peroxide value by Fourier transform infrared spectroscopy. *Journal of the American Oil Chemists Society*, 1994, 71, 921-926.

[18] Wanasundara, U.N., Shahidi, F. Application of NMR spectroscopy to assess oxidative stability of canola and soyabean oils. *Journal of Food Lipids*, 1993, 1, 15-24.

[19] Gu, L., Weng, X. Antioxidant activity and components of Salvia plebeian R. Br.-a Chineese herb. *Food Chemistry,* 2001, 73, 299-305.

[20] Engberg, R.M., Lauridsen, C., Jensen, S.K., Jakobsen, K., Inclusion of oxidised vegetable oil in broiler diets. Its influence on nutrient balance and on the antioxidative status of broilers. *Poultry Science*, 1996, 75, 1003–1011.

[21] Hochgraf, E., Mokady, S., Cogan, U. Dietary oxidized linoleic acid modifies lipid composition of rat liver microsomes and increases their fluidity. *Journal of Nutrition,* 1997, 127, 681–686.

[22] Esterbauer, H., Schaur, R.J., Zollner, H. Chemistry and biochemistry of 4-hydroxynonenal, malonaldehyde and related aldehydes. *Free Radical Biology and Medicine,* 1990, 11, 81-128.

[23] Fang, J., Vaca, L., Valsta, L., Mutanen, M. Determination of DNA adducts of malonaldehyde in humans: Effects of dietary fatty acid composition. *Carcinogenesis*, 1996, 17, 1035-1040.

[24] Shahidi, F., Han, X.Q. Encapsulation of food ingredients. *Critical Reviews in Food Science and Nutrition*, 1993, 33, 501-547.

[25] Heinzelmann, K., Franke, K. Using freezing and drying techniques of emulsions for the microencapsulation of fish oil to improve oxidation stability. *Colloids and Surfaces B: Biointerfaces*, 1999, 12, 223-229.

[26] Klaypradit, W., Huang, Y.W. Fish oil encapsulation with chitosan using ultrasonic atomizer. *LWT-Food Science and Technology*, 2008, 41, 1133-1139.

[27] Drusch, S., Mannino, S. Patent-based review on industrial approaches for the microencapsulation of oils rich in polyunsaturated fatty acid. *Trends in Food Science and Technology,* 2009, 20, 237–44.

[28] Drush, S., GroB, N., Schwarz, K. Efficient stabilization of bulk fish oil rich in long chain polyunsaturated fatty acids. *European Journal of Lipid Science and Technology,* 2008, 110, 351-359.

[29] Serfert, Y., Drusch, S., Schwarz, K. Chemical stabilization of oils rich in long-chain polyunsaturated fatty acids during homogenization, microencapsulation and storage. *Food Chemistry*, 2009, 113, 1106-1112.

[30] Shahidi, F. Antioxidants in food and food antioxidants. *Molecular Nutrition and Food Research,* 2000, 44, 158-163.

[31] Decker, E.A. *Food Lipids:Chemistry, Nutrition and Biotechnology*, eds, Akoh, C.C and D.B.Min., Marcel Dekker, Inc., New York, 1998, p.397.

[32] Reiche, D.W., Lillard, D.A., Eitenmiller, R.R. *Food Lipids:Chemistry, Nutrition and Biotechnology*, eds, Akoh, C.C and D.B.Min., Marcel Dekker, Inc., New York, 1998, 423-448.

[33] Omura, K. Antioxidant synergism between butylated hydroxyanisole and butylated hydroxytoluene. *Journal of the American Oil Chemists Society*, 1995, 72, 1565-1570.

[34] Rupasinghe, H.P.V., Erkan, N., Yasmin, A. Antioxidant protection of eicosapentaenoic acid and fish oil oxidation by polyphenolic enriched apple skin extract. *Journal of Agricultural and Food Chemistry*, 2009, 58, 1233-1239.

[35] Huber, G.M., Rupasinghe, H.P.V., Shahidi, F. Inhibition of oxidation of omega-3 polyunsaturated fatty acids and fish oil by quercetin glycosides. *Food Chemistry*, 2009, 117, 290-295.

[36] Kaitaranta, J.K. Control of lipid oxidation in fish oil with various antioxidative compounds, *Journal of the American Oil Chemists Society*, 1992, 69, 810-813.

[37] Pratt, D.E. *Bailey's Industrial Oil and Fat Products*, ed, Hui, Y.H., John Wiley and Sons, Inc., New York, 1996, 524-545.

[38] Ke, P.J., Nash, D.M., Ackman, R.G. Mackerel skin lipids as an unsaturated fat model system for the determination of antioxidative potency of TBHQ and other antioxidant compounds, *Journal of the American Oil Chemists Society*, 1977, 54, 417-420.

[39] Pazos, M., Alonso, A., Sanchez, I., Medina, I. Hydroxytyrosol prevents oxidative deterioration in foodstuffs rich in fish lipids. *Journal of Agricultural and Food Chemistry*, 2008, 56, 3334-3340.

[40] Pazos, M., Gallardo, J.M., Torres, J.L., Medina, I. Activity of grape polyphenols as inhibitors of the oxidation of lipids and frozen fish muscle, 2005, *Food Chemistry*, 92, 547-557.

[41] Murakami, K., Ito, M., Htay, H.H., Tsubouchi, R., Iwata, S., Yoshino, M. Antioxidant and prooxidant actions of gallic acid derivatives:effect on metal-dependant oxidation of lipids and low density lipoprotein. *Biomedical Research*, 2000, 21, 291-296.

[42] Yoshino, M., Haneda, M., Naruse, M., Htay, H.H., Iwata, S., Tsubouchi, R. Prooxidant action of gallic acid compounds: copper-dependent strand breaks and the formation of 8-hydroxy-2′-deoxyguanosine in DNA. *Toxicology in Vitro*, 2002, 16, 705-709.

[43] Jacobsen, C., Hartvigsen, K., Lund, P., Meyer, A.S., Adler-Nissen, J., Holstborg, J., Holmer, G. Oxidation mechanisms in fish oil enriched mayonnaise: 1. Assessment of propyl gallate as antioxidant by discriminant partial least squares regression analysis. *European Food Research and Technology*, 1999, 210, 13-30.

[44] Farag, R. S., El-baroty, G.S., Basuny, A.M. Safety evaluation of olive phenolic compounds as natural antioxidants. *International Journal of Food Science and Nutrition*, 2003, 54, 159-174.

[45] Kahl, R., Kappus, H.Z. Toxicology of the synthetic antioxidants BHA and BHT in comparison with the natural antioxidant Vitamin E. *Z Lebensm Unters Forsch*, 1993, 196, 329-338.

[46] Verhagen, H., Schilderman, P.A.E.L., Kleinjans, J.C.S. Butylated hydroxyanisole in perspective. *Chemico-Biological Interactions*, 1991, 80, 109-134.

[47] Sarafian, T.A., Kouyoumjian, S., Tashkin, D., Roth, M.D. Synergestic toxicity of Δ^9-tetrahydrocannabinol and butylated hydroxyanisole. *Toxicology Letters,* 2002, 133, 171-179.

[48] Saito, M., Sakagami, H., Fujisawa, S. Cytotoxicity and apoptosis induction by butylated hydroxyanisole (BHA) and butylated hydroxytoluene (BHT). *Anticancer Research,* 2003, 23, 4693-4701.

[49] Jayalakshmi, C.P., Sharma, J.D. Effect of butylated hydroxyanisole (BHA) and butylated hydroxytoluene (BHT) on rat erythrocytes. *Environmental Research*, 1986, 41, 235-238.

[50] Dolatabadi, J.E.N., Kashanian, S. A review on DNA interaction with synthetic phenolic food additives. *Food Research International*, 2010, 43, 1223-1230.

[51] Williams, G.M., Iatropoulos, M.J., Whysner, J. Safety assessment of butylated hydroxyanisole and butylated hydroxytoluene as antioxidant food additives. *Food and Chemical Toxicology*, 1999, 37, 1027-1038.

[52] Hirose, M., Takhashi, S., Ogawa, K., Futakuchi, M., Shirai, T., Shibutani, M., Uneyama, C., Toyodo, K., Iwata, H. Chemoprevention of heterocyclic amine-induced carcinogenesis by phenolic compounds in rats. *Cancer Letters*, 1999, 143, 173-178.

[53] Valenzuela, A., Sanhueza, J., Nieto, S. Cholesterol oxidation. Health hazard and the role of antioxidants in prevention. *Biological Research*, 2003, 36, 291-302.

[54] Slamenova, D., Horvathova, E., Robichova, S., Hrusovska, L., Gabelova, A., Keibl, K., Jakubikova, J., Sedlak, J. Molecular and cellular influences of butylated hydroxyanisole on Chinese hamster V79 cells treated with N-methyl-N'-nitro-N-nitrosoguanidine: antimutagenicity of butylated hydroxyanisole. *Environmental and Molecular Mutagenesis*, 2003, 41, 28-36.

[55] Hirose, M., Ito, T., Takahashi, S., Ozaki, M., Ogiso, T., Nihro, Y., Miki, T., Shitai, T. Prevention by synthetic phenolic antioxidants of 2-amino-3, 8-dimethylimidazo[4,5-f]quinoxaline (MeIQx)- or activated MeIQx-induced mutagenesis and MeIQx-induced rat hepatocarcinogenesis, and role of antioxidant activity in the prevention of carcinogenesis. *European Journal of Cancer Prevention*, 1998, 7, 233-241.

[56] Sherwin, E. R. Oxidation and antioxidants in fat and oil processing. *Journal of the American Oil Chemists Society,* 1978, 55, 809-814.

[57] Packer, L., Weber, S.U., Rimbach, G. Molecular aspects of alpha-tocotrienol antioxidant action and cell signalling. *The Journal of Nutrition*, 2001, 131, 369S–73S.

[58] Tan, B., Saleh, M.H. *Integrated process for recovery of carotenoids and tocotrienols from oil in USPTO 5*, 1992,157,132.

[59] Frankel, E.N., Huang, S.W., Kanner, J., German, J.B. Inferfacial phenomena in the evaluation of antioxidants: bulk oils versus emulsions. *Journal of Agricultural and Food Chemistry*, 1994, 42, 1054-1059.

[60] Lea, C.H., Ward, R.J. Relative antioxidant activities of the seven tocopherols. *Journal of the Science of Food and Agriculture*, 1959, 10, 537-548.

[61] Lea, C.H. On the antioxidant activities of the tocopherols. II. Influence of the substrate, temperature and level of oxidation. *Journal of the Science of Food and Agriculture,* 1960, 11, 212-218.

[62] Kulas, E., Ackman, R.G. Different tocopherols and the relationship between two methods for determination of primary oxidation products in fish oil. *Journal of Agricultural and Food Chemistry,* 2001, 49, 1724-1729.

[63] Kulas, E., Ackman, R.G. Protection of alpha-tocopherol in non-purified and purified fish oil. *Journal of the American Oil Chemists Society*, 2001, 78, 197-203.

[64] Kulas, E., Olsen, E., Ackman, R.G. Effect of α-, γ-, and δ-tocopherol on the distribution of volatile secondary oxidation products in fish oil. *European Journal of Lipid Science and Technology*, 2002, 104, 520-529.

[65] Zuta, P.C., Simpson, B.K., Zhao, X., Leclerc, L. The effect of α-tocopherol on the oxidation of mackerel oil. *Journal of Agricultural and Food Chemistry*, 2007, 100, 800-807.

[66] Chaiyasit, W., McClements, D.J., Decker, E.A. The relationship between the physicochemical properties of antioxidants and their ability to inhibit lipid oxidation in bulk oil and oil-in-water emulsions. *Journal of Agricultural and Food Chemistry*, 2005, 53, 4982-4988.

[67] Vicetti, R., Ishitani, T., Salas, A., Ayala, M. Use of alpha-tocopherol combined with synergists and compared to other antioxidants on the oxidative stability of sardine skin lipids. Journal *of Food Composition and Analysis*, 2005, 18, 131-137.

[68] Horn, A.F., Nielsen, N.S., Jacobsen, C. Additions of caffeic acid, ascorbyl palmitate or γ-tocopherol to fish oil-enriched energy bars affect lipid oxidation differently. *Food Chemistry*, 2009, 112, 412-420.

[69] Huang, S, -W., Frankel, E.N., German, J.B. Antioxidant activity of α- and γ-tocopherols in bulk oils and in oil-in-water emulsions. *Journal of Agricultural and Food Chemistry*, 1994, 42, 2108-2114.

[70] Jung, M.Y., Min, D.B. Effects of oxidized α-, γ-, and δ-tocopherols on the oxidative stability of purified soybean oil. *Food Chemistry*, 1992, 45, 183-187.

[71] Let, M.B., Jacobsen, C., Meyer, A.S. Ascorbyl palmitate,γ-tocopherol and EDTA affect lipid oxidation in fish oil enriched salad dressing differently. *Journal of Agricultural and Food Chemistry,* 2007, 55, 2369-2375.

[72] Hamilton, R.J. Effect of tocopherol, ascorbyl palmitate and lecithin on autooxidation of fish oil. *Journal of the American Oil Chemists Society*, 1998, 75, 813-822.

[73] Shahidi, F, in J. Smish and L.Hong-Shum, eds., *Food Additive Databook*, Blackwell Science, Ltd., Oxford, u.k., 2003, p.75.

[74] Frankel, E.N. Antioxidants in lipid foods and their impact on food quality. *Food Chemistry,* 1996, 57, 51-55.

[75] Jacobsen, C. Effect of ascorbic acid on iron release from the emulsifier interface and on the oxidative flavour deterioration in fish oil enriched mayonnaise. *Journal of Agricultural and Food Chemistry*, 1999, 47, 4917-4926.

[76] Richheimer, S.L., Bailey, D.T., Bernart, M.W., Kent, M., Vininski, J.V., Anderson, L.D. Antioxidant activity and oxidative degradation of phenolic compounds isolated from rosemary. *Recent Research Development in Oil Chemistry*, 1999, 3, 45-58.

[77] Sewalt, V., Robbins, K., Gamble, W. Lipid-soluble antioxidant components of *Rosmarinus officinalis*. *Lipid Technology*, 2005, 17, 106-111.

[78] Aruoma, O.I., Halliwell, B., Aeschbach, R., Loliger, J. Antioxidant and prooxidant properties of active rosemary constituents: carnosol and carnosic acid. *Xenobiotica*, 1992, 22, 257-268.

[79] Perez-Mateos, M., Gomez-Guillen, M.C., Hurtado, J.L., Solas, M.T., Montero, P. The effect of rosemary extract and omega-3 unsaturated fatty acids on the properties of gels made from the flesh of mackerel (Scomber scombrus) by high pressure and heat treatments. *Food Chemistry*, 2002, 79, 1-8.

[80] Medina, I., Gonzalez, M.J., Pazos, M., Della Medaglia, D., Gallardo, J.M., Sacchi, R. Activity of plant extracts for preserving functional food containing n-3- PUFA. *European Food Research and Technology*, 2003, 217, 301-307.

[81] Wada, S., Fang, X. The synergistic antioxidant effect of rosemary extract and α-tocopherol in sardine oil model system and frozen-crushed fish meat. *Journal of Food Process Preservation*, 1992, 16, 263-274.

[82] O'Sullivan, A., Mayr, A., Shaw, N.B., Murphy, S.C., Kerry, J.P. Use of natural antioxidants to stabilize fish oil systems. *Journal of Aquatic Food Product Technology,* 2005, 14, 75-94.
[83] Bhale, S.D., Xu, Z., Prinyawiwatkul, W., King, J.M., Godber, J.S. Oregano and rosemary extracts inhibit oxidation of long-chain n-3 fatty acids in menhaden oil. *Journal of Food Science*, 2007, 72, C504-508.
[84] Cuvelier, M-E., Richard, H., Berset, C. Antioxidant activity and phenolic composition of pilot-plant and commercial extracts of sage and rosemary. *Journal of American Oil Chemist's Society*, 1996, 73, 645-652.
[85] Cuvelier, M-E., Berset, C., Richard, H. Separation of major antioxidants in sage by high performance liquid chromatography. *Sciences des Aliments*, 1994, 14, 811-815.
[86] Nawar, W.W. Lipid in food chemistry, Dekker, New York, 1996.
[87] Hudson, B.J.F., Lewis, J.I. Polyhydroxy flavonoid anti-oxidant for edible oils-Structural criteria for activity. *Food Chemistry*, 1983, 10, 47-55.
[88] Pietta, P.G. Flavonoids as antioxidants. *Journal of Natural Products*, 2000, 63, 1035-1042.
[89] Auger, C., Al-Awwadi, N., Bornet, A., Rouanet, J.M., Gasc, F., Cros, G. Catechins and procyanidins in Mediterranean diets. *Food Research International*, 2004, 37, 233-245.
[90] Balentine, D.A., Wiseman, S.A., Bouwens, L.C.M. The chemistry of tea flavonoids. *Critical Reviews in Food Science and Nutrition*, 1997, 37, 693-704.
[91] Cheng, Q.K., Chen, Z.M. Tea and Health. *Beijing China: Press of Chineese Agricultural Sciences*, 1994.
[92] Wanasundara, U.N., Shahidi, F. Stabilization of seal blubber and menhaden oils with green tea. *Journal of the American Oil Chemists Society*, 1996, 73, 1183-1190.
[93] Shahidi, F., Yang, Z., Saleemi, Z. O. Stabilization of meat lipids with flavonoids and related compounds. *Journal of Food Lipids*, 1993, 1, 69-78.
[94] Husain, S. R., Cillard, J. and Cillard, P. Hydroxy radical scavenging activity of flavonoids. *Phytochemistry*, 1987, 26, 2489-2491.
[95] Chen, C.-W. and Ho, C.-T. Antioxidant properties of polyphenols extracted from green and black teas. *Journal of Food Lipids*, 1995, 2, 35-46.
[96] Zhu, Q.Y., Huang, Y. D.T., Chen, Z.Y. Regeneration of alpha-tocopherol in human low density lipoprotein by green tea catechin. *Journal of Agricultural and Food Chemistry,* 1999, 47, 2020-2025.
[97] Wanasundara, U.N., Shahidi, F. Antioxidant and prooxidant activity of green tea extracts in marine oils. *Food Chemistry*, 1998, 63, 335-342.
[98] Yerlikaya, P., Gokoglu, N. Inhibition effects of green tea and grape seed extracts on lipid oxidation in bonito fillets during frozen storage. *International Journal of Food Science and Technology*, 2010, 45, 252-257.
[99] He, Y., Shahidi, F. Antioxidant activity of green tea and its catechins in a fish meat model system. *Journal of Agricultural and Food Chemistry*, 1997, 45, 4262-4266.
[100] Zhu, Q; Liang, C. P., Cheng, K.W., Peng X., Lo, C.Y., Shahidi, F., Chen, F., Ho C.T., Wang, M. Trapping effects of green and black tea extracts on peroxidation-derived carbonyl substances of seal blubber oil. *Journal of Agricultural and Food Chemistry*, 2009, 57, 1065-1069.
[101] Xia, E.Q., Deng, G.F., Guo, Y.J., Li, H.B. Biological activities of polyphenols from grapes. *International Journal of Molecular Sciences*, 2010, 11, 622-646.

[102] Palma, M., Taylor, L.R. Extraction of polyphenolic compounds from grape seeds with near critical carbon dioxide. *Journal of Chromatography*. A, 1999, 849, 117-124

[103] Pinelo, M., Rodrigez, A.R., Sineiro, J., Senorans, F.J., Reglero, G., Nunez, M.J. Supercritical fluid and solid-liquid extraction of phenolic antioxidants from grape pomace:a comparative study. *European Food Research and Technology*, 2007,226, 199-205.

[104] Yilmaz, Y.; Toledo, R.T. Major flavonoids in grape seeds and skins: Antioxidant capacity of catechin, epicatechin, and gallic acid. *Journal of Agricultural and Food Chemistry,* 2004, 52, 255–260.

[105] Luther, M., Parry, J.. Moore, J., Meng, J.H.., Zhang, Y.F., Cheng, Z.H., Yu, L. Inhibitory effect of chardonnay and black raspberry seed extracts on lipid oxidation in fish oil and their radical scavenging and antimicrobial properties. *Food Chemistry,* 2007, 104, 1065–1073.

[106] Sanchez-Alonso, I.; Borderias, J.; Larsson, K.; Undeland, I. Inhibition of hemoglobin-mediated oxidation of regular and lipid-fortified washed cod mince by a white grape dietary fiber. *Journal of Agricultural and Food Chemistry,* 2007, 55, 5299–5305.

[107] Medina, I., Alcantara, D., Gonza, M.J., Torres, P., Lucas, R., Roque, J., Plou, F.J., Morales, J.C. Antioxidant activity of Resveratrol in several fish lipid matrices:Effect of acylation and glucosylation. *Journal of Agricultural and Food Chemistry*, 2010,58, 9778-9786.

[108] Vinson, J.A., Su, X., Zubik, L., Bose, P. Phenolic antioxidant quantity and quality in foods:fruits. *Journal of Agricultural and Food Chemistry*, 2001, 49, 5315-5321.

[109] Awad, M.A., Jager, A., van Westing, L.M. Flavonoid and chlorogenic acid levels in apple fruit: Characterization of variation. *Scientia Horticulturae*, 2000, 83,249-263.

[110] Tsao, R., Yang, R., Young, J.C., Zhu, H. Polyphenolic profiles in eight apple cultivars using high-performance liquid chromatography (HPLC*). Journal of Agricultural and Food Chemistry*, 2003, 51, 6347-6353.

[111] Wojdylo, A., Oszmianski, J., Laskowski, P. Polyphenolic compounds and antioxidant activity of new and old apple varieties. *Journal of Agricultural and Food Chemistry*, 2008, 56, 6520-6530.

[112] Wolfe, K.L., Liu, R.H. Apple peels as a value added food ingredient. *Journal of Agricultural and Food Chemistry*, 2003, 51, 609-614.

[113] Wolfe, K., Wu, X., Liu, R.H. Antioxidant activity of apple peels. *Journal of Agricultural and Food Chemistry*, 2003, 51, 609-614.

[114] Wanasundara, U.N., Shahidi, F. Stabilization of marine oils with flavonoids. Journal *of Food Lipids*, 1998, 5, 183-196

[115] Montero, P., Gimenez, B., Perez-Mateos, M., Gomez-Guillen., M.C. Oxidation stability of muscle with quercetin and rosemary during thermal and high-pressure gelation. *Food Chemistry*, 2005, 93, 17-23.

[116] Nieto, S., Garrido, A., Sanhueza, J., Loyola, L.A., Morales, G., Leighton, F., Valenzuela. Flavonoids as stabilizers of fish oil: An alternative to synthetic antioxidants. *Journal of the American Oil Chemists Society*, 1993, 70, 773-778.

[117] Rupasinghe, H.P.V., Yasmin, A. Inhibition of oxidation of aqueous emulsions of omega-3 fatty acids and fish oil by phloretin and phloridzin. *Molecules*, 2010, 15, 251-257.

[118] Kahkonen, M.P., Hopia, A.I., Heinonen, M. Berry phenolics and their antioxidative activity. *Journal of Agricultural and Food Chemistry*, 2001, 49, 4076-4082

[119] Kahkonen, M.P., Hopia, A.I., Vuorela, H.J., Rauha, J.P., Pihlaja, K., Kujala, T.S.,, Heinonen, M. Antioxidant activity of plant extracts containing phenolic compounds. *Journal of Agricultural and Food Chemistry*, 1999, 47, 3954-3962.

[120] Nakatani, N., Kikuzaki,H. A new antioxidative glucoside isolated from oregano (*Origanum vulgare* L). *Agricultural and Biological Chemistry*, 1987, 51, 2727-2732.

[121] Kikuzaki, H., Nakatani, N. Structure of a new antioxidative phenolic acid from oregano (Origanum vulgare L). *Agricultural and Biological Chemistry*, 1989,53, 519-524.

[122] Vekiari, S.A., Tzia, C., Oreopoulou, V., Thomopoulos, C.D. *Isolation of natural antioxidants from oregano.* Riv Ital Sost Grasse, 1993, 70,25-28.

[123] Vekiari, S., Oreopoulou, V., Tzia, C., Thomopoulos, C.D. Oregano flavonoids as lipid antioxidants. Journal of the American Oil Chemists Society, 1993, 70, 483-487.

[124] Nakatani N, 'Natural antioxidants from spices', in: *Phenolic Compounds in Foods and Their Effect on Health II, Antioxidants and Cancer Prevention*, ACS Symposium Series, No 507, Huang M-T, Ho C-T and Lee C Y H (eds),Washington,ACS Press, 1992, 72–86.

[125] Tsimidou, M., Papavergou, E., Boskou, D. Evaluation of oregano antioxidant activity in mackerel oil. *Food Research International*, 1995, 28, 431-433.

[126] Sorenson, A-D,M., Nielson, N.S., Jacobsen, C. Oxidative stability of fish oil-enriched mayonnaise based salads. *European Journal of Lipid Science and Technology*, 2010, 112, 476-487.

[127] Yue, X., Xu, Z. Antioxidant capabilities of defatted soy flour extracts, in: *Chemistry, Texture, and Flavor of Soy*, ACS Symposium Series, 1059, Cadwallader, K.R, and Chang, S.K.C (eds) Oxford University Press, 2010, 201-215

[128] Naim, M., Gestetner, B., Zilkah, S., Birk, Y., Bondi A. Soybean isoflavones. Characterization, determination, and antifungal activity. *Journal of Agricultural and Food Chemistry*, 1974, 22, 806–810.

[129] Wang, C., Sherrard, M., Pagadala, S., Wixon, R., Scott R. Isoflavone content among maturity group 0 to II soybeans, *Journal of the American Oil Chemists Society*, 2000, 77 483–487.

In: Fish Oil: Production, Consumption and Health Benefits
Editors: Matthias Van Dijk and Jürgen Vitek ISBN: 978-1-61470-963-3

Chapter VII

Fish Oil

Mohamed.M.Elseweidy
Faculty of Pharmacy-Zagazig University, Egypt

Dietary sources and Biosynthesis pathways represents the main suppliers for the fatty acids needed by the human body for construction of hydrophobic parts of Bio molecules . Various animal and vegetable lipids are ingested, hydrolyzed at least partially by digestive enzymes and absorbed through the intestinal wall to be distributed through the body, first in the lymphatic system and then in the blood stream . To some extent such dietary supply may adjust the composition of fatty acids in the body lipids.

On the other hand, metabolic processes in the tissues of the normal human body can modify the dietary fatty acids and or those that are synthesized in these tissues, to produce almost all the various structures that are needed .For this reason,with one exception the actual composition of the fatty acids supplied in the diet is relatively unimportant. This one exception involves the need for appropriate proportions of the relatively highly unsaturated fatty acids since many higher mammals; including humans are unable to produce fatty acids with double bonds very far towards the end of the molecule either during de novo synthesis or by modification of the dietary acids. Accordingly these fatty acids can provides essential fatty acids and acting also as carriers for oil soluble vitamins like A,D,E,K additionally their intestinal absorption . The oils derived from cold-water fish are unique among all the edible oils and fats. They are an important source of long chain ω-3 or n-3 polyunsaturates.

Fatty acids group referred to as conjugated Linoleic acid are receiving now greater interest due to having health promoting properties. The liver oils from fish such as cod and halibut have an added feature as natural source of highly importance for oil soluble vitamins like A and D.

Two forms of polyunsaturates are considered essential, known as n-3 and n-6, average intake of the former have fallen considerably as compared to the second. This induced more emphasis regarding the need for an adequate intake of performed long chain ω-3 polyunsaturated fatty acids from fish. Dietary 18 c fatty acids (essential fatty acids) were previously referred to as vitamins F1 and F2. These 18 c fatty acids (Linoleic and α linoleic) are converted by a common enzyme system into 20, 22 carbon derivatives. Since the conversion enzymes are the same for both n-3 and n-6 the phenomenon of competitive inhibition occurs. Accordingly, the predominance of one family may deviate the other away from enzyme sites and the conversion process favor the first one. As a result an excess of the dietary ω-6 will inhibit ω-3 conversion to 20, 22 carbons from specifically eicosapentaenoic and Docosahexenoic acids

As illustrated before n−3 fatty acids (popularly referred to as **ω−3 fatty acids** or **omega-3 fatty acids**) are members of a series of essential unsaturated fatty acids that have in common a final carbon–carbon double bond in the *n*−3 position; that is, the third bond from the methyl end of the fatty acid.

Nutritionally important *n*−3 fatty acids include α-linolenic acid (ALA), eicosapentaenoic acid (EPA), and docosahexaenoic acid (DHA), all of which are polyunsaturated. The human body cannot synthesize *n*−3 fatty acids *de novo*, but it has a limited ability to form the "long chain" *n*−3 fatty acids EPA (20 carbon atoms) and DHA (22 carbon atoms) from the "short chain" eighteen-carbon *n*−3 fatty acid ALA.

Essential fatty acids are molecules that cannot be synthesized by the human body but are vital for normal metabolism. One of the two families of these essential fatty acids are the omega-3 fatty acids. Because omega (ω) is the last letter in the Greek alphabet the naming system counts from the last of the carbons to the carbon-carbon double bond. Similarly, the preferred *n*–3 nomenclature uses the letter "*n*" to mean the number of carbon atoms in the chain. If the fatty acid has this third-to-last double bond, it is called an ω–3 ("omega minus 3") fatty acid. Common sources of *n*–3 fatty acids include fish oils and some plant oils such as flaxseed oil.

Chemical structure of alpha-linolenic acid (ALA), an essential *n*−3 fatty acid, (18:3Δ9c,12c,15c, which means a chain of 18 carbons with 3 double bonds on carbons numbered 9, 12 and 15). Although chemists count from the carbonyl carbon (Blue Numbering), physiologists count from the *n* (ω) carbon (red numbering). Note that from the *n* end (diagram right), the first double bond appears as the third carbon-carbon bond (line segment), hence the name "*n*−3". This is explained by the fact that the *n* end is almost never changed during physiologic transformations in the human body, as it is more stable energetically, and other carbohydrates compounds can be synthesized from the other carbonyl end, for example in glycerides, or from double bonds in the middle of the chain.

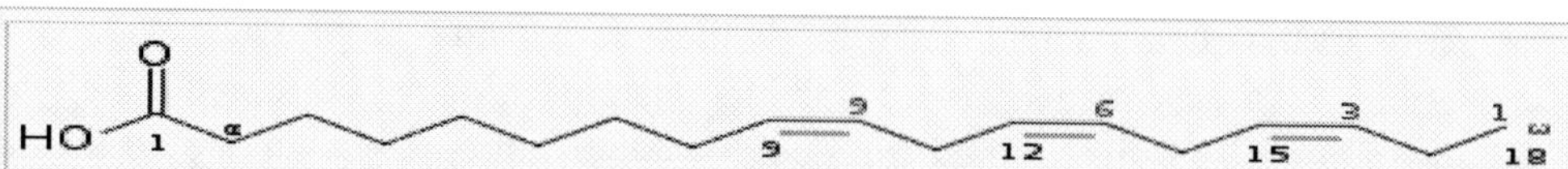

Chemical structure of alpha-linolenic acid (ALA), an essential *n*−3 fatty acid, (18:3Δ9c,12c,15c, which means a chain of 18 carbons with 3 double bonds on carbons numbered 9, 12 and 15). Although chemists count from the carbonyl carbon (Blue Numbering), physiologists count from the *n* (ω) carbon (red numbering). Note that from the *n* end (diagram right), the first double bond appears as the third carbon-carbon bond (line segment), hence the name "*n*−3". This is explained by the fact that the *n* end is almost never changed during physiologic transformations in the human body, as it is more stable energetically, and other carbohydrates compounds can be synthesized from the other carbonyl end, for example in glycerides, or from double bonds in the middle of the chain.

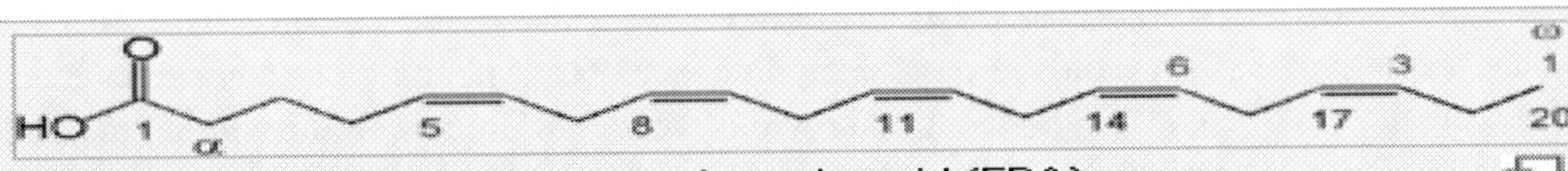

Chemical structure of eicosapentaenoic acid (EPA).

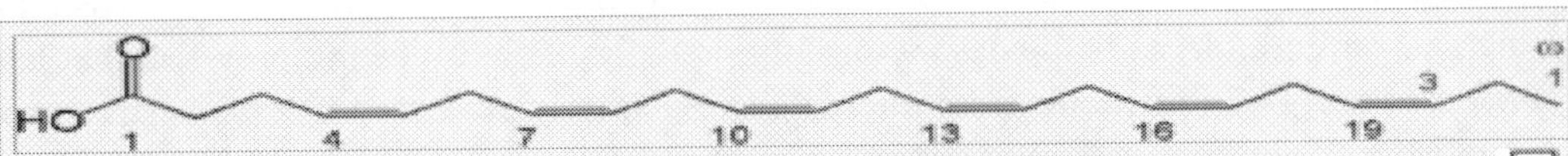

Chemical structure of docosahexaenoic acid (DHA).

The term ***n*−3** (also called **ω−3** or **omega-3**) signifies that the first double bond exists as the **third** carbon-carbon bond from the terminal methyl end (*n*) of the carbon chain.

n−3 fatty acids which are important in human nutrition are: α-linolenic acid (18:3, *n*−3; ALA), eicosapentaenoic acid (20:5, *n*−3; EPA), and docosahexaenoic acid (22:6, *n*−3; DHA). These three polyunsaturates have either 3, 5 or 6 double bonds in a carbon chain of 18, 20 or 22 carbon atoms, respectively. All double bonds are in the *cis*-configuration; in other words, the two hydrogen atoms are on the same side of the double bond.

Most naturally-produced fatty acids (created or transformed in animal or plant cells with an even number of carbon in chains) are in *cis*-configuration.

Like free oxygen radicals, iodine can add to double bonds of docosahexaenoic acid and arachidonic acid forming iodolipids.[1][2][3][4]

List of *N*−3 Fatty Acids

This table lists several different names for the most common *n*−3 fatty acids found in nature.

Common name	Lipid name	Chemical name
Hexadecatrienoic acid (HTA)	16:3 (*n*−3)	*all-cis*-7,10,13-hexadecatrienoic acid
α-Linolenic acid (ALA)	18:3 (*n*−3)	*all-cis*-9,12,15-octadecatrienoic acid
Stearidonic acid (SDA)	18:4 (*n*−3)	*all-cis*-6,9,12,15-octadecatetraenoic acid
Eicosatrienoic acid (ETE)	20:3 (*n*−3)	*all-cis*-11,14,17-eicosatrienoic acid
Eicosatetraenoic acid (ETA)	20:4 (*n*−3)	*all-cis*-8,11,14,17-eicosatetraenoic acid
Eicosapentaenoic acid (EPA)	20:5 (*n*−3)	*all-cis*-5,8,11,14,17-eicosapentaenoic acid
Heneicosapentaenoic acid (HPA)	21:5 (*n*−3)	*all-cis*-6,9,12,15,18-heneicosapentaenoic acid
Docosapentaenoic acid (DPA), Clupanodonic acid	22:5 (*n*−3)	*all-cis*-7,10,13,16,19-docosapentaenoic acid
Docosahexaenoic acid (DHA)	22:6 (*n*−3)	*all-cis*-4,7,10,13,16,19-docosahexaenoic acid
Tetracosapentaenoic acid	24:5 (*n*−3)	*all-cis*-9,12,15,18,21-tetracosapentaenoic acid
Tetracosahexaenoic acid (Nisinic acid)	24:6 (*n*−3)	*all-cis*-6,9,12,15,18,21-tetracosahexaenoic acid

A typical fish oil softgelFish oil is oil derived from the tissues of oily fish. Fish oils contain the omega-3 fatty acids eicosapentaenoic acid (EPA), and docosahexaenoic acid (DHA), precursors of eicosanoids that are known to reduce inflammation throughout the body and are thought to have many health benefits [1].

Fish do not actually produce omega-3 fatty acids, but instead accumulate them from either consuming microalgae that produce these fatty acids, as is the case with fish like herring and sardines, or, as is the case with fatty predatory fish, by eating prey fish that have accumulated omega-3 fatty acids from microalgae. Such fatty predatory fish like shark, sword fish, tilefish, and albacore tuna may be high in omega-3 fatty acids, but due to their position at the top of the food chain, these species can accumulate toxic substances. For this reason, the FDA recommends limiting consumption of certain (predatory) fish species (e.g. albacore tuna, shark, and swordfish) due to high levels of toxic contaminants such as mercury, dioxin, PCBs and chlordane [2].

Fish oil is used as a component in aquaculture feed. More than 50 percent of the world's fish oil used in aquaculture feed is fed to farmed salmon. Fish oil has been studied for treating clinical depression, anxiety, and enhancing the benefits from depression medications. Countries with the highest intake of fish in their diets are correlated with the lowest rates of depression among citizens [3&4].

Fish Oil Production

In 2005, fish oil production declined in all main producing countries with the exception of Iceland. The 2005 production estimate is about 570,000 tonnes in the five main exporting countries (Peru, Denmark, Chile, Iceland and Norway), a 12% decline from the 650,000 tonnes produced in 2004. Peru continues to be the main fish oil producer worldwide, with about one fourth of total fish oil production. Though Peruvian catches of fish, intended to be reduced in 2005, were more or less in line with the 2004 result, fish oil production declined from 350,000 tonnes to 290,000 tonnes, due to lower fat content of the fish. In the recent summer months, the fat content was as low as 2% which compares to 4% in 2004. Despite a 18% decline in production, Peruvian earnings from fish oil exports reached US$156 million in 2005, exceeding the 2004 income by US$6 million. This was due to an increase in fish oil prices [5].

Production process Description: Fish processing includes both Fish canning for human consumption and the production of fish bi products such as meal and oil .Canning itself includes Two methods:

A. Precooking method
B. Raw back method

a) Precooking: The raw fishes are cleaned, cooked before the canning step. It is used typically for larger fish such as Tuna.

b) Raw back: The raw fishes are cleaned, placed in cans before cooking,used for small fish such as Sardines

The byproduct manufacturing segment of the fish industry uses canning or filleting wastes, fish that are not suitable for human consumption to produce fish meal and fish oil.

Caning

A.) Precooking method begins with:

1. Thawing of the fish, eviscerated, washed, cooked using steam oil, hot air or smoke for 1.5- 10 hours depending on the fish size. Such step removes the fish oils, coagulates the protein in the fish to loosen the meat and then cooled for several hours. It may be refrigerated to reduce the time.
2. Head, fins, bones and undesirable meat are removed; the remainder is cut or chooped and placed in cans. Oil, brine and or water are added to the cans which are sealed and pressure cooked before shipment.

B.) Raw back method:

1. It begins with thawing, weighing the fish, washed, possibly brined or nobbed which removes the head,viscera and tail
2. The Fish are placed in cans, cooked, drained and dried.
3. After drying liquid (oil, brine, water, sauce or other) is added to the cans, then sealed, washed and sterilized with steam or hot water.

Fish Byproduct Manufacturing

1. It begins with cooking the fish at 100◦c (lower for some species) in a continuous cooker. This process coagulates the protein and ruptures the cell walls to release water and oil.
2. The mixture may be strained with an auger in a perforated casing before pressing with a screw press.
3. As the fishes are moved along the screw press, the pressure is increased and the volume is decreased.
4. The liquid from the mixture (pressing liquor) is squeezed out through a perforated casing.
5. The pressing liquor which consists of water, oil and some solids is transported to a centrifuge to remove solids.
6. These solids are later returned to the press cake in the drying step.
7. The oil and water are separated using a disc –type centrifuge in the oil separator.
8. The oil is polished by using hot water washes, centrifuged, then sent to an oil – refining operation, the water is removed from the oil (stick water) goes to an evaporation to concentrate the solids .

The press cake, stick water, solids are mixed and sent to either a direct-fired or indirect-fired dryer (steam tube dryer).

A direct-fired dryer consists of a slowly rotating cylinder through which air is heated to about 600◦ C by an open flame, passes through the mishes to evaporate the liquid.

The indirect one is a fixed cylinder with rotating crapers that heat the meal with steam or hot fluids flowing through discs, tubes, coils or the dryer casing itself. Air also passes through the apparatus, but is not heated, flows in the opposite direction to the meal to entrain the evaporated water.

Such process may rquire twice as much time to the direct one procedure . The dried meal is cooled, ground, stored in bulck or in paper, used in animal, pet feeding owing to its high protein content.

The Polished Oil

It is further purified by a process called hardening. First the polished oil is refined by mixing the oil with an alkaline solution in a large stirred vessel. The alkaline solution reacts with free fatty acid in the oil to form insoluble soaps. The mixture is allowed to settle overnight, the cleared oil is extracted off the top, and then washed with hot water to remove any remaining soap.

Bleaching

This is accomplished by mixing the oil with natural clays to remove oil pigment, colored matter at temperature 80-116◦c in either a batch or controlled mode.

Hydrogenation

It is the next step where hydrogenation of the unsaturated fatty acids chain. Nickel catalyst at concentration of 0.05-0.1 percent by weight is added to the oil mixture, heated, stirred and hydrogen is injected into the mixture to react with unsaturated fatty acids chain. The oil is cooled after complete hydrogenation, filtered to remove the nickel.

The hydrogenated oil is refined again before the de oderization step which removes odor and flavor producing chemicals.

De oderization occur in a vacuum chamber where dry oxygen free steam is bubbled through the oil to remove the undesirable chemicals. Volatilization of the undesirable chemical occur at temperature between 170-230◦C. The oil is then cooled to about 38◦C before exposure to air to prevent formation of undesirable chemicals.

Fish oil is obtained by extracting total fish body with food grade ethanol and purified by molecular distillation to remove various contaminants (Figure1). The crude fish oil preparations contain 90% fatty acid triacylglycerols, 2-5% unsaponifiable matter containing sterols, fatty acid-estrified cholesterol, free fatty acids, and minor quantities of fat soluble vitamins. These days fish oil is available in the form of a refined and purified liquid with different flavors (Table 1) [6].

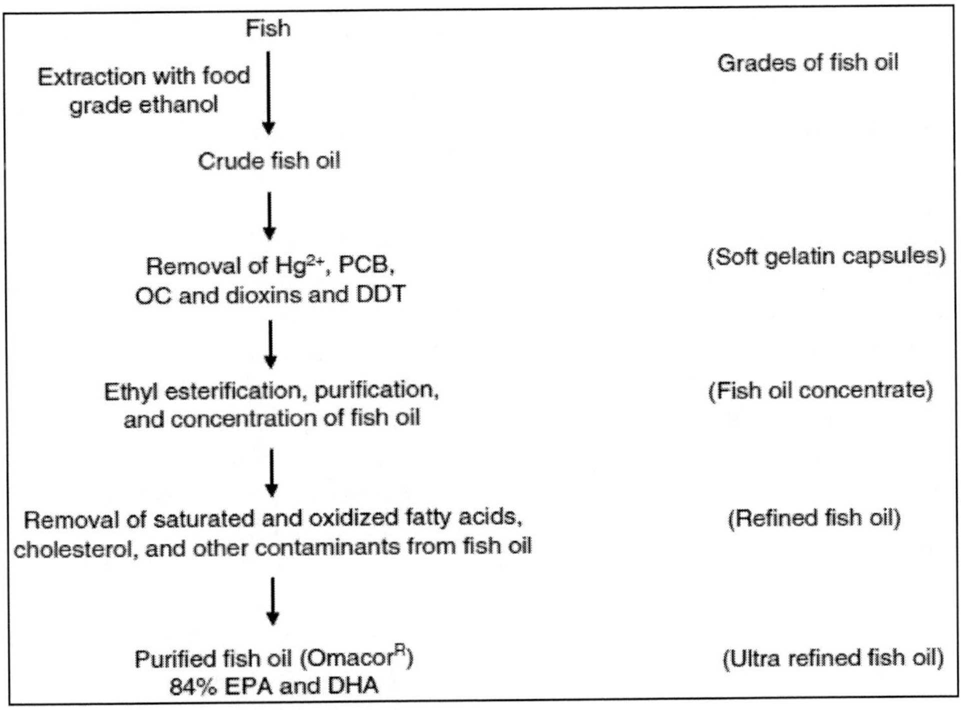

Figure 1. Procedures for the purification of ultrapure fish oil from crude fish oil by molecular distillation.

Table 1. Commercial names and manufacturers of n–3 fatty acid (DHA and EPA) preparations from fish and algal sources

Commercial name	Manufacturer
Purified fish oil	Carlson Laboratories Inc, Arlington Heights, IL, USA
Omegaven™	Kabi Bad Homburg, Germany
Lipoplus™ (LMF541)	B. Braun Melsungen, AG
Omacor™	Reliant pharmaceutical Inc Corner, NJ, USA
Zodin^{R}	Solvary, Takeda, Kuhnil Pharmaceutical Co Ltd, Pierre Fabre Sante, France
DHASCO-S and T	Martek Biosciences Corporation, Columbia, MD, USA
Cardiozen™	Equazen Nutraceuticals, London, UK
DHActive TMCL	Nutrinova, Montpellier, France
Neuramin DHA	AllStar Health, Huntington, CA, USA
O-Mega-Zen^{3}™	Nu Tru Inc, Lincolnwood, IL, USA
Lovaza	GlaxoSmithKline, Philadelphia
Efalex™	Scotia Pharmaceuticals, Scotland, UK
Marinol D-40	Loders Croklaan Lipid Nutrition, Wormerveer, The Netherlands
Vegan omega-3	Deva Nutrition, Chelsea, AL, USA
Krill oil	Jedwards International inc, Quincy, MA, USA

Fish Oil Consumption

Epidemiologic studies have shown a link between total fat consumption and development of chronic degenerative diseases such as cancer [7]. Several studies have reported a positive association between high intake of fat and the incidence of breast, colon, and prostate cancer [8].

Reviews regarding fat ingestion and health revealed that the type of fat consumed also appears to be important in influencing cancer risk; in particular, n-3 polyunsaturated fatty acids (PUFAs) present in oily fish appear to be protective in fish oil (FO) [9].

The present-day Western diet has a ratio of ω-6 to ω-3 fatty acids of about 15:1. The Paleolithic diet on which human beings evolved, and lived for most of their existence, had a ratio of 1:1 and was high in antioxidants [10]. Changes in eating habits, natural versus processed food, and agricultural development within the past 100 to 200 years caused these changes in the ω-6 to ω-3 ratio. The decreased consumption of DHA-enriched foods and increased consumption of ω-6 enriched vegetable oils is responsible for the 15:1 ω-6: ω-3 ratio [11]. The present Western diet promotes the pathogenesis of many chronic diseases such as cardiovascular disease, inflammatory and autoimmune diseases, and neurodegenerative diseases, whereas a diet enriched in ω-3 fatty acids exerts cardioprotective, immunosuppressive, and neuroprotective effects. A lower AA: DHA ratio suppresses the human disorders mentioned above. The American Heart Association recommends that everyone should eat oily fish twice per week and that those with coronary heart disease should consume 1 g/day of EPA plus DHA from oily fish or supplements [12].

Incorporation of ω-3 fatty acids into functional foods is limited by their high susceptibility to oxidative degradation. An oil-in-water emulsion may be amore effectivemethod to deliver ω-3 fatty acids into functional foods [13]. The best sources of dietaryω-3 fatty acids are fishand fishoil. Fish oil is available in the form of a purified liquid in lemon flavor (Carlson Laboratories Inc, Arlington Heights, IL), a 10% fish oil emulsion Omegaven™ (Kabi Bad Homburg, Germany), 20% fish oil emulsion Lipoplus™(MLF541) (B. Braun Melsungen AG), and an FDA approved fish oil preparation Omacor™ (Reliant Pharmaceuticals, Inc., Corner, NJ). Omacor is composed of approximately 90% ω-3 fatty acids (465 mg EPA, 375 mg DHA, and > 60mg other ω-3 fatty acid esters), for a total of > 900mg of ω-3 fatty acids per 1 g capsule. Cardiozen™ (Equazen Nutraceuticals, London,UK) is another fish oil preparation that contains 6 times more EPA than DHA. These fish oil preparations lower plasma triacylglycerol level, increase bleeding time, downregulate gene expression for platelet-derived growth factor, lower blood pressure, decrease the number of endothelial adhesion molecules, improve lipoprotein size, and decrease the risk of cardiovascular and cerebrovascular diseases. Fish oil is well tolerated and has no significantly adverse effects. In neural membranes, EPA and DHA not only affect their physicochemical properties such asmembrane fluidity, permeability, and viscosity, especially in neuronal synapses, but also modulate neurotransmission [14], gene expression [15], activities of enzymes andreceptors, ion channels, and immunity [16]. According to the American Heart Association (AHA), as well as various international organizations, omega-3 fatty acids benefit the heart of healthy people, and those at high risk or suffering cardiovascular disease (CD). In 1996, the AHA released its Science Advisory, "Fish Consumption, Fish Oil, Lipids and Coronary Heart Disease" (Stone, 1996). Since then, important new findings about the benefits of omega-3 fatty acids, especially eicosapentaenoic acid (EPA) and docosohexaenoic acid (DHA) have been reported. The current AHA's dietary guidelines recommend that healthy adults eat at least two servings of fish (particularly fatty fish) per week. The AHA suggests that patients without or with documented CD eat, respectively, a variety of fish (preferably oily) at least twice a week, or to consume about 1 g of EPA+DHA per day, preferably from oily fish. However, the Scientific Statement of the AHA also indicates that fish and seafood is potentially a major source of human exposure to various environmental contaminants. Depending on their stage of life, consumers need also to be aware of the potential health risks of eating fish [17].

Although fish consumption can provide substantial amounts of omega-3 fatty acids, not everyone consumes a sufficient amount of fish to obtain an adequate intake of these important fatty acids, and this is especially true of children [18]. Hence, the interest in the development of other foods, such as dairy products, enriched with fish oil has increased in recent years [19]. Such 'functional foods' could be an effective way to reduce risk factors for several 'lifestyle-related' diseases including CVD, without the need for modification of the consumer's dietary habits in either adulthood or childhood [20].

Consumption of fish oil may protect against cardiovascular disease [21]. Data from observational studies suggest that fish intake is inversely associated with fatal coronary heart disease [22], and randomized controlled trials of dietary fish or fish oil supplementation after myocardial infarction demonstrate a reduction in mortality [23]. These effects are believed to be due to the high amounts of omega-3 fatty acids, eicosapentaenoic acid (EPA) and docosahexaenoic acid (DHA), present in fish oil. EPA and DHA must be obtained from dietary sources and recent guidelines from the American Heart Association recommend the consumption of oily fish at least twice weekly for individuals with and without coronary heart disease [24].

Knowledge about differences in consumer perceptions of health risks and benefits related to fish consumption is important for the development of targeted health interventions associated with dietary choice. Regular fish consumption is part of a healthy diet [25]. However, actual fish consumption levels are often far below dietary advice recommending consumption of two portions per week [26]. Health is an important motive for fish consumption [27], and so health interventions may focus on increasing consumer perceptions of the healthiness of including fish in their diet. Previous research has shown that consumers generally perceive eating fish as healthy. Nevertheless, perceptions of risks associated with fish consumption have a negative influence on fish consumption [28].

Fish consumption is associated with both nutritional benefits and toxicological risks to human health. For example,omega three fatty acids in fatty fish can substantially reduce the risk of cardiovascular disease [29], and fatty fish is an important source of vitamin D compared to other food products, which can improve the development of bones [30]

Dietary intervention studies suggest that a daily fish meal can improve blood pressure (BP); however, such a dietary regimen might be difficult to sustain. Hypertension is one of the causes of cardiovascular disease [31]. Diet plays an important role in the etiology of hypertension, because obesity and nutrient intake are known to affect BP. The BP-lowering properties of ω-3 long-chain polyunsaturated fatty acids (ω-3 LC-PUFA) from fish oil supplements have been thoroughly investigated and confirmed [32], with commonly used doses of 4–5 g of ω-3 LC-PUFAs per day leading to clinically significant reductions in BP. The largest effects are achieved in elderly hypertensives [33]. Several biological mechanisms have been suggested to explain the health benefits of ω-3 LCPUFAs on BP, e.g., changes in phospholipid composition, platelet aggregation, and vasodilatation [34].

Without the use of seafood supplements (fish oil or marine algae), a ω-3 LC-PUFAs intake of 4–5 g/d can hardly be achieved, even if one consumes a daily fish meal. There are relatively few dietary intervention trials that have investigated the effects of daily fish consumption (in contrast to fish oil ingestion) on BP, and some [35] but not all have found BP reduction by fatty fish consumption. Not daily, but still frequent fatty fish consumption, e.g., three times a week, usually provides a daily amount of 1–1.5 g of ω-3 LC-PUFAs and might be sustained easier by less committed seafood eaters than a daily fish meal [36].

Fish Oil Supplements and Safety

Most commercially available fish oils are derived from coldwater fish, primarily menhaden, but also salmon and trout. These oils are rich in the Omega-3 fatty acids eicosapentaenoic acid (EPA) and docosahexaenoic acid (DHA). These two fatty acids are metabolized to series 3 prostaglandins, which can have a significant moderating influence on inflammation. Fish, in turn, obtain EPA and DHA from algae, making super green foods such as marine micro-algae an alternate source of EPA and DHA. Algae may become the dominant source of omega-3 fatty acids as fish populations continue to decline in the world's oceans. Fish oil is readily absorbed as a dietary supplement. After one week of supplementation, increases in omega-3 fatty acids are detectable in the tissues. Tissue elevations in EPA and DHA persist for as long as one to two months after supplementation is discontinued [37]

From a conventional medical perspective, some animals will tend to develop oily coats and large flakes of dander following omega-3 fatty acid supplementation. This condition, known as seborrhoea oleosa, resolves within one to two weeks of discontinuing the supplement. Fish oil supplementation is otherwise very safe at recommended doses. The most common side effect is a fishy odor to the breath or the skin. Omega-3 EFAs may inhibit platelet aggregation (platelets are cells that help in the clotting process) accounting for some clinicians to recommend not using them when other anticoagulant (anti-clotting) medications are used. Fish oil does not seem to cause bleeding problems when it is taken by itself at commonly recommended dosages. Fish oil also does not appear to raise blood sugar levels in people or pets with diabetes, contrary to earlier reports [38].

Beneficial Effects of Fish Oil

The n–3 fatty acids in fish oil markedly effect human health. To achieve a significant increase in human tissues in vivo, intake of high doses of fish oil is required because bioavailability of n–3 fatty acids from fish oil to neural cells involves not only digestion and transport but also metabolism [39]. Furthermore, the efficacy of dietary intervention may also depend upon the health of the individual. For example, patients with gastrointestinal problems may not be able to absorb fish oil supplement. Daily use of n–3 fatty acids (3–5 g/day) by normal individuals may optimize the functions of human heart, brain, lungs, liver, spleen, and kidneys (Fig.2). These fatty acids reduce cardiovascular disease, type 2 diabetes, hypertension, cancer, inflammatory and autoimmune diseases, and neurodegenerative diseases [40]. In human nutritional studies, attempts have been made to increase the consumption of n–3 fatty acid enriched food because Western diet is deficient in n–3 fatty acids and has excessive levels of n–6 fatty acids compared with the diet on which human beings evolved and their genetic patterns are established. Excessive levels of n–6 fatty acids and a very highn–6/ n–3 ratio (20 : 1), as are found in today's Western diets, promote the pathogenesis of inflammatory and autoimmune, and neurodegenerative diseases, whereas increased levels of n–3 fatty acids (a lower n–6/ n–3 ratio) exert suppressive effects and prevent cardiovascular disease, type 2 diabetes, hypertension, cancer, inflammatory and autoimmune diseases, and neurodegenerative diseases. The American Heart Association recommends that everyone should eat oily fish twice per week and that those with coronary heart disease should consume 1 g/day of EPA plus DHA from oily fish or supplements [41].

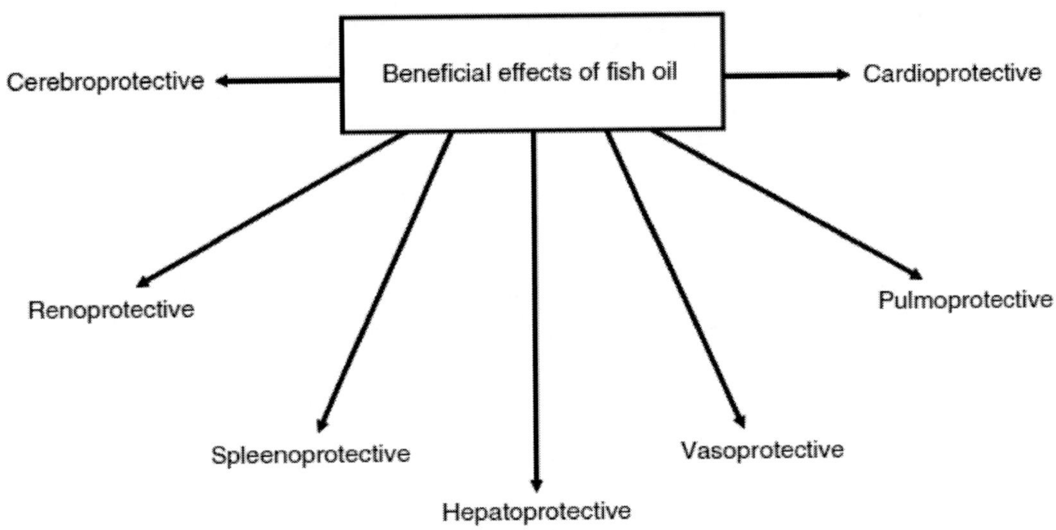

Figure 2. Beneficial effects of fish oil on various organs of human body.

Effects of Fish Oil on Heart

In heart, the incorporation of fish oil constituents, n–3 fatty acids, not only influences the physicochemical properties of membranes (fluidity, permeability) but also modulates the expression of many genes [42]. The n–3 fatty acids reduce proatherogenic cytokines, improve endothelial function, reduce vascular occlusion, and mitigate the course of coronary atherosclerosis. These fatty acids are also needed for vascular smooth muscle cell function [43]. The heart rate is reduced and heart rate variability is increased. An antiarrhythmic effect is also observed at the supraventricular and ventricular level [44]. The n–3 fatty acids also modulate levels of plasma fibrinogen and coagulant factor VII levels [45]. Collective evidence suggests that n–3 fatty acids reduce leukocyte reactivity, atherosclerosis, and thrombosis. In addition, fish oil exerts its effect through several different cellular mechanisms including the effects on lipoprotein metabolism, hemostatic function, platelet/vessel wall interactions, antiarrhythmic actions, and also through the inhibition of proliferation of smooth muscle cells and therefore growth of the atherosclerotic plaque. Fish oil intake also results in moderate reductions in blood pressure and modification of vascular neuroeffector mechanisms. The majority of cardiovascular benefits of fish oil are mediated in the vascular wall and at the vascular endothelium, which plays a central role in the regulation and maintenance of cardiovascular homeostasis and function [46] through the generation of nitric oxide and eicosanoids. In addition to direct effects on contractility, n–3 fatty acids in fish oil may affect atherogenesis via inhibition of vascular smooth muscle cell proliferation at the gene expression level and by modifying the expression of inflammatory cytokines and adhesion molecules [47].

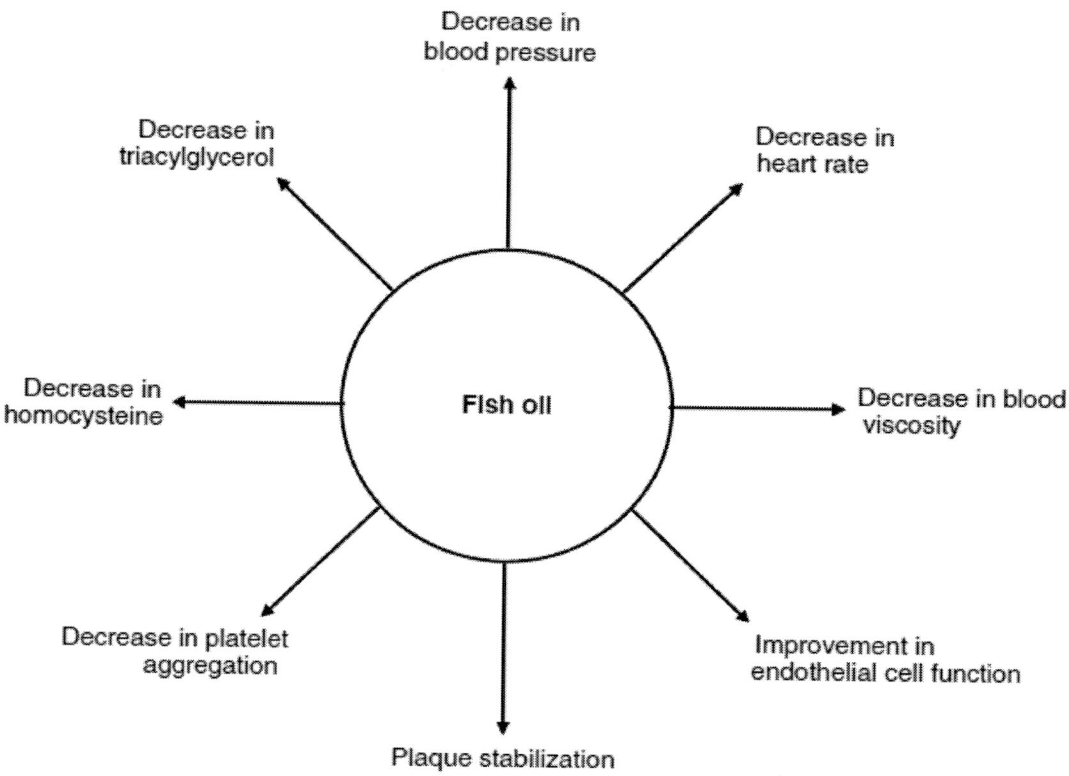

Figure 3. Physiologic and pharmacologic effects of fish oil.

Effects of Fish Oil on Brain

The n–3 fatty acids enter brain from circulation across blood–brain barrier and are incorporated at the sn-2 position of glycerol moiety of glycerophospholipids. They are released through the action of phospholipase A2. The high levels of DHA in the retina and brain gray matter suggests that this fatty acid has important roles in retinal and neural function. Animal studies have shown that depletion of DHA from the retina and brain results in reduced visual function and learning deficits [48]. Aging not only reduces levels of n–3 fatty acids in brain but also decreases neural membrane neuroplasticity. Decline in n–3 fatty acids with age is accompanied by loss of memory and learning. Reduction in n–3 fatty acid levels with age can be restored by DHA supplementation. Molecular mechanism associated with the loss of n–3 fatty acids from neural membrane is not fully understood. However, it is proposed that the loss of DHA with aging may be due to increased activity of plasmalogen-selective PLA2 [49]. This increase in plasmalogen-selective PLA2 is also coupled with the loss of PlsEtn during aging. Dietary supplementation of DHA not only restores the levels of DHA but also increases cerebral choline and acetylcholine levels that improve passive avoidance performance in stroke-prone spontaneously hypertensive rats and also in rat hippocampus during aging [50].

Effects of Fish Oil on Lungs

Lung diseases such as asthma and bronchitis are characterized by continuous inflammation. Thus, factors and drugs that downregulate inflammatory activity may be particularly beneficial for patients with asthma and bronchitis. Treatment of asthmatic subjects with fish oil or n–3 fatty acid supplements results in improved ARA concentrations in neutrophils, reduced neutrophil chemotaxis, reduced leukotriene generation, and reduced airway late response to allergen exposure. However, relevant data are still sparse [51]. Studies in the general adult population indicate that a high fish intake has a beneficial effect on lung function, but the relationship with respiratory symptoms and clinically manifest asthma and bronchitis is less evident [52].

Effects of Fish Oil on Kidneys

The n–3 fatty acid-enriched diet retards the progression of renal diseases in humans and experimental animal models. Thus, administration of n–3 fatty acids reduces proteinuria and ameliorates renal injury in murine lupus nephritis, experimental focal segmental glomerulosclerosis, and other types of renal diseases [53]. Similarly, dietary supplementation of fish oil in dogs produces marked decrease in renal mass, followed by reduction in proteinuria, glomerulosclerosis, tubulointerstitial damage, and progressive loss of renal function [54]. Furthermore, n–3 fatty acid supplementation reduces the progression of IgA nephropathy. In contrast, dogs fed on n–6 fatty acid-enriched diet show progressive deterioration of kidney function associated with proteinuria, hypercholesterolemia, morphologic evidence glomerular and tubulointerstitial injury, and an increased prevalence of end-stage kidney failure. The molecular mechanism associated with n–6 fatty acid-mediated kidney damage and n–3 fatty acid-induced nephroprotection remains unknown [55].

ARA derived lipid mediators are vital for the proper control of renal hemodynamics. The lack of control of ARA-derived mediators can contribute to renal vascular injury and end-stage renal diseases [56]. Three major enzymatic pathways, COX (cyclooxygenase), LOX (lipoxygenase), and EPOX (epoxygenase), are responsible for bioactive eicosanoids. These metabolites, through eicosanoid receptor-mediated mechanism, dilate or constrict the renal vasculature and maintain vascular resistance in the face of changing vasoactive hormones. Renal vascular generation of eicosanoids is altered in pathophysiological conditions such as hypertension, diabetes, metabolic syndrome, and acute renal failure. Collective evidence suggests that n–6-derived vasoactive eicosanoids modulate renal hemodynamics in rats, and early generation of vasoactive eicosanoids may induce glomerular hyperfunction, and subsequent overproduction of thromboxanes is closely associated with the pathogenesis of glomerular damage and proteinuria [57]. In contrast, n–3 fatty acids interfere with the ARA cascade not only by competing for COX and LOX enzymes but also by generating eicosanoids that are less potent than ARA-derived eicosanoids. Studies on the effect of EPA on mesangial cells indicate that EPA modulates PDGF-stimulated proliferation by engendering changes in PDGFstimulated TXA2 synthesis. Fish oil also inhibits mesangial cell activation and proliferation in anti-Thy 1.1 ATS model of mesangial proliferative glomerulonephritis, reduces proteinuria, and decreases histologic evidence of glomerular damage [58].

Potential molecular mechanism underlying the antiproliferative effect of DHA at low doses involves the inhibition of basal and epidermal growth factor (EGF)-stimulated 3H-thymidine incorporation in mesangial cells. At higher doses EPA and DHA equally suppress basal and EGF-stimulated mesangial cells mitogenesis. Low levels of DHA decrease ERK activation by 30%. JNK activity is increased by low-dose DHA, but not by EPA. DHA and EPA have no significant effect on p38 activity. Low dose of DHA inhibits cyclin E activity. DHA upregulates the expression of the cell cycle inhibitor p21, but not p27. EPA has no effect on p21 or p27. It is proposed that the differential effect of low-dose DHA vs EPA in suppressing mesangial cells mitogenesis may be related to downregulation of ERK and cyclin E activity and to induction of p21. Collective evidence suggests that orally administered fish oil, or purifiedDHA, may have a suppressive effect in acute phases or relapses of glomerulopathies, by inhibiting the activation and proliferation of mesangial cells [59].

Effects of Fish Oil on Plasma Lipids

A predominance of small, dense, low-density lipoprotein (LDL) and increased plasma triacylglycerol levels are significant risk for the development of coronary heart disease. Dietary long-chain n–3 fatty acids modulate the levels of triacylglycerols in several ways. They suppress the synthesis of triacylglycerols in the liver by inhibiting the diacyglycerol acyltransferase activity. However its effects on very low-density lipoprotein (VLDL) synthesis and/or VLDL triacylglycerol removal rate via increased lipoprotein lipolysis have not been ruled out. Fish oil ingredients may limit the supply of lipid substrates for triacylglycerol synthesis. The n–3 fatty acids have been reported to increase the sensitivity of certain tissues to the action of insulin. Thus in rat liver, the synthesis and secretion of triacylglycerol and cholesterol ester are reduced by 50–80% in the presence of EPA in comparison with oleic acid. Reduced synthesis of triacylglycerol and cholesterol ester is seen when EPA and oleic acid are given together. EPA causes higher incorporation of 3H water into glycerophospholipids and lower incorporation into triacylglycerol and cholesterol ester as compared with oleic acid. Reduction in synthesis of triacylglycerol and cholesterol ester is also observed when EPA-CoA is given together with oleoyl-CoA, whereas palmitoyl-CoA, stearoyl-CoA, linolenoyl-CoA, and arachidonoyl-CoA have no inhibitory effects. Collectively, prvious studies suggest that n–3 fatty acid-mediated triacylglycerol-lowering effect which redistributes LDL subfractions toward larger and lighter particles, thus providing protection against the generation of atherogenic type of LDL. This effect is more pronounced in carriers of the apoE4 polymorphism [60].

Furthermore, EPA or EPA-CoA also reduces cellular cholesterol esterification by inhibiting the activity of acyl-CoA: cholesterol acyltransferase. The lowered cholesterol esterification induced by EPA also modulates the secretion of VLDL cholesterol ester. The molecular mechanism associated with hypotriglyceridemic effects of fish oil in humans may include the involvement of liver X receptor, hepatocyte nuclear factor-4a (HNF-4 a), farnesol X receptor, and peroxisome proliferator-activated receptors (PPARs). All these receptors are regulated by sterol receptor element binding protein-1c (SREBP-1c), the main genetic switch that modulates lipogenesis. It is proposed that n–3 fatty acids elicit hypotriglyceridemic effects by coordinately suppressing hepatic lipogenesis through reducing levels of SREBP-1c, upregulating fatty oxidation in the liver and skeletal muscle through PPAR activation, and enhancing flux of glucose to glycogen through downregulation of HNF-4α. The net result of these processes is the repartitioning of metabolic fuel from triacylglycerol storage toward oxidation, thereby reducing the substrate available for VLDL synthesis [61]. By simultaneously downregulating genes encoding the proteins that stimulate lipid synthesis and upregulating genes encoding the proteins that stimulate fatty acid oxidation, n–3 fatty acids are more potent hypotriglyceridemic agents than are n–6 fatty acids on a carbon-for-carbon basis. Furthermore, as stated above peroxidation of n–3 fatty acids reduces VLDL secretion through stimulating apolipoprotein B degradation. The n–3 fatty acids may also act by enhancing postprandial chylomicron clearance through reduced VLDL secretion and by directly stimulating lipoprotein lipase activity. It is proposed that the use of fish oil is a valuable clinical tool for the treatment of hypertriglyceridemia [61].

Studies on the Effects of Fish Oil on Hyperlipidemic Apolipoprotein (APO)

E*3-Leiden mice, which have impaired chylomicron and VLDL remnant metabolism, also indicate that fish oil-fed mice show a significant dose-dependent decrease in serum cholesterol (up to –43%) and triacylglycerol levels (up to –60%), mainly due to a reduction of VLDL (–80%). VLDL-apoB kinetic studies indicate that fish oil feeding produces a significant twofold increase in VLDL-apoB fractional catabolic rate (FCR), but hepatic VLDL-apoB synthesis is not affected by fish oil feeding. VLDL–triacylglycerol turnover studies show that fish oil significantly decreases the rate of synthesis of hepatic VLDL–triacylglycerol (–60%). A significant increase in VLDL–triacylglycerol FCR is observed (70%), which is not related to elevation in lipolytic activity. It is suggested that APOE*3-Leiden mice are highly responsive to dietary fish oil and observed strong reduction in serum VLDL is primarily due to an effect of fish oil to decrease hepatic VLDL–triacylglycerol production rate and to increase VLDL-apoB fractional catabolic rate [62]. Collective evidence indicates that the consumption of fish oil is cardioprotective at doses >3 g/day. The cardioprotective effects are due to suppression of fatal arrhythmias rather than stabilization of atherosclerotic plaques. At doses >3 g/day, EPA plus DHA can improve cardiovascular disease risk factors, including decreasing plasma triacylglycerols, blood pressure, platelet aggregation, and inflammation, while improving vascular reactivity. Mainly on the basis of the results of randomized control trials, the American Heart Association recommends for everyone to eat oily fish twice per week and that those with coronary heart disease eat 1 g/day of EPA plus DHA from oily fish or supplements [62].

Effect of Fish Oil on Liver

Fish oil exerts hypolipidemic, antiobesity, and antiinflammatory effects on hepatic lipid metabolism. A slight increase in the serum activity of liver enzymes during n–3 fatty acid supplementation has been reported by several investigators. Treatment of obesity-prone C57BL/6 J mice with 8% fish oilhigh-fat (30%) diet for 5 months results in the loss of body weight as compared to mice fed a 30% triacylglycerol diet without fish oil. In addition to modulating mRNA levels in the liver, fish oil ingestion for 2 weeks upregulates the intestinal mRNA levels of lipid metabolism-related genes such as carnitine palmitoyl transferase 1a, cytochrome P450 4A10, and malic enzyme as compared with mice that are fed with the 30% triacylglycerol diet. Northern blot analysis demonstrate that the expression levels of most lipid metabolism-related genes in the small intestine of mice fed with 8% fish oil diet are comparable to those in the liver. Furthermore, fish oil ingestion also modulates lipid metabolism-related enzyme activity, fatty acid b-oxidation, o-oxidation, and malic enzyme activities in the small intestine of mice fed the 8% fish oil diet compared to mice fed the 30% triacylglycerol-enriched diet. These findings suggest that an upregulation of intestinal lipid metabolism is associated with the antiobesity effect of fish oil [63]. Microarray based expression profiling of genes in rats fed with fish oil and ethanol diet indicates that a large number of genes show significant changes in female livers compared to males. The upregulated genes in female liver are associated with proteosome endopeptidase activity, lipid metabolism, alcohol metabolism, mitochondrial and oxidoreductase activity. The downregulated genes are associated with oxidoreductase activity, chaperone activity, and electron transport activity in the female liver as shown by biological theme analysis. To identify specific regulatory networks of genes operative in promoting liver injury, ingenuity computational pathway analysis has been used. These studies identify a large cluster of genes associated with lipid metabolism, development, cellular growth and proliferation, apoptosis, carcinogenesis, and various signaling pathways [64].

Diet enriched in fish and marine oils also improves serum lipid profiles by suppressing liver X receptor a (LXR a) activity in the liver [65]. Collectively, these studies indicate that dietary fish oil modulates the fatty acid composition of hepatic membranes, plasma lipoprotein cholesterol profile, biliary lipids, and the expression of proteins involved in reverse cholesterol transport. Fish oil reduces plasma HDL cholesterol and increases biliary cholesterol without concomitant modifications in the expression of key genes and proteins involved in reverse cholesterol transport. These findings suggest that functional changes in the activity of these proteins as a consequence of the incorporation of n–3 fatty acids into hepatic membranes and plasma lipoproteins may underlie the effect of fish oil feeding on plasma and hepatic cholesterol metabolism in the rat [66].

Chronic hyperglycemia is an additional risk factor for cardiovascular disease. Diabetes patients have two- to four fold increased risk of dying from complication of cardiovascular disease. Considerable attempts using drugs (statins, fibric acid derivatives, and nicotinic acid) are made to control the dyslipidemia that severely deteriorates the diabetes in patients. Studies on the effect of fish oil on glycemic control of streptozotocin (STZ; 90 mg/kg bodyweight)-treated type 1 diabetic rats, fish oil-treated or untreated nondiabetic rats have indicated that 3 weeks after fish oil treatment, plasma total cholesterol is reduced in both the non-diabetic and the diabetic rats by 35% and 10%, respectively. In non-diabetic and diabetic rats, levels of triacylglycerol are decreased by 69% and 20%, respectively, compared with control rats. Fish oil treatment decreases non-esterified fatty acids (NEFA) by 29% in diabetic rats, but the NEFA levels in non-diabetic rats are not affected. After fish oil treatment in non-diabetic and diabetic rats, platelet aggregation is decreased by 49% and 37%, respectively, and total antioxidant status is increased by 18% and 17%, respectively. Insulin levels are increased by 27% in the fish oil-fed non-diabetic rats, whereas insulin levels are markedly decreased in diabetic rats. Fish oil treatment does not alter glucose levels, but it reduces fructosamine levels by 29% only in fish oil-fed diabetic rats [67]. Collective evidence suggests that fish oil may ameliorate the atherogenic lipid profile, platelet hyperaggregation, and the antioxidative defence of STZ-diabetic rats, and amelioration is independent of the effects of fish oil on glycemic control. Similar results are obtained on noninsulin-dependent diabetic patients on supplementation of n–3 fatty acidsenriched diet. Based on these observations, it is proposed that fish oil treatment decreases vascular complications in diabetes [68].

N–3 Fatty Acids and Bleeding Tendency

The bleeding tendencies of Greenland Eskimos, who consume n–3 fatty acidenriched diet (≥7–10 g/day), have been described by several investigators. Bleeding tendencies include prolonged cutaneous, nose, urinary tract, and obstetric bleedings. Furthermore, Greenland Eskimos show reduced platelet in vitro aggregability, compared with Danish control subjects. This reduction in platelet function has been explained by a shift in eicosanoid metabolism when ARA (20:4n–6) is replaced by EPA (20:5n–3) in platelet membranes. This shift results in the synthesis of thromboxanes and prostacyclins, resulting in more vasodilator and antiaggregatory hemostatic profiles. There is no clinical evidence of an increased bleeding tendency when individuals consumed moderately enriched n–3 PUFA supplemention (2–5 g/day). Collective evidence suggests that daily ingestion of moderate amount of fish oil reduces chances of chronic heart disease, stroke, liver, and kidney diseases independent of the type of fat present in the daily diet [69].

Effect of N–3 Fatty Acids on Blood Pressure

DHA-enriched diet attenuates the development of high blood pressure in spontaneously hypertensive rats. Incorporation of dietary DHA produces changes in the fatty acid composition of the vasculature and organs (aorta, renal artery, plasma, liver, heart, kidney, and lung) involved in the maintenance of blood pressure regulation.. Treatment of DHA-treated stroke-prone spontaneously hypertensive rats (SHRSP) also causes a significant decrease in the levels of total cholesterol, LDL, triglycerides, lipid peroxide, serum creatinine, and blood urea nitrogen as compared with those in non-treated SHRSP, suggesting that DHA-mediated antihypertensive action may be associated with the amelioration of both serum lipid alteration and renal dysfunction in non-treated SHRSP. In addition, DHA-mediated alterations in biophysical properties of membrane and generation of docosanoids may also promote lowering of blood pressure in normal and hypertensive rats [70].

Recommendations for Intake of N-3 Fatty Acids

Commercial preparations of fish oil capsules are available over the counter in drug stores and supermarkets. An excessive use of n–3 fatty acids may produce harmful effects not only due to the effect on enzymic activities but also through their effect on membrane permeability. Recommendations for n–3 fatty acid intake have been made by several international scientific authorities. Thus, Health and Welfare Canada proposes the use of 1.0-1.8 g n–3 fatty acids/day. The International Society for the Study of Fatty Acids and Lipids (ISSFAL) recommends adequate intake of a minimum 0.22 g/day for n–3 fatty acids. British Nutrition Foundation (BNF) suggests a desirable dietary intake of 1.1 g and 1.4 g of n–3 fatty acids for females and males daily. FDA in the United States recommends the use of up to 3 g n–3 fatty acids/day [6].

Conflicts of interest statement

The author declares that there are no conflicts of interest between him and others..

References

[1] Moghadasian MH (May 2008). "Advances in dietary enrichment with n-3 fatty acids". *Critical Reviews in Food Science and Nutrition* 48 (5): 402–10. doi:10.1080/10408390701424303. PMID 18464030.

[2] EPA (2007-01-31). "Fish Consumption Advisories". *http://www.epa.gov/mercury/advisories.htm.* Retrieved 2007-02-08.

[3] Green, Pnina; Hermesh, Haggai; Monselisec, Assaf; Maromb, Sofi; Presburgerb, Gadi; Weizman, Abraham (2006). "Red cell membrane omega-3 fatty acids are decreased in nondepressed patients with social anxiety disorder". *Eur Neuropsychopharmacol* 16 (2): 107–113. doi:10.1016/j.euroneuro.2005.07.005. PMID 16243493.

[4] Yehuda S., Rabinovitz S., Mostofsky D.I. (2005). "Mixture of essential fatty acids lowers test anxiety". *Nutritional Neuroscience* 8 (4): 265–267. doi:10.1080/10284150500445795. PMID 16491653.

[5] 5-"Fish, Levels of Mercury and Omega-3 Fatty Acids". American Heart Association. *http://www.americanheart.org/presenter.jhtml?identifier= 3013797*. Retrieved October 6, 2010.

[6] Farooqui A.A. *Beneficial effect of fish oil in human brain* 2009. Chapter 1, pp. 3,5. Springer Science, USA, ISBN 978-1-4419-0543-7.

[7] Kushi L, Giovannucci E. Dietary fat and cancer. *Am J Med* 2002;113 (Suppl 9B):63S-70S.

[8] Kuriki K, Wakai K, Hirose K, Matsuo K, Ito H, Suzuki T, et al. Risk of colorectal cancer is linked to erythrocyte compositions of fatty acids as biomarkers for dietary intakes of fish, fat, and fatty acids. *Cancer Epidemiol Biomarkers Prev* 2006;15:1791-8.

[9] Riediger ND, Othman RA, Suh M. A systemic review of the roles of n-3 fatty acids in health and disease. *J Am Diet Assoc* 2009;109:668-79.

[10] Cordain, L., Eaton, S.B., Sebastian, A., Mann, N., Lindeberg, S., Watkins, B.A., O'Keefe, J.H., Brand-Miller, J., 2005. Origins and evolution of the Western diet: health implications for the 21st century. *Am. J. Clin. Nutr.* 81, 341–354.

[11] Weylandt, K.H., Kang, J.X., 2005. Rethinking lipid mediators. *Lancet* 366, 618–620.

[12] Simopoulos, A.P., 2006. Evolutionary aspects of diet, the omega-6/omega-3 ratio and genetic variation: nutritional implications for chronic diseases. *Biomed. Pharmacother.* 60, 502–507.

[13] Djordjevic, D., McClements, D.J., Decker, E.A., 2004. Oxidative stability of whey protein-stabilized oil-in-water emulsions at pH 3: potential omega-3 fatty acid delivery systems (Part B). *J. Food Sci.* 69, C356–C362.

[14] Chalon, S., 2006. Omega-3 fatty acids and monoamine neurotransmission. Prostaglandins Leukot. *Essent. Fat. Acids* 75, 259–269.

[15] Deckelbaum, R.J., Worgall, T.S., Seo, T., 2006. n-3 Fatty acids and gene expression. *Am. J. Clin. Nutr.* 83, 1520S–1525S.

[16] Isbilen, B., Fraser, S.P., Djamgoz, M.B.A., 2006. Docosahexaenoic acid (omega-3) blocks voltage-gated sodium channel activity and migration of MDA-MB-231 human breast cancer cells. *Int. J. Biochem. Cell Biol.* 38, 2173–2182.

[17] Kris-Etherton PM, Harris WS, Appel LJ, AHA Nutrition Committee. Omega-3 fatty acids and cardiovascular disease: new recommendations from the American Heart Association. *Arterioscler Thromb Vasc Biol* 2003; 23: 151–2.

[18] Patch CS, Tapsell LC, Mori TA, Meyer BJ, Murphy KJ, Mansour J, et al. The use of novel foods enriched with longchain n-3 fatty acids to increase dietary intake: a comparison of methodologies assessing nutrient intake. *J Am Diet Assoc* 2005; 105:1918-26.

[19] Tricon S, Burdge GC, Jones EL, Russell JJ, El-Khazen S, Moretti E, et al. Effects of dairy products naturally enriched with cis-9, trans-11 conjugated linoleic acid on the blood lipid profile in healthy middle-aged men. *Am J Clin Nutr* 2006; 83:744-53.

[20] Carrero JJ, Martın-Bautista E, Baro′ L, Fonolla′ J, Jimenez J, Boza JJ, et al. Cardiovascular effects of omega-3-fatty acids and alternatives to increase their intake. *Nutr Hosp* 2005; 20: 63-9.

[21] Din JN, Newby DE, Flapan AD.Omega 3 fatty acids and cardiovascular disease-fishing for a natural treatment. *BMJ* 2004; 328:30–5.

[22] He K, Song Y, Daviglus ML, et al. Accumulated evidence on fish consumption and coronary heart disease mortality: a meta-analysis of cohort studies. *Circulation* 2004; 109:2705–11.

[23] Dietary supplementation with n-3 polyunsaturated fatty acids and vitamin E after myocardial infarction: results of the GISSI-Prevenzione trial. Gruppo Italiano per lo Studio della Sopravvivenza nell'Infarto miocardico. *Lancet* 1999; 354:447–55.

[24] Hooper L, Thompson RL, Harrison RA, et al. Risks and benefits of omega 3 fats for mortality, cardiovascular disease, and cancer: systematic review. *BMJ* 2006; 332:752–60.

[25] Gezondheidsraad (2006). Richtlijnen goedevoeding. Availablefrom: *http://www. gezondheidsraad.nl/nl/adviezen/richtlijnen-goede-voeding-2006, http://www. efsa.europa.eu/EFSA/Scientific_Document/comm_ colloque_6_en.pdf.* Accessed June2010.

[26] Welch, A.A.,Lund,E.,Amiano,P.,Dorronsoro,M.,Brustad,M.,Kumle, M.,etal.(2002). Variability of fish consumption within the 10 European countries participating in the European Investigation into Cancer and Nutrition (EPIC) study. *Public Health Nutrition*, 5, 1273–1285.

[27] Verbeke, W.& Vackier,I.(2005). Individual determinants of fish consumption. Application of the theory ofplanned behaviour. *Appetite*, 44, 67–82.

[28] Pieniak, Z.,Verbeke,W., Scholderer,J.,Brunsø, K.,& Olsen, S.O.(2008). Impact of consumers' health beliefs, health involvement and risk perception on fish consumption: A study in five European countries. *British Food Journal*,110, 898–915.

[29] De Goede,J.,Geleijnse,J.M.,Boer,J.M.A.,Kromhout,D.,& Verschuren, W.M.M.(2010). Marine (n-3) fatty acids, fish consumption, and the 10-year risk of fatal and nonfatal coronary heart disease in a large population of Dutch adults with low fish intake. *Journal of Nutrition*, 140, 1023–1028.

[30] Holick, M.F.(2004).Vitamin D. Importance in the prevention of cancers, type 1diabetes, heart disease, and osteoporosis. *American Journal of Clinical Nutrition*, 79, 362–371.

[31] He FJ, MacGregor GA. Salt, blood pressure and cardiovascular disease. *Curr Opin Cardiol* 2007; 22:298–305.

[32] Mori TA. Omega-3 fatty acids and hypertension in humans. *Clin Exp Pharmacol Physiol* 2006; 33:842–6.

[33] Geleijnse JM, Giltay EJ, Grobbee DE, Donders AR, Kok FJ. Blood pressure response to fish oil supplementation: Meta-regression analysis of randomized trials. *J Hypertens* 2002; 20:1493–9.

[34] Engler MB, Engler MM. Docosahexaenoic acid-induced vasorelaxation in hypertensive rats: mechanisms of action. *Biol Res Nurs* 2000; 2:85–95.

[35] Lara JJ, Economou M, Wallace AM, Rumley A, Lowe G, Slater C, et al. Benefits of salmon eating on traditional and novel vascular risk factors in young, non-obese healthy subjects. *Atherosclerosis* 2007; 193:213–21.

[36] Ait-Yahia D, Madani S, Savelli JL, Prost J, Bouchenak M, Belleville J. Dietary fish protein lowers blood pressure and alters tissue polyunsaturated fatty acid composition in spontaneously hypertensive rats. *Nutrition* 2003; 19:342–6.

[37] Hamilton R.J.& Rice R.D. 2007: *Fish oil technology, nutrition and marketing.* Chapter 1 P. 9-27, ISBN 0-9526542-0-2.

[38] Deshpande G, Simmer K. Lipids for parenteral nutrition in neonates. *Curr Opin Clin Nutr Metab Care.* 2011 Mar;14(2):145-50.

[39] Kang Z.B., Ge Y., Chen Z., Cluette-Brown J., Laposata M., Leaf A., and Kang J.X. (2001). Adenoviral gene transfer of Caenorhabditis elegans n-3 fatty acid desaturase optimizes fatty acid composition in mammalian cells. *Proc. Natl. Acad. Sci USA* 98:4050–4054.

[40] Farooqui A.A. (2009). *Hot Topics in Neural Membrane Lipidology*. Springer, New York.

[41] Simopoulos A.P. (2008). The importance of the omega-6/omega-3 fatty acid ratio in cardiovascular disease and other chronic diseases. *Exp. Biol. Med.* (Maywood) 233:674–688.

[42] Deckelbaum R.J., Worgall T.S., and Seo T. (2006). n-3 Fatty acids and gene expression. *Am. J. Clin. Nutr.* 83:1520S–1525S.

[43] Hirafuji M., Machida T., Hamaue N., and Minami M. (2003). Cardiovascular protective effects of n-3 polyunsaturated fatty acids with special emphasis on docosahexaenoic acid. *J. Pharmacol. Sci.* 92:308–316.

[44] von Schacky C. (2006). A review of omega-3 ethyl esters for cardiovascular prevention and treatment of increased blood triglyceride levels. *Vasc. Health Risk Manag.* 2:251–262.

[45] Schmidt E.B. (1997). n-3 fatty acids and the risk of coronary heart disease. *Dan. Med. Bull.* 44:1–22.

[46] Abeywardena M.Y., and Head R.J. (2001). Longchain n-3 polyunsaturated fatty acids and blood vessel function. *Cardiovasc. Res.* 52:361–371.

[47] Verlengia R., Gorjao R., Kanunfre C.C., Bordin S., Martins de Lima T., Fernandes Martins E., Newsholme P., and Curi R. (2004). Effects of EPA andDHAon proliferation, cytokine production, and gene expression in Raji cells. *Lipids*. 39:857–864.

[48] Horrocks L.A., and Farooqui A.A. (2004). Docosahexaenoic acid in the diet: its importance in maintenance and restoration of neural membrane function. Prostaglandins Leukot. *Essent. Fatty Acids* 70:361–372.

[49] Farooqui A.A., Ong W.Y., and Horrocks L.A. (2008) *Neurochemical Aspects of Excitotoxicity*. Springer, New York.

[50] Barcelo-Coblijn G., Kitajka K., Puskas L.G., Hogyes E., Zvara A., Hackler L., Jr., and Farkas T. (2003). Gene expression and molecular composition of phospholipids in rat brain in relation to dietary n-6 to n-3 fatty acid ratio. *Biochim. Biophys. Acta* 1632:72–79.

[51] Romieu I., and Trenga C. (2001).Diet and obstructive lung diseases. *Epidemiol. Rev.* 23:268–287.

[52] Schwartz J. (2000). Role of polyunsaturated fatty acids in lung disease. *Am. J. Clin. Nutr.* 71(1 Suppl):393S–396S.

[53] Donadio J.V., Grande J.P. (2004). The role of fish oil/omega-3 fatty acids in the treatment of IgA nephropathy. *Semin. Nephrol.* 24:225–243.

[54] Brown S.B., Brown C.A., Crowell W.A., Barsanti J.A., Kang C.W., Allen T., Cowell C., and Finco D.R. (2000). Effects of dietary polyunsaturated fatty acids supplementation in early renal insufficiency in dogs. *J. Lab. Clin. Med.* 135:275–286.

[55] Donadio J.V., Grande J.P., Bergstralh E.J., Dart R.A., Larson T.S., and Spencer D.C., (1999). The long-term outcome of patients with IgA nephropathy treated with fish oil in a controlled trial. Mayo Nephrology Collaborative Group. *J. Am. Soc. Nephrol.* 10: 1772–1777.

[56] Imig J.D. (2006). Eicosanoids and renal vascular function in diseases. *Clin. Sci.* 111:21–34.

[57] Hao C.M. and Brever M.D. (2008). Physiological regulation of prostaglandins in the kidney. *Annu. Rev. Physiol.* 70:357–377.

[58] Schmitz P.G., Zhang K., and Dalal R. (2000). Eicosapentaenoic acid suppresses PDGFinduced DNA synthesis in rat mesangial cells: involvement of thromboxane A2. *Kidney Int.* 57:1041–1051.

[59] Yusufi A.N.K., Cheng J., Thompson M.A., Walker H.J., Gray C.E., Warner G.M., and Grande J.P. (2003). Differential effects of low-dose docosahexaenoic acid and eicosapentaenoic acid on the regulation of mitogenic signaling pathways in mesangial cells. *J. Lab. Clin. Med.* 141:318–329.

[60] Griffin B.A. (2001). The effect of n-3 fatty acids on low density lipoprotein subfractions. *Lipids* 36 Suppl: S91–S97.

[61] Davidson M.H., Stein E.A., BaysH.E., Maki K.C.,Doyle R.T., ShalwitzR.A., Ballantyne C.M., Ginsberg H.N., and COMBination of prescription omega-3 with simvastatin (COMBOS) investigators. (2007). Efficacy and tolerability of adding prescription omega-3 fatty acids 4 g/d to simvastatin 40mg/d in hypertriglyceridemic patients: an 8-week, randomized, double-blind, placebo-controlled study. *Clin. Ther.* 29:1354–1367.

[62] Davidson M.H. (2006). Mechanisms for the hypotriglyceridemic effect of marine omega-3 fatty acids. *Am. J. Cardiol.* 98(4A):27i–33i.

[63] Mori T., Kondo H., Hase T., Tokimitsu I., and Murase T. (2007). Dietary fish oil upregulates intestinal lipid metabolism and reduces body weight gain in C57BL/6 J mice. *J Nutr.* 137:2629–2634.

[64] Sharma M.R., Povavarapu R., Roseman D., Eaton E., Kishor P.M., and Nanji A.A. (2008). Increased severity of alcoholic liver injury in female verses male rats: a microarray analysis. *Exp. Mol. Pathol.* 84:46–58.

[65] Zaima N., Sugawara T., Goto D., and Hirata T. (2006). Trans geometric isomers of EPA decrease LXRalpha-induced cellular triacylglycerol via suppression of SREBP-1c and PGC-1beta. *J. Lipid Res.* 47:2712–2717.

[66] Morgado N., Rigotti A., and Valenzuela A. (2005). Comparative effect of fish oil feeding and other dietary fatty acids on plasma lipoproteins, biliary lipids, and hepatic expression of proteins involved in reverse cholesterol transport in the rat. *Ann. Nutr. Metab.* 49: 397–406.

[67] Mahmud I., Hossain A., Hossain S., Hannan A., Ali L., and Hashimoto M. (2004). Effects of Hilsa ilisa fish oil on the atherogenic lipid profile and glycaemic status of streptozotocin treated type 1 diabetic rats. *Clin. Exp. Pharmacol. Physiol.* 31:76–81.

[68] Kesavulu M.M., Kameswararao B., Apparao Ch., Kumar E.G., Harinarayan C.V. (2002). Effect of omega-3 fatty acids on lipid peroxidation and antioxidant enzyme status in type 2 diabetic patients. *Diabetes Metabo.* 28:20–26.

[69] Bang H.O., and Dyerberg N. (1980). The bleeding tendency in Greenland Eskimos. *Dan. Med. Bull.* 27:202–205.

[70] Kimura S. (2000). Antihypertensive effect of docosahexaenoic acid in stroke-prone spontaneously hypertensive rats. Yakugaku Zasshi 120:607–619.

In: Fish Oil: Production, Consumption and Health Benefits ISBN: 978-1-61470-963-3
Editors: Matthias Van Dijk and Jürgen Vitek

Chapter VIII

Stability and Behavior of Omega-3 Food Emulsions

María Soledad Álvarez Cerimedo and María Lidia Herrera
University of Buenos Aires, Faculty of Exact and Natural Sciences
Institute of Chemistry, Environmental Science and Energy (INQUIMAE)- Consejo Nacional de Investigaciones Científicas y Técnicas (CONICET)

Abstract

N-3 Polyunsaturated fatty acids have been shown to have potential beneficial effects for chronic diseases including cancer, insulin resistance and cardiovascular disease. Eicosapentaenoic acid (EPA) and docosahexaenoic acid (DHA) in particular have been studied extensively. In some diets, such as the typical North American diet, intakes of EPA and DHA are typically very low. The fish oil used in this study is a commercial ingredient for the food industry. It is a concentrate from fish oil, mainly salmon, which is recommended for formulation of functional foods such as chocolate, yogurt, jam, pastry filling, salad oil, mayonnaise and dressings. The use of this oil permits food manufacturers to ensure a controlled content of omega-3, EPA, DPA and DHA fatty acids, in the final products and supplies vitamin E. Thus, regarding some of these applications it is very interesting to study its behavior in emulsion systems. In the food industry, stabilization of emulsions is obtained by the addition of proteins. Sodium caseinate is a well-used ingredient because of its functional properties: good solubility and emulsifying properties, high stability during heating, water and fat binding, thickening and gelation. The addition of this protein has a double stabilizing effect since it provokes together with other added surfactants an increase of both viscosity of the continuous phase and stability of the interface. The physicochemical properties of emulsions play an important role in food systems as they directly contribute to texture, sensory and nutritional properties of food. One of the main properties is stability, which refers to the ability of an emulsion to resist changes in its properties over time. Physical instability results in an alteration in the spatial distribution or structural organization of the molecules. Creaming, flocculation, coalescence, partial coalescence, phase inversion, and Ostwald ripening are examples of physical instability. It is important for food scientists to identify the relative importance of each mechanism, the relationship between them, and the factors that influence them, so that effective means of controlling the stability and physicochemical properties of emulsions can be established. Turbiscan MA 2000 is one of the methods used to study emulsion stability. It is a vertical scan analyzer, which allows the optical characterization of any type of dispersion. The reading head is composed of a pulsed near-IR light source and two synchronous detectors: the transmission and the backscattering detectors. The backscattering and transmission profiles as a function of the sample height allow following the physical evolution of this process without disturbing the original system and with good accuracy and reproducibility. Thus, by repeating the scan of a sample at different time intervals, the stability or the instability of dispersions can be studied in detail. The profiles allow calculation of creaming, sedimentation, or phase separation rates, as well as flocculation, and the mechanism making the dispersion unstable can be deduced from the transmission or the backscattering data. The aim of the present work is to investigate the effect of oil-to-protein ratio, sugar concentration on the stability of emulsions formulated with concentrated fish oil as fat phase. Creaming and flocculation kinetics were quantified analyzing the samples with a Turbiscan MA 2000.

Introduction

Emulsions are commonly encountered in food systems. Many traditional food products such as ice cream, low-fat spreads, yoghurt, mayonnaise, cake batters, whipped toppings, dairy creamers and cream liqueurs are some examples of emulsion-based food [1-3]. The physicochemical properties of emulsions play an important role in food systems as they directly contribute to texture, sensory and nutritional properties of food [4-6]. Most dispersed multiphase systems are thermodynamically unstable per se and thus require stabilization. In the food industry, actual stabilization of emulsions is obtained by the addition of proteins. Proteins can stabilize emulsions by lowering the interfacial tension due to their adsorption at the interface. Besides, proteins can form films at the interface, providing electrostatic and steric repulsion between droplets [7]. The caseins, a group of unique milk-specific proteins, represent around 80% of the total protein in the milk of cattle and other commercial dairying species [8]. Casein is widely used as an ingredient since its functional properties include emulsification, water-binding, fat-binding, thickening, and gelation [9-13]. Depending on the product, the caseinate content can range anywhere from <1% to >50% [14]. Casein is of particular importance as an emulsifier because of its ability for rapidly conferring a low interfacial tension during emulsification and because of the strongly amphiphilic characteristics of the major individual caseins [15]. Casein in milk is strongly aggregated into polydisperse protein particles called "casein micelles". The casein micelles are colloidal particles of self-associated casein held together by nanometer-sized clusters of calcium phosphate and sterically stabilized by an outer layer of the glycoprotein *k*-casein [16-17]. Early electron microscopy studies have shown that the micelles have an uneven, raspberry-like appearance, which was interpreted to mean that the micelles are built up from sub-micelles. However in recent studies, the irregularities were considered to be microtubules [18]. The micelles may be dispersed by adding a calcium chelator or also by urea, SDS, high pH or ethanol, indicating that hydrogen bonds, hydrophobic and electrostatic interactions are also involved in micelle integrity [8]. The caseins have been described as rheomorphic proteins, indicating that they adopt molecular structures in solution dictated by the local environment; that is, their structures are flexible enough to "go with the flow" [19-20]. Removing the calcium salts from milk casein and replacing them by sodium salts leads to the production of "sodium caseinate (NaCas)". Commercial NaCas is a variable multicomponent mixture containing four major constituents, α_{s1}, α_{s2}, β, and *k*-casein [21]. NaCas is composed of a soluble mixture of disordered hydrophobic proteins having a strong tendency to associate into small protein particles (casein submicelles, ~ 2.5 x 10^5 daltons), which coexist in equilibrium with the free casein molecules (~2.5 x 10^4 daltons) [15, 22, 23]. In the casein micelle system, the micelle state may be the lowest free-energy state of the system. Of particular interest will be micelle structure and the mechanisms that operate in determining micelle size [24].

The term "emulsion stability" refers to the ability of an emulsion to resist changes in its properties over time: the more stable the emulsion, the more slowly its properties change. An emulsion may become unstable due to a number of different types of physical and chemical processes. Physical instability results in an alteration in the spatial distribution or structural organization of the molecules. Creaming, flocculation, coalescence, partial coalescence, phase inversion, and Ostwald ripening are examples of physical instability. Creaming is the migration of the dispersed phase of an emulsion. The particles float upwards or sink, depending on how large they are and how much less dense or denser they may be than the continuous phase. Flocculation is a process in which individual particles of a suspension form aggregates while coalescence is caused by rupture of the film between two emulsion drops or two foam bubbles. The driving force for coalescence is the decrease in free energy resulting when the total surface area is decreased, as occurs after film rupture. The former process is reversible while the latter lead to bigger particles.

The length of time that an emulsion must remain stable depends on the nature of the food product [25]. Some food emulsions are formed as intermediate steps during a manufacturing process, and therefore only need to remain stable for a few seconds, minutes, or hours (e.g., cake batter, ice cream mix, and margarine premix), whereas others must remain stable for days, months, or even years prior to consumption (e.g., mayonnaise, salad dressings, and cream liqueurs). On the other hand, the production of some foods involves a controlled destabilization of an emulsion during the manufacturing process, for example, margarine, butter, whipped cream, and ice cream [26-35]. The development of an effective strategy to prevent undesirable changes in the properties of a particular food emulsion depends on the dominant physicochemical mechanism(s) responsible for the changes. In practice, two or more of these mechanisms may operate in concert. It is therefore important for food scientists to identify the relative importance of each mechanism, the relationship between them, and the factors that influence them, so that effective means of controlling the stability and physicochemical properties of emulsions can be established [4].

N-3 polyunsaturated fatty acids (PUFA) have demonstrated a wide range of health related benefits including improving heart disease related outcomes, decreasing tumor growth and metastasis, and favorably modifying insulin sensitivity. Alpha-linoleic acid (ALA, 18:3 n-3), the parent fatty acid of the n-3 PUFA family, must be consumed through the diet. ALA is found in leafy vegetables, walnuts, soybeans, flaxseed, and seed and vegetable oils. ALA can be further metabolized to the long chain PUFA eicosapentaenoic acid (EPA; 20:5 n-3) and docosahexaenoic acid (DHA; 22:6 n-3) through a series of desaturation and elongation steps.

However, this is not an efficient process. The International Society for the Study of Fatty Acids and Lipids (ISSFAL) recently released an official statement on the conversion efficiency of ALA to DHA. They concluded that the conversion of ALA to DHA is on the order of 1% in infants, and considerably lower in adults [36]. Alternatively, EPA and DHA can be consumed directly from marine sources. Given the poor conversion efficiency of ALA to its longer-chain counterparts, DHA levels are a concern, particularly for vegetarians and for individuals who do not eat fatty fish [37]. The average per capita intake of DHA plus EPA is approximately 0.1-0.2 g per day in North America and the average per capita intake of ALA in North America is 1.4 g daily [38]. EPA and DHA intake is also low in some European countries and in India, making ALA the principle n-3 PUFA consumed in these regions. The prevalence of cardiovascular disease, insulin sensitivity, and some types of cancer in these countries is elevated in contrast to countries with high fatty fish intake like Japan [39]. If conversion efficiency were the main criteria, then the epidemiological evidence above would suggest that ALA might not confer the same health benefits as its longer chain counter-parts, EPA and DHA.

Trehalose (α-D-glucopyranosyl-α-D-glucopyranoside) is a non-reducing disaccharide of glucose found in several organisms that are able to survive drying. Among saccharides, trehalose is particularly effective in terms of its ability to preserve and maintain activity of biomolecules; it has been shown to protect various proteins, viruses and antibodies during drying. Its capacity to preserve the contents and structure of liposomes has also been demonstrated. This sugar has no toxicity and is currently being used in several industries, such as food, medical, cosmetic, and other bio-industries, to preserve biomaterials under dry conditions against evaporation, oxidation, and chemical reaction. There are several hypotheses that attempt to explain why trehalose is particularly effective in cryopreservation and desiccation protection. Some of them are based upon the interaction of trehalose with biological structures, while others are based upon the interaction of trehalose with water and the thermophysical properties of its aqueous solutions. On one hand, some authors have proposed that the higher glass transition temperature (T_g) of the trehalose/water system (compared to that of other glass-forming mono-and disaccharides) could be responsible for its superior protective properties. Further, they have shown that there is a strong correlation between the protective ability of protective agents and their glass transition temperatures. On the other hand, others have noted that vitrification is not sufficient for preservation. Vitrification alone does not explain why another carbohydrate, dextram, which has a significantly higher glass transition temperature than trehalose, is a much less effective cryoprotectant than trehalose. Regarding trehalose's unique properties and the fact that encapsulation ability is in some extent related to the stability of emulsions before dehydration [40], it is very interesting to investigate the effect of this sugar on emulsion stability. N-3 polyunsaturated fatty acids are susceptible to oxidation; thus taken into account applications, a sugar that has performed well for retaining lipid materials in freeze-drying was selected in this study.

The aim of the present work is to investigate the effect of sodium caseinate or trehalose concentration on the stability of emulsions formulated with concentrated fish oil as fat phase. Creaming and flocculation kinetics were quantified analyzing the samples with a Turbiscan MA 2000.

Description of the Concentrate from Fish Oils

Omega-3, EPA and DHA are long chain essential fatty acids present only in marine species which have to be consumed throughout the whole life, from childhood to senior age due to the multiple benefits they provide to our health, in accordance with the FAO and WHO's recommendations. The fish oil used in this study is a commercial ingredient for the food industry. It is edible liquid oil, a concentrate based on extra-refined and deodorized fish oil, mainly salmon, enriched with Omega-3 fatty acids (EPA/DHA), of yellow color and neutral taste, specially formulated for functional food. It is intended for products such as enriched bakery products (bread, sliced bread, cookies, pies, sweet or salty dough), pastas, ice-creams, edible oils, sausages and meat products, dressings and mayonnaise, and chocolate and margarine. The use of this oil permits food manufacturers to ensure a controlled content of omega-3, EPA, DPA and DHA fatty acids, in the final products and supplies vitamin E.

Table 1. Quality Parameters of the Concentrated from Fish Oils (CFO)

Parameters	Limits	Value	Method
Humidity and impurities	Max 0.3	0.18	AOCS Ca 2b-38
Total ω-3, mg/mL	Min 185	192	AOCS Ce 2-66
EPA, mg/mL	Min 76	82	AOCS Ce 2-66
DHA, mg/mL	Min 82	91	AOCS Ce 2-66
Heavy metals, ppm			
Lead	< 0.1	< 0.01	AOCS Ca 15
Mercury	< 0,1	< 0.004	AOCS Ca 15
Arsenic	< 0.1	< 0.03	AOCS Ca 15
Chromium (VI)	< 0.1	< 0.001	AOCS Ca 15
Pesticides, ppm			
DDT, DDE	< 1.33	ND	AOCS Cd 23
Aldrin	< 0.026	ND	AOCS Cd 23
Dieldrin	< 0.026	ND	AOCS Cd 23
Chlordan	< 0.33	ND	AOCS Cd 23
Mirex	< 0.026	ND	AOCS Ca 15

ND no detectable

Table 2. Fatty Acid (FA) Composition of the Concentrated from Fish Oils (CFO)

Fatty Acid	Percentage (%)
C14:0	11.81
C15:0	2.64
C16:1	2.08
C17:0 branched	2.16
C17:0 linear	2.39
C18:0	6.94
C20:5	10.90
C20:4	4.58
C20:2	3.66
C20:1	7.65
C22:6	7.96
C22:5	5.21
C22:1	5.66
C24:1	2.06

Table 1 shows quality parameters of the concentrate from fish oils (CFO) used in this study and Table 2 shows its FA composition. Only the main FA, that is, the ones with concentrations higher than 1% were included.

Measurements with Turbiscan

Emulsions have been studied by numerous techniques, such as particle sizing, microscopy, and rheology, among others to characterize their physical properties. Most of these techniques involve some form of dilution. This dilution disrupts some structures such as flocs that contribute to destabilization. The ability to study the stability of food emulsions in their undiluted forms may reveal subtle nuances about their stability. A relatively recently developed technique, the Turbiscan method, allows scanning of the turbidity profile of an emulsion along the height of a glass tube filled with the emulsion, following the fate of the turbidity profile over time. These profiles constitute the macroscopic fingerprint of the emulsion sample at a given time. The analysis of the turbidity profiles leads to quantitative data on the stability of the studied emulsions and allows making objective comparisons between different emulsions [41].

Sodium caseinate (NaCas) emulsions stability was analyzed using a vertical scan analyzer Turbiscan MA 2000 (Formulaction, Toulouse, France), which is shown in Figure 1. This equipment allows the optical characterization of any type of dispersion [42-43]. The reading head is composed of a pulsed near-IR light source ($\lambda = 850$ nm) and two synchronous detectors. The transmission detector receives the light, which goes through the sample (0°), while the backscattering detector receives the light back-scattered by the sample (135°). The Turbiscan head acquired *T* and *BS* data every 40 μm along the vertical length of the cell. Therefore, the scan of 60 mm height sample provides patterns, including 1,500 points of measurement, in less than 20 s. Thus, by repeating the scan of a sample at different time intervals, the stability or the instability of dispersions can be studied in detail. The samples were put in a flat-bottomed cylindrical glass measurement cell and scanned from the bottom to the top.

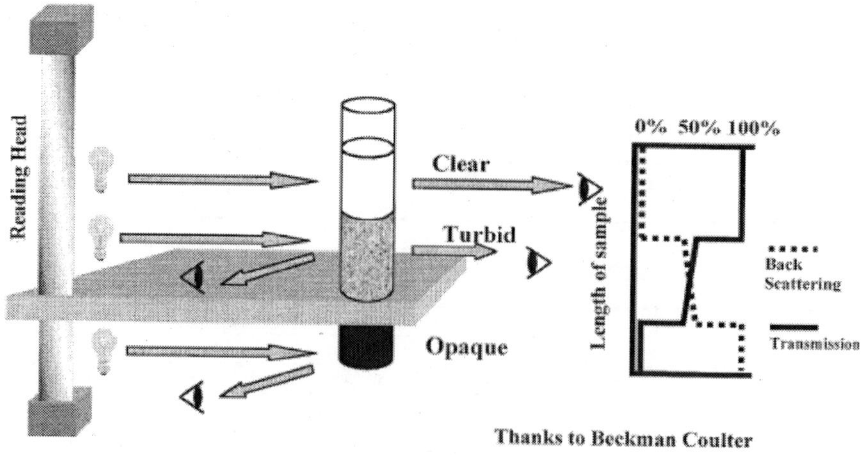

Figure 1. Scheme of the Turbiscan TMA 2000 analyzer.

The backscattering (BS) and transmission (T) profiles as a function of the sample height (total height = 60 mm) were studied in quiescent conditions at 22.5 °C. In this way, the physical evolution of this process is followed with good accuracy and reproducibility [43]. Thus, by repeating the scan of a sample at different time intervals, the stability or the instability of dispersions can be studied in detail. The profiles allow calculation of creaming, sedimentation, or phase separation rates, as well as flocculation, and the mechanism making the dispersion unstable can be deduced from the transmission or the backscattering data [41]. Measurements were performed immediately after preparation of emulsions and at different times for a week. The curves obtained by subtracting the BS profile at t = 0 from the profile at t ($\Delta BS = BS_t - BS_0$), display a typical shape that allows a better quantification of creaming, flocculation and other destabilization processes.

Figure 2 shows as an example a typical profile of an emulsion that destabilized mainly by creaming of small particles in direct and reference mode. Creaming was detected using the Turbiscan as it induced a variation of the concentration between the top and the bottom of the cell. The droplets moved upward because they had a lower density than the surrounding liquid. When creaming takes place in an emulsion, the ΔBS curves show a peak at heights between 0–20 mm. The variation of the peak wide, at a fixed height, during the studied time, can be related to the kinetics of migration of small particles [43]. The creaming destabilization kinetics was evaluated by measuring the peak thickness at 50% of the height at different times (bottom zone). The slope of the linear part of a plot of peak thickness vs. t gives an indication of the migration rate.

For emulsions that destabilize mainly by flocculation, BS mean values (BS_{av}) change with the increase in particle size. Flocculation was followed by measuring the BS_{av} as a function of storage time in the middle zone of the tube. As was theoretically demonstrated [43], the BS intensity decreased as the particle size increased (when particle size is higher than the wavelength (λ) of the incident light). It should be mentioned that if the particle size is lower than λ of the incident light, BS increases with particle size. This phenomenon was used by several authors to determine flocculation kinetics [41, 44]. The optimum zone was the one

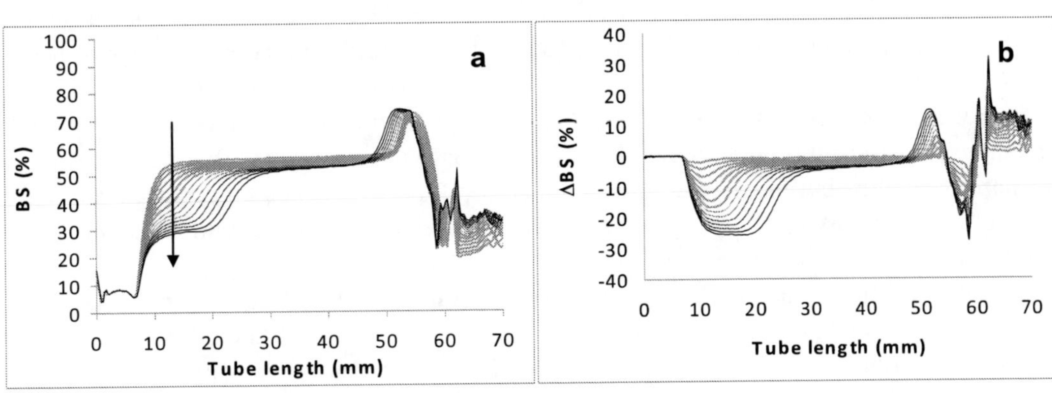

Figure 2. Changes in back scattering (BS), actual and in reference mode profiles, as a function of the tube length with storage time (the emulsion was stored for 1 week, arrow denotes time) in quiescent conditions. It was formulated with 10 wt. % olive oil as fat phase, no trehalose added to the aqueous phase, and a concentration of sodium caseinate (NaCas) of 0.5 wt.%. (a) actual profile of emulsion, (b) profile in reference mode. Tube length 65 mm.

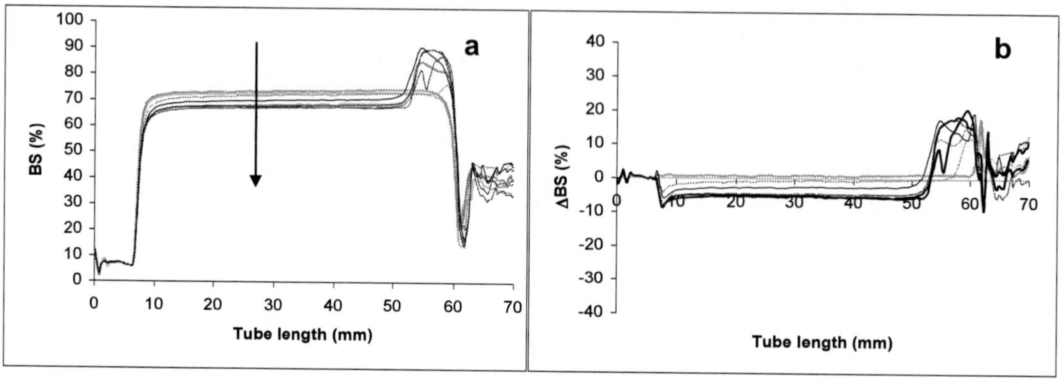

Figure 3. Changes in back scattering (BS), actual and in reference mode profiles, as a function of the tube length with storage time (samples were stored for 1 week, arrow denotes time) in quiescent conditions for the emulsion formulated with 10 wt. % olive oil as fat phase, no trehalose added to the aqueous phase, and a concentration of sodium caseinate (NaCas) of 5.0 wt.%. (a) actual profiles of emulsion (b) profile in reference mode. Tube length 65 mm.

not affected by creaming (bottom and top of the tube), that is, the 20–50 mm zone. Figure 3 shows as an example a typical profile of an emulsion that destabilized mainly by flocculation in direct and reference mode. Actual profile of a flocculated emulsion shows a significant change in BS_{av} in the middle of the tube and has a shape at the top of the tube different of that of migration of individual particles, which is a consequence of the migration of flocs formed during flocculation. In the case of flocculation, the BS profile in reference mode does not show a peak at the bottom of the tube (0-20 mm), which indicates that there is no detectable migration of small particles.

Particle Size Distribution

Figure 4 shows the particle size distribution for the CFO emulsions formulated without trehalose or with 30 or 40 wt.% trehalose and stabilized by different concentrations of NaCas (0.5, 2, and 5 wt.%, a–c). $D_{4,3}$ for emulsions in Figure 4 are reported in Table 3. When the same processing conditions were used, CFO emulsions without trehalose (Figure 4a) showed a monomodal distribution regardless of NaCas concentration. However, 0.5 wt.% NaCas had the narrowest distribution of the three emulsions. $D_{4,3}$ significantly decreased as NaCas concentration increased ($p < 0.05$) indicating that protein concentration limited the fat globule size in this concentration range.

Emulsions with trehalose (Figure 4b-c) and stabilized with 2.0 or 5.0 wt.% NaCas also showed a monomodal distribution. However, 0.5 wt.% NaCas had a shoulder indicative of a second population. $D_{4,3}$ was always smaller than for the emulsions without sugar in the aqueous phase showing that trehalose had strong interactions with the protein influencing droplet size. Distributions for 5 wt.% NaCas emulsions were very narrow with $D_{4,3}$ of 0.30 (b) and 0.29 (c) μm. The shapes were more Gaussian than the formulations without trehalose, which is indicative of a more homogeneous population of droplets.

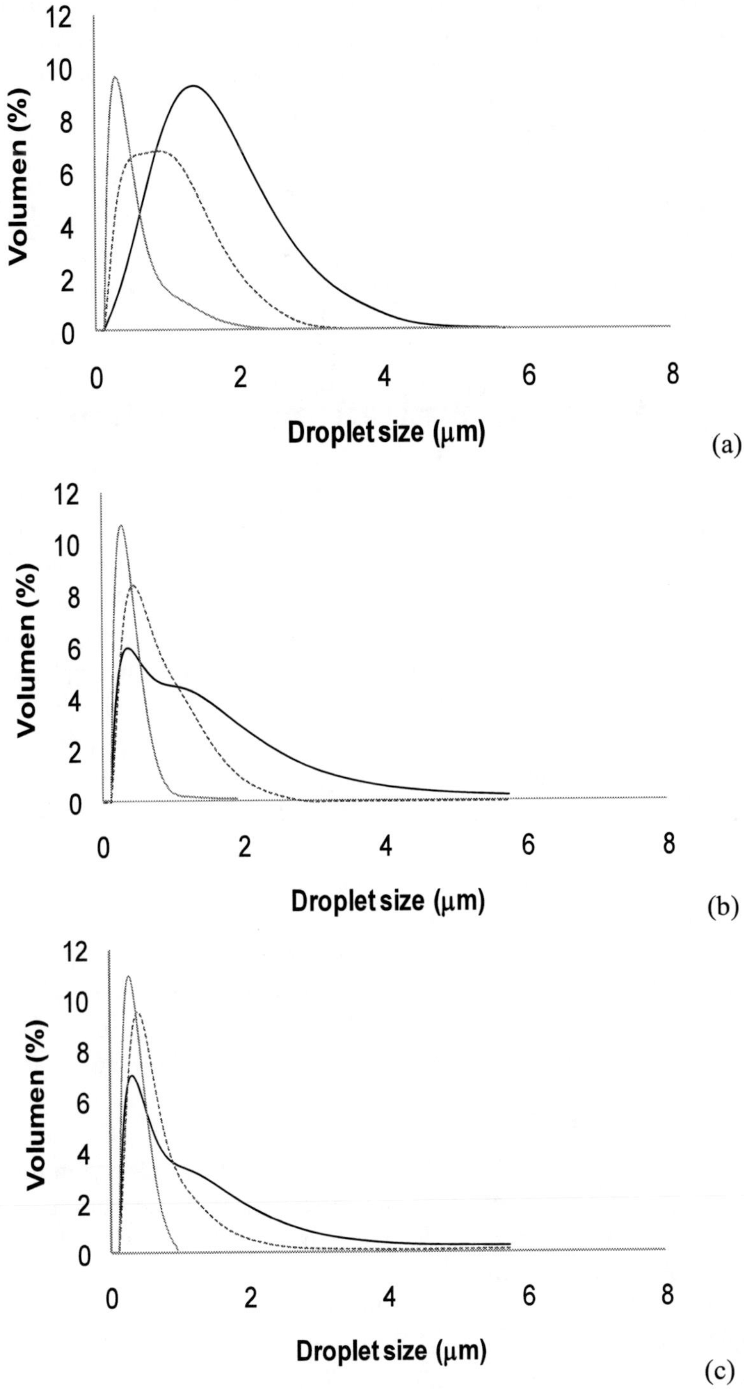

Figure 4. Particle size distribution of emulsions with concentrate from fish oils (CFO) as fat phase and different concentrations of sodium caseinate (black, 0.5 wt.%; 35% black dotted line, 2.0 wt.%; 50% black, 5.0 wt.%): (a) no trehalose added to the aqueous phase, (b) 30 wt.% trehalose, and (c) 40 wt.% trehalose.

Table 3. Volume-weighted mean diameter ($D_{4,3}$, μm) of emulsions formulated with concentrated fish oil (CFO) as fat phase and different concentrations of trehalose or sodium caseinate (NaCas) immediately after preparation

	NaCas (wt.%)		
Sample	0.5	2.0	5.0
Without trehalose	1.22	0.72	0.36
20 wt.% trehalose	0.88	0.63	0.35
30 wt.% trehalose	0.82	0.56	0.30
40 wt.% trehalose	0.80	0.49	0.29

Fish Oil Emulsions Stability

To study the global stability of emulsions the BS profiles were analyzed at different storage times. The main mechanism of destabilization in a given formulation depended on NaCas concentration, that is, to the oil-to-protein ratio (Figure 5). Emulsions formulated with 0.5 wt.% NaCas (O/P 20) destabilized mainly by creaming of individual particles (a). It is noticed from the decrease in BS_t at the bottom of the tube and a concomitant increase of BS_t in the upper zone attributed to the formation of a cream layer. The top of the profile had a shape indicative of the migration of individual particles. However, the clarification degree was still low after 190 h since the serum phase was still optically opaque and no light reached the transmission detector (transmission [h_t % ≈ 0]). All emulsions remained fully turbid along the tube during a week of storage at 22.5°C. Therefore, the transmission profiles were not reported in this study. The BS profiles in reference mode showed a peak at the bottom of the tube (0-20 mm) indicative of creaming destabilization (Figure 5d). Figure 6 shows the kinetics of creaming expressed as peak thickness vs. time for the emulsions in Figures 5d and e. It may be noticed from Figure 6a that the emulsion was stable for 22 h. Then, migration of individual particles started. The slope of the linear region was 0.0318 mm/h.

For the 2 wt.% NaCas (O/P 5) emulsion, the main mechanism of destabilization for the first 30 h was also creaming (Figure 5b and e). However, the significant changes in BS profiles indicated that flocculation/coalescence took place and was the main mechanism of destabilization after 30 h. The BS profiles showed that creaming process occurred with a slower rate than in the case of 0.5 wt.% NaCas. The profiles displayed in the reference mode (Figure 5e) had a peak at the bottom of the tube typical of migration of small particles. However, it is smaller than in Figure 5d, which indicated that destabilization kinetics was slower. As shown in Figure 6b, the slope of the peak thickness vs. time line was 0.0271 mm/h. The increase in NaCas percentage in the emulsions leads to an increase in the stability against creaming. However, the top of BS profile in reference mode (Figure 5e) showed a shaped characteristic of migration of flocculates indicating the presence of a second mechanism of destabilization, that is, flocculation or coalescence.

As evidenced by the BS-profile changes with time, the main destabilization mechanism for emulsions stabilized by more than 2 wt.% NaCas (Figure 5c and f, O/P 2) was flocculation. The profiles showed a great increase in BS at the top of the tube (Figure 5c), which suggested migration of aggregates/flocculates. In addition, during that time, there was also a noticeable decrease in BS_{av} indicative of an increment in the mean diameter particle.

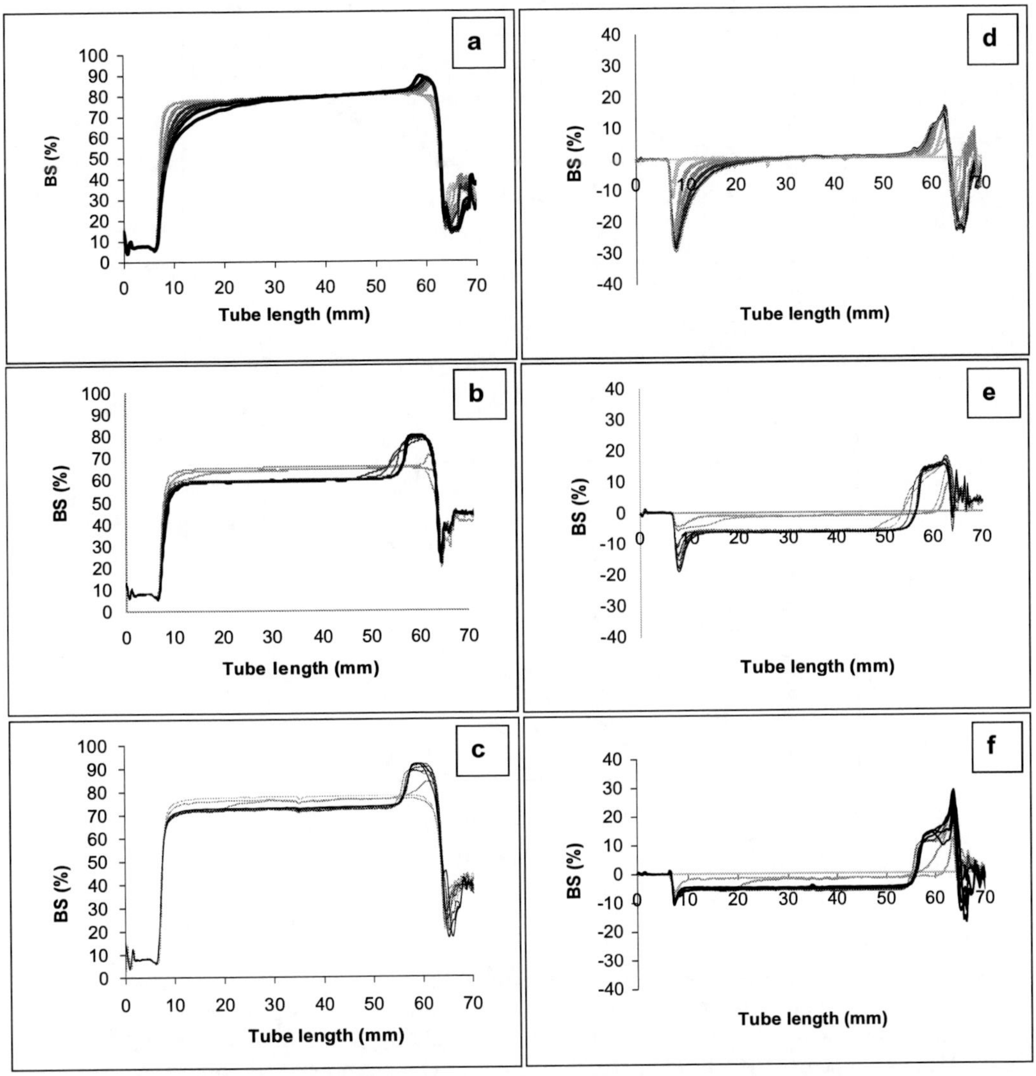

Figure 5. Changes in back scattering (BS) as a function of the tube length with storage time (samples were stored for 1 week, black curve) in quiescent conditions for emulsions with 10 wt. % concentrated from fish oil (CFO) as fat phase, no trehalose added to the aqueous phase, and a concentration of sodium caseinate (NaCas) of 0.5 (a,d), 2.0 (b,e), and 5.0 (c,f) wt.%. a,b, and c, actual profiles (BS); d,e, and f, profiles in reference mode (ΔBS). Tube length 65 mm.

The increase in particle size may be associated to coalescence or flocculation. To distinguish both alternatives $D_{4,3}$ was measured after a week at 22.5 °C in the middle zone of the tube (20–50 mm). The obtained value for 5 wt. % NaCas (0.26 μm) was smaller than emulsion initial value (0.37 μm). Most likely aggregates were separated in the light scattering equipment as consequence of shear forces, exerted during the measurement of particle size in the Mastersizer, which will be sufficient to break-up the weak reversible flocculation. This behavior was previously observed in caseinate-stabilized oil-in-water emulsions [12]. In addition, a lower $D_{4,3}$ value indicated that bigger particles migrated to the top of the tube. This is supported by the shape of the profile (Figure 5c). The obtained $D_{4,3}$ value supported that destabilization occurred by flocculation and not by coalescence.

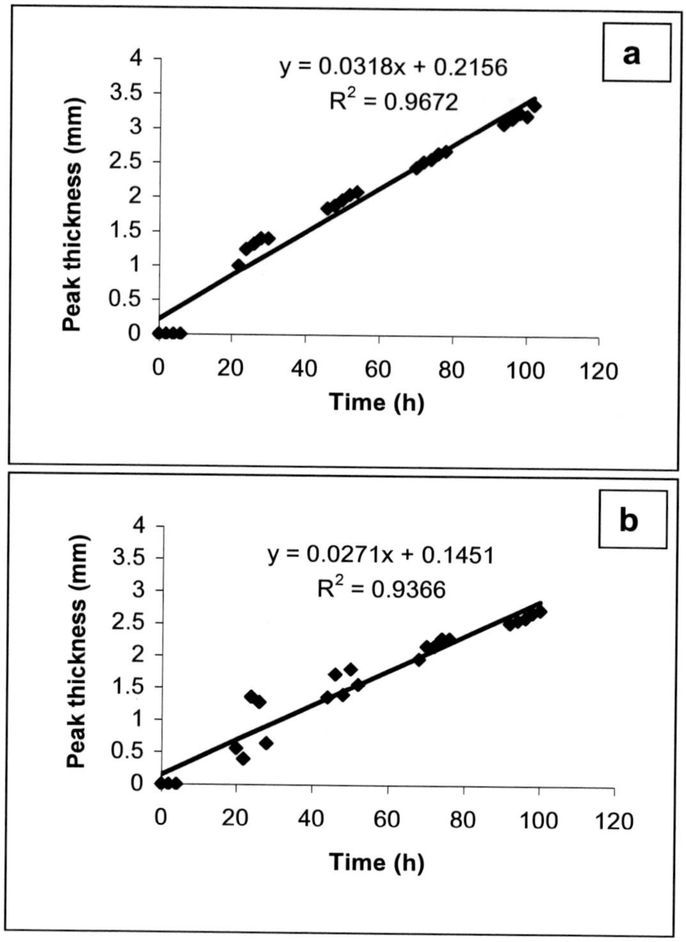

Figure 6. Peak thickness measured at 50% of the height at different times in the bottom zone of the tube, for samples stored in quiescent conditions at 22.5 °C, emulsions with CFO as fat phase, no trehalose added to the aqueous phase, and different concentrations of sodium caseinate: (a) 0.5 wt.%, (b) 2.0 wt.%, monitored over 100 h. Tube length 65 mm. CFO concentrated fish oil.

The BS profiles corresponding to the 5 wt. % emulsion did not show a peak in BS at the bottom of the tube when they were displayed in the reference mode (Figure 5f), which indicated that there was no migration of small particles before emulsion flocculation. On the contrary, there was a dramatic change in stability with an important decrease in BS_{av} indicative of flocculation. The shape of the profile at the top of the tube was a consequence of the migration of flocs formed during flocculation. Thus, the mechanism of destabilization in this case was flocculation followed by creaming of flocs. Flocculation kinetics for emulsion in Figure 5c is shown in Figure 7. The emulsion was stable for an hour and then the BS_{av} changed dramatically. There was a noticeable change for the first 18 h when BS reached an asymptotic value. The 5 wt. % NaCas emulsion had the lowest $D_{4,3}$ value of the three emulsions formulated without trehalose (0.5, 2, and 5 wt. %), which means that this emulsion had the greatest superficial area of all. As the particles are small no migration occurred at the times selected in this study. The fact that migration was very slow and the formation of a great superficial area allowed flocculation to occur.

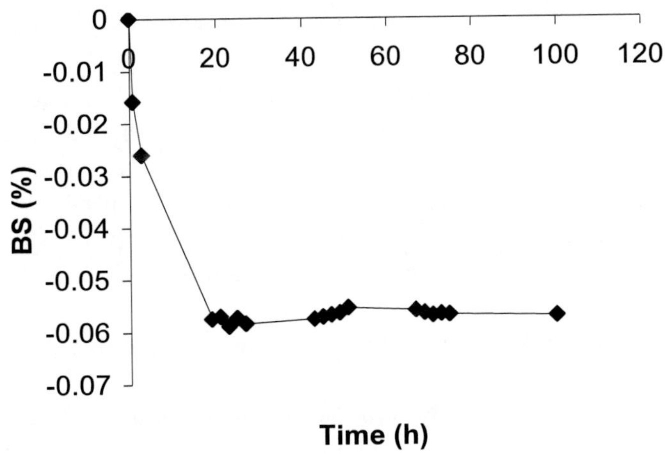

Figure 7. Variation in BS in the 20–50 mm zone monitored over 100 h, for the sample stored in quiescent conditions at 22.5 °C. The emulsion was formulated with CFO as fat phase, no trehalose added to the aqueous phase, and 5.0 wt.% NaCas. Tube length: 65 mm. BS back scattering. CFO concentrated fish oil. NaCas sodium caseinate.

As mentioned, all these samples remained fully turbid during storage, which means that all of them would have been considered stable by visual observation. As an example, Figure 8 shows two Turbiscan tubes containing emulsions without sugar in the aqueous phase. The image was taken after a week at ambient temperature (22.5°C).

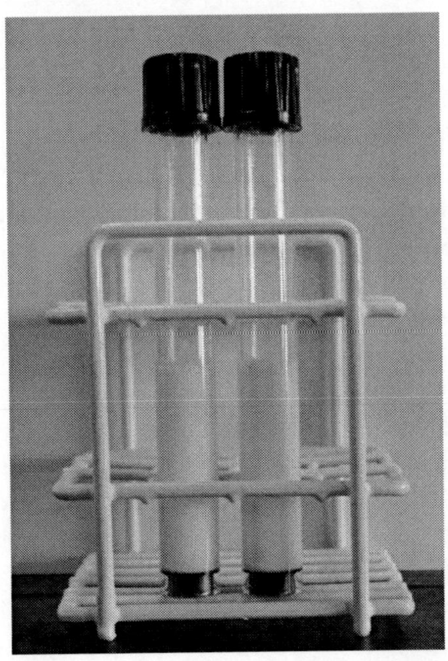

Figure 8. Turbiscan tubes containing emulsions with 10 wt.% concentrated from fish oil (CFO) as fat phase, no trehalose added to the aqueous phase, and a concentration of sodium caseinate (NaCas) of 0.5 (left) and 5.0 (right) wt.%.

Effect of Trehalose Addition on Stability

Figures 9 and 10 show the BS profiles in actual and reference mode as a function of the tube length for emulsions with 30 and 40 wt.% of trehalose added to the aqueous phase, respectively. The 20 wt.% trehalose emulsions showed a behavior similar to the one of emulsions without trehalose. In this case, the main mechanism of destabilization in a given formulation depended on NaCas concentration, that is, on the oil-to-protein ratio. However, the rate of destabilization was markedly lower with addition of sugar. The 5 wt.% NaCas emulsion did not flocculate during a week at 22.5 °C. Its BS remained unchanged during storage showing a great stability. This sample remained fully turbid and in the liquid state [45].

When more sugar (30 or 40 wt.%) was added to the aqueous phase flocculation was suppressed. As may be noticed from Figures 9 and 10 the unique mechanism for destabilization that occurred when emulsions destabilized was creaming.

Figures 9a and d show the behavior of the 0.5 wt.% NaCas emulsion with 30 wt.% trehalose added to the aqueous phase. Both, actual and in reference mode profiles were characteristics of creaming destabilization. As may be noticed, creaming process started after 21 h with a creaming rate of 0.0294 mm/h. This rate was slower than for the emulsion without trehalose.

Figures 9b and e correspond to the 2 wt.% Na Cas emulsion. It is clear from the profiles that BS_{av} did not change significantly with time, as was the case of the same formulation but without sugar added to the aqueous phase. This means that sugar prevent flocculation from occurring. This emulsion destabilized slowly by creaming of small particles. Destabilization process started after 22 h and creaming rate was 0.0271 mm/h.

All these figures showed that the interactions between trehalose and NaCas were positive since as sugar concentration increased, destabilization process slowed down. Trehalose diminished creaming rate and impeded flocculation. The effect seemed to be further than an increase in viscosity. There should be protein-trehalose interactions. Most food emulsions are highly complex systems in terms of both composition and structure and also kinetically and thermodynamically speaking. Particle size is usually modified by interactions among emulsion components. According to Garti [46] droplet size can be smaller if polysaccharides are present with the protein during homogenization, so the rate of creaming can be reduced as long as there is no bridging flocculation. It was also reported that hydrocolloids might display surface activity in addition to effects on hydrodynamic characteristics of emulsions. In our emulsions addition of trehalose decreased $D_{4,3}$ in all cases. Interactions between polysaccharides and proteins are based on hydrogen bond, and dipole-dipole associations, in which the presence of OH-groups plays a predominant role. Besides, in the Biochemistry field, strong interactions between peptides and short oligosaccharides have been recently reported as playing an important role in protein recognition. All the above indicates that sugar-protein interactions are very common. Regarding trehalose special properties described in literature it is not unreasonable to think that trehalose may work as coadjutant in micelle formation and, also, may change the quality of water as a solvent, improving the solvent-protein interaction, leading to smaller particle sizes and more stable emulsions. Although there was a slight increase of viscosity of the continuous phase for addition of trehalose, the fact that particle size was smaller clearly showed that there were sugar-protein interactions playing a key role in stability.

The 5 wt.% Na Cas emulsion was stable showing no changes during storage (Figures 9c and f). The profiles in reference mode clearly showed that no flocculation occurred, as was the case of the same formulation but without sugar in the aqueous phase.

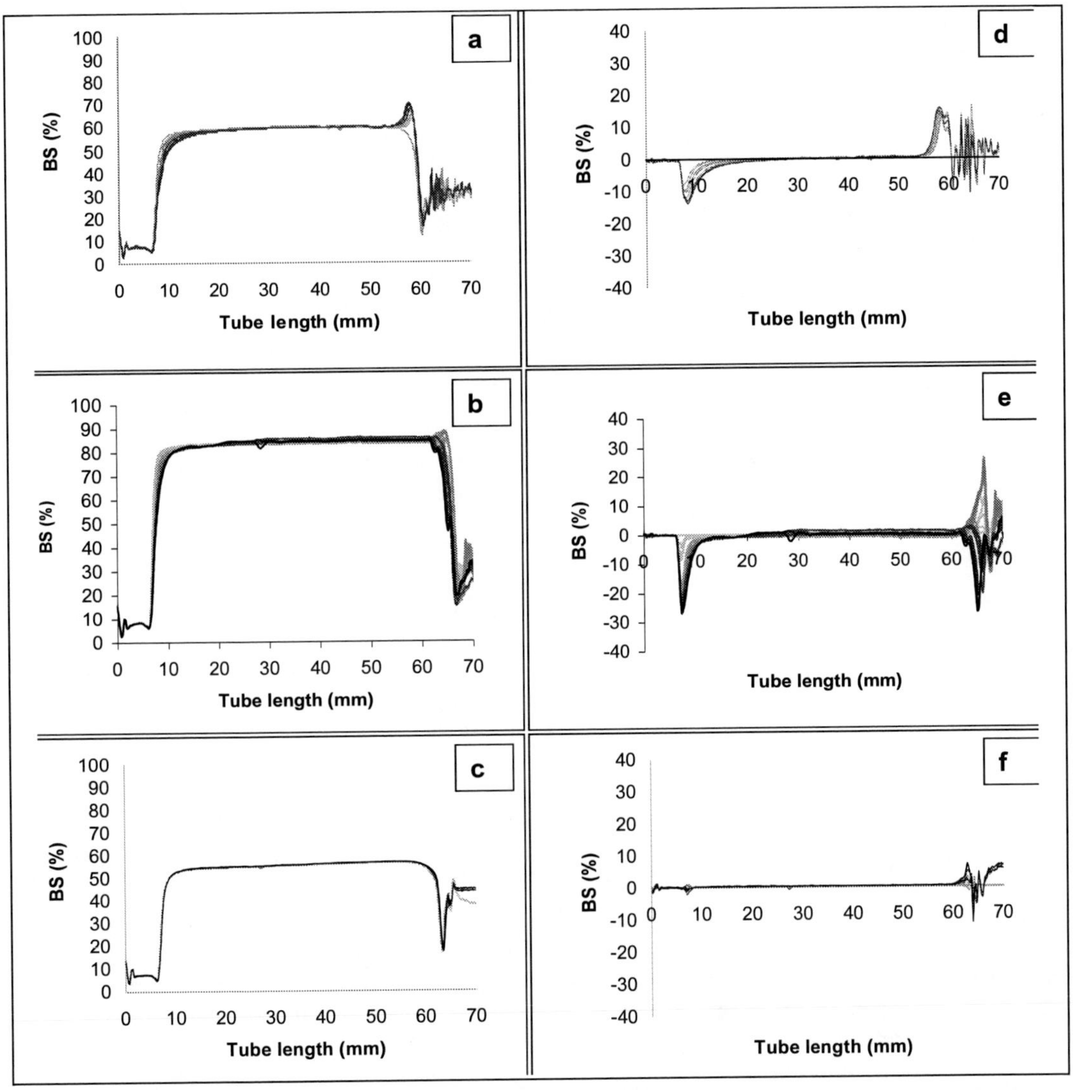

Figure 9. Changes in back scattering (BS) as a function of the tube length with storage time (samples were stored for 1 week, black curve) in quiescent conditions for emulsions with 10 wt. % concentrated from fish oil (CFO) as fat phase, 30% trehalose added to the aqueous phase, and a concentration of sodium caseinate (NaCas) of 0.5 (a,d), 2.0 (b,e), and 5.0 (c,f) wt.%. a,b, and c, actual profiles (BS); d,e, and f, profiles in reference mode (ΔBS).

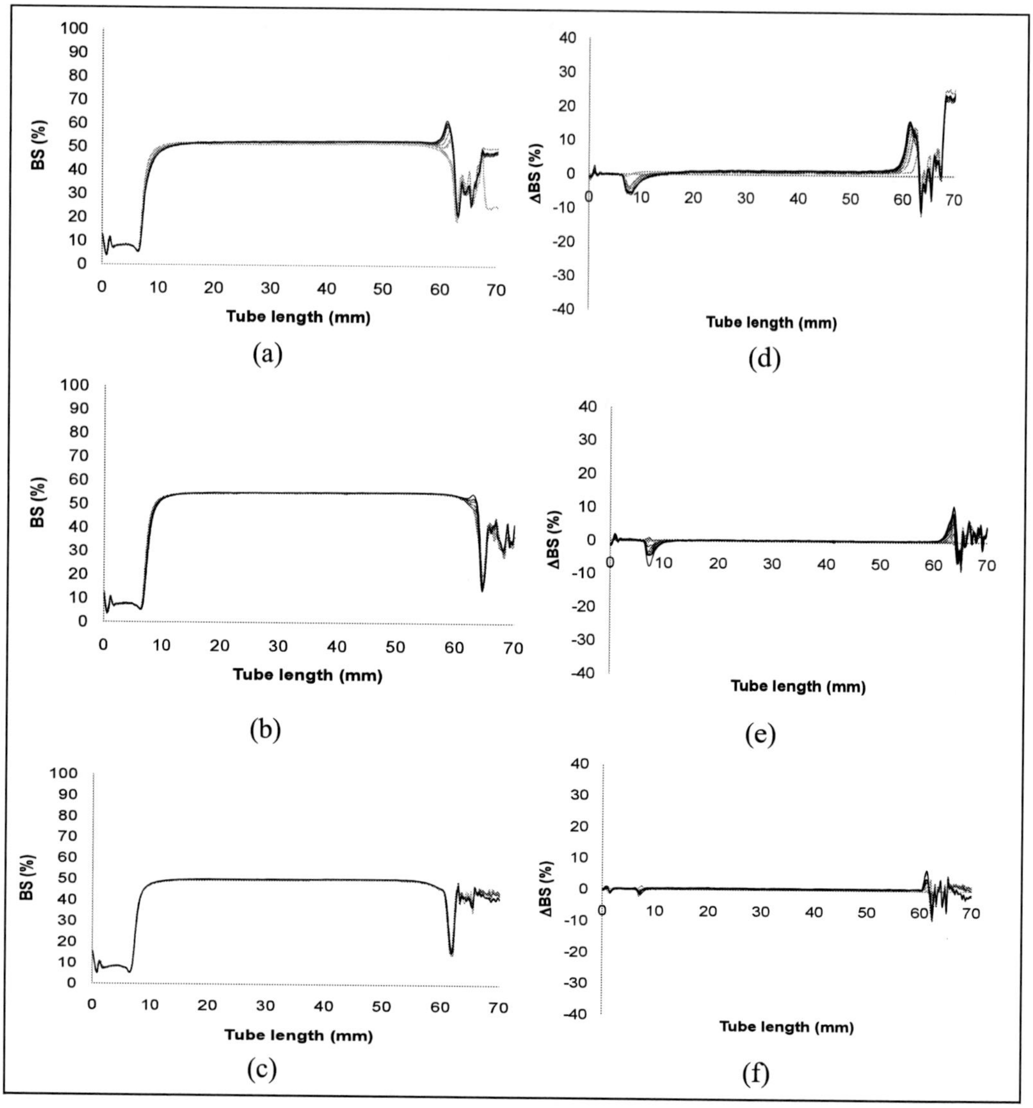

Figure 10. Changes in back scattering (BS) as a function of the tube length with storage time (samples were stored for 1 week, black curve) in quiescent conditions for emulsions with 10 wt. % concentrated from fish oil (CFO) as fat phase, 40% trehalose added to the aqueous phase, and a concentration of sodium caseinate (NaCas) of 0.5 (a,d), 2.0 (b,e), and 5.0 (c,f) wt.%. a,b, and c, actual profiles (BS); d,e, and f, profiles in reference mode (ΔBS).

Emulsions in Figure 10 contained 40 wt.% trehalose added to the aqueous phase. For 0.5 wt.% NaCas (Figures 10a and d) creaming process started after 26 h with a creaming rate of 0.0243 mm/h, significantly slower than for the same emulsion without trehalose. The 2 wt.% Na Cas emulsion (Figure 10b and e) was almost stable. A very slow creaming with a rate of 0.0120 mm/h started after 48 h. Clearly destabilization kinetics was slowly than the one for the same formulation without sugar. In addition, only the creaming process was detected. BS profiles in reference mode indicated that flocculation did not occur after 1 week. The 5 wt.% NaCas emulsion was completely stable (Figure 10c and f) showing no destabilization during storage at 22.5°C.

Effect of Processing Conditions

Figure 11 shows the results of analyzing two tubes corresponding to an emulsion formulated with 5 wt.% NaCas, no trehalose added to the aqueous phase and CFO as fat phase. Both emulsions have the same formulation but they were prepared in different ways. Emulsion in Figure 11a was kept at 60°C during preparation. Then, fat and aqueous phases were mixed using an Ultra-Turrax T8 high-speed blender operated at 20,000 rpm for 1 min to give a coarse dispersion with a $D_{4,3}$ of 12.12 μm. Then, it was further homogenized for 20 min using an ultrasonic liquid processing (Figure 11b) to give a fine emulsion with a $D_{4,3}$ of 0.36 μm.

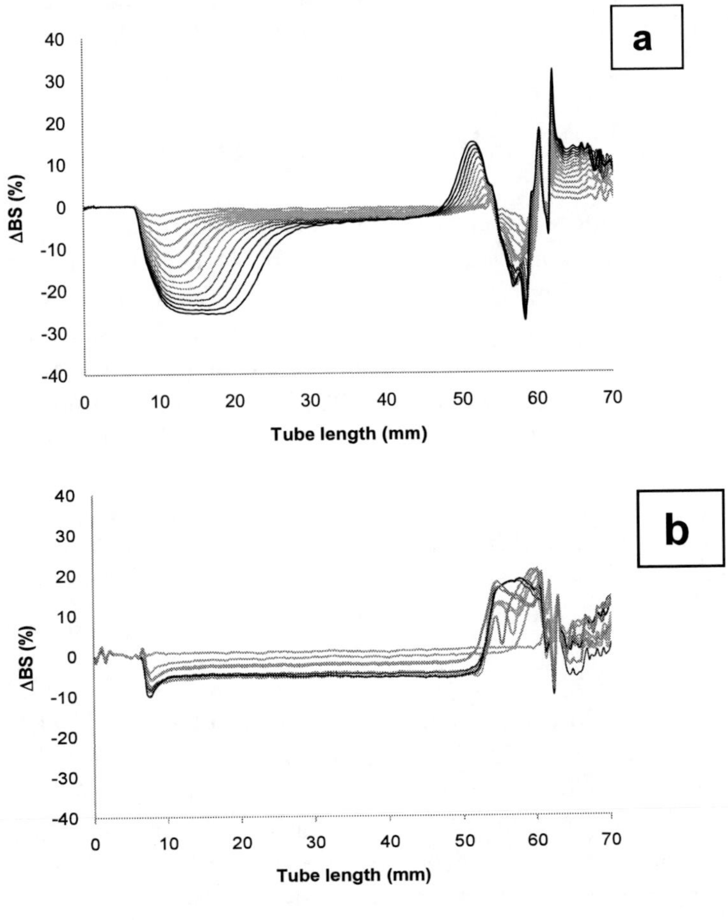

Figure 11. Changes in back scattering (BS) in reference mode profiles as a function of the tube length with storage time (samples were stored for 1 week, arrow denotes time) in quiescent conditions for emulsions with 10 wt.% concentrated from fish oil (CFO) as fat phase, no trehalose added to the aqueous phase, and a concentration of sodium caseinate (NaCas) of 5.0 wt.%. (a) profiles of coarse emulsion, (b) profiles of emulsion further homogenized by ultrasound treatment. Tube length 70 mm.

As may be noticed from Figure 11 the mechanism of destabilization was different in both cases. Figure 11a shows the typical profile of an emulsion that destabilized by creaming of individual particles whereas Figure 11b reports the behavior of an emulsion that destabilized by flocculation. There could be some explanations for the different behavior: it may be related to the aggregation state of the protein in solution, to the different kinetics of creaming and flocculation processes or to the different superficial area due to the different droplet size. In the first case, although the temperature was controlled during the ultrasound treatment and never exceeded 40°C, the protein may have changed the structure. In the second case, it may be pointed out that the creaming process is always faster than flocculation mechanism. If creaming does not occur because particles are small enough to give stability to the studied emulsion, flocculation that has a greater induction time may take place. The last point could be related with the fact that creaming and flocculation occurred for different reasons. Creaming is the result of different densities between continuous and dispersed phases. Flocculation is a consequence of attraction between oil droplets. It may be possible that there could be a minimum interfacial protein amount necessary for flocculation. In any case, these results show the importance of processing conditions in stability behavior.

Microstructure

Figure 12 shows confocal laser scattering microscopy (CLSM) images of emulsions formulated without trehalose and kept at 22.5 °C for 24 h. The images corresponding to emulsions stabilized with 0.5 or 1 wt.% NaCas (Figure 12 a and b) showed a homogeneous droplet distribution. In these images, particles kept their individual shapes. As shown before the 0.5 wt.% NaCas emulsion destabilized mainly by creaming of individual particles. Figure 12a and b are in agreement with Turbiscan results. Creaming mechanism should be expected from emulsion structure. Images show that $D_{4,3}$ decrease with NaCas concentration. Particle size measurement confirmed this result. For Figures 12a and b $D_{4,3}$ were 1.22 and μm, respectively. When protein concentration was 2, 3, 4 or 5 wt.% (Figure 12c, d, e, and f) emulsions presented aggregates/flocculates, which were absent in 0.5 and 1 wt.% emulsions. In these emulsions there were higher protein concentrations in the aqueous phase and formation of flocs. According to the Turbiscan studies these samples destabilized mainly by flocculation.

Figure 13 reports the CLSM images obtained when the 30 wt.% trehalose/10 wt.% CFO emulsions stabilized with different amounts of NaCas were kept at 22.5 °C for 24 h. Figure 13a and b showed that these emulsions also had individual particles homogeneously distributed. In agreement with Turbiscan studies, which indicated that flocculation was less likely to occur when the aqueous phase had trehalose, Figure 13c, d, and e show less formation of flocs and a more homogeneous structure than the corresponding emulsions without trehalose. Surprisingly, a concentration of 5 wt.% NaCas produced an emulsion with a very homogeneous droplet distribution and a very low $D_{4,3}$ (Table 3). In addition to a higher concentration of NaCas in the aqueous phase this emulsion most likely had more protein for the coverage of oil droplet surface. The absence of aggregates/flocculates is in agreement with the great stability of this emulsion as studied by turbiscan. Sugar changed the microstructure of emulsions as well as their stability behavior.

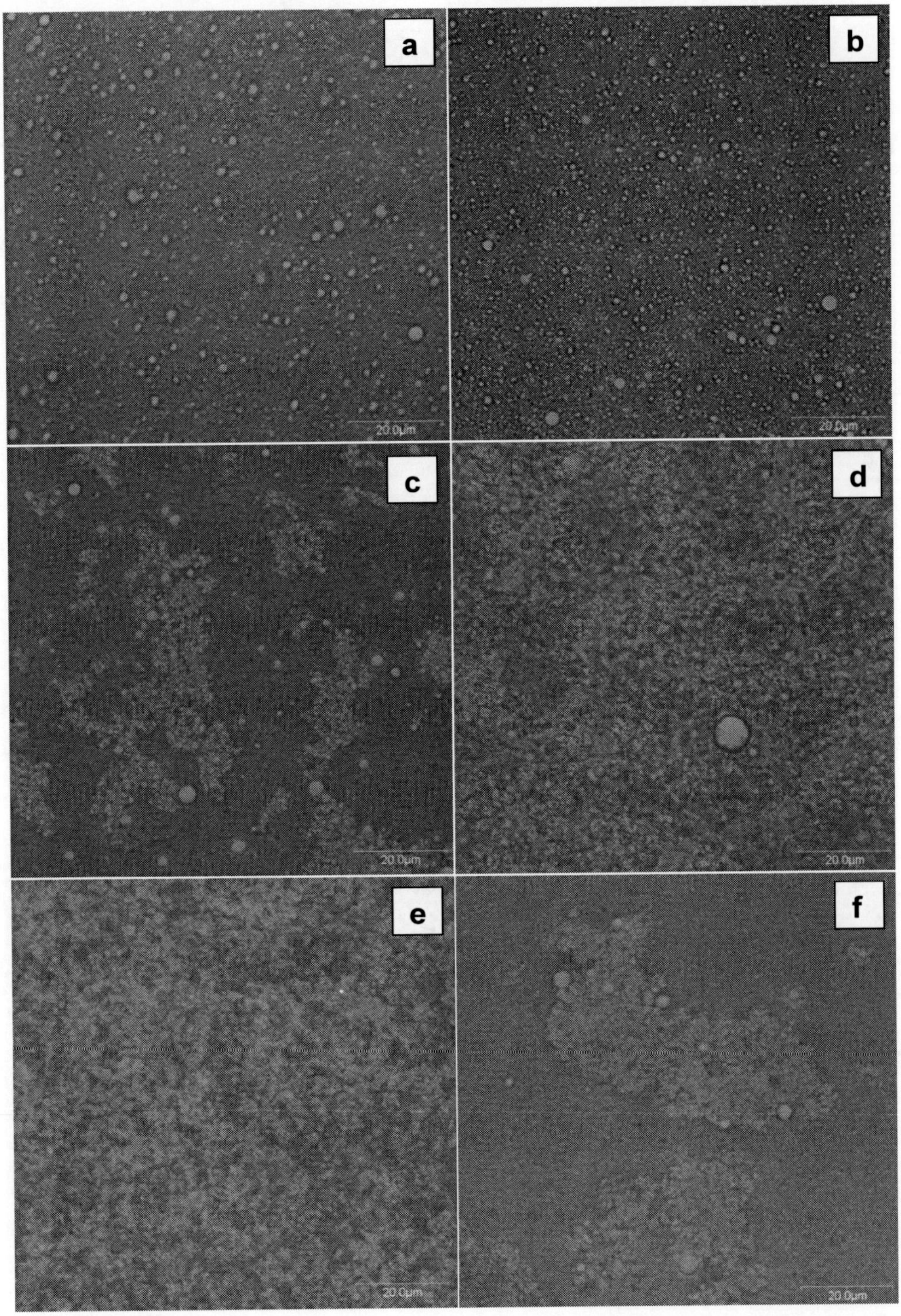

Figure 12. Confocal laser scattering microscopy (CLSM) images of emulsions with 10 wt.% concentrated fish oil (CFO) as fat phase, no trehalose added to aqueous phase, and different concentrations of sodium caseinate (NaCas) kept at 22.5 °C for 24 h: (a) 0.5 wt.%, (b) 1.0 wt.%, (c) 2.0 wt.%, (d) 3.0 wt.%, (e) 4.0 wt.%, and (f) 5.0 wt.%. CFO concentrated fish oil.

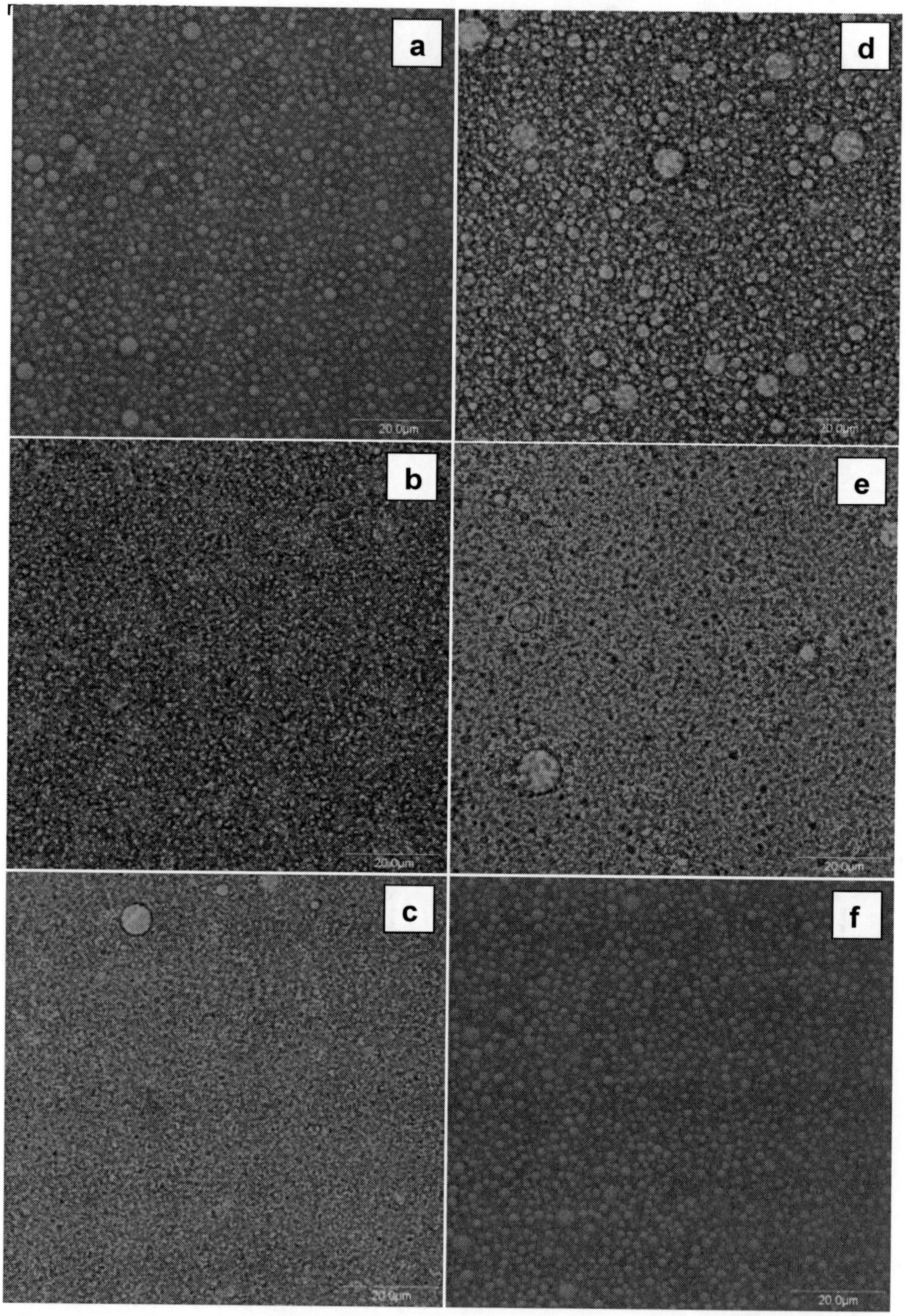

Figure 13. Confocal laser scattering microscopy (CLSM) images of emulsions with 10 wt.% concentrated fish oil (CFO) as fat phase, 30 wt.% trehalose solution as aqueous phase, and different concentrations of sodium caseinate (NaCas) kept at 22.5 °C for 24 h: (a) 0.5 wt.%, (b) 1.0 wt.%, (c) 2.0 wt.%, (d) 3.0 wt.%, (e) 4.0 wt.%, and (f) 5.0 wt.%. CFO concentrated fish oil.

NMR Studies

NMR relaxation properties depend on the spectral density functions, which in turn are sensitive to molecular motion. Spectrometer frequency, molecular size, and internuclear distances are also important parameters. In fact, spectral densities are related to the motional correlation times, which measure the rate of molecular tumbling. These parameters are the basic longitudinal (T_1) and transversal (T_2) relaxation times. NMR relaxation measurements may be used to probe the change of mobility due to structural changes of the sample.

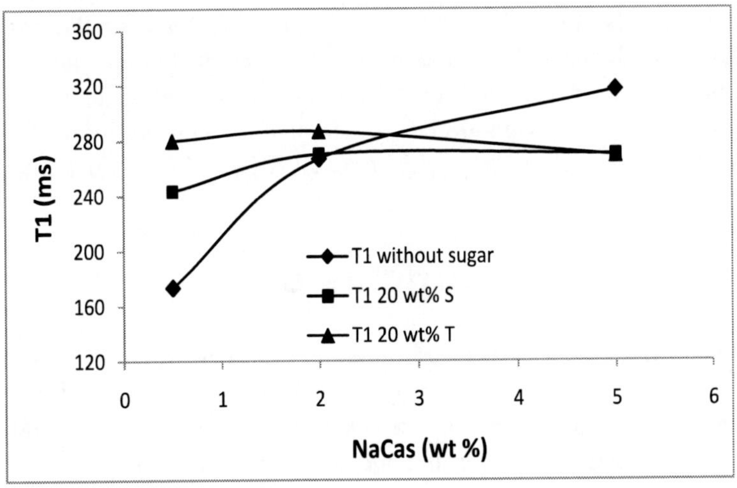

Figure 14. Relaxation time T_2 as a function of NaCas concentration. S: sucrose; T: trehalose. Emulsions were evaluated immediately after preparation.

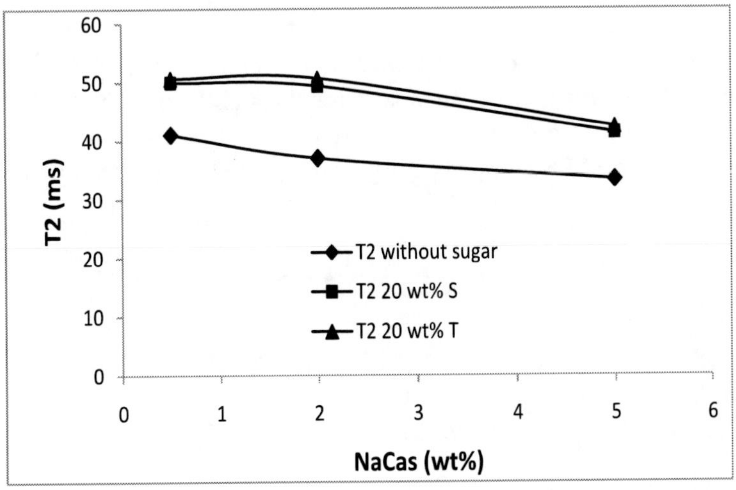

Figure 15. Relaxation time T_1 as a function of NaCas concentration. S: sucrose; T: trehalose. Emulsions were evaluated immediately after preparation.

Figure 14 shows the effect of sucrose or trehalose addition on relaxation longitudinal time T_1 and Figure 15 on relaxation transversal time T_2 for emulsions formulated with 0.5, 2 or 5 wt.% NaCas and 10 wt. CFO. The proton signal from the mobile molecules made the most important contributions to the relaxation times. The protein components that stabilized the interface made only a negligible contribution to the NMR signal. T_1 and T_2 values from low- field NMR appeared to be dominated by the structure of the bulk emulsion. The results showed that sugar displayed surface activity in addition to effects on hydrodynamic characteristics of emulsions, and modified emulsion structure. If sugar had acted only as a thickening agent, shorter T_2 and greater T_1 values would have been expected with addition of sugar for all protein concentrations. The fact that the behavior of T_1 was unexpected, that is, curves obtained for emulsions with sugars crossed the ones for formulations without sugars and had very close values for all NaCas concentrations, indicated changes in structure in the bulk emulsion since T_1 is strongly affected by matrix mobility. T_2 had also an unexpected behavior. Values of T_2 were always higher for emulsions with addition of sugar showing a less restricted mobility, which was the opposite result expected for a thickening agent.

Conclusion

From our results and others discussed in literature, it is clear that the stability of caseinate emulsions was strongly affected not only by the oil-to-protein ratio but also by processing conditions and composition of aqueous phase. The structure of the protein and the interactions protein–sugar played a key role in creaming and flocculation processes.

Acknowledgment

This work was supported by CONICET through Project PIP 11220080101504, by the National Agency for the Promotion of Science and Technology (ANPCyT) through Project PICT 0060, and by the University of Buenos Aires through Project X 451. The authors wish to thank to the Synchrotron Light National Laboratory (LNLS, Campinas, Brazil) for the used of X-ray facilities and the SPES company for providing the concentrated from fish oils.

References

[1] Dickinson, E.; Golding, M. *J. Coll. Interf. Sci.* 1997, *191*, 166-76.

[2] Dickinson, E. *Int. Dairy J.* 1999, *9*, 305-12.

[3] Berli, C. L. A.; Quemada, D.; Parker, A. *Coll. Surf. A: Physicochem. Eng. Aspects* 2002, *203*, 11-20.

[4] Mc Clements, D. J. Food emulsions, principles, practices, and techniques, 2nd ed. CRC Press: New York, NY, 2005; pp 269-339.

[5] Dalgleish, D. G. *Food Hydrocoll.* 2006, *20*, 415-422.

[6] Day L.; Xu, M; Hoobin, P.; Burgar, I.; Augustin, M. A. *Food Chem.* 2007, *105*, 469-79.

[7] van Aken, G. A.; van Vliet, T. 2002. *Langmuir* 2002, *18*, 7364–7370.

[8] Fox, P.F.; Brodkorb, A. *Int. Dairy J.* 2008, *18*, 677-84.

[9] Kinsella, J. E. *Crit. Rev. Food Sci. Nutr.* 1984, *21*, 197-262.

[10] Dickinson, E. *J. Dairy Res.* 1989, *56*, 471-477.

[11] Mulvihill, D. M. In: *Developments in dairy chemistry- 4. Functional Milk Proteins*; Fox, P. F.; Ed.; Elsevier Applied Science: London, UK, 1989; pp 97-130.

[12] Dickinson, E.; Golding, M. *Food Hydrocoll.* 1997, *11*, 13-8.

[13] Tosh, S. M.; Dalgleish, D. G. *J. Dairy Sci.* 1998, *81*, 1840-7.

[14] Dickinson, E.; Golding, M. *J. Coll. Interf. Sci.* 1998, *197*, 133-41.

[15] Dickinson, E. *J. Chem. Soc., Faraday Trans.* 1998, *94*, 1657-1669.

[16] Brinkhuis, J.; Payens, T. A. *J. Biophysical Chem.* 1984, *19*, 75-81.

[17] Holt, C.; Horne, D. S. *Neth. Milk Dairy J.* 1996, *50*, 85-111.

[18] Dalgleish, D. G; Spagnuolo, P. A; Goff, D. G. *Int. Dairy J.* 2004, *14*, 1025-31.

[19] Holt, C.; Sawyer, L. *J. Chem. Soc. Faraday Trans.* 1993, *89*, 2683-92.

[20] Dickinson, E. *Coll. Surf. A: Physicochem. Eng. Aspects* 2006, 288, 3-11.

[21] Jahaniaval, F.; Kakuda, Y.; Abraham, V.; Marcone, M. *Food Res. Int.* 2000, *33*, 637-47.

[22] Waugh, D. F. *Faraday Soc. Discussions* 1958, *25*, 186-92.

[23] Creamer, L. K; Berry, G. D. *J. Dairy Res.* 1975, *42*, 169-83.

[24] Waugh, D. F. In: Milk proteins: Chemistry and molecular biology. McKenzie, H. A.; Ed.; Academic Press: New York, NY, 1971; vol II, pp 3-85.

[25] Dickinson, E, *Introduction to Food Colloids*; Oxford University Press: Oxford, UK, 1992.

[26] Mulder, H.; Walstra, P. *The Milk Fat Globule: Emulsion Science as Applied to Milk Products and Comparable Foods*, Pudoc, Wageningen, The Netherlands. 1974.

[27] Boode, K. *Partial Coalescence in Oil-in-Water Emulsions*, Ph.D. Thesis, Wageningen Agricultural University, Wageningen, The Netherlands. 1992.

[28] Chrysam, M.M. In: *Bailey's Industrial Oil and Fat Products*, *5th Edition*, Hui, Y.H, Ed., John Wiley & Sons: New York, NY, 1996; Vol 3.

[29] Goff, H.D. *Journal of Dairy Science*, 1997, *80*, 2620.

[30] Goff, H.D. (1997). Partial coalescence and structure formation in dairy emulsions, in *Food Proteins and Lipids*, American Chemical Soceity, S. Damodaran, Ed., Plenum Press, NY, p. 137.

[31] Goff, H.D. (2002). Formation and stabilization of structure in ice cream and related products. *Current Opinion in Colloid and Interface Science*, 7, 432.

[32] Goff, H.D. (2003). Ice cream, in *Advanced Dairy Chemistry—1. Proteins*, 3rd ed. Fox, P.F., McSweeney, P.L.H., Eds., Kluwer Academic Publishers, New York, NY, p. 1063.

[33] Walstra, P. (1999). *Dairy Technology: Principles of Milk Properties and Processes*, Marcel Dekker, New York, NY.

[34] Goff, H.D., Hartel, R.W. (2003). Ice cream and frozen desserts, in *Handbook of Food Freezing Techology*, Hui, Y.H., Ed., Marcel Dekker, New York, NY.

[35] Kalnin, D.; Ouattara, M.; Ollivon, M. *Progress in Coll. and Polymer Sci.* 2004, *128*, 207–211.

[36] Brenna, J. T; Salem, N. Jr.; Sinclair, A. J.; Cunnane, S. C. *Prostaglandins Leukot Essent Fatty Acids* 2009, *80*, 85-91.

[37] Chan, J. K; Mc Donald, B. E; Gerrard, J. M.; Bruce, V. M; Weaver, B. J.; Holub, B. J. *Lipids* 1993, *28*, 811-817.

[38] Kris-Etherton, P. M.; Harris, W. S.; Appel, L. J. *Arterioscler Thromb. Vasc. Biol.* 2003, *23*, e20-e30.

[39] Anderson, B. M.; Ma, D. W. L. *Lipids Health Disease* 2009, *8*, 33-52.

[40] Cerdeira, M.; Palazolo, G. G.; Candal, R. J.; Herrera, M. L. *J. Am. Oil Chem. Soc.* 2007, 84, 523–531.

[41] Chauvierre, C.; Labarre, D.; Couvreur, P.; Vauthier, C. *Coll. Polymer Sci.* 2004, *282*, 1097–1104.

[42] Pan, L. G.; Tomás, M. C.; Añón, M. C. *J. Surf. Detergents*, 2002, *5*, 135–143.

[43] Mengual, O.; Meunier, G.; Cayré, I.; Puech, K.; Snabre, P. *Talanta* 1999, *50*, 445–456.

[44] Palazolo, G. G.; Sorgentini, D. A.; Wagner, J. R. *Food Hydrocoll.* 2005, *19*, 595–604.

[45] Álvarez Cerimedo, M. S.; Huck Iriart, C.; Candal, R. J.; Herrera, M. L. *Food Res. Int.* 2010, *43*, 1482-93.

[46] Garti, N. In: *Physical Properties of Lipids*. Marangoni, A. G.; Narine, S. S.; Eds.; Marcel Dekker, Inc: New York, NY, 2002; pp 265-386.

In: Fish Oil: Production, Consumption and Health Benefits
Editors: Matthias Van Dijk and Jürgen Vitek
ISBN: 978-1-61470-963-3

Chapter IX

Inflammation and Diets Rich in Fish and Soybean Oil

Vera Lucia Flor Silveira[ab]***, Karina Vieira de Barros***[a]***,***
Roberta Araujo Navarro Xavier[a] ***and Marta Wolhers***[a]
[a] Department of Physiology, Federal University of São Paulo, São Paulo, SP, Brazil
[b] Department of Biological Sciences, Federal University of São Paulo,
Diadema, SP, Brazil

Introduction

The Omega 3 polyunsaturated fatty acids (w-3 PUFA or n-6 PUFA) from fish oil are known not only because its essentiality, but because their unquestionable anti-inflammatory effect. This effect has put the fish oil on the top of the list of the most studied oil in the world. The anti-inflammatory effect of fish oil has been observed in a variety of inflammatory diseases, such as colitis, asthma and cardiovascular disease. Fatty acids are components of cell membranes, which are important for maintaining cellular homeostasis and intercellular communication. Several studies have shown that changes in diet composition may alter the lipid composition of membrane phospholipids, altering their functionality (Calder 2002).

The relationship between inflammatory response and fatty acids (FAs), especially in regard to polyunsaturated fatty acids (PUFA), has been investigated on the last years. One reason for this interest, comes from the fact that arachidonic acid (AA), n-6 PUFA, which is a precursor of eicosanoids, substances that have important and inflammatory properties, is derived directly from dietetic vegetable oils sources such as soybean, corn and sunflower or indirectly formed from linoleic acid (18:2 n-6) or gamma-linolenic acid (18:3 n-6).

On the other hand, epidemiological studies have shown that the Eskimos population, large consumers of eicosapentaenoic acid (EPA) and docosahexaenoic acid (DHA), both polyunsaturated n-3, have low incidence of inflammatory and immunological diseases (Kromman & Green 1980). Since the report of this finding, a number of researchers have documented the beneficial effects of n-3 PUFA (rich in EPA and DHA) on acute and chronic inflammatory conditions (Wu & Meydani 1998, Harbidge 1998). These effects were considered to result mainly from a modification in the production of inflammatory mediators (cytokines, chemokines, and costimulatory molecules) and the suppression of inflammatory leukocytes (neutrophils, lymphocytes, macrophages, and dendritic cells).

Biological Roles of PUFA

PUFA are involved in regulating lipid metabolism and in processes involving the transport of lipids to the target tissue. We can quote as examples of such activities, the inhibiting role of n-3 and n-6 PUFA in hepatic triacylglycerol synthesis, which causes an effect in decreasing plasma triglyceride levels and the role of low density cholesterol and linoleic acid. Rahman et al. (2001), for example, demonstrated that supplementing the diet with linoleic acid increases the β-oxidation in the liver, promoting decrease in plasma triglyceride levels in OLETF rat strain.

Furthermore, PUFA are important components of the membranes in all cells, representing 50% of the membrane structure. The nature of fatty acids into membrane phospholipids contributes to its fluidity and is believed to play a regulatory role in the activity of proteins present in this membrane. Phospholipids are also sources of second messengers such as diacylglycerol, phosphatidic acid, inositol triphosphate, ceramide and AA, which are responsible for signaling events that are originally from the membrane to the cytosol and the nucleus, promoting an appropriate cellular response.

N-3 PUFA enriched diets promotes an increase in the fluidity of the membranes of macrophages, while diets rich in n-6 PUFA have the opposite effect. These changes in membrane fluidity are associated with decreased binding affinity of tumor necrosis factor (TNF), activity of GTPase in the production of cAMP, modulation of cytokines release (Tapp et al. 1997), has also implications in cell depolarization and in control of ion channels (Zeng et al. 1998). For example, AA causes rapid membrane depolarization, an effect that seems to be associated with calcium influx (Chow et al. 1991).

An important functional role of PUFA with 20 carbons, is a substrate for the synthesis of the mediators family known as eicosanoids (prostaglandin (PG), tromboxanes (TX), leukotrienes (LT), lipoxins (LX), etc.), which are oxygenated and derived from fatty diom-g-linolenic AA and EPA. Although some PUFA with 20 carbon atoms serve as precursors of eicosanoids, AA is usually the main substrate for their synthesis. This occurs because the membrane of most cells contains large amounts of AA, compared with other potential precursors of eicosanoids (including EPA). The AA found in cell membranes can be mobilized by various phospholipase (PL) enzymes kind, but mainly by phospholipase A2 (PLA2) (Calder 1997). The metabolism of AA by cyclooxygenase (COX) increases PG and TX Series 2. There are two isoforms of COX: COX-1 is a constitutive enzyme and COX-2 is induced in stimulated inflammatory cells and responsible for the sharp increase in PG. The metabolism of AA by 5-lipooxigenase (LIPOX) results in the increase of hydroxy and hydroperoxy derivatives and LT Series 4 (Zurier 1991).

Eicosanoids act as mediators (e.g PGE2 causes pain), modify the response to other mediators (e.g., PGE2 enhances the pain caused by Bradykinin) and act as regulators of other processes such as platelet aggregation, blood coagulation, leukocyte chemotaxis, inflammatory cytokine production and immune function (Bjorksten 1989).

PGE2 has a number of pro-inflammatory effects, including fever, increase in vascular permeability, vasodilatation and increase in the formation of edema and pain caused by other agents such as Bradykinin and Histamine (Form & Averback 1993). However, PGE2 suppresses the production of TNF-alpha, interleukin-1 (IL-1), IL-2, interferon-γ (IFN-γ), lymphocyte proliferation, the activity of natural killer cells and this sense would have an immunosuppressive action. TXA2 promotes, among other effects, platelet aggregation and adhesion of leukocytes. The LTB4 increases vascular permeability, local blood flow, production of reactive oxygen species, TNF-α, IL-1 and IL-6. It is a potent chemotactic agent for leukocytes and induces the release of lysosomal enzymes (Hang & Dale 1995). In inflammatory conditions there are increased levels of eicosanoids derived from AA.

When incorporated into membrane phospholipids, EPA inhibits the oxidation of AA by COX (Obata et al. 1999), being the preferred substrate of COX and LIPOX, with consequent formation of PG and TX series 3 and series 5 LT (Sane et al. 2000), less potent eicosanoids in the inflammatory process (Lee et al. 1984, Goldman et al. 1983). Thus, consumption of fish oil rich in EPA, decreases the production of PGE2, TXA2 and LTB4 and can potentially reduce platelet aggregation, coagulation and leukocyte chemotaxis, and modulate the production of inflammatory cytokines and immune function. This has been demonstrated in cell cultures, animals and human volunteers (Calder 2003).

Arntzen et al. (1988) found significant reduction in basal production of PGE2 and PGF2 in cells after in vitro supplementation with n-3 PUFA, EPA and DHA. Already with AA supplementation, the basal production of PGE2 increased 432.3% compared to control. Raedestorff et al. (1996) also found reduced levels of LTB4 and PGE2 in animals supplemented with EPA and DHA, compared to animals fed a diet rich in n-6 PUFA. The reduction of the generation of AA-derived mediators that accompanies the consumption of fish oil, has been associated with beneficial effects of n-3 PUFA on inflammatory conditions (Calder, 1997). Recent studies suggest that the metabolism of EPA by COX increases the release of a new series of anti-inflammatory eicosanoids (Serhan et al. 2000).

Besides the decrease of eicosanoids derived from AA, the n-3 PUFA have other actions, associated or not with this reduction, which may be important for the antiinflammatory effect of FAs (Miles & Calder 1998, Calder 2002). In that sense it was shown that n-3 PUFA decrease the production of non-lipid inflammatory mediators such as IL-1, IL-6, TNF and tissue factors derived from monocytes, macrophages or endothelial cells stimulated (Calder 2002). Priante et al. (2002) showed that AA stimulates the production of IL-1 α and β in cultured human osteoblasts while EPA inhibits at least 50% the induction of these cytokines by AA.

Inflammatory Response

The innate immune system is the first line of defense against invading microorganisms. This instantaneous response is mediated by macrophages and polymorphonuclear leukocytes that are recruited into the injured tissues in response to certain stimuli or pathogens. These cells, due to the presence of receptors that recognize pathogens, are able to identify in different microorganisms, specific classes of molecules with known molecular patterns associated with pathogens (Takeda et al. 2003). In humans, a special form of transmembrane proteins, called receptors like Toll (Toll-like receptors, TLRs) trigger, after recognition of specific antigens, a series of reactions that culminate in the activation of transcription factor, called nuclear factor kappa B (NF-κB). This promotes the increased expression of several genes involved in inflammatory response (Medzhitov et al. 1997). Occurs at the same time stimulating the production of T lymphocytes by the acquired immune system, which is responsible for antigen-specific mechanism of host defense response that includes cell-mediated immune antibodies (Medzhitov et al. 1997).

Monocytes initially characterized as quiescent cells of the immune system, secrete large amounts of inflammatory mediators. In that case, it was found that fatty acids and glucose activate via NF-κB in monocytes, raising the production of proinflammatory cytokines (Dickinson et al. 2007). Moreover, activation of the transcription factor PPAR-γ counter-regulates the activity of NF-κB, reducing the production of proinflammatory cytokines by monocytes and increasing apoptosis of this cell type (Dickinson et al. 2007).

NF-κB is activated as a result of the sequential phosphorylation and degradation of Iκ-B. The free NF-κB is translocated to the nucleus, where it activates IL-2 gene transcription by binding to the NF-κB. Denys et al. (2005) demonstrated that n-3 PUFA suppress IL-2 gene expression by inhibiting the membrane recruitment of protein kinase C alfa (PKC-α) and blocking the nuclear translocation of NF-κB involved in T-Cell proliferation. Novak et al. (2002) also demonstrated that murine treated with n-3 supplementation, significantly decreased Iκ-B phosphorylation and subsequently the transduction cascade, reducing NF-κB activity and consequently proinflammatory cytokine transcription.

PUFA and Acute Inflammation

Inflammation is a body's response to injury tissues, which can be triggered by mechanical stimuli, chemical, microbial invasion or due to hypersensitivity reactions. This response includes complex processes that involve the immune system cells and biological mediators (Rankin et al. 2004).

The acute phase response is characterized by increased blood flow, vascular permeability, accumulation of fluid, leukocytes and inflammatory mediators. The chronic phase is characterized by the development of immune responses specific humoral and cellular for pathogen (s) present (s) at the site of injury (Saadi et al. 2002).

The inflammatory response can be nonspecific, for example, phagocytosis of bacteria or scraps, secretion of proteolytic enzymes, production of reactive oxygen species (ROS) and secretion of molecular modulators. It may also be immune mediated where there is participation of lymphocytes and antigen-presenting cells. This second type is closely associated with the initiation and maintenance of chronic inflammations (Pompeia et al. 1999).

In our laboratory it was found that both diets rich in n-3 PUFA and n-6 PUFA (which promote the release of potent inflammatory eicosanoids) promote, on the model of rat paw edema induced by carrageenan, reduced inflammatory response and increased plasma concentration of corticosteroids, potent anti-inflammatory mediators (Silveira et al. 1995). As adrenalectomy abolished the effect of anti-inflammatory diets, the decreased inflammatory response in both groups was attributed to high levels of corticosteroids observed and possible changes in cytokines and / or other mediators corticosteroid dependent.

Over out control inflammation is now considered a central component in many chronic diseases. Wohlers et al. (2005) again showed that both diets increased corticosteroid levels and the anti-inflammatory cytokine, IL-10, and reduced plasma kallikrein, bradykinin and nitric oxide (NO) from inflammatory exudates, H_2O_2 and NO released by stimulated macrophages. The diets promoted also a decrease in the pro-inflammatory cytokines, IL-1 and IL-6, analyzed on exudate and serum (Wohlers et al. 2007).

Pufas and Chronic Diseases

Inconsistencies on different type of dietary fatty acid recommendation seem to be related to the difficulty of interpretation from scientific evidence (Smit et al. 2009). Several evidence are available, including that from the randomized controlled trials (RCTs), prospective cohort studies, retrospective case-control studies, ecological studies, cross-sectional studies, case series or reports and animal studies. The creation of fatty acids dietary guidelines, it is fundamentally important for the upper and lower knowledge level that has to be consumed daily.

In experimental colitis, we have demonstrated that a normal fat diet, with balance on n-3/n-6 PUFA ratio (Soybean and fish oil mixture, 2:1), is able to change the colon fatty acid incorporation, protects against lose weight, and reduces disease activity index. The diet decreased the myeloperoxidase activity, suggesting a reduced neutrophil infiltration in colon tissue, increased IL-10 and protecting against DNA damage, when compared to colitic rats that received a control diet with 11:1 n-6/n-3 ratio. In colitis we could observe that the mixture of fish and soybean oil (2:1) in the diet was better than the use of fish oil as an exclusive source of fat (Barros et al. 2010).

Fish or soybean oil rich-diets likewise exerted a potential anti-inflammatory effect upon the experimental asthma, decreasing lung inflammatory process. Total and differential cell counts, IL-4 and IL-5 cytokines and bradykinin were reduced; while NO was increased. Lipoxin A4 and corticosterone were also increased in the soybean group. The beneficial anti-inflammatory action of diets was related to the reduction of Th2 response, balance between bradykinin and NO and the alterations in the lipoxin A4 and corticosterone levels (Navarro Xavier et al. 2010 a, b).

N-3/N-6 Ratio

An ideal balance between different types of PUFA in the diet has been studied. The n-6/n-3 ratio found in the Paleolithic man was estimated at 1:1 to 5:1, while today this ratio is around 20:1 to 50:1. The prevalence of n-6 PUFA in western diets has many causes, including new technologies that focus on cereal-based foods rich in n-6 and poor in n-3 PUFA, culminating with the impoverishment of their contents in beef, eggs and milk, the higher consumption of vegetable oils with high content of n-6 PUFA, strongly recommended by physicians in the 60 and 70, by being able to lower cholesterol levels, and the reduced presence of n-3 PUFA in fish creation in relation to fish that feeds mainly on phytoplankton. It is suggested that in an ideal diet, intake of n-6 exceeds that of n-3, there are controversies regarding the optimal ratio, which ranges from 4:1 to 14:1 (Holman et al. 1998).

However, in most western populations the n-3 PUFA consumption is not enough to maintain health and prevent diseases (Elmadfa and Kornsteiner 2009). Also, it is necessary a multidisciplinary work involving researchers, policy-makers and the food industry in order to translate the science and dietary guidelines for PUFA into practical coherent dietary recommendation and high quality products that allow people to improve the fat quality of their diets and benefit their health (Calder 2010).

Sufficient intakes of PUFA during childhood are required for optimal growth and development and for prevention of the onset of chronic disease in later life. Consumption of a healthy diet that includes PUFA throughout the life is important to maintain cardiovascular and possibly also cognitive and immune health (WHO/FAO 2003).

Polymorphisms

The relationship between genetic and environment has been recognized as base of knowledge among disease and health. On the last two decade, considering advances in molecular biology has been demonstrated that genetics factors determine diseases susceptibility, while environment determine if genetically susceptible individuals will be affected (Simopoulos et al. 2008, Paolini-Giacobini et al. 2003). In this context, the nutritional aspects are being considered as one of the most important environmental factors (Simopoulos et al. 2008). Several studies have shown mechanisms which genes may influence the metabolism of nutrients as well as mechanisms that nutrients can influence gene expression (Simopoulos et al. 2008, Paolini-Giacobini et al. 2003, Calder 2007). With advances in science, and emphasis on studies of nutrigenomics and nutrigenetics, it has been shown that certain nutrients can influence the inflammatory response, accelerating or regressing time curing diseases (Simopoulos et al. 2008, Paoloni-Giacobino et al. 2003, Heller et al. 2002, Weiss et al. 2002, Mayer et al. 2003).

It is well known that not all individuals respond to nutritional therapy (NT) in the same way. For any nutrient used in NT it is possible to find individuals with good response, poor response or non-responders. Due to the considerable individual variability, large number of patients is necessary in studies of nutritional intervention (Paolini-Giacobini et al. 2003). The variation in the intensity of the inflammatory response in chronic diseases, including sepsis, and also the longevity of life in the elderly have been associated with single nucleotide polymorphisms (SNPs) (Visentainer et al. 2003, Nakada et al. 2005, Mira et al. 1999, Cederholm et al. 2007). These polymorphisms are present in regulatory regions of genes that encode pro-inflammatory cytokines may affect the transcription rate and synthesis of cytokines (Visentainer et al. 2003), may alter the immunological and inflammatory responses. Population differences in frequency of alleles in genes that encode cytokines, may contribute to the incidence of different diseases (Carvalho-Silva et al. 2001).

Regarding this, some studies have shown that genetic variability in FADS1-FADS-2 gene cluster encoding delta-5 (D5D) and delta-6 (D6D) desaturases has been associated with plasma long-chain PUFA and lipid levels in adults (Bokor et al.2010). Desaturases and elongases catalyse the conversion of PUFAs in humans. The D5D and D6D desaturases are known to be the key enzyme of this pathway. Both desaturases are expressed in a majority of human tissue, with the highest levels in liver but also with major amounts in brain, heart and lungs. The hypothesis that they play a key role in inflammatory diseases is strengthened by functional studies in mice, where selective D5D and D6D inhibitors showed an anti-inflammatory response.

Several single nucleotid polimophism (SNP) in FADS genes were reported in humans, and some showed association between FADS SNPs and fatty acids in serum or plasma phospholipids, erythrocyte membrane and adipose tissue (Schaeffer et al. 2006; Malerba et al. 2008; Rzehak et al. 2009) demonstrating that theses concentration are influenced not only by diet, but to a large extent also genetic variants common in the world population (Koletzko et al. 2011).

Resolution of Inflammation

The inflammatory response is designed to remove the inciting stimulus and resolve tissue damage. However, excessive inflammatory response can cause local tissue damage and remodelling, which may lead to a significant and chronic injury. Therefore acute inflammation in healthy individuals is self-limited and has an active termination program (Seki et al. 2009). In the past, was believed that this termination program was a passive mechanism but, nowadays is known that the process of resolution inflammation is an active and well controlled event, in part due by the formation of newly endogenous mediators that acts as local autacoids stimulating proresolving mechanisms (Serhan 2007, Gilroy et al. 2004). These proresolving mediators are derived from essential fatty acids that include lipoxins (Lx) from arachidonic acid (AA) and resolvins (Rv) and protectins from eicosapentaenoic acid (EPA) and docosahexaenoic acid (DHA) (Gilroy et al. 2004) that are biosynthesized in inflammatory exudates during spontaneous resolution.

Lipoxins were first described in 1984 by Serhan and co-workers, being the first mediators recognized to have dual anti-inflammatory and pro-resolution activities (Serhan & Savill 2005, Simopoulos 2008). The Lipoxins (LXA4 and LXB4) are lipoxygenase-derived eicosanoids enzymatically from AA, n-6 PUFA, which is released and mobilized, during inflammation (Samuelsson 1987) and has potent actions *in vivo* and *in vitro*. In humans, they are biosynthesized via transcellular metabolic events during leucocyte interactions with mucosal cells, that is, epithelium of the gastrointestinal tract or bronchial tissue, and within the vasculature during platelet–leucocyte interactions (Serhan 2007). The murine dorsal air pouch was used to determine the formation and roles of endogenous LXA4 in the resolution of acute inflammation (Levy et al. 2001).

It is important to know that to reach the resolution phase, the onset of the inflammatory response have to occur, since within the inflammatory exudate, arachidonate-derived eicosanoids changed from initial production of prostaglandins (PGs) and leukotrienes (LTs) to lipoxins, as part of resolution. Lipoxins signal macrophages to enhance engulfment of apoptotic (Godson 2000), are also potent chemoattractants, but in a non-philogistic manner as they activate infiltration of mononuclear cells without stimulating release of proinflammatory chemokines or activation of pro-inflammatory gene pathways and products (Serhan 2007).

Omega 3-PUFA has long been known to be important in maintaining organ function and health and even in reducing the incidence of infection and inflammation (Serhan et al. 2002, Arita el al. 2005, Burr & Burr 1973, Galli & Rise 2009, Riediger et al. 2009, Kasuga et al. 2008).

Originally, it was hypothesized that fish oils demonstrate their anti-thrombotic, immuno-regulatory and anti-inflammatory bio-actions by inhibiting PGs and LTs synthesis (De Caterina 1983). But since the discovery of novel proresolving compounds released from EPA and DHA, that are responsible for eliciting these immuno-modulatory effects, a new look has been given to the Omega 3-PUFA.

First identified in the resolving exudate of a mouse dorsal air pouch or peritonitis model (Serhan et al. 2000, Serhan et al. 2002, Lu et al. 2005, Serhan et al. 2009), these naturally occurring bioactive lipid mediators are termed Rvs (derived from 'resolution phase interaction products'), protectins and maresins (derived from 'macrophage mediator in resolving inflammation'). All these n-3 PUFA-derived products possess stereo specific and potent anti-inflammatory and immuno-regulatory actions that are protective in vitro and in vivo (Serhan 2008a, Serhan 2008b). RvE1 and RvE2 can be produce by conversion of 18R-HEPE released from endothelial cells to leukocytes for subsequent by 5-LOX, via a 5(6) epoxide-containing intermediate (Arita et al. 2005a). RvE1 is spontaneously produced in healthy subjects, with levels increasing after treatment with either aspirin or EPA (Arita et al. 2005b). Interestingly, microbial and mammalian cytochrome P450 enzymes are also involved in generating E-series Rvs. They convert EPA in 18-HEPE, which can then be transformed by human neutrophils into either RvE1 or RvE2. Besides RvE1 was discovery recent, it has been demonstrated in several animal models of inflammatory diseases, as a potent counter regulatory actions that protect against leukocyte-mediated tissue injury and excessive proinflammatory gene expressions, *in vitro* and *in vivo* (Periodontal disease model, Inflammatory bowel disease model, Asthma model, Hypoxia-induced retinopathy model, zymosan induced peritonites), being neutrophils, dendritic cells, macrophages and adhesion molecules, target cells of RvE1 (Seiki et al. 2009).

RvE1 exerts its effects by acting via at least two distinct G protein coupled receptors: CMKLR1 receptor expressed predominantly on monocytes/macrophages and plasmacytoid dendritic cells that mediate cell migration (Samson et al. 1998, Wittamaer et al. 2003, Cash et al. 2008), and the LTB4 receptor 1 (BLT1). Studies have established that RvE1 binds to the human BLT1 with relatively lower affinity than CMKLR1 (Arita et al. 2007). RvE1 effectively competes with LTB4 for BLT1 binding to functionally antagonize LTB4-mediated responses. The RvE2 actions are also receptor-mediated, yet the molecular identity of the RvE2 receptor has not been established (Uddin & Levy 2001).

On the other hand, DHA is also a substrate for the production of D series Rvs. The two major classes of D-series resolvins have been named resolvins (RvD1 to RvD4) and pirin-triggered (AT) resolvins (AT-RvD1 to AT-RvD4) (Serhan et al. 2004). Specific binding sites for RvD1 were recently identified on human leukocytes (Krishnamoorthy et al. 2010). RvD1 interacts with phagocyte GPCR-32 as a potent agonist to signal for pro-resolving actions and can directly activate ALX/FPR2 with high affinity and is as equipotent as LXA4. The ALX/FPR2 receptor is up regulated during experimental airway inflammation and lung injury to serve as a mechanism for LX-mediated catabasis (Levy et al. 2002, Bonnans et al. 2006).

In addition to LXs, this receptor may also has important roles for RvD1's pro-resolving actions in the airway and is the subject of ongoing research. ALX/FPR2 expression is relatively decreased in eosinophils and neutrophils in severe asthma (Planaguma et al. 2008), raising the possibility that this condition represents a deficit in pro-resolving signalling. PD1 is also a DHA product that is decreased during acute exacerbations of asthma and the bronchoprotective actions of PD1 have recently been demonstrated in a murine model of allergic asthma *in vivo* (Levy et al. 2007).

The proresolving actions of maresins have recently been demonstrated during the resolution of murine peritonitis *in vivo* (Serhan et al. 2009) and have not yet been examined in the context of pulmonary inflammation.

To better understand the role of specialized mediators in the resolution phase, relevant parameters of resolution indices were introduced (more information in Bannenberg et al. 2005, Schwab et al. 2007). These indices track neutrophilic infiltration, their maxima, and the duration of their presence at inflammatory sites and within exudates. In this scenario, LXA4 acts as STOP signals blocking the LTB4 actions (Serhan & Sevill 2005).

Rvs and protectins reduce the amplitude of neutrophilic infiltration, but also shortened the resolution interval, which reflects on the duration of the resolution phase (Seki et al. 2010). Considering that, many anti-inflammatory therapies in use such as nonsteroidals, anti-inflammatory drugs, etc, were developed to reduce the initiation and amplitude of an inflammatory event along with the reduction of the cardinal signs of inflammation, which can actually lead to an enhanced duration of the inflammatory response (Serhan 2010). This happen because, especially in the case of COX-2 inhibitors (Gilroy et al. 1999), which block PG formation, is relevant to resolution. Bringing the idea that anti-inflammatories can be toxicity for resolution, affecting it by blocking key steps in this process, thus prolonging inflammation (Chiang et al. 2008, Gilroy et al. 1999), which can be rescued by administration of LXA4, RvE1 and PD2 (Schwab et al. 2007). On the other hand, stables analogs of glucocorticoids do stimulate macrophage uptake of apoptotic neutrophils (Heasman et al. 2003) and via Anexin A1, has demonstrated a role in the resolution by stimulating the Lx receptor (Perretti & D'Acquisto 2009), but are ultimately immunosuppressive. Additionally, COX-2 inhibitors can delay resolution by blocking the formation of Rvs and other proresolving mediators (Serhan 2010).

Besides inflammatory models used to test newly anti-inflammatory drugs is not effective to test a proresolving agent, since anti-inflammatory drugs are traditionally tested for efficacy during the first hours of onset and their ability to trigger proresolution parameters is never investigated. As a result, there is now, a necessity of drugs that mimic the mode of action of endogenous proresolution mediators to drive ongoing inflammation down to a proresolution pathway (Navarro-Xavier et al. 2010 c). For this purpose a new strategy was presented by Navarro-Xavier and co-workers (2010) based on the increasing understanding of the resolution pathways to help to identify novel drugs for their ability to switch inflammation off and restore homeostasis. The use of this system also allows discrimination between the actions of resolving macrophages and processes, such as efferocytosis (Serhan et al. 2010).

In summation, the identification of the main cellular events and the molecular pathways that predicts the switch off inflammation and the beginning of resolution is a key step to the treatment of chronic inflammatory diseases, where the specialized mediators of the resolution phase, Lx, Rvs and PDs have an important role. This field is entering to an exciting period of development of many novel therapeutic approaches to inflammation.

References

Arita M, Bianchini F, Aliberti J, Sher A, Chiang N, Hong S, et al. Stereochemical assignment, antiinflammatory properties, and receptor for the omega-3 lipid mediator resolvin E1. *J Exp Med.* 201:713–22, 2005b.

Arita M, Clish CB, Serhan CN. The contributions of aspirin and microbial oxygenase to the biosynthesis of anti-inflammatory resolvins: novel oxygenase products from omega-3 polyunsaturated fatty acids. *Biochem Biophys Res Commun.* 338:149–57, 2005a.

Arita M, Ohira T, Sun YP, Elangovan S, Chiang N, Serhan CN. Resolvin E1 selectively interacts with leukotriene B4 receptor BLT1 and ChemR23 to regulate inflammation. *J Immunol.* 178:3912–7, 2007.

Arntzen KJ, Brekke OL, Vatten L and Austgulen R. Reduced Production of PGE2 and PGF2 from decidual cells cultures suplemented with n-3 polyunsaturated fatty acids. *Prostaglandins & Other Lipid Mediators.* 56: 183-195, 1988.

Bannenberg GL, Chiang N, Ariel A, Arita M, Tjonahen E, Gotlinger KH, Hong S, Serhan CN: Molecular circuits of resolution: formation and actions of resolvins and protectins. *J Immunol.* 174:4345–4355, 2005.

Barber RC, Aragaki CC, Rivera-Chavez FA, Purdue GF, Hunt JL, Horton JW. TLR4 and TNF-alpha polymorphisms are associated with an increased risk for severe sepsis following burn injury. *J Med Genet.* 41:808-13, 2004.

Barros KV, Xavier RA, Abreu GG, Martinez CA, Ribero ML Gambero A, Carvalho PO, Nascimento CM, Silveira VL. Soybean and fish oil mixture protects against DNA damage and decrease colonic inflammation in rats with dextran sulfate sodium (DSS). *Lipids Health Dis.* 68:8-14, 2010.

Bjorksten B. Fatty acids and inflammatory responses: Is there a connection? *Acta. Pediatric. Scand. Suppl.* 351: 76-79, 1989.

Bokor S, Dumont J, Spinneker A, Gonzalez-Gross M, et al. Single nucleotide polymorphisms in the FADS gene cluster are associated with delta-5 and delta-6 desaturase activities estimated by serum fatty acid ratios. *J Lipid Res.* 51(8):2325-33, 2010.

Bonnans C, Fukunaga K, Levy MA, Levy BD. Lipoxin A(4) regulates bronchial epithelial cell responses to acid injury. *Am J Pathol.* 168:1064–72, 2006.

Burr GO, Burr MM. A new deficiency disease produced by the rigid exclusion of fat from the diet. *Nutr Rev.* 31:248–9, 1973.

Calder PC. Dietary modifications with lipids. *Proc Nutr Soc.* 61: 345-358, 2002.

Calder PC. Effects of fatty acids and dietary lipids on cell of the immune system. *Proc. Nutr Soc.* 55: 127-150, 1996.

Calder PC, Immunomodulation by omega-3 fatty acids. *Prostaglandins Leukot Essent Fatty Acids.* 77:327-35, 2007.

Calder PC. Long-chain n-3 fatty acids and inflammation: potential application in surgical and trauma patients. *Braz J Med Biol Res.* 36: 433-446, 2003.

Calder PC. N-3 polyunsaturated fatty acids and immune cell function. *Adv. Enzyme Regul.* 37: 197-237, 1997.

Calder PC, Dangour AD, Diekman C, et al. Essential fats for future health. Proceedings of the 9th Unilever Nutrition Symposium, 26–27 May 2010. *European Journal of Clinical Nutrition.* 64: S1–S13, 2010.

Carvalho-Silva DR, Santos FR, Rocha J & Pena S.D. The phylogeography of Brazilian Y-chromosome lineages. *American Journal of Human Genetics*. 68:281-289, 2001.

Cash JL, Hart R, Russ A, Dixon JP, Colledge WH, Doran J, et al. Synthetic chemerin-derived peptides suppress inflammation through ChemR23. *J Exp Med*. 205:767–75, 2008.

Cederholm T, Persson M, Anderson P et al. Polymorphisms in cytokine genes influence long-term survival differently in elderly male and female patients. *Journal of Internal Medicne*. 262:215-223, 2007.

Chiang N, Schwab JM, Fredman G, Kasuga K, Gelman S, Serhan CN: Anesthetics impact the resolution of inflammation. *PLoS ONE*. 3:e1879, 2008.

Chow SC, Sisfontes L, Jondal M, Bjorkhem I. Modification of membrane phospholipid fatty acyl composition in a leukemic T cell line: effects on receptor mediated intracellular Ca2+ increase. *Biochim Biophys Acta*. 92: 358-66, 1991.

De Caterina R, Caprioli R, Giannessi D, Sicari R, Galli C, Lazzerini G, et al. n-3 fatty acids reduce proteinuria in patients with chronic glomerular disease. *Kidney Int*. 44:843–50, 1993.

Denys A, Hichami A, and Khan NA. n-3 PUFAs modulate T-cell activation via protein kinase C-α and -£ and the NF- kB signaling pathway. *Journal of Lipid Research*. 46, 2005.

Dickinson S, Hancock DP, Petocz P, Ceriello A, Brand-Miller J. High-glycemic index carbohydrate increases nuclear factor-kappaB activation in mononuclear cells of young, lean healthy subjects. *Am J Clin Nutr*. 87:1188-93, 2008.

Elmadfa I, Kornsteiner M. Fats and fatty acid requirements for adults. *Ann.Nutr. Metab*. 55: 56-75, 2009.

Form DM, Averback R. PGE2 and angiogenesis. *Proceedings of the society of Experimental Biology and medicine*. 172: 214-218, 1993.

Galli C, Rise P. Fish consumption, omega 3 fatty acids and cardiovascular disease. The science and the clinical trials. *Nutr Health*. 20:11–20, 2009.

Gilroy DW, Colville-Nash PR, Willis D, Chivers J, Paul-Clark MJ, Willoughby DA: Inducible cycloxygenase may have anti-inflammatory properties. *Nat Med*. 5:698–701, 1999.

Gilroy DW, Newson J, Sawmynaden P, Willoughby DA, and Croxtall JD. A novel role for phospholipase A2 isoforms in the checkpoint control of acute inflammation. *FASEB J*. 18: 489–498, 2004.

Godson C, Mitchell S, Harvey K, Petasis NA, Hogg N, Brady HR.Cutting edge: lipoxins rapidly stimulate nonphlogistic phagocytosis of apoptotic neutrophils by monocyte-derived macrophages. *J Immunol*. 164:1663–7, 2000.

Goldman DW, Pickett WC, and Goetzl EJ. Human neutrophil chenotatic and degranulating activities of leukotriene B5 derived from eicosapentaenopic acid. *Biochem. Biophys. Res. Commun*. 117: 282-288, 1983.

Hang HP, Dale MM. *Farmacologia*. 3 ed. Guanabara Koogan, 1995.

Harbidgel LS. Dietary w-6 e w-3 fatty acids in immunity and autoimmune disease. *Proc Nutr Soc*. 57:555-62,1998.

Heasman SJ, Giles KM, Ward C, Rossi AG, Haslett C, Dransfield I: Glucocorticoid-mediated regulation of granulocyte apoptosis and macrophage phagocytosis of apoptotic cells: implications for the resolution of inflammation. *J Endocrinol*. 178:29–36, 2003.

Heller AR, Fischer S, Rossel T et al. Impact of n-3 fatty acid supplemented parenteral nutrition on haemostasis patters after major abdominal surgery. *Brit J Nutr.* 87:S95-S101; 2002.

Holman RT. The slow discovery of the importance of n-3 essential fatty acids in human health. *J. Nutr.* 128: 427S-433S, 1998.

Kasuga K, Yang R, Porter TF, Agrawal N, Petasis NA, Irimia D, Toner M, Serhan CN. Rapid appearance of resolvin precursors in inflammatory exudates: novel mechanisms in resolution. *J Immunol.* 15;181(12):8677-87, 2008.

Kelley D, and Daudu PA. Fat intake and immune response. *Prog Food Nutr Sci.* 17: 17-63, 1993.

Koletzko B, Lattka E, Zeilinger S, Illig T, Steer C. Genetic variants of the fatty acid desaturase gene cluster predict amounts of red blood cell docosahexaenoic and other polyunsaturated fatty acids in pregnant women: findings from the Avon Longitudinal Study of Parents and Children. *Am J Clin Nutr.* 93(1):211-9, 2011.

Krishnamoorthy S, Recchiuti A, Chiang N, Yacoubian S, Lee CH, Yang R, et al. Resolvin D1 binds human phagocytes with evidence for proresolving receptors. *Proc Natl Acad Sci USA.* 107:1660–5, 2010.

Kromann N, and Green A. Epidemiological studies in the Upernavik district, Greenland. Incidence of some chronic diseases, 1950-1974. *Acta. Med. Scand.* 208 (5): 401-6, 1980.

Lee TH, Mencia-Huerta JM, Shih C, Corey EJ, Lewis RA, and Austen KF. Characterization and biologic properties of 5, 12- dihydroxy derivatives of eicosapentaenoic acid. *J. Biol. Chem.* 259: 2383-2389, 1984.

Levy BD, Clish CB, Schmidt B, Gronert K, Serhan CN. Lipid mediator class switching during acute inflammation: signals in resolution. *Nat Immunol.* 2:612–19, 2001.

Levy BD, De Sanctis GT, Devchand PR, Kim E, Ackerman K, Schmidt BA, et al. Multi-pronged inhibition of airway hyper-responsiveness and inflammation by lipoxin A(4). *Nat Med.* 8:1018–23, 2002.

Levy BD, Lukacs NW, Berlin AA, Schmidt B, Guilford WJ, Serhan CN, et al. Lipoxin A4 stable analogs reduce allergic airway responses via mechanisms distinct from CysLT1 receptor antagonism. *FASEB J.* 21:3877–84, 2007.

Lu Y, Hong S, Tjonahen E, Serhan CN. Mediator-lipidomics: databases and search algorithms for PUFA-derived mediators. *J Lipid Res.* 46:790–802, 2005.

Malerba G, Schaeffer L, Xumerle L, et al. SNPs of the FADS gene cluster are associated with polyunsaturated fatty acids in a cohort of patients with cardiovascular disease. *Lipids*, 2008.

Mayer K, Gokorsc S, Fegbeutel C, Hattar K et al. Parenteral nutrition with fish oil modulates cytokine response in patients with sepsis. *Am J Resp Crit Care Med.* 167:1321-1328; 2003.

Medzhitov R, Janeway CA. Innate immunity: the virtues of a nonclonal system of recognition. *Cell.* 91: 295-8, 1997.

Miles EA, and Calder PC. Modulation of immune function by dietary fatty acids.Proceed *Nutr.Soc.* 57: 277-292, 1998.

Mira JP, Cariou A, et al. Association of TNF2, a TNF-α promoter polymorphism, with septic shock susceptibility and mortality- A multicenter study. *JAMA.* 11(1):282, 1989.

Molto-Puigmart C, Plat J, Mensink RP, et al. FADS1 FADS2 gene variants modify the association between fish intake and the docosahexaenoic acid proportions in human milk. *Am J Clin Nutr*. 91:1368–76, 2010.

Nakada T, et al. Influence of toll-like receptor 4, CD14, tumor necrosis factor, and interleukine-10 gene polymorphisms on clinical outcome in Japanese critically ill patients. *J Surg Reserch*. 129:322-328, 2005.

Navarro Xavier RA, Pedreira de Castro MA, Abreu GG, Andrade IS, Silveira VLF. Fish oil or soybean oil-rich diet in experimental asthma: Immunodulatory and anti-inflammatory effect. In *.9th Conference of the International Society for the Study of Fatty Acids and Lipids (ISSFAL),* Maastricht, Netherlands, 2010 a.

Navarro Xavier RA, Barros KV, Abreu GG, Silveira VF. Inflammatory mediators are modified by soybean (PUFA n-6) or fish (PUFA n-3) oil-rich diets: antiinflammatory effect upon the development of experimental asthma. In *9th Conference of the International Society for the Study of Fatty Acids and Lipids (ISSFAL)*, Maastricht, Netherlands, 2010 b.

Navarro Xavier RA, Newson J, Silveira VLF, Farrow SN, Gilroy DW, Bystrom J. A new strategy for the identification of novel molecules with targeted proresolution of inflammation properties. *J Immunol*. 184:1516–1525, 2010 c.

Novak TE, Babcock TA, Jho DH, et al. NF-kB inhibition by w-3 fatty acids modulates LPS-stimulated macrophage TNF-a transcription. *Am J Physiol Lung Cell Mol Physiol*. 284:84-9, 2003.

Obata T, Nagakura T, Masaki T, Maekawa K, and Yamashita K. Eicosapentaenoic acid inhibits prostaglandin D2 generation by inhibiting cyclo-oxigenase-2 in cultured human mast cells. *Clin. Exper. Allergy*. 29: 1129-1135, 1999.

Otani S, Oda S, Sadahiro T, Nakamura M, Watanabe E, Nakada TA, Abe R, Tokuhisa T, Hirasawa H. Clinical application of cytokine-related gene polymorphism analysis using a newly developed DNA chip in critically ill patients. *Clin Biochem*. 42:1387-93, 2009.

Paoloni-Giacobino A, Grimble R, and Pichard C. Genomic interactions with disease and nutrition. *Clin Nutr*. 22:507-514, 2003.

Planaguma A, Kazani S, Marigowda G, Haworth O, Mariani TJ, Israel E, et al. Airway lipoxin A4 generation and lipoxin A4 receptor expression are decreased in severe asthma. *Am J Respir Crit Care Med*. 178:574–82, 2008.

Perretti M, D'Acquisto F. Annexin A1 and glucocorticoids as effectors of the resolution of inflammation. *Nat Rev Immunol*. Jan;9(1):62-70, 2009.

Pompéia C, Lopes LR, Miyasaka CK, Procópio J, Sannomiya P. Effect of fatty acids on leukocyte function. *Med. Res*. 33 (11): 1255-68, 2000.

Pot GK, Geelen A, Majsak-Newman G, et al. Increased Consumption of Fatty and Lean Fish Reduces Serum C-Reactive Protein Concentrations but Not Inflammation Markers in Feces and in Colonic Biopsies. *J Nutri*. 140: 371-6, 2010.

Priante G, Bordin L, Musacchio E, Clari G, and Baggio B. Fatty acids and cytokine mRNA expression in human osteoblastic cells: a specific effect of arachidonic acid. *Clin. Sci*. 102: 403-409, 2002.

Raedestorff D, Pantzem, Bachmannh H, Moser U. Anti-inflammatory properties of docosahexaenoic and eicosapentaenoic acids in Phorbol-Ester Induced Mouse Ear Inflammation. *Int Arch Immunol*. 111: 284-290, 1996.

Rahman SM, Wang Y, Yotsumoto H, Cha J, Han S, Inoue S, Yanagita T. Effects of conjugated linoleic acid on serum leptin concentration, body-fat accumulation, and beta-oxidation on fatty acid in OLEFT rats. *Nutrition*. 17(5): 385-390, 2001.

Rankin Ja. Biological mediators of acute inflammation. *AACN Clin Issues*. 15(1): 3-17, 2004.

Riediger ND, Othman RA, Suh M, Moghadasian MH. A systemic review of the roles of n-3 fatty acids in health and disease. *J Am Diet Assoc*. 109:668–79, 2009.

Rios DLS, Cerqueira CCS, Bonfim-Silva R, et al. Interleukine-1 beta and interleukine-6 gene polymorphism associoations with angiographically assessed coronary artery disease in Brazlians. *Cytokine*. 20:292-296, 2010.

Rivera-Chavez FA, Peters-Hybki DL, Barber RC, O'Keefe GE. Interleukin-6 promoter haplotypes and interleukin-6 cytokine responses. *Shock* 20:218-23, 2003.

Roos B, Mavrommatis Y, Brouwer IA. Long-chain n-3 polyunsaturated fatty acids: new insights into mechanisms relating to inflammation and coronary heart disease. *British Journal of Pharmacology*. 158: 413-28, 2009.

Rzehak P, Heinrich J, Klopp N, et al. Evidence for an association between genetic variants of the fatty acid desaturase 1 fatty acid desaturase 2 (FADS1 FADS2) gene cluster and the fatty acid composition of erythrocyte membranes. *Br J Nutr*. 101:20–6, 2009.

Saadi S, Wrenshall LE, Platt JL. Regional manifesttions and control of the immune system. *FASEB J*. 16(8):849-56. 2002.

Samson M, Edinger AL, Stordeur P, Rucker J, Verhasselt V, Sharron M, et al. ChemR23, a putative chemoattractant receptor, is expressed in monocytederived dendritic cells and macrophages and is a coreceptor for SIV and some primary HIV-1 strains. *Eur J Immunol*. 28:1689–700, 1998.

Samuelsson B, Dahlen SE, Lindgren JA, Rouzer CA, Serhan CN. Leukotrienes and lipoxins: structures, biosynthesis, and biological effects.*Science*. 237:1171–6, 1987.

Sane S, Baba M, Kusano C, Shirao K, Andoh T, Kamada T, and Aikou T. Eicosapentaenoic acid reduces pulmonary edema in endotoxemic rats. *J. Surg. Res*. 93: 21-27, 2000.

Schaeffer L, Gohlke H, Muller M, et al. Common genetic variants of the FADS1 FADS2 gene cluster and their reconstructed haplotypes are associated with the fatty acid composition in phospholipids. *Human Molecular Genetics*. 15 (11): 1745–1756, 2006.

Schwab JM, Chiang N, Arita M, Serhan CN: Resolvin E1 and protectin D1 activate inflammation-resolution programmes. *Nature*. 447:869–874, 2007.

Seki H, Fukunaga K, Arita M, Arai H, Nakanishi H, Taguchi R, Miyasho T, Takamiya R, Asano K, Ishizaka A, Takeda J, Levy BD: The anti-inflammatory and proresolving mediator resolvin E1 protects mice from bacterial pneumonia and acute lung injury. *J Immunol*. 184:836–843, 2010.

Seki H, Tani Y, Arita M. Omega-3 PUFA derived anti-inflammatory lipid mediator resolvin E1. *Prostaglandins Other Lipid Mediat*. 89(3-4):126-30, 2009.

Serhan CN. Controlling the resolution of acute inflammation: a new genus of dual anti-inflammatory and proresolving mediators. *J Periodontol*. 79:1520–6, 2008a.

Serhan CN. Novel lipid mediators and resolution mechanisms in acute inflammation: to resolve or not? *Am J Pathol*. 177(4):1576-91, 2010.

Serhan CN. Resolution phases of inflammation: novel endogenous anti-inflammatory and pro-resolving lipid mediators and pathways. *Annu. Rev. Immunol*. 25: 101–137, 2007.

Serhan CN. Systems approach with inflammatory exudates uncovers novel anti-inflammatory and pro-resolving mediators. *Prostaglandins Leukot Essent Fatty Acids.* 79:157–63, 2008b.

Serhan CN, Arita M, Hong S, Gotlinger K. Resolvins, docosatrienes, and neuroprotectins, novel omega-3-derived mediators, and their endogenous aspirin-triggered epimers. *Lipids*. 39:1125–32, 2004.

Serhan CN, Clish CB, Brannon J, Colgan SP, Chiang N, Gronert K. Novel functional sets of lipid-derived mediators with antiinflammatory actions generated from omega-3 fatty acids via cyclooxygenase 2-nonsteroidal antiinflammatory drugs and transcellular processing. *J Exp Med.* 192:1197–204, 2000.

Serhan CN, Clish CB, Brannon J, Colgan SP, Gronert K, and Chiang N. Anti-microinflammatory lipid signals generated from dietary n-3 fatty acids via cyclooxygenase-2 and transcellular processing: a novel mechanism for NSAID and n-3 PUFA therapeutic actions. *J. Phisiol. Pharmacol.* 51: 643-654, 2000.

Serhan CN, Hong S, Gronert K, Colgan SP, Devchand PR, Mirick G, et al. Resolvins: a family of bioactive products of omega-3 fatty acid transformation circuits initiated by aspirin treatment that counter proinflammation signals. *J Exp Med.* 196:1025–37, 2002.

Serhan CN, Sevill J. Resolution of inflammation: the beginning programsthe end. *Nat Immunol.* 6:1191–7, 2005.

Serhan CN, Yang R, Martinod K, Kasuga K, Pillai PS, Porter TF, et al. Maresins: novel macrophage mediators with potent antiinflammatory and proresolving actions. *J Exp Med.* 206:15–23, 2009.

Silveira VLF, Limões EA, Nunes DW. Participation of adrenal gland in the anti-inflammatory effect of polyunsaturated diets. *Mediators of Inflammation*. 4: 359-363, 1995.

Simopoulos AP. The importance of the omega-6 / omega-3 fatty acid ratio in cardiovascular disease and other chronic diseases. *ExpBiolMed*(Maywood). 233:674–88, 2008.

Smit LA, Mozaffarian D, Willett W. Review of fat and fatty acid requirements and criteria for developing dietary guidelines. *Ann Nutr Metab.* 55: 44–5, 2009.

Takeda K, Kaisho T, Akira S. Toll-like receptors. *Annu. Rev. Immunol.* 21: 335–376, 2003.

Tappia OS, Ladha S, Clark DC, Grimble RF. The influence of membrane fluidity; TNF receptor binding, cAMP production and GTP-ase activity on macrophage cytokine production in rats fed a variety of fat diets. *Mol. Cell Biochem.* 166: 135-43, 1997.

Uddin M, Levy BD. Resolvins: natural agonists for resolution of pulmonary inflammation. *Prog Lipid Res*. 50(1):75-88, 2011.

Visentainer JEL, Lieber SR, Persoli LBL, Vigorito AC, Aranha FJP, Eid KAB, et al. serum cytokine levels and acute graft-versus-host disease after HLA-identical hematopoietic stem cell transplantation. *Experimental Hematology*. 31:1044, 2003.

Weiss G, Meyer F, Mathies B, Pross M, et al. Immunomodulation by perioperative administration of n-3 fatty acids. *Brit J Nutr.* 87:S89-S94, 2002.

Wittamer V, Franssen JD, Vulcano M, Mirjolet JF, Le Poul E, Migeotte I, et al. Specific recruitment of antigen-presenting cells by chemerin, a novel processed ligand from human inflammatory fluids. *J Exp Med.* 198:977–85, 2003.

WHO/FAO. Diet, nutrition and the prevention of chronic diseases: report of a joint *WHO/FAO expert consultation*. Geneva 2003.

Wohlers M; Navarro Xavier RA; Oyama LM; Ribeiro EB; Nascimento CMO; DE Casarini; Silveira VLF. Effect of fish or soybean oil-rich diets on bradykinin, kallikrein, nitric oxide, leptin, corticosterone and macrophages in carrageenan stimulated rats. *Inflammation*, v. 29, p. 17-25, 2005.

Wohlers M, Xavier RAN, Silveira VLF. Effect of soybean and fish oil-rich diets on in vivo release of catecholamines and cytokines. *Ann Nutr Metab*. 51(1): 284-515, 2007.

Wu D, Mura C, Beharka AA, Nim Ham S, Paulson KE, Hwang D, Meydani SN. Age-associated increase in PGE2 synthesis and COX activity in murine macrophages is reversed by vitamin E. *Am J Physiol*. 275: C661-C668, 1998.

Zeng Y, Han X, Sclesinger P, Gross RW. Nonesterified fatty acids induce transmembrane monovalent cation flux: host-guest interactions as determinants of fatty acid-induced ion transport. *Biochemistry*. 37: 9497-508, 1998.

Zurier B. Essential fatty acids and inflammation. *Ann Rheum Dis*. 50 (11):745-6, 1991.

In: Fish Oil: Production, Consumption and Health Benefits
Editors: Matthias Van Dijk and Jürgen Vitek ISBN: 978-1-61470-963-3

Chapter X

The Combined Effects of Omega-3 Fatty Acids and Exercise on Cardiovascular Disease Risk and Mortality

Rodney G. Bowden and M. Renée Umstattd Meyer
Department of Health, Human Performance and Recreation,
School of Education, Baylor University, Waco, Texas, U. S.

Abstract

Myocardial infarction associated with atherosclerosis is the leading cause of death globally. Novel therapies are needed to reduce the rates of mortality and morbidity associated with cardiovascular disease (CVD). Previous study findings suggest omega-3 fatty acids (FO) may have a beneficial effect on risk for CVD and its associated morbidity and mortality rates. Both docosahexaenoic acid (DHA) and eicosapentaenoic acid (EPA) have demonstrated positive effects on cholesterol levels, inflammatory markers, blood pressure, endothelial dysfunction, resting hear rate, and arrhythmia. Study authors have reported positive effects on low-density lipoprotein cholesterol (LDL), high-density lipoprotein cholesterol (HDL), triglycerides, and emerging risk factors of LDL particle number and LDL size. Additionally, various study outcomes have demonstrated an effect of n-3 on inflammatory markers such as Interleukin-6 (IL-6), Interleukin-1beta (IL-1β), and Tumor Necrosis Factor-alpha (TNF-α). Many of these same effects have been reported for individuals who regularly engage in aerobic exercise including a decreased heart rate and additional improvements in heart rate variability. The primary inflammatory markers associated with exercise have been improved levels of IL-6, IL-1 β, TNF-α, and C-reactive protein (CRP). Therefore exercise may contribute to the reduction of vascular and inflammatory diseases, more specifically CVD. Recently, studies have emerged attempting to understand the effects of combining exercise and supplementing FO on mortality and morbidity associated with CVD. Findings have ranged from increased performance during exercise to improving heart function or heart rate variability, decreasing resting heart rates, and improving lipid and inflammatory profiles. Most importantly there has been emerging evidence that the combination of exercise and FO supplementation may have a synergistic effect when combined. Though little is known among the general public and health practitioners about this combination of therapy on the reduction in heart disease, a growing body of research has addressed this issue. Therefore the purpose of this chapter will be to explore the literature to address what effects combining exercise and FO supplementation have on CVD. Specifically we will address issues of cholesterol, inflammation, heart rate variability, blood pressure, and general health markers of CVD.

Exercise and CVD Risk and Mortality

Exercise and physical activity are well supported mechanisms in the promotion of health and prevention of disease. Regular physical activity and exercise have consistently been linked with lower mortality rates across the lifespan; chronic disease prevention, reduction, and management; and improved mental capability, depressive states, psychological health, independence, balance, bone and muscular strength, and overall quality of life. Additionally, evidence supports lower mortality and morbidity rates for those who are moderately active on a regular basis as compared with those who are the least active (U.S. Department of Health and Human Services [USDHHS], 1996). Chronic diseases associated with regular physical activity and exercise, benefits associated with cardiovascular health, cardiovascular disease (CVD), and related morbidity and mortality are undeniable (Carlson et al., 1999; Haskell et al., 2007; Mazzeo et al., 1998; Pate et al., 1995; Physical Activity Guidelines Advisory Committee [PAGAC], 2008; USDHHS, 1996).

Clarification between the terms exercise and physical activity are necessary before continuing. While these terms are often used interchangeably, they differ in definition and at times in their association with cardiovascular health and CVD prevention and reduction. Physical activity is defined as "any bodily movement produced by the contraction of skeletal muscle that increases energy expenditure above a basal level" (PAGAC, 2008, p. C-1). Exercise on the other hand is considered a sub-category of physical activity and is defined as any physical activity that is "planned, structured, and repetitive and purposive in the sense that the improvement or maintenance of one or more components of physical fitness is the objective" (Caspersen, Powell, & Christenson, 1985). Physical fitness is defined as "the ability to carry out daily tasks with vigor and alertness, without undue fatigue and with ample energy to enjoy leisure-time pursuits and meet unforeseen emergencies" (USDHHS, 1996, p. 20). The following are regularly recognized improvement or maintenance components of physical fitness: cardiorespiratory endurance; skeletal muscular endurance, strength, and power; flexibility; balance; movement speed; reaction time; and body composition (PAGAC, 2008). However, in reference to most research regarding the relationship between physical activity and CVD and cardiovascular health, aerobic exercise and resistance exercise are most commonly applied and referenced. Aerobic exercise is an effective means for improving cardiorespiratory endurance by primarily using the aerobic energy producing systems for energy while improving the capacity and efficiency of these systems (PAGAC, 2008). Resistance training is also referred to as strength training, muscular strength, muscular endurance, and muscle-strengthening activities and is exercise aimed to increase skeletal muscle strength, endurance, power, and mass (PAGAC, 2008).

When considering research examining the exact benefits of exercise and physical activity with regards to cardiovascular health and CVD prevention, evidence supports several consistent effects on CVD risk factors including cholesterol, both low-density lipoprotein cholesterol (LDL) and high-density lipoprotein cholesterol (HDL), triglycerides (TG), inflammation, blood pressure, heart rate variability, and other general health markers of CVD.

Exercise, Cholesterol, and Triglycerides

Information regarding the relationship between cholesterol and physical activity and exercise is vast, as cholesterol, specifically low serum concentrations of high-density lipoprotein (HDL) cholesterol and elevated low-density lipoprotein (LDL) cholesterol and TG levels are consistently related with increased risk of CVD, CVD related mortality, and more specifically atherosclerosis and coronary artery disease (USDHHS, 1996; PAGAC, 2008; Durstine et al., 2001). Research also consistently supports a positive relationship between aerobic exercise and HDL cholesterol where increased rates of exercise are related with increases in HDL cholesterol, therefore allowing for protection against atherosclerosis by improving the reverse cholesterol transport system and the return of cholesterol to the liver for elimination. Recently, a meta-analysis substantiated the claim that aerobic exercise is significantly related with increased HDL cholesterol levels, but noted that this is only at a modest level (2.53 mg/dL). This meta-analysis concluded that volume of exercise is the most important indicator of achieving exercise-related HDL effects, where a minimum level of approximately 120 minutes of exercise per week (10-12 metabolic equivalent [MET] hours per week) is required to obtain HDL cholesterol benefits (Kodama et al., 2007; PAGAC, 2008). In general, research also supports a significant inverse relationship between exercise and serum TG suggesting that increased rates of exercise are related with decreased serum TG levels. Levels of aerobic exercise required to incur reductions in TG are similar to levels required for HDL benefits and research suggests that sustained changes in TG are related with moderate intensity exercise versus vigorous intensity activity (PAGAC, 2008). It should be noted that some studies suggest that women are more resistant to the effect of exercise on TG levels, although this finding is not conclusive.

While exercise is supported as a significant mechanism for positive changes in both HDL cholesterol and TG, it is not generally related with LDL cholesterol reduction. In a few studies that have demonstrated slight support for this relationship, exercise-related benefits for LDL cholesterol tend to require slightly greater volumes of aerobic exercise (12 MET-hours per week) than required for HDL and TG benefits (PAGAC, 2008). Additionally, one relatively recent study found that in comparison to a sedentary control group, whose LDL cholesterol levels increased over time, that an exercise intervention group's LDL cholesterol levels did not change (Slentz et al., 2007), suggesting a meaningful benefit. However, further research is needed to fully understand the possible relationship between aerobic exercise and LDL cholesterol levels (PAGAC, 2008).

Exercise and Inflammation

The role of inflammation has been increasingly recognized as an indicator in the onset and progression of many chronic diseases including CVD (Beavers, Brinkley, & Nicklas, 2010; O'Connor & Irwin, 2009; Walsh et al., 2011). While inflammation is a natural and necessary biological response of the immune system, prolonged states of inflammation have been linked to increased health risk and are recognized as predictors of mortality and disability even in the absence of disease (Beavers et al., 2010). Research specifically supports the relationship between consistent slight elevation of inflammatory markers and atherosclerosis, heart failure, CVD, diabetes, cancer, coronary heart disease, insulin resistance, metabolic syndrome, sarcopenia, arthritis, osteoporosis, chronic obstructive pulmonary disease, dementia, and depression to name a few (Beavers et al., 2010; Walsh et al., 2011). Several specific inflammatory biomarkers are consistently related with CVD-related risk, with C-reactive protein (CRP) being the most frequently studied and associated. In addition to the consistently strong relationship seen between CRP and both CVD and cardiovascular health, several other inflammatory markers have emerged as prospective CVD risk factors, including interleukin-6 (IL-6), tumor necrosis factor alpha (TNF-α), interleukin-1 Beta (IL-1β), interleukin-15 (IL-15), and interleukin 8 (IL-8); however, it is not well understood if any of these markers are better indicators of inflammation than the others, or if there is increased risk with elevation of multiple markers. With the growth of evidence linking inflammation and chronic disease, including CVD, research examining the potential role of behavioral factors is warranted.

The association between physical activity and inflammation is regularly recognized and strongly supported with growing evidence linking various inflammatory biomarkers with exercise and physical activity. Although the underlying mechanisms acting in this relationship are not fully understood, two hypothesized mechanisms are fat mass and the establishment of an anti-inflammatory environment through each exercise session (Walsh et al., 2011). A recent literature review included 19 observational studies examining the relationship of inflammatory biomarkers and self-reported physical activity, 9 observational studies examining the relationship between inflammatory biomarkers and aerobic fitness, and 12 randomized control trials examining interventional effects of aerobic exercise and inflammatory biomarkers. The study summarizes the current findings from both observational and interventional studies supporting the role of aerobic exercise and physical activity in controlling and reducing inflammation. Specific study findings demonstrate aerobic exercise and/or physical activity as inversely associated with CRP concentration, IL-6, TNF-α, IL-8, tumor necrosis factor receptor-1 (sTNFR1), and tumor necrosis factor receptor-2 (sTNFR2) among other inflammatory markers (Beavers et al., 2010).

Since fat mass is a strongly supported correlate of inflammatory biomarkers and physical activity and exercise, fat mass is supported as one possible mechanism by which the relationship between exercise and inflammation is operating. To better understand the independent role of exercise in inflammation several studies have controlled for fat mass in analyses. Although not unanimously across studies, the relationship between tested inflammatory markers and physical activity remained significant in the majority of studies controlling for body mass index (BMI), thus supporting an independent effect of physical activity and/or aerobic exercise on inflammation (Beavers et al., 2010). Thus, it is safe to conclude that current research supports the relationship between physical activity and aerobic exercise and inflammatory biomarkers, even after controlling for measures of fat mass.

Exercise and Heart Rate Variability

Another cardiovascular adaptation produced by exercise is an increase in heart rate variability (HRV). Heart rate variability (HRV) is recognized as an important risk factor associated with chronic disease, including CVD and cardiovascular health, where reduced HRV is related with increased CVD risk and associated negative health outcomes. Research supports a significant relationship between a heart rate that is variable and responsive and increased health, including decreased risk and management of CVD, diabetes, chronic heart failure, myocardial infarction, and unstable angina (Carter, Banister, & Blaber, 2003; Routledge, Campbell, McFetridge-Durdle, & Bacon, 2010). With the innate onset of decreasing HRV and parasympathetic control of heart rate with age, the commonly recognized positive relationship between exercise and HRV is encouraging. Specifically, exercise engagement is related with decreased risk of chronic disease and CVD via an increase in HRV. Through the influence of long-term endurance exercise on autonomic nervous system activity, increases in HRV, increases in parasympathetic activity, and decreases in sympathetic activity are realized. The relationship between HRV and exercise is supported in both healthy patients and those with chronic disease. A recent review examined interventions to increase HRV and concluded with supporting exercise as a means to improve HRV in myocardial infarction, chronic heart failure, and revascularization patients. Two supported mechanisms by which this could be explained were presented: (1) through increased vagal tone and (2) through decreased sympathetic activity, whereby it is postulated that vagal modulation is improved via exercise through mediation by angiotensin II and nitric oxide (Routledge et al., 2010).

Exercise and Blood Pressure

High blood pressure is a strong predictor of CVD onset and mortality across the lifespan, including coronary heart disease, ischemic stroke, and peripheral vascular disease (USDHHS, 1996; PAGAC, 2008). Although blood pressure rates have declined since the mid 1900's, no significant declines have occurred in the past decade, with 30% of all U.S. adults reporting high blood pressure in 2008 (Yoon, Ostchega, & Louis 2010). The Surgeon General's report on physical activity (1996) and the Physical Activity Guidelines Advisory Committee report (2008) both review numerous meta-analyses examining the relationship between blood pressure and physical activity. In summary, studies consistently report a significant and strong relationship between aerobic exercise and reductions in systolic and diastolic blood pressure in adults, whereby aerobic exercise is defined by bouts of 40 minutes at a moderate-to-high intensity for 3-5 times per week (a sum of 800 MET-minutes of aerobic exercise / week). Although not as conclusive, additional and more recent evidence also supports the ability of progressive resistance exercise to reduce systolic and diastolic blood pressure (PAGAC, 2008). One recent and robust meta-analysis examining the effects of aerobic exercise and resting blood pressure involved hypertensive, prehypertensive, and normotensive adults and included 72 studies. This meta-analysis concluded that average resting blood pressure reductions ranged from 2-5 mmHG for resting systolic blood pressure and 2-3 mmHG for resting diastolic blood pressure, where hypertensive participants reported greater reductions as compared to pre- and normotensive participants (Cornelissen & Fagard, 2005). To place this into a public health perspective as presented in the Physical Activity Guidelines Advisory Committee report (2008), it has been estimated that reductions in population resting systolic blood pressure by as little as 2 mmHg could reduce coronary heart disease, stroke, and all-cause mortality rates by 4%, 6%, and 3% respectively, and a reduction of 5 mmHg would reduce mortality by 9%, 14%, and 7% respectively (PAGAC, 2008). Additionally, regular physical activity has also demonstrated an inverse relationship with blood pressure in hypertensive people (USDHHS, 1996).

Exercise and Obesity and Overweight

The primary general health marker of CVD that has not been directly addressed yet is that of overweight and obesity. The relationship with overweight and obesity with CVD-related morbidity and mortality, increased risk of hypertension related morbidity, dyslipidemia, coronary heart disease, stroke, and overall mortality is well established. Physical activity and exercise are also consistently related with the prevention and treatment of obesity and overweight (Haskell et al., 2007; PAGAC, 2008; USDHHS, 1996). In addition to CVD-related associations, obesity and overweight are also related with increased risk of type 2 diabetes, gallbladder disease, osteoarthritis, sleep apnea, respiratory problems, inflammation, and various cancers (PAGAC, 2008). Beginning in the 1990s obesity and overweight were labeled and identified as significant and growing risk factors globally. Although recommendations for the prevention of obesity and overweight were voiced in the 1990s, the incidence of overweight and obesity has continued to surge across the lifespan, thus impacting and increasing the risk for CVD and other associated chronic diseases. U.S. age-adjusted prevalence rates of overweight and obesity for men are currently 72.3% and 32.2%, respectively, with women reporting 64.1% and 35.5%, respectively (Flegal, Carroll, Ogden, & Curtin, 2010). Research strongly supports a dose-response relationship between physical activity and weight loss; however the relationship between weight stability and physical activity is less conclusive. As summarized by the Physical Activity Guidelines Advisory Committee Report (2008), most trials support a dose of physical activity ranging from 13-26 MET-hours per week to achieve a 1% - 3% weight loss, in which 13 MET-hours per week is described as 150 minutes of walking per week that is being conducted at a 4 mile/hour pace. However, research also strongly concludes that dietary interventions are necessary to achieve greater weight loss.

Fish Oil

Research regarding the consumption of omega-3 fatty acids (FO) has been conducted for approximately the last four decades. Findings in the early 1970s in Greenland Eskimos suggested beneficial effects on cardiovascular disease risk leading to numerous studies trying to elucidate the effects (Eslick, Howe, Smith, Priest, & Bensoussan, 2009) in animal and human models, observational studies, and randomized controlled trials. Research findings have suggested that FO helps to reduce cardiovascular risk by controlling endothelial dysfunction, lowering of systemic inflammation, improving insulin sensitivity, improving circulatory function, and improving TG, LDL, HDL, and other lipoprotein levels (Kelly, 2010). These effects are primarily associated with two fatty acids, eicosapentaenoic acid (EPA) and docosahexaenoic acid (DHA) which have also been associated with antiarrhythmic and antithrombotic effects and a decrease in cardiovascular mortality (Lin et al., 2010). Both EPA and DHA are essential nutrients that must be obtained from food and are regularly found in fatty fish such as salmon, herring, sardines, and tuna, but is also in over-the-counter FO supplements (McAnulty et al., 2010). Recently, the FDA has approved Lovaza, a prescription FO that contains 80-90% fatty acids (Plaisance, Grandjean, & Mahurin, 2009). EPA and DHA are reported to inhibit regulatory enzymes and cytokines such as diacylglycerol transferase, fatty acid synthase, acetyl coenzyme transferase, and lipoprotein lipase (Plaisance et al., 2009). It has been suggested that few American adults consume enough fatty fish in their diet to have sufficient levels of EPA and DHA and therefore a viable alternative is FO supplements. The latest safety guidelines by the American Heart Association suggest 3-4 g/day of fish oil containing both EPA and DHA is a maximum dosage that should be used (Eslick et al., 2009).

Fish Oil and Inflammation

Systemic inflammation in humans has been measured through CRP, IL-6, TNF-α, and IL-1β in research studies. Inflammatory processes are caused by environmental factors, genetic influences, infections, and injury (Zabel, Ash, King, Naslund, & Bauer, 2010). Primarily, endothelial injuries occur through increased blood pressure, cigarette smoking, oxidized lipoproteins, and hyperglycemia primarily associated with type II diabetes, metabolic syndrome, overweight, and obesity (Ramel, Martinez, Kiely, Bandarra, & Thorsdottir, 2010). Increased inflammation may cause downstream effects such as unstable plaques, thromboses, and emboli increasing risk for a myocardial infarction. Most studies that have reported on the effects of FO and inflammation have focused primarily on patients with chronic inflammation such as end-stage renal disease (ESRD), chronic kidney disease (CKD), diabetes, and CVD with changes in inflammation measured primarily by CRP (Bowden, Jitomir, Wilson, & Gentile, 2009). This may be due to FO supplementation being less effective in controlling inflammation in apparently healthy populations with low levels of systemic inflammation. One exception is that some study authors who have used fatty fish rather than FO supplements have reported positive outcomes in healthy populations. But in populations with chronic inflammation and existing cardiovascular disease many see a significant benefit with both FO supplementation and fatty fish consumption (Ohsawa et al., 2008). Most studies that have reported effects of FO on inflammation were between 8 weeks and 6 months in duration with results in those using FO supplements that contained both EPA (between 100-2000 mg/dL) and DHA (between 100-760 mg/dL). The changes in inflammatory markers may have occurred through a decreased lymphocyte proliferation and cytokine production (Bowden et al., 2009). Finally, a dose-response relationship regarding FO supplementation and inflammation has yet to be established, but most published work suggests the need to have both DHA and EPA in the supplements to have the greatest effect. It should be noted that fatty fish provides both DHA and EPA in sufficient quantities to elucidate an effect on inflammation levels as measured by CRP suggesting that FO supplementation may not be necessary in an apparently healthy population (Pot et al., 2010).

Fish Oil and Lipids

Though there are some equivocal findings in relation to FO and the prevention of cardiovascular disease, published studies have suggested FO may help to decrease LDL, LDL particle number, LDL size, TG, and increase HDL (Eslick et al., 2009). To date there have been four major systematic reviews of FO and cardiovascular disease benefits (Balk et al., 2006; Eslick et al., 2009; Hooper, et al., 2006; Lewis, Lookinland, Beckstrand, & Tiedeman, 2004). The most comprehensive is Eslick et al. (2009) who reported on 16,511 subjects and reported a clinically significant reduction in TG levels, minor effects on HDL (increased levels) and LDL (increased levels), and no effects reported regarding total cholesterol. Balk et al. (2006) reported on 7,803 subjects with virtually the same outcomes with no effects on total cholesterol, improved TG and HDL levels, and an increase in LDL levels. Hooper et al. (2006) reported on 36,913 subjects ascertaining the effects of FO on both cardiovascular disease and cancer. The study authors reported no effects on cardiovascular events or reduction in cardiovascular related mortality and did not report findings specifically related to lipids. Finally, a review was conducted by Lewis et al. (2004) and reported only on changes in TG levels with a reduction when consuming FO.

Additionally, reports from individual randomized controlled trials suggest significant decreases in cholesterol with participants who had hypertriglyceridemia with the exception of one study where participants were already consuming a large amount of fatty fish prior to the implementation of the study. Another recent review, though not systematic in reference selection, also reported that recent FO study outcomes suggest the smallest effects of FO on TG are more likely to occur in participants who have normal TG levels. Finally it should be noted that individual studies have reported positive changes in all lipoproteins including HDL, LDL, VLDL, TG, and novel risk factors such as LDL particle number and LDL size. Consequently the role of FO in the control of lipids levels is yet to be fully elucidated (Eslick et al., 2009).

Fish Oil and Exercise

Cardiovascular disease is the leading cause of death globally and novel approaches are needed to help control risk, mortality, and morbidity. As evidenced by numerous studies, FO helps to control inflammation and cholesterols levels and exercise helps to lower lipids levels through increased HDL and decreased TG and possibly LDL. Additionally, aerobic exercise can improve glucose tolerance, increase insulin sensitivity, and enhance fat oxidation (Boss, Lecoultre, Ruffieux, Tappy, & Schneiter, 2010). Most recently, there is emerging evidence that FO supplementation and fatty fish in the diet may help as well in fat oxidation, gene expression that effects key enzymes in fatty acid transportation and oxidation (Hill, Buckley,

Murphy, & Howe, 2007), increasing the production of lipoprotein lipase (which helps to regulate LDL and other cholesterol lipoproteins)and acetyl-CoA, and controling inflammatory cytokines, suggesting there needs to be an examination beyond the independent effects of exercise and FO to ascertain if there are any additive or synergistic effects in metabolic and cardiovascular health. Therefore it is intuitive that approaches that combine both FO and exercise should be examined (Kelly 2010). To date there have been a number of published studies regarding the combination of FO and aerobic exercise with equivocal findings.

Studies of Exercise, Fish Oil, and Lipids

Warner, Ullrich, Albrink, and Yeater (1989) followed 34 hyperlipidemic participants for twelve weeks while supplementing their diets with 50 ml/d of FO and requiring exercise three days a week (aerobic exercise). No effects were reported regarding HDL, total cholesterol, or TG, but significant improvement occurred with LDL and apolipoprotein-B during the study. Brilla and Landerholm (1990) studied the effects of combining FO and exercise in healthy, sedentary males (19-34 years old). Participants consumed 4g/d of FO and exercised aerobically for 60 minutes three days a week for ten weeks. No changes were reported in lipid values in the exercise and FO group compared to the control (no exercise or FO).

Another early study (Dunstan et al., 1997) had participants supplement their diet with FO and engage in aerobic exercise for eight weeks. When exercise and FO were combined there was a significant decrease in triglycerides that was 24% greater than exercise alone and 75% greater than FO alone. This is one of the few studies reporting positive results regardless of the risk classification of the participants. However, it should be noted that study participants were diabetics who more than likely had elevated levels of lipids, inflammation, and obesity prior to the start of the study.

A more recent study conducted by Hill et al. (2007) supplemented either 6 grams of tuna FO a day or placebo for twelve weeks, with the exercise group walking or running 3 times a week for 45 minutes at 75% of their max heart rate. The groups that supplemented their diet with FO had significant positive changes in TG and HDL. Additionally, the combination of FO and exercise reduced LDL cholesterol and apolipoprotein B (a proxy for LDL particle number) in participants who were hyperlipidemic that was greater than in the FO only group. Yet no significant effects were reported for cholesterol values for either the moderate intensity exercise group only or the FO and exercise group in normolipemic participants. These equivocal findings within this study may be explained by a dose-response relationship and the demographics of the study population. The FO groups consumed 260 mg/d of DHA but only 60 mg/d of EPA. Some of the latest studies suggest the need for increased levels of EPA with a ratio of EPA-DHA of 5:1 (DeFina, Marcoux, Devers, Cleaver, & Willis, 2011) with doses as high as 2000 mg/d for EPA. Therefore Hill's study (2007) did not have enough EPA in their FO supplement to elicit an effect on lipids beyond what occurred through exercise in the healthy participants. Normolipemic individuals may have a sufficient level of lipoprotein lipase which may not be enhanced beyond the benefits of aerobic exercise. This supports previous research that FO may be beneficial for those in disease states such as ESRD, CKD, or diabetes, but may not be beneficial for apparently healthy populations.

Exercise, Fish Oil, and Inflammation

Much of the research regarding FO and exercise and the regulation of inflammation has been conducted in well trained, athletic populations. An early study (Ernst, Saradeth, & Achhammer, 1991) used FO supplements with 1.75 g/day of EPA and 1.05 g/day of DHA with lowered inflammatory cytokines prior to exercise and post exercise in a group of apparently healthy participants who were not active. The same effects occurred in well-trained elite swimmers (Andrade, Ribeiro, Bozza, Costa Rosa, & do Carmo, 2007) who supplemented FO for six weeks (1.8g/d). Conversely, Hill et al. (2007) supplemented FO (2.4g/day of EPA and DHA) or placebo in fifty participants for twelve weeks. Supplements were consumed after each strenuous exercise session in a group of trained cyclists. There was no attenuation of plasma levels of inflammatory cytokines (CRP, TNF-α, and IL-6) when compared to placebo in participants supplementing FO. Though few studies have examined the effects of FO, exercise, and inflammation, the greatest attenuation of inflammatory cytokines may occur in diseased populations, as apparently healthy and well conditioned populations may have enhanced ability to control the inflammatory response. It is worth noting that Hill et al. (2007) used FO supplements that contained low doses of EPA, again suggesting the need to conduct more studies with higher doses of EPA and suggesting that inflammation may be more likely attenuated based on a dose-response relationship of EPA/DHA and in diseased populations.

Postprandial Effects of Fish Oil and Exercise

Another aspect of measuring the effects combining FO and aerobic exercise could be when lipids and inflammatory cytokines are measured. Recent studies (Plaisance, et al., 2009) have suggested that combining therapies may have the greatest impact on lipids and inflammation postprandial requiring more research on non-fasted participants. One study (Thomas, Liu, Linden, & Rector, 2007) reported that after supplementing 4g/d of FO for three weeks that TG were decreased by 33% in those with fasting hypertriglyceridemia but that postprandial triglyceride levels were not changed. The authors further stated that the failure to control postprandial concentration of lipids may be due to FO reducing a normal postprandial triglyceride effect found routinely in study participants who engage in aerobic exercise. The converse could also be possible when combining FO and exercise. Lipids may be normal when fasted, but postprandial lipids could be elevated due to increased fatty acid oxidation and increased levels of lipoprotein lipase production. In other words, the positive effects elucidated by exercise could in fact be overcome through the supplementation of FO. FO may be controlling a postprandial TG response and therefore may provide an effect on LDL, VLDL, LDL particle number, and specifically LDL size during a fasting state. Since postprandial lipids are controlled through exercise and FO, fasting lipids may also be more regulated and may cause there to be little benefit to combining FO and exercise if lipids are measured in a fasting state. Since fasting levels of lipids occur primarily in the morning, normally most people have postprandial effects occurring throughout the day suggesting a new avenue of research to understand how FO and exercise may affect lipid levels and inflammation when the therapies are combined in apparently healthy and disease populations. There may seemingly be no benefit when combining therapies, because most of the beneficial effects may occur outside the normal window of a screening (i.e. in fasted state prior to engaging in aerobic exercise for the day). This could also help to explain why most benefits may occur in diseased populations such as ESRD, CKD, diabetes, and CVD, as TG and VLDL production can be dysfunctional in chronic disease, especially when in conjunction with elevated levels of inflammation, by a poorly controlled regulation of lipoprotein lipase. Because both exercise and FO can enhance lipoprotein lipase activity, those individuals with low levels of lipoprotein lipase (ESRD, diabetics, and CKD patients) may experience downstream effects of enhanced lipid control mechanisms and therefore have positive effects of combining therapies that would not be seen in an apparently healthy population that do not have problems in lipid metabolism, lipoprotein lipase regulation, and/or inflammation.

Fish Oil, Exercise, and Obesity and Overweight

Obesity and overweight are commonly associated with inflammation, increased blood pressure, abnormal lipids, and insulin resistance. Both exercise and FO are associated with controlling these risk factors. More importantly, recent evidence suggests that FO and exercise can enhance fat oxidation and may help provide a means for weight control when combined (Boss, et al., 2010). In the only study that includes both exercise only and FO only control groups, Hill et al. (2007) followed 81 overweight participants for 22 weeks while supplementing their diet with FO and starting an aerobic exercise program. In both the exercise only and the FO only groups a significant reduction in body fat occurred. However, additional body fat reduction did not occur in the FO and exercise group. The most recent study (DeFina, et al., 2011) had an exercise only group compared to an exercise and FO group. Both groups exercised 150 minutes a week for 24 weeks. Both groups lost >5% of their body weight, and there was not additional weight and/or body fat loss with the addition of FO. Present findings regarding FO and exercise on weight loss suggest that the addition of FO in the diet or in combination with exercise is not beneficial for weight loss.

Fish Oil, Exercise, and Heart Rate Variability

Little work has been reported regarding the combination of exercise, fish oil, and HRV. FO, and specifically EPA and DHA, can increase parasympathetic tone which can attenuate the release of TNF-alpha and IL-6, while exercise can enhance parasympathetic tone and assist in the product of interleukin-10 (IL-10), an anti-inflammatory cytokine, which in turn can positively affect HRV. The combination of both FO and exercise may help to increase HRV and protect against ventricular arrhythmias and CVD (Das, 2000; Ismail, 2005). The only published study regarding the effects of combining FO and exercise on HRV was conducted by Ninio, Hill, Howe, Buckley, and Saint (2008). Participants (N=65) consumed 6 g/d of FO that was primarily comprised of DHA (1.56 g/d of DHA, 0.36/d of EPA) or placebo for twelve weeks while exercising three days a week for 45 minutes at 75% of their age-predicted maximum. HRV was followed in 46 patients, with an increase in parasympathetic activity and improved HRV, resting heart rate, and exercise heart rate when compared to the placebo group.

Conclusions

At the very least, studies that have reported no additional benefits from combining exercise and FO suggest both of these therapies affect the same mechanisms, cytokine regulation, and enzymatic control (Plaisance, et al., 2009). Because inflammatory, lipid, and fat oxidative pathways are enhanced by exercise and FO, the reductions that occur may not necessarily be aided by combing therapies in apparently healthy populations. Lastly, there have been no effects reported with FO, exercise, and exercise/sport performance (Buckley, Burgess, Murphy, & Howe, 2009). Where the combination of therapies may prove beneficial is with participants and patients who have elevated lipids, elevated inflammatory cytokines, and other comorbid conditions such as ESRD, CKD, diabetes, and existing CVD that can be controlled through behavioral and nutritional interventions.

References

Andrade, P. M. M., Ribeiro, B. G., Bozza, M. T., Costa Rosa, L. F. B., & do Carmo, M. G. T. (2007). Effects of the fish-oil supplementation on the immune and inflammatory responses in elite swimmers. *Prostaglandins, Leukotrienes, and Essential Fatty Acids, 77*, 139-145.

Balk, E. M., Lichtenstein, A. H., Chung, M., Kupelnick, B., Chew, P., & Lau, J. (2006). Effects of omega-3 fatty acids on coronary restenosis, intima–media thickness, and exercise tolerance: A systematic review. *Atherosclerosis 184*, 237–246

Beavers, K. M., Brinkley, T. E., & Nicklas, B. J. (2010). Effect of exercise training on chronic inflammation. *Clinica Chimica Acta: International Journal of Clinical Chemistry, 411*(11-12), 785-93.

Boss, A., Lecoultre, V., Ruffieux, C., Tappy, L., & Schneiter, P. (2010). Combined effects of endurance training and dietary unsaturated fatty acids on physical performance, fat oxidation and insulin sensitivity. *British Journal of Nutrition, 103*, 1151–1159.

Bowden, R. G., Jitomir, J., Wilson, R. L., & Gentile, M. (2009). Over the counter omega-3 fatty acid supplementation significantly changes lipid levels in end-stage renal disease patients. *Journal of Renal Nutrition, 19*(4), 259-266.

Brilla, L. R., & Landerholm, T. E. (1990). Affiliation effect of fish oil supplementation and exercise on serum lipids and aerobic fitness. *The Journal of sports medicine and physical fitness, 30*(2), 173-80.

Buckley, J. D., Burgess, S., Murphy, K. J., & Howe, P. R. C. (2009). DHA-rich fish oil lowers heart rate during submaximal exercise in elite Australian rules footballers. *Journal of Science and Medicine in Sport, 12*, 503-501.

Carlson J. E., Ostir G. V., Black S. A., Markides, K. S., Rudkin, L., & Goodwin, J. S. (1999). Disability in older adults. 2: Physical activity as prevention. *Behavioral Medicine,24*(4),157-168.

Carter, J. B., Banister, E. W., & Blaber, A. P. (2003). The effect of age and gender on heart rate variability after endurance training. *Medicine & Science in Sports & Exercise, 35*(8), 1333-1340.

Caspersen, C. J., Powell, K. E., & Christenson, G. M. (1985). Physical activity, exercise, and physical fitness: definitions and distinctions for health-related research. *Public Health Report, 100*(2), 126-131.

Cornelissen, V. A., & Fagard, R. H. (2005). Effects of endurance training on blood pressure, blood pressure-regulating mechanisms, and cardiovascular risk factors. *Hypertension, 46*(4), 667-675.

Das, U. N. (2000). Beneficial effect(s) of n-3 fatty acids in cardiovascular diseases: but, why and how? *Prostaglandins, Leukotrienes, and Essential Fatty Acids, 63*(6), 351-62.

DeFina, L. F., Marcoux, L. G., Devers, S. M., Cleaver, J. P., & Willis, B. L. (2011). Effects of omega-3 supplementation in combination with diet and exercise on weight loss and body composition. *American Journal of Clinical Nutrition, 93*, 455-462.

Dunstan, D. W., Mori, T. A., Puddey, I. B., Beilin, L. J., Burke, V., Morton, A. R., & Stanton, K. G. (1997). The independent and combined effects of aerobic exercise and dietary fish intake on serum lipids and glycemic control in NIDDM. A randomized controlled study. *Diabetes Care, 20*(6), 913-21.

Durstine, J. L., Grandjean, P. W., Davis, P. G., Ferguson, M. A., Alderson, N. L., & DuBose, K. D. (2001). Blood lipid and lipoprotein adaptations to exercise: A quantitative analysis. *Sports Medicine, 31*(15), 1033-1062.

Ernst, E., Saradeth, T., & Achhammer, G. (1991). N-3 fatty acids and acute-phase proteins. *European Journal of Clinical Investigation, 21*, 77-82.

Eslick, G. D., Howe, P. R., Smith, C., Priest, R., & Bensoussan, A. (2009). Benefits of fish oil supplementation in hyperlipidemia: A systematic review and meta-analysis. *International Journal of Cardiology, 136*(1), 4-16.

Flegal, K. M., Carroll, M. D., Ogden, C. L., & Curtin, L. R. (2010). Prevalence and trends in obesity among US adults, 1999-2008. *JAMA: the Journal of the American Medical Association, 303*(3), 235-241.

Haskell, W. L., Lee, I., Pate, R. R., Powell, K. E., Blair, S. N., Franklin, B. A., … Bauman, A. (2007). Physical activity and public health: Updated recommendations for adults from the American College of Sports Medicine and the American Heart Association. *Medicine and Science in Sports and Exercise, Special Reports*, 1423-1434.

Hill, A. M., Buckley, J. D., Murphy, K. J., & Howe, P. R. C. (2007). Combining fish-oil supplements with regular aerobic exercise improves body composition and cardiovascular disease risk factors. *American Journal of Clinical Nutrition, 85*, 1267–1274.

Hooper, L., Thompson, R. L., Harrison, R. A., Summerbell, C. D., Ness, A. R., Moore, H. J., … Davey Smith, G. (2006). Risks and benefits of omega 3 fats for mortality, cardiovascular disease, and cancer: Systematic review. *British Medical Journal, 332*(7544), 752-760.

Ismail, H. M. The role of omega-3 fatty acids in cardiac protection: An overview. (2005). *Frontiers in Bioscience: A Journal and Virtual Library, 10*, 1079-1088.

Kelly, R. B. (2010). Diet and exercise in the management of hyperlipidemia. *American Family Physician, 81*(9), 1097-1104.

Kodama, S., Tanaka, S., Saito, K., Shu, M., Sone, Y., Onitake, F., … Sone, H. (2007). Effect of aerobic exercise training on serum levels of high-density lipoprotein cholesterol: A meta-analysis. *Archives of Internal Medicine, 167*(10), 999-1008.

Lewis, A., Lookinland, S., Beckstrand, R. L., & Tiedeman, M. E. (2004). Treatment of hypertriglyceridemia with omega-3 fatty acids: A systematic review. *Journal of the American Academy of Nurse Practitioners, 16*(9), 384-395.

Lin, C. Y., Chen, P. C., Kuo, H. K., Lin L. Y., Lin J. W., & Hwang, J. J. (2010). Effects of obesity, physical activity, and cardiorespiratory fitness on blood pressure, inflammation, and insulin resistance in the National Health and Nutrition Survey 1999-2002. *Nutrition, Metabolism, and Cardiovascular Diseases: NMCD, 20*(10), 713-719.

Mazzeo, R. S., Cavanagh, P., Evans, W. J., Fiatarone, M., Hagberg, J., McAuley, E., & Startzell, J. (1998). ACSM position stand on exercise and physical activity for older adults. *Medicine & Science in Sports & Exercise, 30*(6), 992-1008.

McAnulty, S. R., Nieman, D. C., Fox-Rabinovich, M., Duran, V., McAnulty, L. S., Henson, D. A., Jin, F., & Landram, M. J. (2010). Effect of n-3 fatty acids and antioxidants on oxidative stress after exercise. *Medicine & Science in Sports & Exercise, 42*(9S), 1704-1711.

Ninio, D. M., Hill, A. M., Howe, P. R., Buckley, J. D., & Saint, D. A. (2008). Docosahexaenoic acid-rich fish oil improves heart rate variability and heart rate responses to exercise in overweight adults. *British Journal of Nutrition 100*, 1097-1103.

O'Connor, M. F., & Irwin, M. R. (2010). Links between behavioral factors and inflammation. *Clinical Pharmacology and Therapeutics, 87*(4), 479-482.

Ohsawa, M., Itai, K., Onoda, T., Tanno, K., Sasaki, S., Nakamura, M., Ogawa, A., … Okayama, A. (2008). Dietary intake of n-3 polyunsaturated fatty acids is inversely associated with CRP levels, especially among male smokers. *Atherosclerosis, 201*, 184–191.

Pate, R., Pratt, M., Blair, S., Haskell, W. L., Macera, C. A., Bouchard, C., … Wilmore, J. H. (1995). Physical activity and public health: A recommendation from the Centers for Disease Control and Prevention and the American College of Sports Medicine. *JAMA: the Journal of the American Medical Association, 273*(5), 402-407.

Plaisance, E. P., Grandjean, P. W., & Mahurin, A. J. (2009). Independent and combined effects of aerobic exercise and pharmacological strategies on serum triglyceride concentrations: A quality review. *The Physician and Sportsmedicine, 37*(1), 11-19.

Physical Activity Guidelines Advisory Committee (PAGAC). (2008). *Physical Activity Guidelines Advisory Committee Report, 2008.* Washington, DC: U.S. Department of Health and Human Services. Retrieved from http://www.health.gov/PAGuidelines/Report

Pot, G. K., Geelen, A., Majsak-Newman, G., Harvey L. J., Nagengast, F. M., Witteman, B. J., … Kampman, E. (2010). Increased consumption of fatty and lean fish reduces serum c-reactive protein concentrations but not inflammation markers in feces and in colonic biopsies. *Journal of Nutrition, 140*(2), 371–376.

Ramel, A., Martinez, J. A, Kiely, M., Bandarra, N. M., & Thorsdottir, I. (2010). Effects of weight loss and seafood consumption on inflammation parameters in young, overweight and obese European men and women during 8 weeks of energy restriction. *European Journal of Clinical Nutrition, 64*, 987–993.

Routledge, F. S., Campbell, T. S., McFetridge-Durdle, J. A., & Bacon, S. L. (2010). Improvements in heart rate variability with exercise therapy. *The Canadian Journal of Cardiology, 26*(6), 303-312.

Slentz, C. A., Houmard, J. A., Johnson, J. L., Bateman, L. A., Tanner, C. J., McCartney, J. S., … Kraus, W. E. (2007). Inactivity, exercise training and detraining, and plasma lipoproteins. STRRIDE: A randomized controlled study of exercise intensity and amount. *Journal of Applied Physiology, 103*(2), 432-442.

Thomas, T. R., Liu, Y., Linden, M. S., & Rector, R. S. (2007). Interaction of exercise training and n-3 fatty acid supplementation on postprandial lipemia. *Applied Physiology Nutrition and Metabolism, 32*(3), 473-480.

U.S. Department of Health and Human Services (USDHHS). Centers for Disease Control and Prevention and Health Promotion. (1996). *Physical Activity and Health: A Report of the Surgeon General*. Retrieved from http://www.cdc.gov/nccdphp/sgr/index.htm

Walsh, N. P., Gleeson, M., Shephard, R. J., Gleeson, M., Woods, J. A., Bishop, N. C., … Simon P. (2011). Position statement. Part one: Immune function and exercise. *Exercise Immunology Review, 17*, 6-63.

Warner, J. G. Jr, Ullrich, I. H., Albrink, M. J., & Yeater, R. A. (1989). Combined effects of aerobic exercise and omega-3 fatty acids in hyperlipidemic persons. *Medicine & Science in Sports & Exercise, 21*(5), 498-505.

Yoon, S. S., Ostchega, Y., & Louis, T. (2010). *Recent Trends in the Prevalence of High Blood Pressure and its Treatment and Control, 1999–2008. NCHS Data Brief.* U.S. Department of Health and Human Services (USDHHS). Centers for Disease Control and Prevention and Health Promotion. Atlanta, GA. Retrieved from http://www.cdc.gov/nchs/data/databriefs/db48.pdf

Zabel, R., Ash, S., King, N., Naslund, E., & Bauer, J. (2010). Gender differences in the effect of fish oil on appetite, inflammation and nutritional status in haemodialysis patients. *Journal of Human Nutrition and Dietetics, 23*, 416–425.

In: Fish Oil: Production, Consumption and Health Benefits
Editors: Matthias Van Dijk and Jürgen Vitek
ISBN: 978-1-61470-963-3

Chapter XI

Nutrition for Consciousness

Alfred Ordman*

Biochemistry Program, Beloit College, Beloit, Wisconsin, U. S.

Abstract

Richard Dawkins has written "The evolution of the capacity to simulate seems to have culminated in subjective consciousness. Why this should have happened is, to me, the most profound mystery facing modern biology." In writing this review of recent research on fish oil, I invite you to consider another exciting mystery of modern science that depends upon fish oil, consciousness. Omega-3 (n-3) fatty acids are essential in the human diet for the brain to function. From a biochemical perspective, it is clear how DHA, the longest omega-3 fatty acid, which is found in FO (fish oil found in cold water fish), plays an essential role in brain function. Using epidemiological studies of people, scientists have discovered that those who consume FO have a lower risk for dementia. In biochemical analyses of molecules that are necessary for the brain, researchers have elucidated how FO provides flexibility for dendritic mobility. We now know that dietary nutrients produce metabolic signals similar to hormones. This review provides vocabulary and structures necessary to understand some important fatty acids, and presents fats in the brain related to FO. It describes the origin of those fatty acids in algae and their functions in fish and humans. DHA in FO activates at least two areas in the brain that reduce appetite and increase basic metabolic rate. I review other nutrition studies done during recent years that demonstrate that FO is important for both brain function and weight regulation. These studies demonstrate the benefit for humans of a daily intake of FO from before conception through senescence to maintain optimal health.

* Alfred "Roc" Ordman email: ordman@beloit.edu

I. Introduction

After being involved in nutrition research for decades, my interest in human aging has grown to include vitamin C, calcium, weight loss, and most recently, consciousness. These two latest topics have made me realize how vital a basic understanding of the biochemistry of fish oil is to healthy longevity. If it were not for fish oil, we would not be conscious. So I begin by exploring what consciousness is. I then consider how to obtain good nutrition for consciousness, of which a primary requirement is fish oil. Next, I go through basic chemistry, biochemistry, and functions of fish oil, and finally review the latest research on the role of DHA in weight control.

II. What is Consciousness?

There are many research questions about fish oil to be explored, including its key role in consciousness. Richard Dawkins has written "The evolution of the capacity to simulate seems to have culminated in subjective consciousness. Why this should have happened is, to me, the most profound mystery facing modern biology" (Dawkins, 1976).

Daniel Dennett (1991), who is a leader in consciousness theory, views consciousness as a cohesive mental synthesis from multiple neuronal firings. Often consciousness is considered a single central processor in the brain. But Dennett suggests the entire brain assembles our ability to make choices. Parallel processing by different neuronal networks, like computer parallel processing, provides cerebral time traveling, that integrates past experiences with future possibilities.

A. Evolution of Consciousness and Free Will

In considering why consiousness has evolved in humans, I assume that there must be a selective advantage that it has provided. As I consider whether to take a fish oil supplement regularly, it is via consciousness that I am able to consider my choices. Will it help my brain maintain its function? Might it help me maintain a healthy weight? In reaching this decision, I realize that the key reason for which consciousness would be selected is that it allows me to exercise free will, to make a subjective choice based on the evidence. On the one hand, as a scientist I accept that we live in a deterministic universe, where cause and effect govern every decision. Under these circumstances, I cannot imagine how free will can exist, as all decisions are based on previous causes of experience and environment. But if all decisions are automatic and do not require conscious contemplation and decision-making, then I cannot imagine what selective advantage consciousness has provided. Until someone provides a better explanation, I hypothesize that because we have evolved consciousness, we must have free will.

B. Definition of Consciousness

Parfit (1987) argues for the Bundle Theory of consciousness (and mentions that the Buddha was the first bundle theorist [Blackmore, 2004]). Bundle theory states that we cannot explain the unit of consciousness as a property of a single person, but rather as a series of mental states and events. A similar idea of consciousness is held by Daniel Dennett. "The Multiple Drafts model makes "writing it down" in memory criterial for consciousness: that is *what it is* for the "given" to be "taken" ... There is no reality of conscious experience independent of the effects of various vehicles of content on subsequent action (and hence, of course, on memory)." (Dennett, 1991).

These ideas have led to my operational definition of consciousness. At its most basic level, consciousness is simply the sum of the electrical discharges occurring throughout the nervous system of a being at any given instant. However, once a level of consciousness where learning is possible has been reached, consciousness can be defined as the level of expression of mRNAs being produced that facilitate axon and dendrite elongation. That lengthening results in long-term facilitation. That is what leads to memory formation (Izquierdo, 1997). Although protocols and technologies do not yet exist or have not been published to measure these values, I forsee a future when an instrument can measure the sum of all nervous impulses at any given instant, or assay the level of the appropriate mRNAs. Then it will be easy to compare activities like sleeping or concentrating to see which increases the instanteous impulse level, and thus one's level of consciousness.

C. How to Provide Nutrition for Consciousness

What is necessary to nourish ourselves for optimal consciousness? Discoveries have expanded in the field of nutrition through long-term studies like the Physicians and Nurses Health Studies. Walter Willett published *Eat, Drink and Be Healthy* in 2001 (Willett, 2001), a book that revealed that the Food Pyramid issued by the United States Department of Agriculture (USDA, 1994) did not help people to stay healthy. His scientifically based food pyramid, the Willett Pyramid, provides validated recommendations about nutrition. In contrast, the next USDA food pyramid of 2001 (USDA, 2011) has also been replaced. Below are suggestions in addition to a healthy diet to consider for consciousness:

1. Exercise – A significant change in the Willett Pyramid, and subsequently the USDA pyramid, is that exercise is fundamental to good nutrition. Since then, numerous studies have demonstrated the link between exercise and retention of mental function. For example, Nynke de Jong (2001) demonstrated that even amongst frail elderly, exercise prolonged neuropsychological functioning. In model systems, endurance exercise has been shown to be effective partly by reducing free radical damage and promoting mitochondrial rejuvenation (Safdar, 2011).

In a 2005 Symposium on obesity (Spiegel, 2005), it was reported that in the US obesity causes about 1,400,000 deaths per year and costs $117 billion. The executive summary states "65% of US adults are overweight or obese. The solution may seem simple: 'get people to eat less and exercise more.' " There it was reported that the average person should get 30 min of daily exercise to remain healthy, 60 min to control weight, and 90 min to lose weight.

2. Sex – The National Institute of Aging has been running a caloric restriction project with *Rhesus* monkeys who are now 18 to 35 years old. One of the only clearly identified biomarkers of aging found in those colonies as of 2005 was a decrease in the time spent thinking about sex, reflected in observable behaviors like autoeroticism (Butler, 2004; Ordman, 2005). In 2008, one of the signaling pathways originating in the gonads was identified, explaining how this connects to longevity (Xie, 2008). In addition, testosterone levels have been shown to be important in maintaining cognitive abilities in aging humans (Asthana, 2004).

3. Meditation – Many studies have revealed that meditating regularly has benefits for various cognitive abilities. Researchers report that certain regions in the brains of long-term meditators were larger (Wheeler, 2009). Five days of meditation practice reduced stress, increased immunity, and increased attention (Tang, 2007). The findings of a study of long term and novice meditators demonstrated that even a short program in mindfulness meditation produces demonstrable positive effects on brain and immune function (Davidson, 2003). Sitting meditation seems to be an effective intervention in the treatment of adverse physiologic, psychosocial, and behavioral conditions among youth (Black, 2009). Another study indicates how meditation can alter circuitry in the brain (Lutz, 2008). The mental expertise to cultivate positive emotion alters the activation of brain circuits. Those circuits are linked to emotional stimuli and increased levels of empathy.

4. Longevity via telomeres – In 1961, Leonard Hayflick discovered the limited ability of non-cancerous eukaryotic cells to divide (Hayflick, 1961, Olovinikov, 1996). For humans, the Hayflick limit is about 70 cell divisions. In 2009, Elizabeth Blackburn received the Nobel Prize for her work on telomerase and telomeres. Her work involves telomeres and meditation, and how people under stress have shortened telomeres (Epel, 2009). Telomeres are repetitive sequences of DNA at the ends of chromosomes necessary for proper function of DNA genes. In humans, the sequence is TTAGGG. At fertilization this sequence repeats for about 15,000 base pairs, at birth 10,000, then decreasing about 50 bp per year, until at a length of 5,000 cells become senescent. Telomeres explain why the Hayflick limit is reached, causing cellular senescence. Because telomeres shorten after each cell division, replicating cells eventually enter senescence. Telomerase is the enzyme that can lengthen telomeres, but it is normally inactive except in cancer cells, which are able to replicate indefinitely. Telomerase activity and telomere length appear to be associated with micronutrient levels. For instance, evidence from *in vitro* studies of human fibroblasts suggests that magnesium may affect the longevity of telomeres (Killilea, 2008). Vitamin D may also affect telomere length, as measured in peripheral blood leukocytes. Serum vitamin D concentrations in 2160 female twins aged 18–79 years (mean age: 49.4), indicated that leucocyte telomere length (LTL) was correlated with age ($r = -0.40$, $P < 0.0001$) while serum vitamin D concentrations showed a weak positive association with longer LTL ($r = 0.07$, $P = 0.0010$) and this finding persisted even after adjustment for age ($r = 0.09$, $P < 0.0001$) and other variables that independently could affect LTL (age, season of vitamin D measurement, menopausal status, use of hormone replacement therapy, and physical activity). In addition to the effects of micronutrients, there is some evidence that lifestyle may affect telomerase production. A low-fat diet (primarily vegetables, soy protein) and supplements including fish oil, selenium, and vitamins C and E, and stress management procedures including yoga and meditation, were associated with increased telomerase activity in 29-84% of subjects. This improvement was attributed to decreases in LDL cholesterol as well (Richards, 2007). Regular exercise appears to be associated with reduced telomere erosion in both mice and humans, at least in the leukocytes and blood vessel walls (Mead, 2008; Werner, 2009).

D.Food for thought

a. Choline - *Choline* (fig. 1E) is a dietary component essential for the structural integrity and signaling functions of cell membranes. It directly affects cholinergic neurotransmission and lipid transport from the liver, and it is the major source of methyl groups in the diet. Betaine, one of choline's metabolites, participates in the methylation of homocysteine to form methionine (Baker, 1984). Severe choline deficiency adversely affects cellular methylation and DNA integrity, with potentially serious implications for disease risk (Shin, 2010). Higher dietary intakes of choline and betaine in the Greek population reduce inflammation as assessed by several biomarkers in blood (Zeisel, 2008). In many mammals, including baboons, prolonged (weeks to months) ingestion of a diet deficient in choline but adequate, though limited, in methionine and folate, has consequences that include hepatic, renal, pancreatic, memory, and growth disorders (Zeisel, 2005). Papers presented at a 2009 symposium on methyl donors considered 3 specific nutrients: methyl donors folate and choline, iodine, and docosahexaenoic acid (DHA; 22:6n–3), all nutrients for which there was new evidence for increased dietary importance during pregnancy and lactation and all of which are important for neurodevelopment of the fetus and infant (Greer, 2009). Choline concentrations were also negatively associated with anxiety symptoms but not with depression symptoms (Bjelland, 2009).

b. DHA - “The risk for dementia, a major contributor to incapacitation and institutionalization, rises rapidly as we age, doubling every 5 y after age 65. Tens of millions of new Alzheimer's disease (AD) and other dementia cases are projected as elderly populations increase around the world, creating a projected dementia epidemic for which most nations are not prepared. DHA may help suppress insulin/neurotrophic factor signaling deficits, neuroinflammation, and oxidative damage that contribute to synaptic loss and neuronal dysfunction in dementia. We advocate early intervention in a prodromal period with nutrigenomically defined subjects with an appropriately designed nutritional supplement, including DHA and antioxidants” (Cole, 2010).

The Journal of Nutrition and American Journal of Clinical Nutrition have been publishing more than 50 studies per year on DHA, many about fetal mental development during pregnancy and dementia during aging. For example, DHA deficiency is associated with Prefrontal Cortex Neuropathology in Recurrent Affective Disorders (McNamara, 2010), with dementia (Cole, 2010), cognitive functioning (Muldoon, 2010), and neurodegeneration (Zhang, 2010). The latter study is especially interesting because it highlights signaling by DHA. As opposed to just providing molecular building blocks and calories, nutrients over the past decade have been recognized to be signaling molecules, similar to hormones. Nutrients can cause changes in DNA and other nucleotide and protein expression and activation, as will be discussed in section IV. E. Weight Control.

c. Weight control - The inverse association between fish and prevalent dementia is unlikely to result from poorer dietary habits among demented individuals. Meat consumption was higher in those with a diagnosis of dementia (Albanese, 2009). 25% of adults are obese; this increases their risk of cardiovascular disease, diabetes, cancer, and other health problems.

"This process involves brain areas that control appetite and energy metabolism" (Wisse, 2007). The review of literature regarding the overconsumption of energy and excess body mass suggests poorer academic achievement during development and greater decay of brain structure and function, accompanied by increased cognitive aging during older adulthood in the obese. A similar review of research on energy expenditure through the adoption of increased physical activity suggests that exercises contribute to increased cognitive health and function (Burkhalter, 2011). We hypothesize that DHA exerts a wide array of effects on geriatric diseases via changing expression of genes for many regulators (Cha, 2001). The deposition of excess fat into proinflammatory sites promotes diabetes and most other serious diseases associated with obesity (including myocardial infarction, stroke, and dementia) (Roth, 2011). Long-term obesity and long-term underweight in adulthood are associated with lower cognitive scores in late midlife. Public health messages should promote a healthy weight at all ages (Sabia, 2009).

III. Basic Vocabulary

Figures 1 to 3 show the chemical structures important to the functions of fish oil. Figure 1A shows one of the main fatty acids humans use to store energy, long carbon chains ending in a carboxylic acid. These are saturated with energetic non-polar C-C and C-H bonds that are oxidized to provide electrons for the electron transport chain in mitochondria to produce ATP. When there are double bonds present, which provide carbons not saturated with hydrogen, the fatty acid is unsaturated, as in figure 1B. Biochemists and nutritionists use different vocabularies to designate the position of the double bond. c8:1(5c) signifies a fatty acid with 8 carbons and one double bond, which is in the cis configuration beginning at the 5th carbon counting from the carboxyl group. This nomenclature permits designation of the numerous fatty acids found in nature and the laboratory.

Nutritionists designate fatty acids counting from the opposite end of the carboxylic acid. This is relevant physiologically for two reasons. First, humans are not able to synthesize sufficient or perhaps any omega-3 and omega-6 fatty acids *de novo* (Gerster, 1998; Arterburn, 2006), and must obtain them from the diet. Second, omega-3 and omega-6 fats generally have opposing effects on metabolic processes related to maintaining health (Farina, 2011). Omega-3 fatty acids are essential in the diet and are metabolized to produce fluid cell membranes, anti-inflammatory molecules, and a variety of signaling molecules, as described in the section on functions below. Omega-6 fatty acids have the opposite effect, producing pro-inflammatory molecules.

Figures 1B-D show a simple omega-3 fatty acid, and the two major fatty acids associated with fish oil, commonly referred to as EPA and DHA. Alpha-linolenic acid, c18:3(n-3) found in flax and other vegetarian sources can be enzymatically converted by humans to EPA (c20) and to DHA (c22) by humans. However, the metabolic process is so slow in people that dietary sources of DHA are essential for good health. "[M]ost studies in humans have shown that whereas a certain, though restricted, conversion of high doses of ALA to EPA occurs, conversion to DHA is severely restricted. The use of ALA labelled with radioisotopes suggested that with a background diet high in saturated fat, conversion to long-chain metabolites is approximately 6% for EPA and 3.8% for DHA. With a diet rich in n-6 PUFA, conversion is reduced by 40 to 50%. It is thus reasonable to observe an n-6/n-3 PUFA ratio not exceeding 4-6. Restricted conversion to DHA may be critical since evidence has been increasing that this long-chain metabolite has an autonomous function, e.g. in the brain…" (Gerster, 1998). The other two molecules required to construct the fat necessary for nerve cell membranes are choline (fig. 1E), which has now been designated as a vitamin (Food and Nutrition Board, 1998), and glycerol (fig. 1F).

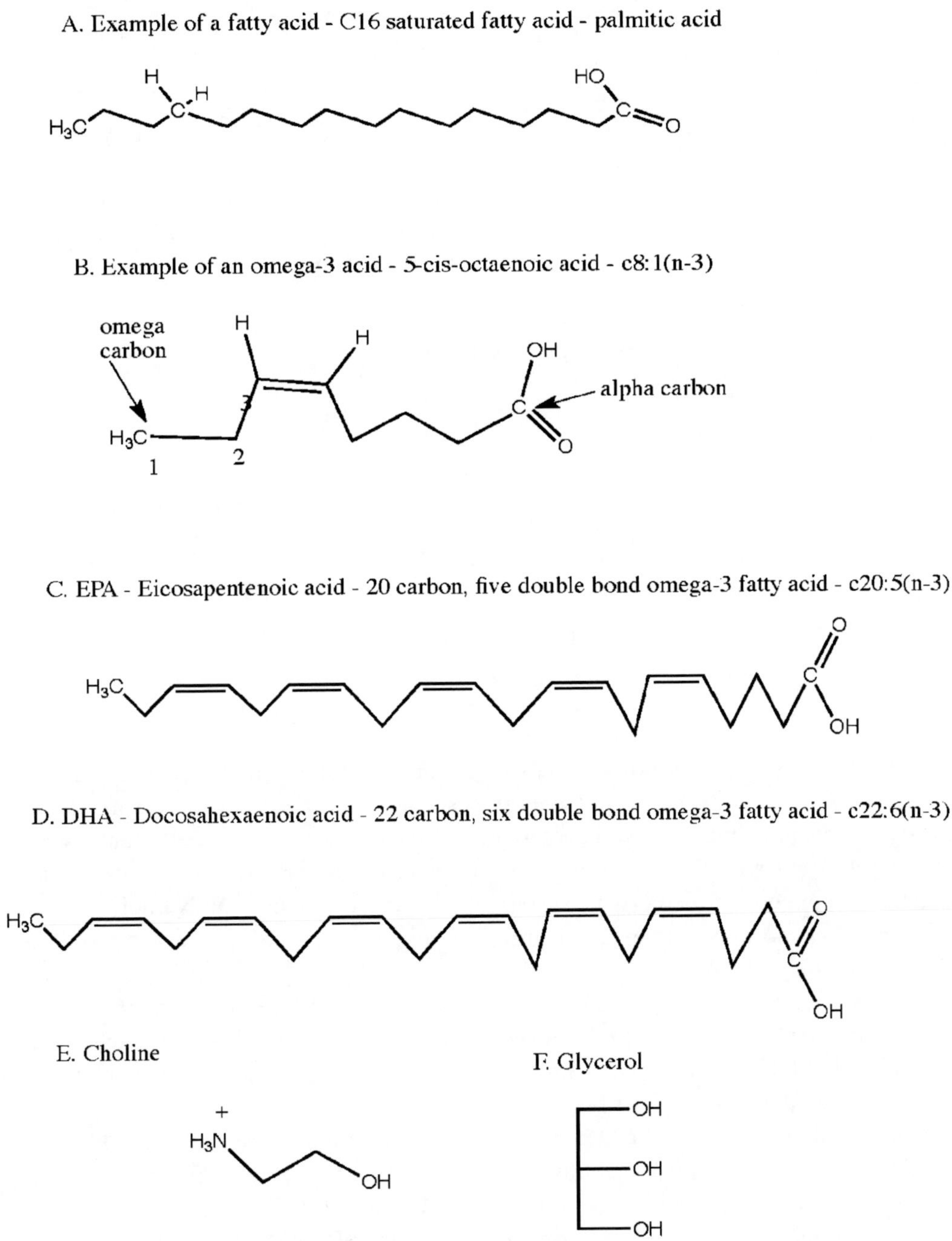

Figure 1. Components of Fats in Nerve Membranes.

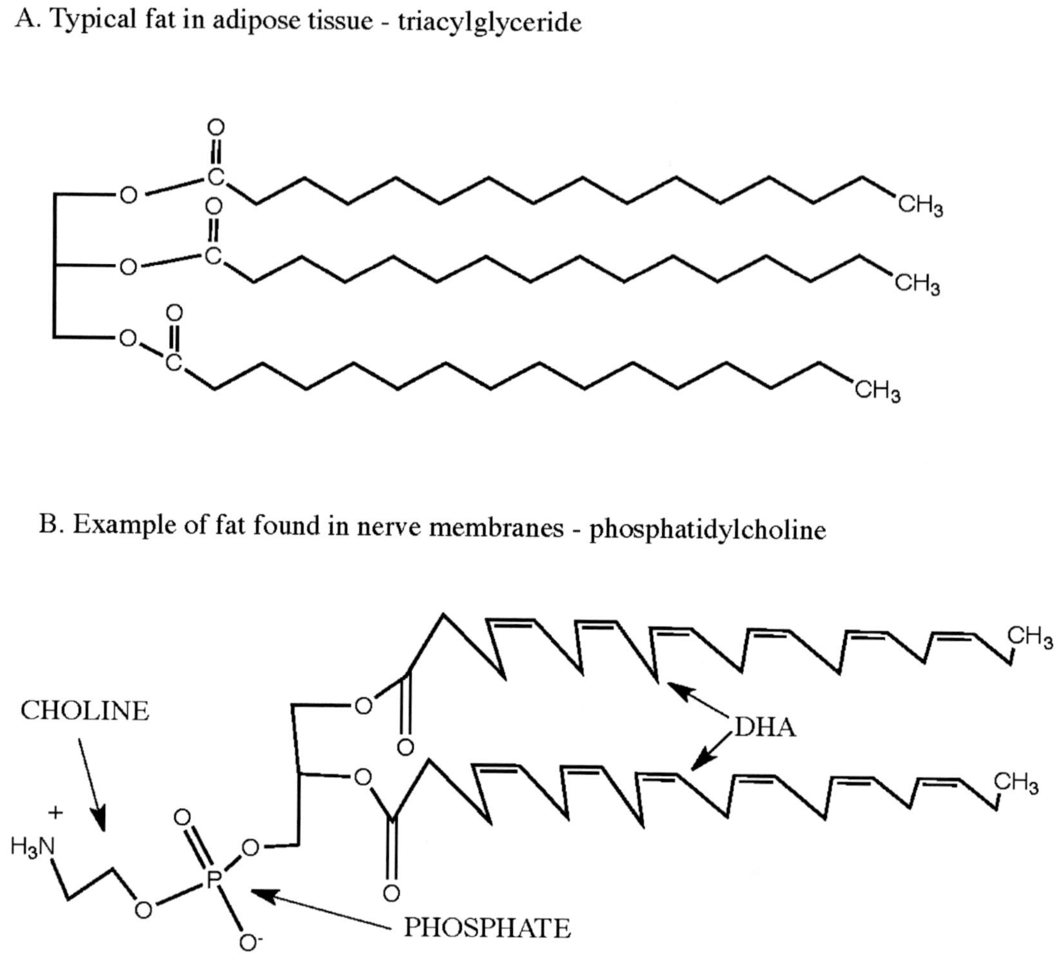

Figure 2. Structure of Fats.

Figure 2 shows how the molecules in Fig. 1 are assembled into fats or lipids. Fig. 2A shows how fatty acids are stored for energy reserves, esterified onto glycerol. These fats, triacylglycerides, predominantly store saturated fatty acids. By contrast, cell membrane lipids are diacylglycerides with C3 of the glycerol bonded to phosphate and then usually one of 3 other ligands. For cells of the nervous system, this ligand is predominantly choline, as shown in Fig. 2B. The phosphocholine "head group" is highly polar, while the fatty acid "tails" provide a non-polar region.

Figure 3 diagrams how the phosphatidylcholine molecules assemble into the lipid bilayer of a cell membrane. Two layers of lipid surround cells, with protein pores and receptors embedded in the bilayer using polar amino acids for the interior and non-polar ones at the exterior to embed the protein in the bilayer.

Figure 3 also diagrams the advantage of polyunsaturated fatty acids (PUFAs) for facilitating membrane fluidity. Saturated fats (fig. 2A) are regular in structure, readily crystallize, and so can be relatively solid at room temperature (RT), as is the case with butter, nutritionally commonly derived from 4-legged animal fat. Vegetable and fish oils are PUFAs (fig. 2B) and are more difficult to crystallize, remaining liquid at RT.

The highly unsaturated DHA (fig. 1D) esterified into fat (fig. 2B) provides the fluidity needed for growth and mobility of nerve axons and dendrites. In fig. 3B, the outer cell membranes of the axon and dendrite grow closer by producing more membrane. At the synapse, flexibility and growth of the membrane is essential for long-term facilitation of nerve impulses leading to memory formation (Scott, 1989).

A. Structure of lipid bilayer

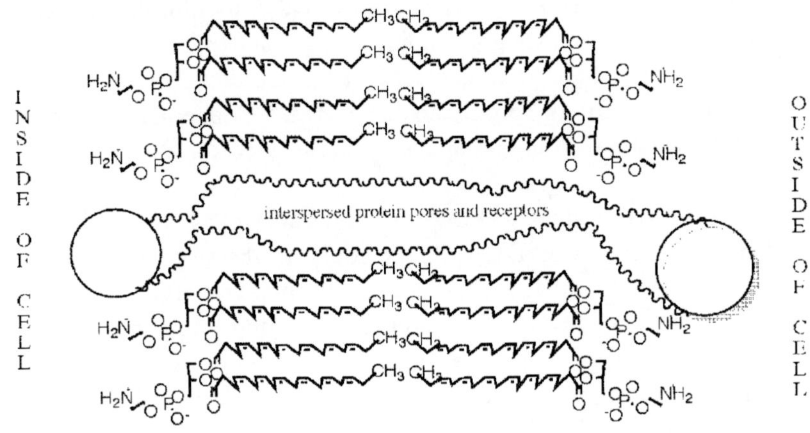

B. Neuronal cell membrane - Repeated nerve stimulation causes decrease in synapse gap causing long term faciliation.
NT=neurotransmitter

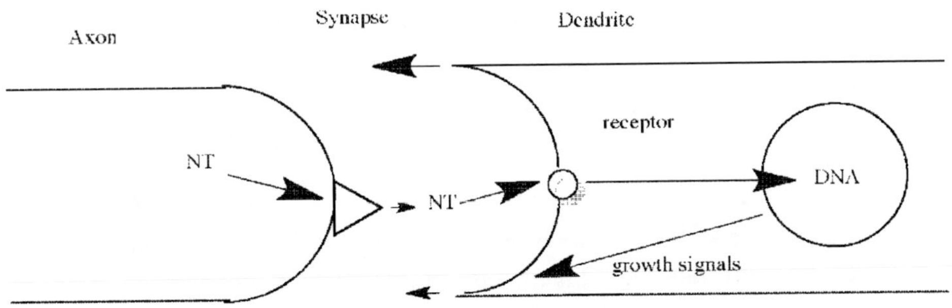

Figure 3. Structure of membranes.

IV. Functions of Fish Oil

A. Sources of Fish Oils

1. *De novo* in people - Neurons are unable to produce DHA, and only the liver may have the potential to produce a small amount of it *de novo* from shorter omega-3 fatty acids (Scott, 1989). However, more recent research indicates that little can be provided even this way.

Plasma alpha-linolenic acid (alpha-LNA, 18:3n-3) and linoleic acid (LA, 18:2n-6) do not contribute significantly to the brain content of docosahexaenoic acid (DHA, 22:6n-3) or arachidonic acid (AA, 20:4n-6), respectively, and neither DHA nor AA can be synthesized *de novo* in vertebrate tissue. Therefore, measured rates of brain cell membrane growth are based solely on incorporation of circulating DHA and AA into brain tissue. None is made *in situ*. (Rapoport, 2007).

2. *De novo* in fish - Unlike most terrestrial animals, marine fishes cannot synthesize DHA *de novo* from precursor molecules. For successful larval fish culture, broodstock must be fed proper amounts of DHA to spawn good quality eggs, and prey for larval fish have to be enriched with oil containing DHA. In the natural marine ecosystem, algae and, to a lesser extent, bacteria, are the major producers of DHA. Copepods and other crustaceans accumulate DHA by feeding on algae, and fish larvae feed on these zooplankton (Masuda, 2003).

3. *De novo* in blue green algae - Only a small number of algae species are used to make supplements that contain EPA and DHA. Algae contain substantially lower concentrations of EPA and DHA than fish, as do their respective oil supplements. Some seaweeds, such as wakame, contain EPA but not DHA. Some algae, including popular blue-green algae (more strictly cyanobacteria), contain a good balance of ALA and LA but negligible amounts of EPA and DHA. They are not therefore comparable to fish oils. Algae of the genus *Schizochytrium* contain significant levels of DHA and have therefore been selected for supplement manufacture (Li, 2009).

B. Function of Fish Oil in Fish

The concentration of EPA and DHA varies substantially between warm and cold water dwelling fish (Kris-Etherton, 2002). The higher omega-3 content is necessary to maintain flexibility of cell membranes at colder temperatures. The melting point of DHA is -44°C, while of EPA it is -53.5°C. By contract, the saturated fat in fig. 1A melts at 62.9°C.

C. Composition of Fish Oil

Because of the variation in omega-3 content of fish, fish oil capsules state the quantity of EPA and DHA. Generally fish oil supplements contain about 1 g of various oils from about 3.5 oz of cold water fish (MedlinePlus, 2011). Few complete analyses of fish oil have been done (Saify, 2003). A regular 1 g fish oil softgel usually contains 300 mg of the omega-3 fatty acids, 180 mg EPA and 120 mg DHA. It is the DHA that is vital for neuronal membranes.

D. Function pf Fish Oil in Brain

1. Composition of human brain

A human brain weights about 1.35 kg, and contains about 100 billion neurons. The brain is about 77% water, 10-12% lipids, and 8% protein (McIlwain, 1985). The brain is the fattiest organ of the body, being nearly 70% phospholipids, esp. phosphatidyl choline (fig. 3). DHA is the major fatty acid, constituting 40% of the PUFAs in the brain, and 50% of the neuronal membranes (Singh, 2005). EPA is found only in trace amounts (Arterburn, 2006).

2. Function

The fluidity of DHA at standard temperature and pressure permits dynamics of nerve channels for ion transport, synaptic transport of neurotransmitters, the reconfiguration of synapses between axons and dendrites, and synaptic remodeling to control short and long-term facilitation for learning (Fujita, 2001). The manner by which neurons function remains controversial, and the neuron doctrine of signals moving linearly from the axon of one neuron to dendrite of the next has become controversial (Bullock, 2005). Neurons in infants and teenagers contain about 100,000 dendrites each, which are pruned to approximately 10,000 about 3 years later (Thagard, 2010).

E. Weight Control

1. Introduction to nutrient signaling

Our understanding of the role of nutrients has changed substantially since the late 20th century. In addition to providing molecular structures and calories, nutrients are now known to signal key physiologic functions, cellular responses including transcription and translation of DNA that can change metabolic rates, and even trigger apoptosis (Bhalla and Iyengar, 1999; Hardwick, 1999).

Once this was recognized, three signaling pathways relevant to weight regulation were discovered. *Cota* (2006) demonstrated that branched chain amino acids (BCAAs) regulate food intake via the mTOR pathway (Sabatini, 1994). Two behaviors were initiated in the brain of rats, one region decreasing appetite and the other increasing basal metabolic rate. Then Hsu (2006) discovered that oleic acid, c18:1(9c), regulates the metabolism of apidocytes. When serum oleic acid levels are raised, adipocytes slow the rate of absorbing fatty acids, decrease the synthesis of triglycerides, and increase the hydrolysis of fats, secreting fatty acids into the serum.

2. Effect of DHA on weight loss

One mechanism by which DHA can reduce the risk of chronic disease is its ability, as an omega-3 fatty acid, to reduce the level of inflammation. Omega-3 fatty acids are converted into anti-inflammatory molecules, and dietary DHA is especially effective in reducing coronary heart disease, rheumatoid arthritis, psoriasis, asthma, and inflammatory bowel disorders (Mori, 2004).

It was known that DHA prevents cardiovascular disease by decreasing obesity (Cha, 2001). Compared with controls fed high (n-6) fatty acid diets [high (n-6) group], the livers of male and female mice fed DHA [high (n-3) group] contained six- ($P < 0.001$) and fivefold ($P < 0.001$) more DHA, respectively. The high (n-3) group had less white adipose tissue [35.3% in males ($P < 0.001$) and 27.3% in females ($P < 0.001$)].

With the discovery of nutrient signaling, Kim (2006) discovered that in culture, DHA also blocks differentiation and triggers apoptosis in pre-adipocytes. In addition, in fully differentiated adipocytes, DHA increased the rate of lipolysis compared to controls.

To determine concentrations that might be effective in the human diet for weight reduction, I tried levels of fish oil, olive oil (which is 85% oleic acid), and BCAAs in a double-blind clinical trial pilot study with college-age and mature adults (Ordman, 2008). Although the pilot study was only funded for a two week trial, and used fish oil rather than concentrated DHA, it was found that 1 or 2 g of fish oil, BCAAs, and olive oil taken twice daily before breakfast and dinner were well tolerated, and had the potential to promote weight loss through nutrient signaling, preventing the rebound effect induced by traditional dieting using reduced caloric intake (Villaverde, 2008).

V. Intake and Dosage

The intake of omega-3 fatty acids has fallen dramatically over the past century, from 31 to 22% of highly unsaturated fatty acid intake (Harris, 2011).

Given the many benefits attributed to fish oil, and specifically DHA, it is interesting to note the dosages used in research studies. The US Food and Drug Administraton states that a food product must contain 160mg DHA/serving to be labeled "High in DHA" (FDA, 2007). In 2006, Stephensen reported that the American Heart Association recommended that those at risk for cardiovascular disease consume 1 to 3g/d of EPA and DHA as supplements. As most commercial fish oil supplements contain a total of only 0.3g of EPA and DHA combined, the AHA dosage can require up to 10 fish oil tablets per day.

In June 2006, the American Journal of Clinical Nutrition published a supplement on n3 Fatty Acids: Recommendations for Therapeutics and Prevention. Johnson (2006) reported "Our own unpublished observations from the Framingham Heart Study suggest that ≥180 mg/d of dietary DHA (≈2.7 fish servings/wk) is associated with an ≈50% reduction in dementia risk." This dose corresponds to one commercial 1g capsule daily. For people over 60, 2g daily is more commonly used in studies. An epidemiological study of people age 70-74 found that those with an intake over 10g of fish/d had much higher cognitive scores (Nurk, 2007). A review of fish oil trials (Wang, 2006) showed significant benefit for many conditions, including dementia. The largest trial followed 11,324 patients with recent myocardial infarction for 3.5 y in Italy and reported that people eating 0.85 g EPA+DHA/d, compared with controls, significantly reduced the relative risk of all-cause mortality, cardiac death, and sudden death by 21%, 35%, and 45%, respectively (Marchioli, 1999, 2002). Finally, in my weight loss study, men who took 2g of fish oil twice a day were more likely to lose weight than those who took 0 or 1g. Young women were more likely to see a benefit with 2g, but mature women over 40 saw no effect after only 2 weeks, and a future trial would be more likely to obtain statistically significant results if tablets with much higher amounts of only DHA were used.

Table 1. Fish Oil Dosages

Group	Condition	Dosage Used	Reference
United States	For general health	650 mg DHA+EPA/d = 2 g fish oil/d	National Institutes of Health
At risk for heart disease	To reduce risk of heart disease	1-3 g EPA+DHA/d = 3-10 g fish oil/d	AHA, Stephensen, 2006
Framingham	To reduce risk of dementia	1 g fish oil/d	Johnson, 2006
Over 70	To reduce risk of dementia	10 g fish/d	Nurk, 2007
Men	To promote weight loss	2 g fish oil/d	Ordman, 2008

VI. Conclusion

How the world will find ways to provide these essential nutrients without depleting fish populations will remain an exciting research challenge. Fish oil, and specifically DHA, is at the junction of many exciting developments in current research. In neuroscience, DHA plays an essential role in neuronal membranes, and thus consciousness. In nutrition, as essential nutrients in the human diet, EPA and DHA are necessary to reduce inflammation. In controlling obesity, DHA is an essential signaling molecule controlling processes related to lipid metabolism, hunger, and cell differentiation and survival.

References

Albanese, E., Dangour, A.D, Uauy, R., Acosta, D., Guerra, M., Guerra, S.S., Huang, Y., Jacob, K.S., de Rodriguez, J.L., Noriega, L.H., Salas, A., Sosa, A.L., Sousa, R.M., Williams, J., Ferri, C.P., Prince, M.J. (2009). Dietary fish and meat intake and dementia in Latin America, China, and India: a 10/66 Dementia Research Group population-based study. *Am J Clin Nutr* 90: 392-400.

Arterburn, L.M., Hall, E,B., Oken, H. (2006). Distribution, interconversion, and dose response of n–3 fatty acids in humans. *Am J Clin Nutr* 83: S1467-1476S.

Asthana, S., Bhasin, S., Butler, R.N., Fillit, H., Finkelstein, J., Harman, S.M., Holstein, L., Korenman, S.G., Matsumoto, A.M., Morley, J.E., Tsitouras, P., Urban, R. (2004). Masculine Vitality: Pros and Cons of Testosterone in Treating the Andropause. *J Gerontol A Biol Sci Med Sci* 59: M461-M465.

Baker, H., Frank, O., Chen, T., Feingold, S., DeAngelis, B., Baker, E. (1984). Vitamin content of some normal human brain segments. *J Neurosci Res*. 11:419-35.

Bhalla, U.S., Iyengar, R. (1999). Emergent Properties of Networks of Biological Signaling Pathways. *Science* 283: 381-387.

Bjelland, I., Grethe, S. T., Vollset, S.E., Konstantinova, S., Ueland, P.M. (2009). Choline in anxiety and depression: the Hordaland Health Study. *Am J Clin Nutr* 90:1056-1060.

Black, D.S., Milam, J., Sussman, S. (2009). Review Article: Sitting-Meditation Interventions Among Youth: A Review of Treatment Efficacy. *Pediatrics* 124: e532-e541.

Blackmore, S. (2004) *Consciousness: An introduction*. Oxford Univ. Press, New York.

Brefczynski-Lewis, L.A., Johnstone, T., Davidson, R.J. (2008). Regulation of the Neural Circuitry of Emotion by Compassion Meditation: Effects of Meditative Expertise. *PLoS ONE* 3(3): e1897.

Bullock, T.H., Michael, V. L., Bennett, D.J., Josephson, R., Marder, E., Fields, R.D. (2005). The Neuron Doctrine, Redux. *Science* 310: 791 - 793.

Burkhalter, T.M., Hillman, C.H. (2011). A Narrative Review of Physical Activity, Nutrition, and Obesity to Cognition and Scholastic Performance across the Human Lifespan. *Adv Nutr* 2:201S-206S.

Butler, R.N., Sprott, R., Warner, H., Bland, J., Feuers, R., Forster, M. (2004). Biomarkers of aging: from primitive organisms to humans. *J Gerontol Biol Sci* 59: B560-7.

Cha, S.H., Fukushima, A., Sakuma, K., Kagawa, Y. (2001). Chronic Docosahexaenoic Acid Intake Enhances Expression of the Gene for Uncoupling Protein 3 and Affects Pleiotropic mRNA Levels in Skeletal Muscle of Aged C57BL/6NJcl Mice. *J. Nutr.* 131:2636-2642.

Cole, G.M., and Frautschy, S.A. (2010). DHA May Prevent Age-Related Dementia, *J. Nutr.* 140: 869-874.

Cota. D., Prouix, K., Blake Smith, K.A., Kozma, S.C., Thomas, G., Woods, S.C., Seeley, R.J. (2006). Hypothalamic mTOR Signaling Regulates Food Intake. *Science* 312: 927-930.

Davidson, R.J., Kabat-Zinn, J., Schumacher, J., Rosenkranz, M., Muller, D., Santorelli, S.F., Urbanowski, F., Harrington, A., Bonus, K. and Sheridan, J.F., (2003). Alterations in Brain and Immune Function Produced by Mindfulness Meditation. *Psychosomatic Medicine* 65: 564-570.

Dawkins, R. (1976). *The Selfish Gene*. Oxford Univ. Press, Oxford.

Dennett, D. (1991). *Consciousness Explained*. Little, Brown & Co., New York.

Epel, E., Daubenmier, J., Moskowitz, J.T., Folkman, S., Blackburn, E. (2009). Can Meditation Slow Rate of Cellular Aging? Cognitive Stress, Mindfulness, and Telomeres. *Annals of the New York Academy of Sciences* 1172: 34–53.

Farina, E.K., Kiel, D.P., Roubenoff, R., Schaefer, E.J., Cupples, L.A., Tucker, K.L. (2011). Protective effects of fish intake and interactive effects of long-chain polyunsaturated fatty acid intakes on hip bone mineral density in older adults: the Framingham Osteoporosis Study. *Am J Clin Nutr* 93:1142-1151.

FDA. (2007). Federal Register Notice of Proposed Rulemaking (Food Labeling) 72 FR 66103 November 27, 2007: Food Labeling: Nutrient Content Claims; Alpha-Linolenic Acid, *Eicosapentaenoic Acid, and Docosahexaenoic Acid Omega-3 Fatty Acids, Volume 72,* Number 227.

Food and Nutrition Board, Institute of Medicine. (1998). *Dietary Reference Intakes: Thiamin, Riboflavin, Niacin, Vitamin B-6, Vitamin B-12, Pantothenic Acid, Biotin, and Choline.* Washington, DC: National Academy Press, pages 390-422.

Fujita,S., Ikegaya, Y., Nishikawa, M., Nishiyama, N., Matsuki, N. (2001). Docosahexaenoic acid improves long-term potentiation attenuated by phospholipase A2 inhibitor in rat hippocampal slices. *Br J Pharmacol* 132: 1417–1422.

Gerster, H. (1998). Can adults adequately convert alpha-linolenic acid (18:3n-3) to eicosapentaenoic acid (20:5n-3) and docosahexaenoic acid (22:6n-3)?. *Int. J. Vitam. Nutr. Res.* 68 (3): 159–173.

Greer, F.R. (2009). Introduction, Symposium: Methyl Donors, Iodine, and Docosahexaenoic Acid-Is Maternal Supplementation Beneficial? *AJCN* 89: 661S- 687S.

Hardwick, J.S., Kuruvilla, F.G., Tong, J.K., Shamji, A.F., Schreiber, S.L. (1999). Rapamycin-modulated transcription defines the subset of nutrient-sensitive signaling pathways directly controlled by the Tor proteins. *Proc Natl Acad Sci U S A*. 96: 14866–14870.

Harris, W.S., Klurfeld, D.M. (2011). Twentieth-century trends in essential fatty acid intakes and the predicted omega-3 index: evidence versus estimates. *Am J Clin Nutr* 93: 907-908.

Hayflick, L., Moorhead, P.S. (1961). The serial cultivation of human diploid cell strains. *Exp Cell Res* 25: 585–621.

Hsu, S., Huang, C. (2006). Reduced Fat Mass in Rats Fed a High Oleic Acid–Rich Safflower Oil Diet Is Associated with Changes in Expression of Hepatic PPAR and Adipose SREBP-1c–Regulated Genes. *J. Nutr*. 136:1779-1785.

Izquierdo, I., Medinab, J.H. (1997). Memory Formation: The Sequence of Biochemical Events in the Hippocampus and Its Connection to Activity in Other Brain Structures. *Neurobiology of Learning and Memory* 68: 285-316.

Johnson, E.J., Schaefer, E.J. (2006). Potential role of dietary n–3 fatty acids in the prevention of dementia and macular degeneration. *Am J Clin Nutr* 83: S1494-1498S.

Killilea, D.W., Ames, B.N. (2008). Magnesium deficiency accelerates cellular senescence in cultured human fibroblasts. *PNAS US*, 105: 5768-5773.

Kim, H., Della-Fera, M., Lin, J., Baile, C.A. (2006). Docosahexaenoic Acid Inhibits Adipocyte Differentiation and Induces Apoptosis in 3T3-L1 Preadipocytes. *J. Nutr*. 136:2965-2969.

Kris-Etherton, P.M., Harris, W.S., Appel, L.J. (2002). AHA Scientific Statement. Fish consumption, fish oil, omega-3 fatty acids, and cardiovascular disease. *Circulation* 106: 2747–57.

Li, M.H., Robinson, E.H., Tucker, C.S., Manning, B.B., Khoo, L. (2009). Effects of Dried Algae Schizochytrium Sp., A Rich Source of Docosahexaenoic Acid, on Growth, Fatty Acid Composition, and Sensory Quality of Channel Catfish Ictalurus Punctatus. *Aquaculture*. 292:232-236.

Marchioli R. (1999). Dietary supplementation with n–3 polyunsaturated fatty acids and vitamin E after myocardial infarction: results of the GISSI-Prevenzione trial. *Lancet* 354:447–55.

Marchioli, R., Barzi. F., Bomba, E., Chieffo, C., Di Gregorio, D. (2002). Early protection against sudden death by n–3 polyunsaturated fatty acids after myocardial infarction: time-course analysis of the results of the Gruppo Italiano per lo Studio della Sopravvivenza nell'Infarto Miocardico (GISSI)-Prevenzione. *Circulation* 105:1897–903.

Masuda, R. (2003). The critical role of docosahexaenoic acid in marine and terrestrial ecosystems: from bacteria to human behavior in The Big Fish Bang. *Proceedings of the 26th Annual Larval Fish Conference*. Ed. Howard I. Browman and Anne Berit Skiftesvik, Institute of Marine Research, Postboks 1870 Nordnes, N-5817, Bergen, Norway.

McIlwain, H. and Bachelard, H.S. (1985). *Biochemistry and the Central Nervous System*. Churchill Livingstone, Edinburgh.

McNamara, R.K. (2010). DHA Deficiency and Prefrontal Cortex Neuropathology in Recurrent Affective Disorders. *J. Nutr*. 140: 864-868.

Mead, M.N. (2008). Molecular biology: telomerase tells on lifestyle. *Environmental Health Perspectives,* 116: 521.

Mori, T.A., Lawrence, J., Beilin, L.J. (2004). Omega-3 fatty acids and inflammation. *Current Atherosclerosis Reports* 6: 461-467.

Muldoon, M.F., Ryan, C.M., Sheu, L., Yao, J.K., Conklin, S.M., Manuck, S.B. (2010). Serum Phospholipid Docosahexaenonic Acid Is Associated with Cognitive Functioning during Middle Adulthood. *J. Nutr*. 140: 848-853.

Nurk, E., Drevon, C.A., Refsum, H., Solvoll, K., Vollset, S.E., Nygård, O., Nygaard, H.A., Engedal, K.,Tell, G.S., Smith, A.D. (2006). Cognitive performance among the elderly and dietary fish intake: the Hordaland Health Study. *Am J Clin Nutr* 86:1470-1478.

Nynke de Jong, M., Paw, C.A., JM, Lisette, J.M., de Groot, C.P.G.M., Rutten, R.A.M., Swinkels, D.W., Kok, F.J., van Staveren, W.A. (2001). "Nutrient-dense foods and exercise in frail elderly: effects on B vitamins, homocysteine, methylmalonic acid, and neuropsychological functioning. *Am J Clin Nutr* 73: 338-346.

Olovnikov, A.M. (1996). Telomeres, telomerase, and aging: Origin of the theory. *Experimental Gerontology* 31: 443-448.

Ordman, A.B., Colman, R.J., Kemnitz, J.W. (2005). Selection of Aging Biomarkers in Primates: Caloric Restriction of Rhesus Monkeys. *http://chemistry.beloit.edu/Ordman/posters/postinds/zpostrocresch.htm*, accessed April 8, 2011.

Ordman, A.B. (2008). Pilot study for an age- and gender-based nutrient signaling system for weight control. *AGE* 30, 201-208.

Parfit, D. (1987). *Divided minds and the nature of persons*. In C. Blakemore and S. Greenfield (eds) Mindwaves. Oxford: Blackwell, 19-26.

Rapoport, S.I., Rao, J.S., Igarashi, M. (2007). Brain metabolism of nutritionally essential polyunsaturated fatty acids depends on both the diet and the liver. *Prostaglandins Leukot Essent Fatty Acids* 77:251-61.

Richards, J.B., Valdes, A.M., Gardner, J.P., Paximadas, D., Kimura, M., Nessa, A., Lu, X. (2007). Higher serum vitamin D concentrations are associated with longer leukocyte telomere length in women. *Am. J. Clin. Nutr*. 86:1420–5.

Roth, J., Szulc, A.L., Danoff, A. (2011). Energy, evolution, and human diseases: an overview. *Am J Clin Nutr* 93:875S-883S.

Sabatini, D.M., Erdjument-Bromage, H., Lui, M., Tempst, P., Snyder, S.H. (1994). RAFT1: A mammalian protein that binds to FKBP12 in a rapamycin-dependent fashion and is homologous to yeast TORs. *Cell* 78, 35.

Sabia, S., Kivimaki, M., Shipley, M.J., Marmot, M.G., Singh-Manoux, A. (2009). Body mass index over the adult life course and cognition in late midlife: the Whitehall II Cohort Study. *Am J Clin Nutr* 89:601-607.

Safdar, A., Bourgeois, J.M., Ogborn, D.I., Little, J.P., Hettinga, B.P., Akhtar, M., Thompson, J.E., Melov, S., Mocellin, N.J., Kujoth, G.C., Prolla, T.A., Tarnopolsky, M.A. (2011). Endurance exercise rescues progeroid aging and induces systemic mitochondrial rejuvenation in mtDNA mutator mice. *Proc Natl Acad Sci U S A* 108:4135-40.

Saify, Z.S., Shamim, A., Khan, K.M., Perveen, S., Ayattollahi, S.A.M., Hassan, S., Arif, M., Haider, S.M., Ahmad,F., Siddiqui, S., ZarrarKhan, M. (2003). A Study on the Fatty Acid Composition of Fish Liver Oil from Two Marine Fish, Eusphyra blochii and Carcharhinus bleekeri. *Turk J Chem* 27: 251 - 258.

Scott, B.L., Bazan, N.G. (1989). Membrane docosahexaenoate is supplied to the developing brain and retina by the liver. *Proc. Natl. Acad. Sci. U.S.A*. 86: 2903–2907.

Shin, W., Yan, J., Abratte, C.M., Vermeylen, F., Caudill, M.A. (2010). Choline Intake Exceeding Current Dietary Recommendations Preserves Markers of Cellular Methylation in a Genetic Subgroup of Folate-Compromised Men. *J. Nutr.* 140: 975-980.

Singh, M. (2005). Essential Fatty Acids, DHA and Human Brain. *Indian J Pediatr* 72: 239-242.

Spiegel, A.M., Alving, B.M. (2005). Executive summary of the Strategic Plan for National Institutes of Health Obesity Research. *Am J Clin Nutr* 2005 82: 211S-214S.

Charles B Stephensen, C.B., Kelley, D.S. (2006). The innate immune system: friend and foe. *Am J Clin Nutr* 83:187-188.

Tang, Y., Yinghua M., Wang, J., Fan, Y., Feng, S., Lu, Q., Yu, Q., Sui, D., Rothbart, M.K., Fan ||, M., Posner, M.I. (2007). Short-term meditation training improves attention and self-regulation. *PNAS* 104: 17152-56.

Thagard, P. (2010). *The Brain and the Meaning of Life*. Paul Thagard, Princeton Univ. Press.

USDA. (1992). Food Guide Pyramid. *http://fnic.nal.usda.gov/nal_display/index.php?info_center=4&tax_level=3&tax_subject=256&topic_id=1348&level3_id=5729*, accessed May 9, 2011.

USDA. (2005). Food Guide Pyramid. *http://www.mypyramid.gov/index.html*, accessed May 9, 2011.

Villaverde, C., Ramsey, J.J., Green, A.S., Asami, D.K., Yoo, S., Fascetti, A.J. (2008). Energy Restriction Results in a Mass-Adjusted Decrease in Energy Expenditure in Cats That Is Maintained after Weight Regain. *J. Nutr.* 138:856-860.

Wang, C., Harris, W.S., Chung, M., Lichtenstein, A.H., Balk, E.M., Kupelnick, B., Jordan, H.S., Lau, J. (2006) n–3 Fatty acids from fish or fish-oil supplements, but not α-linolenic acid, benefit cardiovascular disease outcomes in primary- and secondary-prevention studies: a systematic review. *Am J Clin Nutr* 84: 5-17.

Werner, C., Fürster, T., Widmann, T., Pöss, J., Roggia, C.,, Hanhoun, M., Scharhag, J., Büchner, N., Meyer, T., Kindermann, W., Haendeler, J., Böhm, M., Laufs, U. (2009). Physical Exercise Prevents Cellular Senescence in Circulating Leukocytes and in the Vessel Wall. *Circulation* 120 (24): 2438–47.

Wheeler, M. (2009). How to build a bigger brain. NeuroImage, *http://www.eurekalert.org/pub_releases/2009-05/uoc--htb051209.php*, accessed April 10, 2011.

Willett, W.C., Skerrett, P.J. (2001). *Eat, Drink, and Be Healthy: The Harvard Medical School Guide to Healthy Eating*. Free Press, New York.

Wisse, B.E., Kim, F., Schwartz, M.W. (2007). An Integrative View of Obesity. *Science* 318: 928-929.

Xie, T. (2008). Burn Fat, Live Longer. *Science* 322: 865-866.

Zeisel, S.H. (2005). Choline, homocysteine, and pregnancy. *Am J Clin Nutr* 82: 719-720.

Zeisel, S.H. (2008). Is there a new component of the Mediterranean diet that reduces inflammation? *Am J Clin Nutr* 87: 277-278.

Zhang, C., Bazan, N.G. (2010). Lipid-Mediated Cell Signaling Protects against Injury and Neurodegeneration. *J. Nutr.* 140: 858-863.

In: Fish Oil: Production, Consumption and Health Benefits ISBN: 978-1-61470-963-3
Editors: Matthias Van Dijk and Jürgen Vitek

Chapter XII

Fish Oils, Omega-3 Fatty Acids and Male Fertility

C. A. Castellano[1], I. Audet[2], J. P. Laforest[3] and J. J. Matte[2]

[1]Faculty of Medicine and Health Sciences, Department of Physiology and Biophysics, Université de Sherbrooke, Sherbrooke, QC, Canada

[2]Dairy and Swine Research and Development Centre, Agriculture and Agri-Food Canada, 2000 College Street, P.O. Box 90, Lennoxville STN, Sherbrooke, QC, Canada

[3]Faculty of Agriculture and Agri-Food Sciences, Department of animal sciences, Université Laval, Quebec, QC, Canada

Over the last three decades, the potential role of omega-3 polyunsaturated fatty acids on health and disease has been a worldwide center of attention. In the western typical diet, the omega-6 to omega-3 fatty acid ratio is at least 10 to 1, likely due to the high prevalence of vegetable oils (such as soybean oil, corn oil and sunflower oil) rich in omega-6 fatty acid. Since excessive amounts of omega-6 fatty acids contribute to rising incidence of many chronic diseases such as cardiovascular disease and whereas increasing omega-3 fatty acid intake cause a protective effect, a more balanced omega-6 to omega-3 fatty acid ratio is recommended (omega-6 to omega-3 fatty acid ratio between 1 to 1 and 3 to 1). A good natural source of omega-3 polyunsaturated fatty acid is seafood and particularly fish oil. Fish and marine products contain two major omega-3 polyunsaturated fatty acids – eicosapentaenoic acid (EPA) and docosahexaemoic acid (DHA) - both of which appear to be beneficial for cardiovascular prevention, immune function, inflammatory response, infant development and mental health. Fish oils may also improve female fertility (ovulatory processes, premature birth and lactation).

Although there is a large amount of information available on fish oil, omega-3 fatty acid supplement and their pleiotropic beneficial effects on global health, it is sometimes misleading and not always support by scientific findings, in particular in the case of male reproductive health. Therefore, this review considers the role played by fish oils supplement in male fertility, with large references to human and various animal models (pig, horse, cattle, fowl, rabbit and sheep).

Many of the male fertility problems can be related to oligospermia (a low sperm count) or a poor sperm quality (cell with abnormal shape or low motility). In the management of male fertility, omega-3 polyunsaturated fatty acids like others nutrients (vitamins, minerals, zinc, etc.) play a key role in reproductive health.

Sperm cells require highly polyunsaturated fatty acids, in particular a high proportion of DHA to provide optimal cell membrane fluidity essential to sperm motility and fertilization success (acrosomal reaction and oocyte penetration). Some studies have suggested that subfertility could be related to the low DHA sperm content. As reported in human, in pig, and several others animal models, fish oil diet can alter significantly sperm fatty acid composition by increasing DHA and EPA content and modify omega-6 to omega-3 fatty acid ratio.

Some studies have underlined the potential benefit of fish oil supplement on sperm count. However this effect is more controversial since a diet rich in energy or in proteins also increase sperm production. In fact, dietary omega-3 polyunsaturated fatty acids can affect male fertility directly by modifying sperm membrane composition but also indirectly through various mechanisms: prostaglandin synthesis, steroid metabolism and gene expression.

In parallel to the benefit of consuming fish oil is the concern about potential harmful effects on male reproductive health. Because of his high polyunsaturated fatty acid content, sperm cells have a strong oxidative potential. In normal conditions, there is a balance between the generation of oxidants and antioxidant defense mechanisms. Dietary fish oil can induce an additional oxidative stress to the cell which is detrimental for sperm membrane fluidity and DNA integrity. In fact, it is suggested that any fish oil supplementation should be accompanied by antioxidants like vitamins E and C.There is also evidence that adding omega-3 polyunsaturated fatty acid to the diet can influence prostaglandin synthesis which could have an effect on testosterone secretion. Because chemicals such as PCB, pesticides, and sex hormones are fat-soluble, fish and fish oil can also be a dietary source of contaminants that may have deleterious effect on male reproduction.

In conclusion, dietary fish oil may help to improve male fertility by increasing omega-3 polyunsaturated fatty acids in sperm cells and would be most beneficial with sperm of initial poor quality. However, a particular attention must be taken in regard to antioxidant supplementation.

Introduction

In the collective mind, terms such as “omega-3”, “DHA”, “EPA” and “fish/fish oil” are generally associated with health benefits. Oily cold-water fish are the main dietary source of omega-3 fatty acids eicosapentaenoic acid (EPA) and docosahexaenoic acid (DHA). These fatty acids have important biological functions including primary roles in cell membranes and in eicosanoid metabolism. Indeed, there are evidences that omega-3 polyunsaturated fatty acids are essential nutrients for infant development. Also their positive roles in reducing cardiovascular risk, arthritis, cancer as well as improving mental health have been widely documented in human and animals studies for the last three decades [1]. Furthermore, omega-3 fatty acids may have specific health benefits in female reproduction [2]. A little less is known about the roles of omega-3 fatty acids in male reproduction. This review based on animal models and human studies will focus on the potential benefits as well as harmful effects of fish oil supplementation on male fertility.

Metabolism of Polyunsaturated Fatty Acids

Polyunsaturated fatty acids (PUFA) are classified into two main groups on the basis of their chemical structure, omega-3 and omega-6, according the localisation of the first double bond from the methyl (omega) end of the fatty acid in 3 or 6 carbons, respectively. Linoleic acid (LNA, 18:2n-6) is the most common PUFA and is abundant in vegetable oils. Alpha-linolenic acid (ALA, 18:3n-3) is found mainly in green leafy vegetables [3]. In human and others mammals, LNA and ALA cannot be synthesized *de novo*, and must be provided by the diet. Longer-chains PUFA (20-22-carbon fatty acids), such as arachidonic acid (20:4n-6, ARA), eicosapentaenoic acid (20:5n-3, EPA) and docosahexaenoic acid (22:6n-3, DHA), are produced from the metabolism of LNA and ALA through series of elongation and desaturation reactions within the tissues (Figure 1), mainly in the liver [4]. However enzymatic conversion efficiencies vary considerably among species and tissues [5]. According to some authors [6, 7], an active conversion of EPA to DHA is observed specifically in rat testicular tissue. In human, this metabolic activity is relatively low compared to rats [8]. Moreover, it appear that general fatty acid metabolism is relatively inefficient in humans with <1% of ALA transformed into DHA [9]. Present evidence indicates that 20-22-carbon fatty acids should be obtained directly from nutrition. Arachidonic acid occurs primarily in animal fat whereas EPA and DHA are found in large proportions (up to 30%) in fish oils [3].

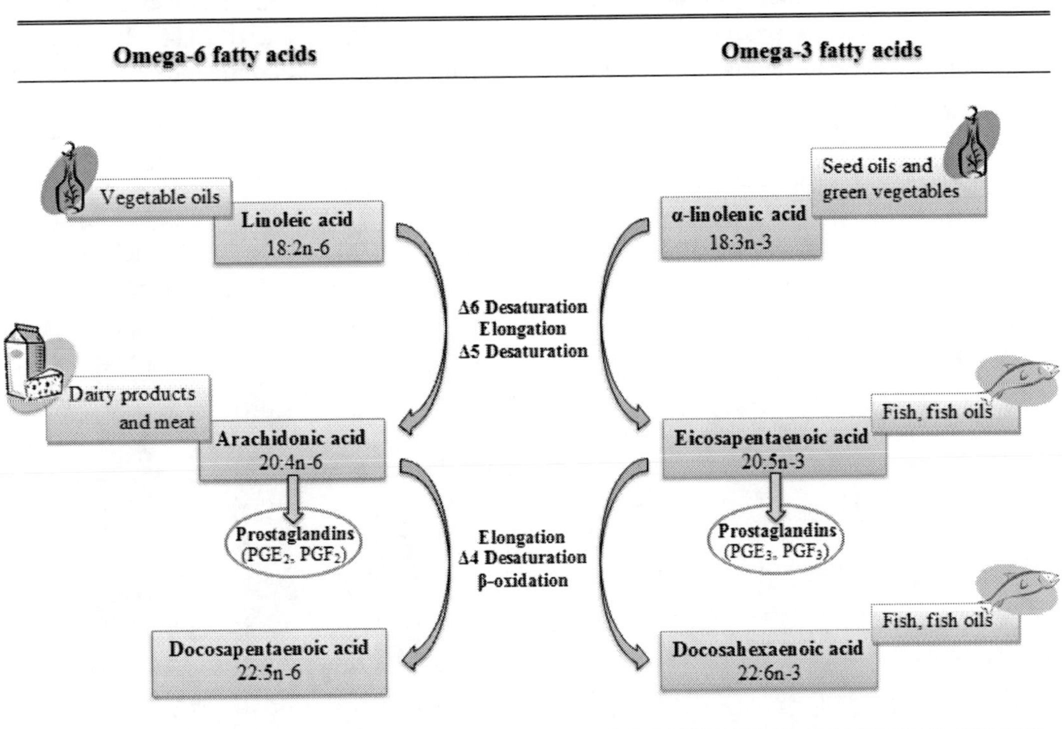

Figure 1. Metabolism of omega-3 and omega-6 polyunsaturated fatty acids.

Lipid Composition of Testicular Tissue and Spermatozoa

In all mammalian cell membranes, fatty acids are structural component. Although a large diversity of fatty acid pattern is observed in various tissues, including varying chain lengths and degrees of unsaturation, a common aspect is the presence of significant levels of long chain polyunsaturated fatty acids (20-24 carbons). Even if the exact role of these particular fatty acids is not completely understood, it is well accepted that long chain PUFA contribute to cell membrane structure and function [10]. In human tissues, omega-3 fatty acid DHA and omega-6 fatty acid ARA are the most abundant but have different patterns of distributions [11]. In the majority of tissues, as liver and muscle, ARA is the predominant fatty acid (<10%) and DHA proportions do not exceed 5% (Figure 2). However, specific tissues such as neural (brain and retina) and testicular tissues, are particularly rich in DHA (up to 22% in retina) [12-14]. Fats in testes and spermatozoa contain up to 65% of long chain PUFA mostly arachidonic acid (AA, 20:4n-6), docosapentaenoic acid (DPA, 22:5n-6) and DHA with species-specific variability in these fatty acids [15, 16]. Omega-6 fatty acids dominate in testis of rat [17], hamster [18], rabbit [19], and others rodents whereas omega-3 fatty acids are relatively abundant in testis of human [20, 21], ram [22], bull [23] and boar [24]. A similar fatty acid pattern can be observed in mammalian semen (Table 1). In human sperm along with several others species (monkey, bull, ram) omega-3 fatty acid DHA is mainly present whereas in stallion, dog and rodents omega-6 fatty acid DPA is the principal fatty acid. Boar sperm shows a more balance profile with high proportions of DPA and DHA [15, 25]. Sperm in avian species (rich in omega-6 fatty acids) is peculiar with a predominance of arachidonic acid (20:4n-6) and docosatetraenoic acid (22:4n-6) [26, 27].

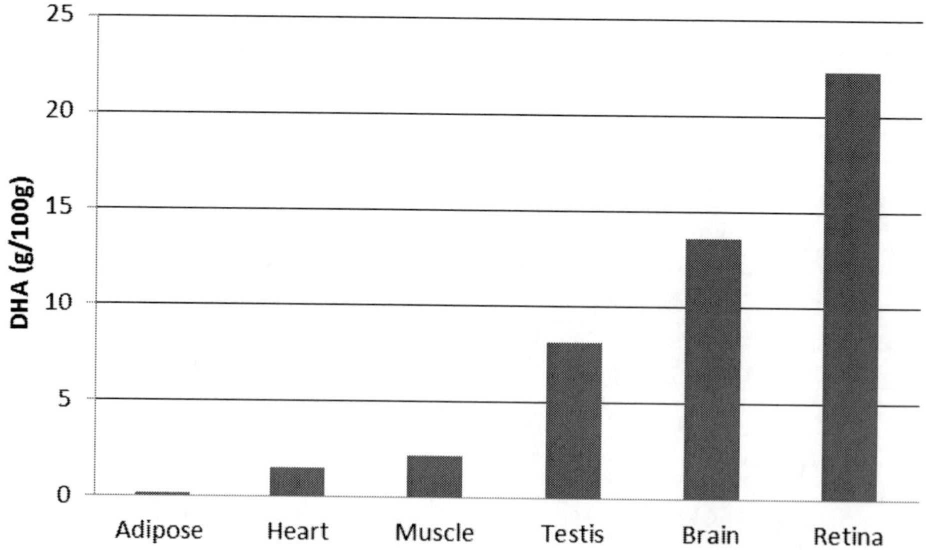

Figure 2. Fatty acid concentration of DHA (g/100g of total fatty acids) in various human tissues. References : adipose tissue [28]; muscle [29] ; heart [30]; testis [20]; brain [13]; retina [14].

Table 1. Major polyunsaturated fatty acids (% total fatty acids) of phospholipid fraction present in spermatozoa of various species

Species	LNA 18:2n-6	ARA 20:4n-6	DPA 22:5n-6	DHA 22:6 n-3
Rhesus monkey	5.4	9.1	nd	23.9
Man	4.0	5.0	nd	35.2
Ram	1.7	4.5	nd	61.4
Bull	3.9	3.5	nd	61.3
Boar	2.1	3.2	27.9	37.7
Rabbit	4.8	nd	39.0	nd
Dog	3.2	6.6	28.4	3.9
Chicken	1.8	6.2	1.0	2.3
Stallion	--	18.2	17.0	7.59

LNA : linoleic acid ; ARA : arachidonic acid ; DPA : docosapentaenoic acid ; DHA : docohexaenoic acid ; nd : not determined. References : rhesus monkey [31]; man, ram, bull, boar and rabbit [15]; dog [32]; chicken [33]; stallion [34].

Roles of PUFA in Male Reproduction

The essential role of polyunsaturated fatty acids in male reproduction has been confirmed by many studies with experimental animals. In 1930, Burr and Burr were the first to report one of the consequences of polyunsaturated fatty acid deficiency is male infertility. In their experimental study, rats fed with a PUFA deficient diet show an impairment of reproduction [35]. Since this observation, several authors established in rat [36, 37], rabbit [19] and cat [38] that testes degeneration and subsequent infertility occurred in absence of unsaturated fatty acids. Bourre et al. [39] reported that an omega-3 fatty acid dietary deficiency in adult rat affected testis content with a progressive decline of DHA. A same negative effect of an omega-6 fatty acid deficiency on fertility of males chicken was observed [40]. Furthermore, several studies in human established a correlation between polyunsaturated fatty acid content and male fertility. A lower proportion of total omega-3 fatty acids in particular DHA is found in infertile spermatozoa [41, 42].

Membrane Properties of Spermatozoa

Sperm plasma membrane plays a key role in the fertilization process including acrosome reaction and sperm-oocyte interactions [43, 44]. A high percentage of polyunsaturated fatty acids is present in human and in mammalian spermatozoa [15, 45]. It has been suggested that the unusual composition and organisation in the sperm membrane may have an influence on several physical properties of the cell membrane including membrane order (fluidity) and membrane microdomain [46, 47]. As already highlighted by Lenzi et al. [48], some analogy can be made among the specific polyunsaturated fatty acid composition of membrane sperm (especially DHA), its capacity to react promptly to stimuli and other very active membrane cells such as nerve cells. Membrane fluidity/flexibility, which is required for the success of the membrane fusion events associated with fertilization, are directly related to the degree of unsaturation and the length of the carbon chain [49]. Fluidity is also important for the motility of sperm tails. Evidences of an association between polyunsaturated fatty acid content and sperm motility have been provided in monkeys [50], in men [51] and in chickens [52]. Furthermore, Conquer et al. [53] observed that sperm cells from infertile individuals with low sperm motility (refered as asthenozoospermic) contain less DHA.

Energy Source for Sperm Cell

Glycolysis is the preferential metabolic pathway generating energy for the male gamete [54]. However, sperm cells are able to use others energy substrates such as pyruvate, lactate and fatty acids. The possible use of fatty acid from lipid membrane degradation as metabolic substrate has been underlined in bull [55], ram [56], aries [57] and boar [58]. Moreover, some sea urchin studies show that this invertebrate sperm is able to use the endogenous fatty acids for its energy metabolism [59].

Eicosanoid Precursors

Some particular 20-carbon fatty acids (ARA, EPA) in cell membrane can serve as precursor for number of active hormone-like compounds referred as eicosanoids [60]. The eicosanoids include prostaglandins, thromboxanes, leukotrienes and lipoxins. As reviewed by Abayasekara and Wathes [61], prostaglandins are involved in many reproductive functions. In female reproduction, prostaglandins have an effect on follicular development, ovulation, corpus luteum function, luteolysis and lactation. In male reproduction, studies in rodent and in human supported the essential role of prostaglandins (PG) in the events leading to fecundation [62, 63]. In human semen, PGE and PGF are the major prostaglandin types [64]. Prostaglandins play a role in spermatogenesis [65] and sperm fertility [66]. Seminal PGE concentrations were correlated with sperm motility [67]. Moreover, prostaglandins can modulate testosterone biosynthesis. As already reported in goldfish by Wade et al. [68], prostaglandin-E_2 (a product of the metabolism of omega-6 fatty acid ARA) can stimulate testosterone production whereas PGE_3 (derived from omega-3 fatty acid EPA) is recognized as inhibitory regulator of steroidogenesis.

Fish Oil Supplementation and Male Reproduction

As previously discussed, polyunsaturated fatty acids are determinant in sperm fertility. Polyunsaturated fatty acids can influence reproductive processes through various mechanisms mainly related to sperm membrane and prostaglandin metabolism [2]. Furthermore, it is well accepted that the proportions of polyunsaturated fatty acids ingested through the diet is reflected in cell membrane composition [69]. Infertile men show a suboptimal nutritional intake of omega-3 fatty acids [70] and DHA (22:6n-3) sperm content is correlated with sperm motility in human [51] and others mammals. Therefore, there is a considerable interest to study the relationship between male infertility and polyunsaturated fatty acid dietary supplementation. Because fish oils are a major dietary source of omega-3 fatty acids (DHA and EPA), several experiments in human and livestock animals have been conducted to evaluate their effects in fertility. As show in Figure 3, the quantities of EPA and DHA can vary among fish species.

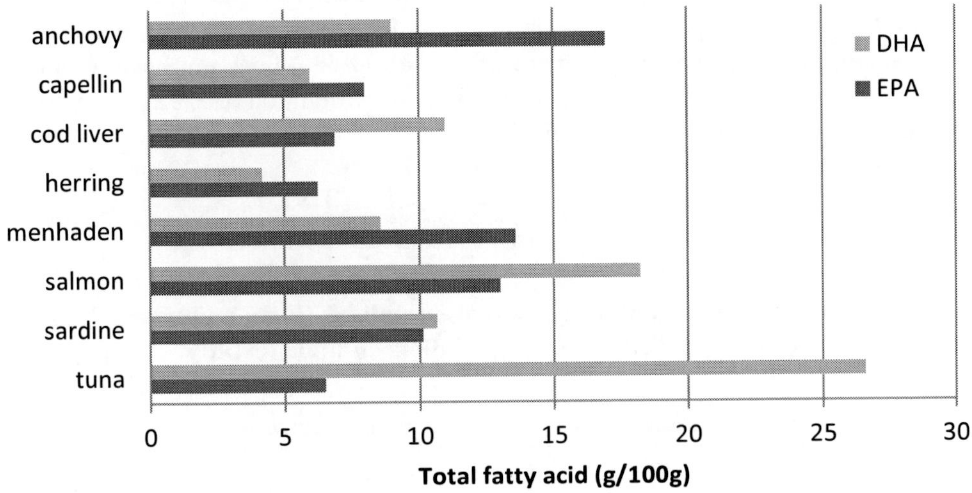

Figure 3: Proportions of EPA and DHA in fish oils (in regard of species, season, fish diet and processing methods, omega-3 fatty acid amounts can vary). References: anchovy and capelin [71]; cod liver, herring, menhaden, salmon and sardine [72]; tuna [73].

Consequences on Sperm Membrane Composition

Fatty acid composition of bird sperm, particularly rich in omega-6 fatty acids, clearly contrasts with sperm of mammalian species and seems to be more resistant to tissue fatty acid modulation by dietary fat sources [74]. Nevertheless, as reported in many domestic animals (chicken [74, 75], rabbit [76], stallion [77], boar [78], ram[79]) and in humans [80], fish oil diets resulted in a partial remodelling of the membrane fatty acid profile of spermatozoa, mainly in inducing an increase in the proportion of omega-3 fatty acids (DHA 22:6n-3) in parallel with an equivalent decrease in the proportions of omega-6 fatty acids (ARA 20:4n-6 and DPA 22:4n-6).

Consequences on Sperm Production

Many studies were conducted in poultry to evaluate the effect of different fatty acids on sperm production. Overall, results are inconsistent. Surai et al. [81] reported that 5% of tuna orbital oil prevented the natural decrease in the chicken number of sperm with aging. Nevertheless, two other studies did not present any alteration of sperm total number in chicken fed a fish oil supplementation [82-84].

In the majority of mammalian models, there is no evidence of any improvement of sperm production with a fish oil supplementation (Table 2). In human, whereas Schramm et Luley [85] observed an increase of total sperm number but not related to a dietary effect (season effect), Knapp [80] did not see any effect of sperm counts for subjects receiving 50 ml of menhaden oil. In bull, total sperm output was not affected by dietary treatment (100 g DHA-enrichment from salmon oil) [86]. In boar, tuna oil or menhaden supplementation did not increase sperm production [87, 88]. In rabbit [76, 89], fish oil do not increase sperm concentration. In goat, a dietary supplement of fish oil (2.5%) does not have a significant effect on sperm concentration [90]. Nevertheless, in ram the addition of 3% anchovy oil in the diet increases the number of total sperm [79].

Consequences on Sperm Quality and Fertility

Table 2. Summary of experimental trials in mammalians (farm animals and human) assessing the effects of fish oil diets on male fertility

Study	Species	Daily dose	Duration	Outcomes
Castellano et al. (2010)	Boar (n=34)	2.2% animal fat, 2.4% menhaden oil or 2.4% tuna oil	30 weeks	Sperm production, motility and morphology were unaffected
Samadian et al. (2010)	Ram (n=8)	3% anchovy oil	13 weeks	Sperm motility was higher in fish oil group
Gholami et al. (2010)	Bull (n=19)	1% salmon oil*	12 weeks	Fresh sperm motility and viability parameters were improved.
Gliozzi et al. (2009)	Buck (n=52)	1.5 % fish oil	19 weeks	Semen quality parameters were not affected by the dietary treatments.
Dolatpanah et al. (2008)	Goat (n=16)	2.5% fish oil	≈10 weeks	Semen quantity and quality parameters did not differ between control and fish oil
Brinsko et al. (2005)	Stallion (n=8)	1.7% fish oil*	14 weeks	Sperm motion characteristics in fresh semen were unaffected by treatment.
Mitre et al. (2004)	Boar (n=13)	1.6% shark liver oil*	4 weeks	Sperm motility was improved by 2.9%
Rooke et al. (2001)	Boar (n=10)	2.7% tuna oil*	6 weeks	Sperm progressive motility and normal morphology were increased
Paulenz et al. (1995)	Boar (n=8)	2.7% cod liver oil*	9 weeks	There were no significant differences in the non-return rates (4-25 days)
Diaz-Fontdevila and Bustos-Obregon (1993)	Buck (n=20)	7.8% fish oil	8 weeks	Proportion of sperm to undergo acrosome reaction was decreased
Knapp (1990)	Man (n=10)	50 ml menhaden oil	4 weeks	Sperm counts and motility were not altered during the study
Schramm and Luley (1989)	Man (n=10)	9 g of fish oil	12 weeks	Sperm number increase but not a therapeutic effect (= annual changes)

* Estimated value from daily intact

Controversial results were reported for the effect of a supplementation of dietary fish oils on semen quality parameters (motility, morphology, and fertilizing ability). Studies with birds [75, 82, 91-93], bulls [86], and boars [87, 94] have reported benefits of fish oils on male reproductive capacity. Other studies in humans [80], fowls [83], rabbits [76], goat [90] and boars [78, 88, 95], however, did not report any effect of fish oil supplementation on semen quality. Nevertheless, interesting data can be found in regard of poor-quality sperm problems. In turkey [92], Blesbois et al. suggested that increasing the dietary of omega-3 fatty acids can sustain the reproductive capacity of older male turkeys. Moreover, in ram a 3% of anchovy oil supplementation attenuated the decreasing of ram semen quality over season [79]. In stallion, two studies reported a potential positive effect on initially poor-quality ejaculates [96, 97].

Fish Oil and Antioxidants Complement

The high number of double bonds in PUFA makes them very susceptible to oxidative damage induced by reactive oxygen species (ROS) [98]. Since mammalian sperm are rich in PUFA, there is growing evidence that excessive ROS generation play a key role in the ethiology of male infertility [99]. Reactive oxygen species are produced by sperm cells themselves through cell aerobic metabolism. In normal condition, sperm generation of ROS are controlled through a battery of ROS scavengers (antioxidants)[100] and are needed for sperm to acquire fertilizing ability [101, 102]. However, providing PUFA through diet increases ROS generation and unbalanced the oxidative cellular homeostasis. *In vitro*, addition of PUFA such as ARA and DHA is associated with an increase of ROS generation, an oxidative damage leading to a decrease in sperm motility [103]. *In vivo*, Cerolini et al. [84] reported that birds receiving 1% fish oil diet (without addition of antioxidant) showed a decrease in sperm concentration. Major antioxidants such as vitamin E and vitamin C have shown benefits for male subfertility [104, 105]. Vitamin E is a well-documented antioxidant and has been shown to inhibit ROS induced membrane damage [106].

Fish Oil Contaminants and Male Fertility

There is major concern in reproductive health since several scientific studies reported the potential risk of environmental chemicals for male fertility in terms of semen quality [107] and testosterone concentrations [108]. Indeed, fish tissue may be contaminated by myriad of lipophilictoxicants including dioxins, polychlorinated biphenyls (PCB), heavy metals (mercury), and synthetic estrogens [109, 110].

Mercury compounds are known to produce deleterious effects on male fertility in experimental animals [111] and men [112]. Decreases in sperm motility have been reported in methyl mercury exposed monkeys [113] and mouses [114]. In men, infertility was associated to higher blood mercury and seafood consumption [115]. Since methyl mercury has high bioaccumulation potential, very high concentrations of mercury may be found in fish tissue, in particular predatory fish such as swordfish and shark [116].

Available data indicate that cod liver oil may contain higher concentrations of PCB and dioxin compared to other fish oils [117, 118]. In pig sperm, an inverse association between PCB and semen quality, with reduced sperm motility/viability was reported [119]. As reviewed by Meeker and Hauser [120], major human studies show a detrimental effect of PCB on semen quality, specifically on sperm motility. However, as reported in a recent US study, consuming fish oil supplements, compared to fish meal, may lower PCB exposure [121]. Furthermore, there are continued advances in refining processes (decontamination) for fish oils to improve supplement safety while preserving nutritional quality [122-124].

Conclusion

Effects of dietary supplementation of fish oils (rich in omega-3 fatty acids) on male reproduction are still unclear. Responses to fish oil diet vary in function of the animal model, the design of the experiment, the type and the period of supplementation. However, fish oil supplementation would be most beneficial in initial situations where sperm quality is poor. It appears that dietary omega-3 fatty acids may help to improve male fertility by increasing omega-3 polyunsaturated fatty acids in sperm content and, hence, enhancing the sperm fluidity membrane essential for fertilization. Nevertheless, a particular attention should be paid to the adequate intake of antioxidants such vitamin E in order to prevent the potential oxidative damage of sperm membranes related to consumption of fish oil. Moreover some fish oils (not highly refined) may be contaminated by mercury and chemicals like polychlorinated biphenyls which are potentially harmful for male fertility.

References

[1] Yashodhara, B.M., et al., Omega-3 fatty acids: A comprehensive review of their role in health and disease. *Postgraduate Medical Journal*, 2009. 85(1000): p. 84-90.

[2] Wathes, D.C., D.R.E. Abayasekara, and R.J. Aitken, Polyunsaturated fatty acids in male and female reproduction. *Biol Reprod*, 2007. 77(2): p. 190-201.

[3] Gunstone, F., ed. *Fatty Acid and Lipid Chemistry*. 1996, Blackie Academic & Professional: Glasgow (UK). 251.

[4] Hughes, C.L. and T.R. Dhiman, Dietary compounds in relation to dietary diversity and human health. *Journal of Medicinal Food,* 2002. 5(2): p. 51-68.

[5] Barceló-Coblijn, G. and E.J. Murphy, Alpha-linolenic acid and its conversion to longer chain n-3 fatty acids: Benefits for human health and a role in maintaining tissue n-3 fatty acid levels. *Progress in Lipid Research*, 2009. 48(6): p. 355-374.

[6] Sebokova, E., et al., Alteration of the lipid composition of rat testicular plasma membranes by dietary (n-3) fatty acids changes the responsiveness of Leydig cells and testosterone synthesis. *J Nutr,* 1990. 120(6): p. 610-618.

[7] Retterstøl, K., et al., A comparative study of the metabolism of n-9, n-6 and n-3 fatty acids in testicular cells from immature rat. *Biochimica et Biophysica Acta - Lipids and Lipid Metabolism*, 1998. 1392(1): p. 59-72.

[8] Retterstøl, K., et al., Studies on the metabolism of essential fatty acids in isolated human testicular cells. *Reproduction*, 2001. 121(6): p. 881-887.

[9] Brenna, J.T., et al., α-Linolenic acid supplementation and conversion to n-3 long-chain polyunsaturated fatty acids in humans. *Prostaglandins Leukotrienes and Essential Fatty Acids*, 2009. 80(2-3): p. 85-91.

[10] Jump, D.B., The Biochemistry of n-3 Polyunsaturated Fatty Acids. *Journal of biological chemistry*, 2002. 277(11): p. 8755-5758.

[11] Arterburn, L.M., E.B. Hall, and H. Oken, Distribution, interconversion, and dose response of n-3 fatty acids in humans. *American Journal of Clinical Nutrition,* 2006. 83(6).

[12] Coniglio, J.G., Testicular lipids. *Prog Lipid Res*, 1994. 33(4): p. 387-401.

[13] Carver, J.D., et al., The relationship between age and the fatty acid composition of cerebral cortex and erythrocytes in human subjects. *Brain Research Bulletin,* 2001. 56(2): p. 79-85.

[14] Van Kuijk, F.J.G.M. and P. Buck, Fatty acid composition of the human macula and peripheral retina. *Investigative Ophthalmology and Visual Science,* 1992. 33(13): p. 3493-3496.

[15] Poulos, A., A. Darin-Bennett, and I.G. White, The phospholipid-bound fatty acids and aldehydes of mammalian spermatozoa. *Comp Biochem Physiol B*, 1973. 46(3): p. 541-9.

[16] Bieri, J.G. and E.L. Prival, Lipid composition of testes from various species. *Comp Biochem Physiol,* 1965. 15(3): p. 275-282.

[17] Chanmugam, P.S., M.D. Boudreau, and D.H. Hwang, Dietary (n-3) fatty acids alter fatty acid composition and prostaglandin synthesis in rat testis. *J Nutr,* 1991. 121(8): p. 1173-1178.

[18] Whelan, J., et al., Dietary arachidonate enhances tissue arachidonate levels and eicosanoid production in Syrian hamsters. *J Nutr*, 1993. 123(12): p. 2174-2185.

[19] Ahluwalia, B., G. Pincus, and R.T. Holman, Essential fatty acid deficiency and its effects upon reproductive organs of male rabbits. *J Nutr,* 1967. 92(2): p. 205-214.

[20] Coniglio, J.G., W.M. Grogan Jr, and R.K. Rhamy, Lipid and fatty acid composition of human testes removed at autopsy. *Biol Reprod,* 1975. 12(2): p. 255-259.

[21] Coniglio, J.G., W.M. Grogan Jr, and R.K. Rhamy, Lipids of human testes removed at orchidectomy. *J Reprod Fertil,* 1974. 41(1): p. 67-73.

[22] Scott, T.W., J.K. Voglmayr, and B.P. Setchell, Lipid composition and metabolism in testicular and ejaculated ram spermatozoa. *Biochem J,* 1967. 102(2): p. 456-461.

[23] Neill, A.R. and C.J. Masters, Fatty acid incorporations and lipid compositions of mature and immature bovine testes. *Int J Biochem*, 1974. 5(2): p. 137-156.

[24] Castellano, C., et al., Fish oil diets alter the phospholipid balance, fatty acid composition, and steroid hormone concentrations in testes of adult pigs. *Theriogenology*, 2011. In press.

[25] Johnson, L.A., V.G. Pursel, and R.J. Gerrits, Total phospholipid and phospholipid fatty acids of ejaculated and epididymal semen and seminal vesicle fluids of boars. *Journal of animal science,* 1972. 35(2): p. 398-403.

[26] Howarth, B., Jr., D. Torregrossa, and W.M. Britton, The phospholipid content of ejaculated fowl and turkey spermatozoa. *Poult Sci,* 1977. 56(4): p. 1265-8.

[27] Kelso, K.A., et al., Lipid and antioxidant changes in semen of broiler fowl from 25 to 60 weeks of age. *J Reprod Fertil,* 1996. 106(2): p. 201-6.

[28] Katan, M.B., J.L. Harryvan, and P. van de Bovenkamp, n-3 fatty acids in human fat tissue aspirates are stable for up to 6y. *European Journal of Clinical Nutrition*, 2003. 57(7): p. 816-818.

[29] Andersson, A., et al., Fatty acid composition of skeletal muscle reflects dietary fat composition in humans. *American Journal of Clinical Nutrition,* 2002. 76(6): p. 1222-1229.

[30] Harris, W.S., et al., Omega-3 fatty acids in cardiac biopsies from heart transplantation patients: Correlation with erythrocytes and response to supplementation. *Circulation*, 2004. 110(12): p. 1645-1649.

[31] Lin, D.S., et al., Unique lipids of primate spermatozoa: Desmosterol and docosahexaenoic acid. *Journal of Lipid Research,* 1993. 34(3): p. 491-499.

[32] Darin Bennett, A., A. Poulous, and I.G. White, The phospholipids and phospholipid bound fatty acids and aldehydes of dog and fowl spermatozoa. *Journal of Reproduction and Fertility,* 1974. 41(2): p. 471-474.

[33] Surai, P.F., et al., Fatty acid composition, glutathione peroxidase and superoxide dismutase activity and total antioxidant activity of avian semen. *Comparative Biochemistry and Physiology - B Biochemistry and Molecular Biology,* 1998. 120(3): p. 527-533.

[34] Chow, P.Y.W., I.G. White, and B.W. Pickett, Stallion sperm and seminal plasma phospholipids and glycerylphosphorylcholine. *Animal Reproduction Science,* 1986. 11(3): p. 207-213.

[35] Burr, G.O. and M.M. Burr, On the nature and role of the fatty acids essential in nutrition. *J Biol Chem*, 1930. 86: p. 587-621.

[36] Evans, H., S. Lepkovsky, and E. Murphy, Vital need of the body for certain unsaturated fatty acids. VI. Male sterility on fat-free diets. *J. Biol. Chem*., 1934. 106: p. 445-451.

[37] Leat, W.M.F., et al., Effect of dietary linoleic and linolenic acids on testicular development in the rat. *Quarterly Journal of Experimental Physiology,* 1983. 68(2): p. 221-231.

[38] MacDonald, M.L., et al., Effects of linoleate and arachidonate deficiencies on reproduction and spermatogenesis in the cat. *Journal of Nutrition,* 1984. 114(4): p. 719-726.

[39] Bourre, J.M.E., et al., Dietary α-linolenic acid deficiency in adult rats for 7 months does not alter brain docosahexaenoic acid content, in contrast to liver, heart and testes. *Biochimica et Biophysica Acta - Lipids and Lipid Metabolism*, 1992. 1124(2): p. 119-122.

[40] Lillie, R.J. and H. Menge, Effect of linoleic acid deficiency on the fertilizing capacity and semen fatty acid profile of the male chicken. *Journal of Nutrition*, 1968. 95(2): p. 311-315.

[41] Zalata, A.A., et al., The fatty acid composition of phospholipids of spermatozoa from infertile patients. *Mol Hum Reprod,* 1998. 4(2): p. 111-8.

[42] Gulaya, N.M., et al., Phospholipid composition of human sperm and seminal plasma in relation to sperm fertility. *Arch Androl*, 2001. 46(3): p. 169-175.

[43] Ladha, S., Lipid heterogeneity and membrane fluidity in a highly polarized cell, the mammalian spermatozoon. *Journal of Membrane Biology*, 1998. 165(1): p. 1-10.

[44] Flesch, F.M. and B.M. Gadella, Dynamics of the mammalian sperm plasma membrane in the process of fertilization. *Biochim Biophys Acta*, 2000. 1469(3): p. 197-235.
[45] Parks, J.E. and D.V. Lynch, Lipid composition and thermotropic phase behavior of boar, bull, stallion, and rooster sperm membranes. *Cryobiology*, 1992. 29(2): p. 255-266.
[46] Stubbs, C.D. and A.D. Smith, The modification of mammalian membrane polyunsaturated fatty acid composition in relation to membrane fluidity and function. *Biochimica et Biophysica Acta (BBA) - Reviews on Biomembranes,* 1984. 779(1): p. 89-137.
[47] Stillwell, W. and S.R. Wassall, Docosahexaenoic acid: Membrane properties of a unique fatty acid. *Chemistry and Physics of Lipids*, 2003. 126(1): p. 1-27.
[48] Lenzi, A., et al., Lipids of the sperm plasma membrane: from polyunsaturated fatty acids considered as markers of sperm function to possible scavenger therapy. Hum Reprod Update, 1996. 2(3): p. 246-56.
[49] Israelachvili, J.N., S. Marcelja, and R.G. Horn, Physical principles of membrane organization. Quarterly Reviews of Biophysics, 1980. 13(2): p. 121-200.
[50] Connor, W.E., et al., Uneven distribution of desmosterol and docosahexaenoic acid in the heads and tails of monkey sperm. *Journal of Lipid Research,* 1998. 39(7): p. 1404-1411.
[51] Nissen, H.P. and H.W. Kreysel, Polyunsaturated fatty acids in relation to sperm motility. *Andrologia*, 1983. 15(3): p. 264-9.
[52] Cerolini, S., et al., Lipid manipulation of chicken semen by dietary means and its relation to fertility: A review. *World's Poult Sci J*, 2003. 59(1): p. 65-75.
[53] Conquer, J.A., et al., Fatty acid analysis of blood serum, seminal plasma, and spermatozoa of normozoospermic vs. asthenozoospermic males. *Lipids*, 1999. 34(8): p. 793-9.
[54] Miki, K., Energy metabolism and sperm function. *Society of Reproduction and Fertility supplement*, 2007. 65: p. 309-325.
[55] Lardy, H. and P. Phillips, Phospholipids as a source of energy for motility of bull spermatozoa. *American Journal of Physiology - Endocrinology and Metabolism,* 1941. 134: p. 542-548.
[56] Hartree, E.F. and T. Mann, Phospholipids in mammalian semen. *J Reprod Fertil,* 1960. 1: p. 23-9.
[57] Neill, A.R. and C.J. Masters, Metabolism of fatty acids by ovine spermatozoa. *Journal of Reproduction and Fertility*, 1973. 34(2): p. 279-287.
[58] Jones, A.R. and L.A. Chantrill, Oxidative metabolic activity of boar spermatozoa: a system for assessing anti-glycolytic activity of potential inhibitors in vitro. *Reproduction, Fertility and Development*, 1989. 1(4): p. 357-367.
[59] Mita, M., I. Yasumasu, and M. Nakamura, Endogenous substrate for energy metabolism and ultrastructural correlates in spermatozoa of the sea urchin Diadema setosum. *Molecular Reproduction and Development,* 1995. 40(1): p. 103-109.
[60] Benatti, P., et al., Polyunsaturated fatty acids: biochemical, nutritional and epigenetic properties. *Journal of American College of Nutrition,* 2004. 23(4): p. 281-302.
[61] Abayasekara, D.R.E. and D.C. Wathes, Effects of altering dietary fatty acid composition on prostaglandin synthesis and fertility. *Prostaglandins Leukot Essent Fatty Acids,* 1999. 61(5): p. 275-287.

[62] Joyce, C.L., et al., Evidence for a role of cyclooxygenase (prostaglandin synthetase) and prostaglandins in the sperm acrosome reaction and fertilization. Journal of Andrology, 1987. 8(2): p. 74-82.

[63] Roy, A.C. and S.S. Ratnam, Biosynthesis of prostaglandins by human spermatozoa in vitro and their role in acrosome reaction and fertilization. Molecular Reproduction and Development, 1992. 33(3): p. 303-306.

[64] Samuelsson, B., Isolation and identification of prostaglandins from human seminal plasma. J. biol. Chem., 1963. 238: p. 3229-323.

[65] Conte, D., M. Nordio, and F. Romanelli, Role of seminal prostaglandins in male fertility. II. Effects of prostaglandin synthesis inhibition on spermatogenesis in man. *Journal of Endocrinological Investigation,* 1985. 8(4): p. 289-291.

[66] Isidori, A., D. Conte, and G. Laguzzi, Role of seminal prostaglandins in male fertility. I. Relationship of prostaglandin E and 19-OH prostaglandin E with seminal parameters. *Journal of Endocrinological Investigation,* 1980. 3(1): p. 1-4.

[67] Gottlieb, C., et al., Effect of prostaglandins on human sperm function in vitro and seminal adenosine triphosphate content. *Fertility and Sterility*, 1988. 49(2): p. 322-327.

[68] Wade, M.G., et al., Release and steroidogenic actions of polyunsaturated fatty acids in the goldfish testis. *Biol Reprod*, 1994. 51(1): p. 131-139.

[69] Lands, W.E.M., Long-term fat intake and biomarkers. *American Journal of Clinical Nutrition*, 1995. 61(3 SUPPL.).

[70] Christophe, A., et al., Fatty acid composition of sperm phospholipids and its nutritional implications. Middle East Fertility Society Journal, 1988. 3(SUPPL. 1): p. 46-53.

[71] Sargent, J.R., Fish oils and human diet. *British Journal of Nutrition,* 1997. 78(SUPPL. 1): p. S5-S13.

[72] USDA Nutrient Data Laboratory. USDA National Nutrient Database. 2010 12/02/2010 [cited 2011 May 5]; Available from: *http://www.ars.usda.gov/ba/bhnrc/ndl.*

[73] Klinkesorn, U., et al., Chemical transesterification of tuna oil to enriched omega-3 polyunsaturated fatty acids. *Food Chemistry*, 2004. 87(3): p. 415-421.

[74] Kelso, K.A., et al., The effects of dietary supplementation with docosahexaenoic acid on the phospholipid fatty acid composition of avian spermatozoa. *Comparative Biochemistry and Physiology - B Biochemistry and Molecular Biology,* 1997. 118(1): p. 65-69.

[75] Blesbois, E., et al., Effect of dietary fat on the fatty acid composition and fertilizing ability of fowl semen. *Biology of Reproduction*, 1997. 56(5): p. 1216-1220.

[76] Gliozzi, T.M., et al., Quality and lipid composition of spermatozoa in rabbits fed DHA and vitamin E rich diets. *Theriogenology*, 2009. 71(6): p. 910-919.

[77] Harris, M.A., et al., Stallion spermatozoa membrane phospholipid dynamics following dietary n-3 supplementation. *Anim Reprod Sci,* 2005. 89(1-4): p. 234-7.

[78] Paulenz, H., et al., A preliminary study on the effect of dietary supplementation with cod liver oil on the polyunsaturated fatty acid composition of boar semen. *Veterinary Research Communications*, 1995. 19(4): p. 273-284.

[79] Samadian, F., et al., Effects of dietary n-3 fatty acids on characteristics and lipid composition of ovine sperm. *Animal*, 2010. 4(12): p. 2017-2022.

[80] Knapp, H.R., Prostaglandins in human semen during fish oil ingestion: evidence for in vivo cyclooxygenase inhibition and appearance of novel trienoic compounds. *Prostaglandins*, 1990. 39(4): p. 407-423.

[81] Surai, P.F., et al., Effect of long-term supplementation with arachidonic or docosahexaenoic acids on sperm production in the broiler chicken. Journal of Reproduction and Fertility, 2000. 120(2): p. 257-264.

[82] Zaniboni, L., R. Rizzi, and S. Cerolini, Combined effect of DHA and α-tocopherol enrichment on sperm quality and fertility in the turkey. *Theriogenology*, 2006. 65(9): p. 1813-1827.

[83] Bongalhardo, D.C., S. Leeson, and M.M. Buhr, Dietary lipids differentially affect membranes from different areas of rooster sperm. *Poult Sci.*, 2009. 88(5): p. 1060-1069.

[84] Cerolini, S., et al., Effect of docosahexaenoic acid and α-tocopherol enrichment in chicken sperm on semen quality, sperm lipid composition and susceptibility to peroxidation. *Theriogenology*, 2006. 66(4): p. 877-886.

[85] Schramm, P. and C. Luley, Fischöl und spermiogenese [Fish oil and spermiogenesis]. *Aktuelle Dermatologie,* 1989. 15(11): p. 321-323.

[86] Gholami, H., et al., Effect of feeding a docosahexaenoic acid-enriched nutriceutical on the quality of fresh and frozen-thawed semen in Holstein bulls. *Theriogenology*, 2010. 74(9): p. 1548-1558.

[87] Rooke, J.A., C.C. Shao, and B.K. Speake, Effects of feeding tuna oil on the lipid composition of pig spermatozoa and in vitro characteristics of semen. *Reproduction*, 2001. 121(2): p. 315-322.

[88] Castellano, C.A., et al., Effect of dietary n-3 fatty acids (fish oils) on boar reproduction and semen quality. *J Anim Sci,* 2010. 88(7): p. 2346-2355.

[89] Diaz-Fontdevila, M. and E. Bustos-Obregon, Cholesterol and polyunsaturated acid enriched diet: Effect on kinetics of the acrosome reaction in rabbit spermatozoa. *Molecular Reproduction and Development,* 1993. 35(2): p. 176-180.

[90] Dolatpanah, M.B., et al., Effects of dietary fish oil on semen quality of goats. *Asian-Australasian Journal of Animal Sciences*, 2008. 21(1): p. 29-34.

[91] Hudson, B.P. and J.L. Wilson, Effects of Dietary Menhaden Oil on Fertility and Sperm Quality of Broiler Breeder Males. *Journal of Applied Poultry Research,* 2003. 12(3): p. 341-347.

[92] Blesbois, E., et al., Effects of n - 3 polyunsaturated dietary supplementation on the reproductive capacity of male turkeys. *Theriogenology*, 2004. 61(2-3): p. 537-549.

[93] Al-Daraji, H.J., et al., Effect of dietary supplementation with different oils on productive and reproductive performance of quail. *International Journal of Poultry Science,* 2010. 9(5): p. 429-435.

[94] Mitre, R., et al., Oral intake of shark liver oil modifies lipid composition and improves motility and velocity of boar sperm. *Theriogenology*, 2004. 62(8): p. 1557-1566.

[95] Castellano, C.A., et al., Dietary omega-3 fatty acids (fish oils) have limited effects on boar semen stored at 17 °C or cryopreserved. *Theriogenology*, 2010. 74(8): p. 1482-1490.

[96] Brinsko, S.P., et al., Effect of feeding a DHA-enriched nutriceutical on the quality of fresh, cooled and frozen stallion semen. *Theriogenology*, 2005. 63(5): p. 1519-1527.

[97] Elhordoy, D., N. Cazales, and G. Costa, Effect of dietary supplementation with DHA on the quality of fresh, cooled and frozen stallion semen. *Animal Reproduction Science*, 2008. 107: p. 319.

[98] Aitken, R.J., D. Harkiss, and D.W. Buckingham, Analysis of lipid peroxidation mechanisms in human spermatozoa. *Molecular Reproduction and Development,* 1993. 35(3): p. 302-315.

[99] Aitken, R.J. and M.A. Baker, Oxidative stress, sperm survival and fertility control. *Molecular and Cellular Endocrinology*, 2006. 250(1-2): p. 66-69.

[100] Agarwal, A. and L.H. Sekhon, The role of antioxidant therapy in the treatment of male infertility. *Human Fertility,* 2010. 13(4): p. 217-225.

[101] de Lamirande, E., et al., Reactive oxygen species and sperm physiology. *Reviews of Reproduction,* 1997. 2(1): p. 48-54.

[102] de Lamirande, E. and C. O'Flaherty, Sperm activation: Role of reactive oxygen species and kinases. *Biochimica et Biophysica Acta - Proteins and Proteomics,* 2008. 1784(1): p. 106-115.

[103] Aitken, R.J., et al., Cis-unsaturated fatty acids stimulate reactive oxygen species generation and lipid peroxidation in human spermatozoa. *Journal of Clinical Endocrinology and Metabolism,* 2006. 91(10): p. 4154-4163.

[104] Comhaire, F.H., et al., The effects of combined conventional treatment, oral antioxidants and essential fatty acids on sperm biology in subfertile men. *Prostaglandins Leukotrienes and Essential Fatty Acids,* 2000. 63(3): p. 159-165.

[105] Sheweita, S.A., A.M. Tilmisany, and H. Al-Sawaf, Mechanisms of male infertility: Role of antioxidants. *Current Drug Metabolism*, 2005. 6(5): p. 495-501.

[106] Traber, M.G. and J. Atkinson, Vitamin E, antioxidant and nothing more. *Free Radical Biology and Medicine,* 2007. 43(1): p. 4-15.

[107] Carlsen, E., et al., Evidence for decreasing quality of semen during past 50 years. *British Medical Journal,* 1992. 305(6854): p. 609-613.

[108] Travison, T.G., et al., A population-level decline in serum testosterone levels in American men. *Journal of Clinical Endocrinology and Metabolism,* 2007. 92(1): p. 196-202.

[109] Sidhu, K.S., Health benefits and potential risks related to consumption of fish or fish oil. *Regulatory Toxicology and Pharmacology*, 2003. 38(3): p. 336-344.

[110] Hauser, R., The environment and male fertility: Recent research on emerging chemicals and semen quality. *Seminars in Reproductive Medicine,* 2006. 24(3): p. 156-167.

[111] Khera, K.S., Reproductive capability of male rats and mice treated with methyl mercury. *Toxicology and Applied Pharmacology,* 1973. 24(2): p. 167-177.

[112] Popescu, H.I., Poisoning with alkylmercury compounds. *British Medical Journal*, 1978. 1(6123): p. 1347.

[113] Mohamed, M.K., T.M. Burbacher, and N.K. Mottet, Effects of methyl mercury on testicular functions in Macaca fascicularis monkeys. *Pharmacology and Toxicology,* 1987. 60(1): p. 29-36.

[114] Rao, M.W., Effects of methylmercury on mouse epididymis and spermatozoa. *Biomedica Biochimica Acta,* 1989. 48(8): p. 577-582.

[115] Choy, C.M.Y., et al., Infertility, blood mercury concentrations and dietary seafood consumption: A case-control study. *BJOG: An International Journal of Obstetrics and Gynaecology*, 2002. 109(10): p. 1121-1125.

[116] Smith, K.L. and J.L. Guentzel, Mercury concentrations and omega-3 fatty acids in fish and shrimp: Preferential consumption for maximum health benefits. *Marine Pollution Bulletin*, 2010. 60(9): p. 1615-1618.

[117] Fernandes, A.R., et al., Dioxins and polychlorinated biphenyls (PCBs) in fish oil dietary supplements: Occurrence and human exposure in the UK. *Food Additives and Contaminants,* 2006. 23(9): p. 939-947.

[118] Martí, M., et al., Persistent organic pollutants (PCDD/Fs, dioxin-like PCBs, marker PCBs, and PBDEs) in health supplements on the Spanish market. *Chemosphere*, 2010. 78(10): p. 1256-1262.

[119] Campagna, C., et al., Effects of an environmentally relevant organochlorine mixture and a metabolized extract of this mixture on porcine sperm parameters in vitro. Journal of Andrology, 2009. 30(3): p. 317-324.

[120] Meeker, J.D. and R. Hauser, Exposure to polychlorinated biphenyls (PCBs) and male reproduction. *Systems Biology in Reproductive Medicine*, 2010. 56(2): p. 122-131.

[121] Ashley, J.T.F., et al., Evaluating daily exposure to polychlorinated biphenyls and polybrominated diphenyl ethers in fish oil supplements. *Food Additives and Contaminants - Part A Chemistry, Analysis, Control, Exposure and Risk Assessment,* 2010. 27(8): p. 1177-1185.

[122] Oterhals, Å. and E. Nygård, Reduction of persistent organic pollutants in fishmeal: A feasibility study. *Journal of Agricultural and Food Chemistry*, 2008. 56(6): p. 2012-2020.

[123] Kawashima, A., et al., Removal of dioxins and dioxin-like PCBs from fish oil by countercurrent supercritical CO2 extraction and activated carbon treatment. *Chemosphere*, 2009. 75(6): p. 788-794.

[124] Gibon, V., et al., How to reduce the rate of environmental pollutants in fish oils without affecting nutritional characteristics? *Comment réduire le taux de contaminants environnementaux dans les huiles de poisson sans en affecter les caractéristiques nutritionnelles?,* 2010. 17(4): p. 227-231.

In: Fish Oil: Production, Consumption and Health Benefits ISBN: 978-1-61470-963-3
Editors: Matthias Van Dijk and Jürgen Vitek

Chapter XIII

Review of the Current Production of Omega-3 Concentrates*

Nuria Rubio-Rodríguez, Sagrario Beltrán and María Teresa Sanz
Dpto Biotechnology & Food Science, University of Burgos, Spain

Abstract

Since, at the end of the ´80s, epidemiological studies began to establish a certain relationship between a high fatty fish consumption and a low incidence of cardiovascular diseases in Nordic people, the amount clinical and biological essays about polyunsaturated fatty acids (PUFA), especially omega-3 fatty acids, has greatly increased, being voluminous the current available information related to their biochemical mechanisms of action, biological effects and health implications. Nowadays, nobody doubts about the importance of omega-3 fatty acids, especially EPA and DHA, in human diet, which recommended daily intakes have been established by several nutritionist committees all over the world. As a consequence, the demand of omega-3 enriched products and nutraceuticals has grown up noticeably, especially in those societies with a diet based a on high consumption of seed oils and meat, which has promoted the development of plenty of novel strategies and competitive methods for producing, on large scale, the high quality omega-3 concentrates requested for both food and pharmaceutical industries.

This chapter is proposed as an overview of the current situation of omega-3 fatty acids. Firstly, a brief introduction about essential fatty acids, focusing on the most relevant clinical studies published in the last 10 years about their role in human health. The last part of the chapter reviews the state-of-the-art of fish oil and omega-3 production processes on large scale, with an emphasis on the scientific articles and patents published from 2000 to 2010 and distinguishing two main groups: conventional methods based on physical and chemical processes and alternative methods based on the use of supercritical fluid technologies. In addition, a short compilation of different fish oil and omega-3 concentrates currently available in the market is presented.

* This Chapter has been partially published in the Journal of Innovative Food Science and Emerging Technologies (Rubio-Rodríguez and others 2010).

Nomenclature

AA	Arachidonic Acid
ALA	Alpha-Linolenic Acid
AV	Anisidine Value
BHA	Butylated hydroxyanisole
BHT	Butylated hydroxytoluene
CHD	Cardiovascular Heart Disease
CP	Critical Point
DGLA	Dihomo-Gamma Linolenic Acid
DHA-EE	Docosahexaenoic Acid (Ethyl ester)
DPA	Docosapentaenoic Acid (n-3)
EDTA	Ethylenediaminetetraacetic acid
EPA-EE	Eicosapentaenoic Acid (Ethyl ester)
FAEE	Fatty Acid Ethyl Ester
FAO	Food and Agriculture Organisation
FFA	Free Fatty Acid
GC	Gas Ghromatography
GLA	Gamma-Linolenic acid
GOED	Global Organization for EPA and DHA
HPLC	High Pressure Liquid Chromatography
ISSFAL	International Society for the Study of Fatty Acids and Lipids
LA	Linoleic Acid
LC-PUFA	Long Chain Polyunsaturated Fatty Acids
MUFA	Monounsaturated Fatty Acid
P	Pressure (MPa)
P_c	Critical Pressure (MPa)
P_r	Reduced Pressure (dimensionless)
PCBs	Polychlorinated biphenyls
PCDDs	Polychlorinated dibenzo-para-dioxins
PCDFs	Polychlorinated dibenzofurans
PGSS	Particles from Gas Saturated Solutions
PUFA	Polyunsaturated Fatty Acid
PV	Peroxide Value
RESS	Rapid Expansion of Supercritical Solutions
SAS	Supercritical Anti Solvent precipitation
$SC\text{-}CO_2$	Supercritical Carbon Dioxide
SCF	Supercritical Fluid
SFA	Saturated Fatty Acids
SFC	Supercritical Chromatography
SFE	Supercritical Fluid Extraction
SFEE	Supercritical Fluid Extraction of Emulsions
SFF	Supercritical Fluid Fractionation
SSI	Supercritical Solvent Impregnation
T	Temperature (K)
T_c	Critical Temperature (K)
T_r	Reduced Temperature (dimensionless)
TAG	Triacylglycerides
TP	Triple Point
UFA	Unsaturated Fatty Acids

WHO	World Health Organization
WHO-TEQ	World Health Organization Toxic Equivalent
Greek Letters	
ρ	Density (kg / m^3)
ρ_c	Critical density (kg / m^3)
ρ_r	Reduced density (dimensionless)

1. Omega-3 Fatty Acids: Reasons for Being Interesting

Abstract

Omega-3 fatty acids have been very often the subject of scientific research in the last years, being numerous the studies developed about their biological effects and health implications.

In this Section, a description of the role of essential fatty acids in the organism and the influence of omega-3 fatty acids in human health is presented, as well as the requirements of these fatty acids on human diet.

1.1. Introduction to Essential Fatty Acids

Fatty acids are organic compounds formed by a hydrocarbonated chain and a carboxylic group that is normally bounded with glycerol forming acylglycerides (mono-, di- or triglycerides).

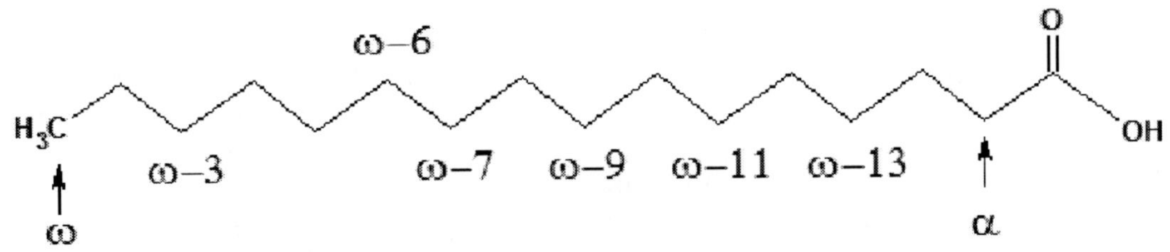

Figure 1. Common carbon positions in the hydrocarbonated chain of fatty acids.

The most common fatty acids in nature are reported in Table 1. They are classified according to the number of unsaturations (number of double bounds in the hydrocarbonated chain) as saturated (SFA), monounsaturated (MUFA) or polyunsaturated fatty acids (PUFA); or according to the position of the first C-C double bound as omega-3, -6, -7, -9, -11 or 13 fatty acids, where the term omega, expressed as "ω" or "n", is related to the carbon position further from the functional group –COOH, as shown in Figure 1.

The human body is able to synthesize SFA such palmitic acid (C16:0) and MUFA of the n-7 and n-9 series such as palmitoleic acid (C16:1n-7) or oleic acid (C18:1n-9). However, it cannot produce fatty acids with a C-C double bound in the position n-6 or n-3 of the hydrocarbonated chain such as linoleic acid (C18:2n-6, LA) or α-linolenic acid (C18:3n-3,

ALA), which are considered essential fatty acids in human nutrition and must be taken directly for the diet.

Table 1. Common fatty acids in human diet.

Type		Common name	Carbon number	Double bounds C-C	Formula
SFA		Butyric	4	0	C4:0
		Caproic	6	0	C6:0
		Caprilic	8	0	C8:0
		Capric	10	0	C10:0
		Lauric	12	0	C12:0
		Myristic	14	0	C14:0
		Palmitic	16	0	C16:0
		Stearic	18	0	C18:0
		Araquidic	20	0	C20:0
		Behenic	22	0	C22:0
		Lignoceric	24	0	C24:0
MUFA	ω 9	Palmitoleic	16	1	C16:1n-9
		Oleic	18	1	C18:1n-9
		Gadoleic	20	1	C20:1n-9
	ω 11	Gondoic	20	1	C20:1n-11
	ω 13	Erucic	22	1	C22:1n-13
PUFA	ω 6	Linoleic	18	2	C18:2n-6
		γ-Linolenic	18	3	C18:3n-6
		Dihomo- γ-Linolenic	20	3	C20:3n-6
		Araquidonic	20	4	C20:4n-6
	ω 3	α-Linolenic	18	3	C18:3n-3
		Stearidonic	18	4	C18:4n-3
		EPA	20	5	C20:5n-3
		DPA	22	5	C22:5n-3
		DHA	22	6	C22:6n-3

LA and ALA are the parent of omega-6 and omega-3 fatty acids respectively and, from them, other omega-6 such as arachidonic acid (C20:4n-6; AA) or omega-3, as eicosapentaenoic acid (C20:5n-3; EPA), docosapentaenoic acid (C22:5n-3, DPA) and docosahexaenoic acid (C22:6n-3, DHA), can be synthesized in the human body by a series of enzymatic reactions based on desaturation and elongation of the hydrocarbonated chain (*see* Figure 2). Nevertheless, since LA and ALA compite for the same enzymes, a high level of LA in the organism, related to a high consumption of vegetable oils, means a lower conversion of ALA in EPA and DHA, and, for that reason, these omega-3 fatty acids are considered essential fatty acids too.

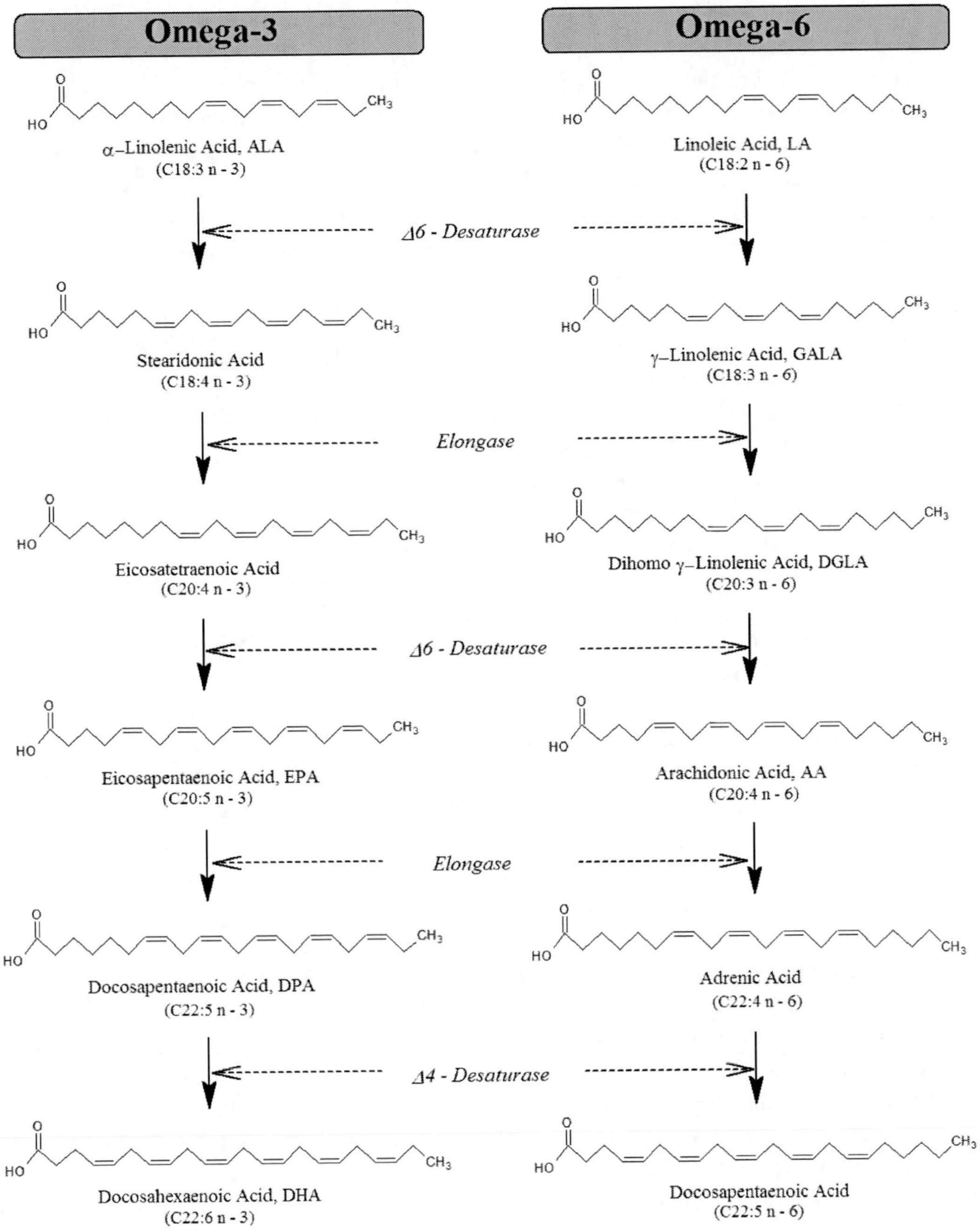

Figure 2. Metabolic pathways for the synthesis of omega-3 and omega-6 fatty acids (*adapted from* (*Simopoulos*, 1991)).

1.2. Omega-3 Fatty Acids and Human Health

The implications of fatty acids in human health have been the subject of many scientific articles and reviews in the last years. One of the most complete compilations of scientific research on this subject can be found in the book edited by Chow (*Chow*, 2000) and one of the most recent review articles on dietary fat and cancer risk has been published by Chen et al. (Chen and others 2007).

Specifically dealing with omega-3 fatty acids, there is also plenty of research. Their importance in human health was realized in the ′80s when several authors (Dyerberg, 1986; Kromann and Green, 1980) published epidemiological studies showing the relation between an omega-3 enriched diet and the prevention of some diseases like myocardial infarction or bronchial asthma. Subsequently, an enormous number of epidemiological and clinical studies have deal with the effect of omega-3 PUFA, especially EPA and DHA, in human health and the mechanism by which this effect takes place.

In this section, we will only mention the latest review articles that compile most of the research done on this subject and summarise the conclusions to clarify the real effect of omega-3 PUFA in human health.

Ruxton et al. published a general review in 2005 on the impact of long chain (LC) n-3-PUFA on human health. They concluded that, there is strong evidence of the clinical benefit of this type of n-3 PUFA on cardiovascular diseases or rheumatoid arthritis, although further studies are needed to show the benefits for other inflammatory conditions as asthma, cystic fibrosis, bowel diseases or their role in mental illnesses (Ruxton and others 2005).

The effect of LC n-3 PUFA when treating asthma has been recently reviewed by Reisman et al. (Reisman and others 2006).

Zulfakar et al. have reviewed the works that have examined the potential use of n-3 PUFA in psoriasis (Zulfakar and others 2007).

Several recent reviews have studied the influence of omega-3 PUFA on bowel diseases (Diamond and others 2008; Razack and Seidner, 2007; Turner and others 2008).

The application of omega-3 fatty acids in the treatment and prevention of mental illnesses (Clayton and others 2007; Horrobin and others 1991; Mazza and others 2007; McNamara, 2006; Ross and others 2007; Song and Zhao, 2007; Stillwell and Wassall, 2003) and on the prevention of several types of cancer (Calviello and others 2007 ; Chen et al., 2007; MacLean and others 2006) has also been widely reviewed.

The latest overview found about the effect of omega-3 fatty acids in rheumatoid arthritis was published in 1998 (Ariza-Ariza and others 1998) although there is a more recent one (EC) not published in English (Stancík and others 2006).

Several recent reviews on cardiovascular effects have also been recently published (Biscione and others 2007; Das, 2008; Tziomalos and others 2007; von-Schacky and Harris, 2007).Von Schacky & Harris proposed the omega-3 index (percentage of EPA + DHA of total fatty acids in red blood cells) as a risk factor for sudden cardiac death and concluded that this index should be higher than 8 % (von-Schacky and Harris, 2007).There are also several studies that propose the mechanisms by which the omega-3 PUFA act in humans (Horrobin et al., 1991; Massaro and others 2007; Shaikh and Edidin, 2008; Stillwell and Wassall, 2003).

All this scientific activity regarding long chain omega-3 PUFA usually ends up by advising an intake of this type of PUFA, either through the natural food products that contain them or as a supplement in the diet for beneficial effects on health (*Lands*, 2008). Moreover, nutrition experts have suggested that an n-6:n-3 fatty acid ratio of 5:1 or less is desired in order to maintain a good human health (*WHO/FAO*, 1994), and other expert committees have proposed specific recommendations of EPA and DHA intakes in different population sectors such as healthy adults, pregnant and lactating women, patients with cardiovascular heart disease (CHD) or patients with high triacylglyceride levels in blood (*see* Table 2).

1.3. Omega-3 Fatty Acids in Human Diet

Fish, and especially oily fish from *Scombridae*, *Clupeidae* and *Salmonidae* families, is the most important natural source of omega-3 EPA and DHA in the foodstuff portion (*see* Table 3); whereas seed oils such as sunflower oil, are the main source of omega-6 (*see* Table 4).

Table 2. Daily intakes recommendations for EPA and DHA

Population Sector	Recommendation	Expert Committee	Reference
Healthy Adults	500 Mg EPA + DHA / Day	ISSFAL	(Cunnane And Others 2004)
Pregnant And Lactating Women,	200 Mg DHA / Day	Perinatal Lipid Intake Working Group	(Koletzko And Others 2007)
Patients With CHD	1 G EPA + DHA / Day (*)	American Hearth Asociation	(Kris-Etherton And Others 2002)
Patients With High Triglyceride Level	2-4 G / Day (*)	American Hearth Asociation	(Kris-Etherton Et Al., 2002)

(*) Under Medical Supervision.

Nowadays food habits in western society are characterized by a high consumption of meat, seed oils, fast food (pizzas, hamburgers…) and snack food (cakes, biscuits…), that contain a large amount of saturated fatty acids and a low proportion of omega-3 fatty acids (*Fernández-SanJuan*, 2000). Comparing the composition of fast food, consumed mostly by young people, with typical Japanese food (Kamei and others 2002) or Mediterranean food (Ambring and others 2006), both of them with a large amount of fish, it can be observed that the n-6:n-3 ratio in blood, in people who consume Japanese or Mediterranean food, is close to 2:1, while in people who consume fast food, it can reach values up to 25:1, much higher than desired.

Table 3. EPA and DHA content in some species of fish. Adapted from literature (Mataix and Gil, 2005)

Species	Common name	g/100 g of foodstuff portion	
		C20:5n-3 (EPA)	C22:6n-3 (DHA)
Scomber scombrus	mackerel	1.10	2.56
Mullus surmuletus	red mullet	0.91	1.66
Sardina pilchardus	sardine	0.62	1.12
Salmo salar	salmon	0.50	1.00
Thunnus thinnus	ton	0.24	0.98
Engraulis encrasicolus	anchovy	0.14	0.80
Pagellus bogaraveo	sea bream	0.12	0.61
Gadus morrhua	cod	0.23	0.47
Merluccius merluccius	hake	0.10	0.54
Conger conger	conger eel	0.15	0.43
Luvarus imperialis	swordfish	0.15	0.30
Galeorhinus geleus	dogfish	0.04	0.30

In some cases, maintaining a good omega-3/omega-6 ratio through fish consumption is quite difficult, since it requires changing the nutritional habits, or even impossible when it involves an allergic reaction. Furthermore, the consumption of marine fishes like salmon, sardine, tuna, anchovy, mackerel or hake, sometimes is questioned due to the presence of toxic compounds such heavy metals as copper or mercury, or organic pollutants as PCBs or dioxins (Domingo and others 2007).

Table 4. Lipids (g / 100 g oil) in different kind of seed and fish oils. Adapted from Mataix et al. (Mataix and Gil, 2005)

Oil	SFA	MUFA	PUFA	n-3	n-6	n-6/ n-3
Sunflower	12.0	20.5	67.5	0.10	63.2	632
Corn	14.5	29.9	55.6	0.90	50.4	56
Soya	15.6	21.2	63.2	7.30	51.5	7.05
Palm	47.8	37.1	15.1	0.30	10.1	33.66
Olive	14.3	73.0	12.7	0.70	7.8	11.14
Cod liver	22.6	20.7	56.8	19.8	0.9	0.04
Herring	21.3	56.6	22.1	11.9	12	1.01
Salmon	19.9	17.0	63.1	35.3	1.06	0.03
Sardine	30.4	14.5	55.1	28.1	2.2	0.07

In the last years, many products enriched with n-3, like nutritional supplements or functional foods, have been developed in order to maintain a a good n-6:n-3 ratio in the diet with a low fish consumption. Nowadays, the market offers a wide variety of commercial food products enriched with omega-3 including bread and bakery products, milk and derivatives, spreadable fats, eggs, juices and soft drinks, meat and poultry products, etc. (Kolanowski and Laufenberg, 2006).

The increment in the production of omega-3 supplements and enriched food products involves a higher demand of omega-3 concentrates with a good quality at low cost. Therefore, the study of novel and more competitive omega-3 production processes has acquired a great interest both in the food and the pharmaceutical industries.

The most important natural sources of omega-3 PUFA are marine organisms (fish, seafood, algaes…), that are fed, directly or indirectly, from marine phytoplankton, the primary producer of omega-3 in the trophic chain. Nowadays, the majority of commercial omega-3 concentrates derive from fish or fish by-products, and its production involve several steps, i.e.: fish oil extraction, refining, concentration, stabilization and / or formulation (*see* Figure 3).

Conventional processes, based on physical and/or chemical methods, are the most common methods carried out in the current industrial production of omega-3. However, recent studies have shown that supercritical fluid technology could be interesting in omega-3 processing, since it allows avoiding the use of high temperatures, which prevent omega-3 oxidation, and minimising the use of organic solvents.

In next sections, omega-3 processing by both conventional methods and supercritical fluid technology are reviewed.

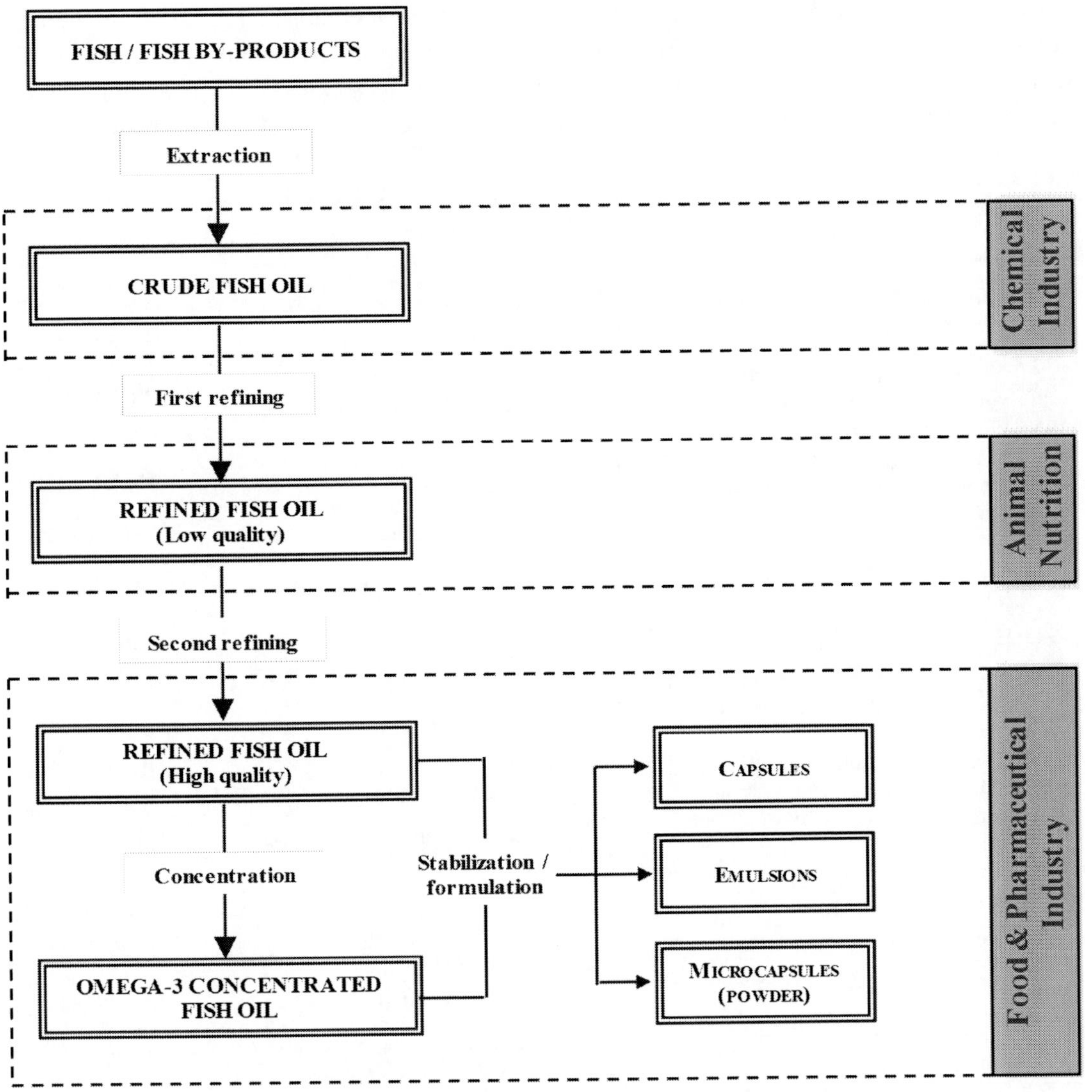

Figure 3. Scheme of fish oil production from fish and fish by-products..

2. Production of Omega-3 Fatty Acids from Fish Oil: State-of-the Art

Abstract

Due to their benefits for human health, the production of omega-3 fatty acids has acquired a great importance in the last years, especially in the food and the pharmaceutical industries.

This Section accounts for both, the current methods and the most recent advances, related to the several stages of omega-3 processing from fish and fish-by-products, i.e., extraction, refining, concentration, formulation and / or stabilization. In the first part, a review of conventional procedures based on physical and chemical methods is provided, including a compilation of commercial fish oil and omega-3 concentrates available nowadays in the market. The last part of the Section is focused on the recent studies developed about the use of supercritical fluid technologies in the production of both fish oil and omega-3 concentrates.

Table 5. Main patents about fish oil extraction published in the twenty and twenty-first centuries

Year	Title	Inventors	Patent number
1901	Process of extracting oil from fish or other material	E.R. Edson	US689472
1930	Process of recovering oil from fish livers and other similar materials	A.W. Owe	US1742666
1932	Fish oil extraction	S. Hiller	US1840715
1933	Method and process of extracting oil and moisture from fish press cake	W.T. Conn	US1903503
1938	Improvements in and relating to the production of fish-liver	Non available	GB0486277
1939	Process and apparatus for the extraction of oil from fish-liver	Non available	GB0500645
1943	Improved method of obtaining oil form fish livers	Non available	GB0558290
1952	Production of oil and proteins from fish	Non available	GB0664827
1952	Improvements in the extraction of oil from fish-liver	Non available	GB0675661
1966	Production of pharmaceutical oil from fish-oil	E. Potter	GB1026359
1967	Method of recovering fish oil	Non available	GB1070128
1976	Process for producing improved fish meal, and fish oil by-product	D.B. Vincent	US3959518
1982	Process for recovering meal and oil from raw fish	P. Bladh	US4344976
1987	Purified fish oil and its production	T. Wakabayashi, and S. Nagahama	JP62093234
1988	Production of fish liver oil containing high units of vitamins	M. Morimitsu	JP63290823
1989	Process for producing protein-rich fish meal and/or fish oil	Y. Shirakawa, Y. Minowa, T. Azumi, and J. Hisano	EP0301795
1990	Method for extracting oil from fish offal	F. Eriksson	WO9008179
1995	Fish oil having decreased fish odour and a method for preparing the same	H. Konishi, I. Riverside, K. Tatsumi, and N. Sato	EP0665287
1996	A method for recovering fish oil having low cholesterol content from fat fish.	A. Oterhals,	WO9608547
1998	Production of high-quality fish oil and high-quality edible extract from head of bonito	N. Koichi	JP10225275
2001	Method and plant for extracting fish oil ad resulting products	P. Barrier, and J.Y. Rousseau	US6214396
2001	Process for producing edible quality refined fish oil	J.B. Crowther, B.H. Booth, and D.D. Blackwell	WO014158
2007	A process for the production of oil and protein from fish waste	J.B. Cloughley	GB2428682
2007	Process for the separation of anchovy meat and anchovy oil	L. B. Tae and C.B. Soo	KR100718551
2008	Method from preparing high-purity edible fish oil from coarse fish oil	S. Yong	CN 101297708
2010	Method for extracting crude fish oil in leftovers of tilapia	B. Yang et al.,	CN101768507

2.1. Conventional Methods in Omega-3 Production

2.1.1. Extraction of Crude Fish Oil

Natural fish oil, or crude fish oil, is the lowest quality fish oil obtained directly from whole fish or fish by-products. This oil is not suitable for human consumption, but is used in the chemical industry as well as raw material for high quality fish oil and omega-3 fatty acids.

Historically, crude fish oil is produced from the antiquity by Nordic towns that used it as fuel in lamps.

At the beginning of the 19th century, US began to produce crude fish oil from menhaden, using a process with two steps: fish cooking and rock-weighted pressing. Around 1850, this type of press was replaced by mechanical screw presses and later by hydraulic presses. Since the beginning of the 20th century, numerous patents have been published to describe new extraction apparatuses and/or to improve the yield of the extraction, the quality of the fish oil extracted and the profitability of the process for industrial purposes, especially using fish by-products as raw material (*see* Table 5).

Nowadays, crude marine oil extraction is usually carried out in fish meal and oil plants by pressing or centrifuging fish or fish by-products previously cooked, although alternative methods based on the protein digestion with a protease have been also proposed in the literature in order to avoid the use of high temperatures and improve oil quality.

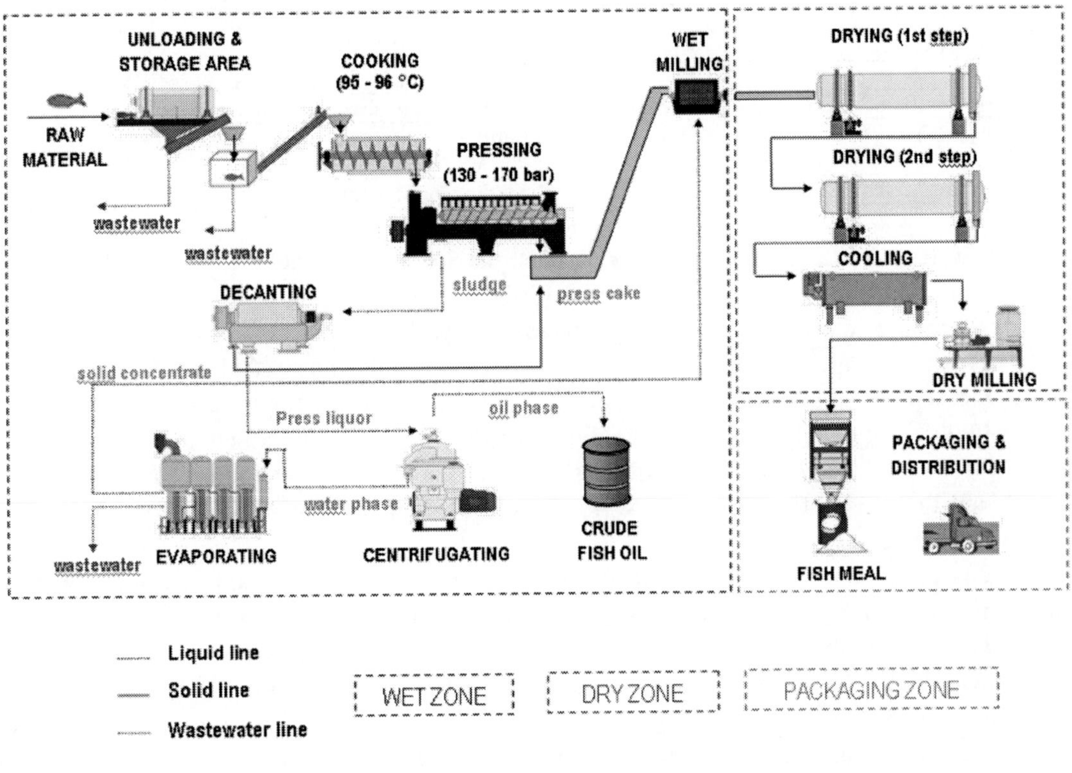

Figure 4. Industrial process for crude oil extraction in fish meal and oil plants. Adapted from www.copeinca.com.pe/.

i. Production of Fish Oil in Fish Meal Plants

The traditional process to obtain crude fish oil from whole fresh fish such capelin or mackerel at industrial scale is the wet pressing method, as described by the Food and Agriculture Organization of the United Nations (*FAO*, 1986).

This process involves the production of fish oil and fish meal through several steps, i.e. cooking of the raw material, pressing of the cooked material and final filtration or centrifugation to recover the oil from the micelle (*see* Figure 4). The use of a 3-phase centrifuge can greatly simplify the separation stages after cooking.

Following this process, several companies, mainly located in Europe, South America and Asia, produce crude fish oil from different types of fish and fish by-products (*see* Table 6).

Table 6. Industrial plants for crude fish oil extraction in Europe

Company	Country	Raw material
Triple Nine Fish Protein	Denmark	Sand eel, sprat, blue whiting, Norway pout, horse mackerel
Havsbrún Ltd.	Faroe Islands (Denmark)	Norwegian pout, capelin, blue whiting
SR-Mjöl HF.	Iceland	Capelin, herring, blue whiting
Vereinigte Fischmehlwerke Cuxhaven GmbH & Co KG	Germany	Pollock, rosefish, plaice, herring
Agro-Fish	Poland	Herring, sprat, spotted silver carp, mackerel, cod
ARTABRA, S.A.	Spain	Whole fish mixed with by-products of canned fish
Copeinca ASA	Peru	Anchovy
Salmonoil	Chile	Salmon and trout by-products
Pesquera Pacific Star, S.A.	Chile	Sardine, scad, anchovy, salmon by-products
Janatha Fish Meal & Oil Products	India	Sardine
Raj Fish Meal & Oil Products	India	Sardine, pink perch

In the last years, several studies have been carried out in order to improve the fish oil quality through improving the raw material freshness and avoiding or minimising the use of high temperatures during the extraction process.

Focussing on the influence of the raw material, Chantachum et al. published a study about the separation of oil from tuna heads by a wet reduction method (Chantachum and others 2000). They studied both the yield and the quality of the oil extracted from precooked (100 ºC for 60 min) and non-precooked fish at different heating temperatures and times, and concluded that the optimum results were achieved when heating at 85 ºC for 30 min and without precooking.

Aidos et al., also reported the oil production from herring by-products using a method consisting of mincing the raw material (16 mm), cooking it in a heat exchanger (8 min at 95 ºC) and recovering the oil in a three-phase decanter (4 min at 95 ºC) with good results (Aidos and others 2001). Moreover, they focused on the influence of by-product freshness (Aidos and others 2003) and the different process parameters (cooking temperature, pumping speed to the heat exchanger and decanter speed) on fish oil quality (Aidos et al., 2003). They concluded that herring by-products have good storage stability and that the main variables that influence oil quality are the separation speed of the decanter and the pumping speed.

ii. Fish Oil Extraction by Enzymatic Methods

The use of enzymes in fish oil extraction is fairly recent but it has become a good alternative to traditional methods, since it can be simpler and cheaper regarding investment cost and energy expense. Besides, this technology requires neither organic solvents nor high temperatures (*Rolle*, 1998). These advantages have promoted the research on the use of enzymatic technology to release lipids from fish avoiding the use of solvents and high temperatures.

Liaset et al. studied the enzymatic hydrolysis of salmon frames with proteases and the composition of the different fractions obtained after separation by centrifugation. They reported that this process enables to obtain omega-3 enriched oil with a good recovery (about 77 %) as well as several interesting products such as peptides or essential amino acids (Liaset and others 2003).

Linder et al. developed another enzymatic method to extract oil from ground salmon heads at middle temperature (55 ºC) using different commercial enzymes: a protease (Alcalase), an exo-peptidase (Neutrase) and an endo-peptidase (Flavourzyme). They concluded that the highest oil recovery (17.4 % after 2 h) was obtained by using Alcalase, being close to the recovery obtained by the Bligh & Dyer method (20 %) (Linder and others 2005).

Šližyte et al., studied the enzymatic hydrolysis of mixtures of cod by-products using Flavourzyme and Neutrase respectively. They studied the influence of the composition and state of the substrate on the yield and composition of the hydrolysis products (oil fraction, hydrolysed protein, sludge and emulsion) (Daukšas and others 2005) and on the chemical composition of the lipid phase (Daukšas et al., 2005). The same authors, (Daukšas et al., 2005), also studied the influence of initial heating of the raw material and on the yield and the chemical composition of the oil extracted by enzymatic hydrolysis of cod by-products using other enzymes such as Alcalase and Lecitase.

Liu et al. proposed an enzymatic process based on a proteolytic extraction of oil from crude tuna heads followed by an urea complexation step, obtaining a mixture of DHA and EPA with a purity of 85.02 % and a yield of 25.10 % (Liu and others 2006).

Gbogouri et al. studied the enzymatic hydrolysis of fresh salmon heads, with Alcalase, Neutrase and Protamex concluding that Alcalase was the most efficient enzyme regarding oil yield. They also found phospholipids to be more effective carriers of LC-PUFA (Gbogouri and others 2006).

Most recently, Al-Sayed Mahmoud et al., have reported a similar study about the enzymatic extraction of oil from rainbow trout roe by using Alcalase, Neutrase and Protamex respectively (Al-Sayed-Mahmoud and others 2008). They also found Alcalase to be the enzyme that leads to the highest oil recovery.

The general conclusion reached by the authors that have studied fish oil extraction by using enzyme technology is that this technology yields better oil than thermal treatments.

iii. Other Physico-Chemical Methods for Fish Oil Extraction

Fish oil extraction based on protein precipitation has been also proposed in the literature (Okada and Morrissey, 2007). This method replaces the cooking step by a pH adjustment to the isoelectric point of the protein of the raw material, and has shown good results for extracting oil from high-oil pelagic species such as sardine, although the main drawback is that several acids (hydrochloric, citric and tartraric acid) and salts (calcium citrate and calcium tartrate) are required.

2.1.2. Fish Oil Refining

Crude fish oil obtained directly in fish meal and oil plants are characterized by a high free fatty acid content and other impurities that limit its use in animal or human nutrition. Therefore a subsequent refining step must be carried out in order to aim the quality standards established by the British Pharmacopoeia (*BP*, 2008) or the Global Organization for EPA and DHA (*GOED*, 2006) (*see* Table 7).

The conventional oil refining process involves different physical and chemical methods aimed to remove impurities (free fatty acids, glycerides, phospholipids, sterols, pigments…), toxic compounds (heavy metals, dioxins, PCBs…) and smelly compounds, depending on the final use of the refined fish oil, that is, animal feeding or human nutrition.

In the last years, the demand of health food-grade or pharmaceutical-grade aimed to human nutrition has increased noticeably, and nowadays several companies produce it all over the world (*see* Table 8) following the quality standards required. The most common refining methods used are reviewed below.

Table 7. Specifications for fish oil aimed to human nutrition established by GOED (*GOED*, 2006) and British Pharmacopeia (*BP*, 2008)

Parameter	Specification	Unit
Acid value	Max. 3	mg KOH / g
Peroxide value (PV)	Max. 10	mq O_2 / kg
Anisidine value (AV)	Max. 20	---
PCDDs/PCDFs	Max 2	pg (WHO-TEQ) / g
Dioxine-like PCBs	Max. 3	pg (WHO-TEQ) / g
Lead, Pb	Max 0.1	mg / kg
Cadmiun, Cd	Max 0.1	mg / kg
Mercury, Hg	Max. 0.1	mg / kg
Inorganic arsenic, As	Max. 0.1	mg / kg

Table 8. Industrial production of health-grade and pharmaceutical-grade fish oil

Country	Company	Product
Iceland	Lysi	Cod liver oil, salmon oil, tuna oil
Norway	Denomega	Anchovy oil
United Kingdom	Seven Seas	Cod liver oil
France	Winterisation Europe	Fish oil, cod liver oil
Spain	GSN	Salmon oil
Spain	Solgar	Cod liver oil
Spain	Nutrytec	Salmon oil
Canada	Enerex	Salmon oil
USA	Lamberts	Herring oil, mackered oil, cod liver oil
USA	NewChapter	Salmon oil
New Zealand	Xtend-life	Hoki oil

iv.Removing Impurities and Contaminants

The main procedure to remove fish oil impurities involves several steps such as degumming, to separate phospholipids; neutralization or deacidification, to clear free fatty acids and decrease oil acidity and bleaching to absorb pigments.

This process presents several drawbacks since it implies the use of chemical products (alkalis), that contaminate the environment, and some neutral oil losts, mainly in oils with high free fatty acid content.

Physical refining processes, based on the application of superheated steam under low pressure have been proposed as alternative to remove free fatty acids and volatile compounds. However, these methods require a preliminary step of chemical refining and, due to the use of high temperatures, they are not suitable for thermolabile oils such as fish oil (Čmolík and Pokorný, 2000).

Physical adsorption on activated carbon has been proposed recently to remove contaminants, such as dioxins and PCBs, from fish (Maes and others 2005; Oterhals and others 2007)

v. Removing smelly compounds

Oil deodorization is also an important process stage, especially in crude fish oils, which are usually characterized by a fishy odour that reduces their sensory quality and limits their application in the food industry.

Traditional oil deodorization is based on the application of high temperatures (Čmolík and Pokorný, 2000). This method is also applied to fish oil although several studies have demonstrated that, at a temperature above 180 ºC, an important PUFA degradation, involving the formation of many undesirable compounds such as polymers, PUFA isomers, mono and di-trans and cyclic fatty acids monomers, is produced (Fournier and others 2006).

Alternative methods based on vacuum steam distillation at low temperatures followed by a treatment in a silica gel column (Chang and others 1989), adsorption with a resin (Nishimoto and Nagagawa, 1996) or treatment with diatomaceous earth (Yoshikazu and others 1997), have been proposed for removing smelly compounds from fish oil.

2.1.3. Omega-3 Concentration

Concentrated fish oil is a refined fish oil subjected to modification in order to increase the amount of omega-3 to at least 600 mg omega-3 / g oil, usually in form of ethyl esters.

The majority of the industrial processes for production of omega-3 concentrates on large scale involve a first step of marine oil extraction from marine organisms, followed by concentration and stabilization steps.

In the last years many processes have been developed to isolate, fractionate or concentrate n-3 PUFA from fish oil, although the majority of them are referred to omega-3 ethyl esters formed by the esterification or saponification of triglycerides with ethanol.

Nowadays, these methods are used by several companies to produce omega-3 concentrates both with pharmaceutical and nutraceutical quality and with different amounts of EPA and DHA (*see* Table 9). However, the main drawback of these procedures is that the natural triglyceride form is lost during the process.

Table 9. Commercial omega-3 concentrated fish oils

Company	Process	Product	Chemical Form	Omega-3
Croda	PureMax Molecular Distillation Technology	Incromega DHA500TG SR	TAG	≤ 100 mg/g EPA Min 500 mg/g DHA
		Incromega EPA500TG SR	TAG	Min 500 mg/g EPA ≤ 60 mg/g DHA
		Incromega TG3322	TAG	Min 33 % EPA Min 22 % DHA
		Incromega E3322	EE	Min 33 % EPA Min 22 % DHA
		Incromega E7010	EE	Min 70 % EPA ≤ 10 % DHA
		Incromega DHA 700E SR	EE	≤ 10 % EPA Min 70 % DHA
Huatai	Multi-stages short-path distillation	Omega-3 H API	EE	Min 400 mg/g EPA Min 340 mg/g DHA
		Omega-3 H Ultra Purity EPA700	EE/TAG	Min 700 mg/g EPA
		Omega-3 H Ultra Purity DHA700	EE/TAG	Min 700 mg/g DHA
		Omega-3 H Ultra Purity	EE/TAG	Min 75 – 5 % EPA Min 5 - 75 % DHA
		Omega-3 H EPA rich	EE/TAG	Min 60 – 30 % EPA Min 15 – 30 % DHA
		Omega-3 H DHA rich	EE/TAG	Min 20 – 10 % EPA Min 40 – 50 % DHA
Pronova biopharma	Urea complexation / molecular distillation	Omacor	EE	55 % EPA 45 % DHA

Several authors, as Mishra et al. (Mishra and others 1993) or Shahidi & Wanasundara (Shahidi and Wanasundara, 1998) have reported a summary of the traditional methods to purify omega-3 fatty acids, i.e. chromatography, vacuum or molecular distillation, low-temperature crystallization, urea complexation, as well as other new processes based on the use of enzymes or supercritical fluids.

vi. Traditional concentration procedures

The most common methods to concentrate omega-3 from fish oil on large scale are molecular distillation and urea complexation.

- *Molecular distillation* implies two main steps: esterification of fatty acids as ethyl esters (EE) and separation of the EE at a low temperature and vacuum according to their molecular weight.
- *Urea complexation* involves the formation of a solution of FFA and urea in a mixture of ethanol / water (95 : 5 %) at 60 °C. The solution is then cooled at room temperature in order to obtain an urea complex slurry, which includes preferentially the saturated fatty acids (SFA), and a liquid phase, formed mainly by unsaturated fatty acids (UFA). Therefore, UFA are easily separated from SFA through gravity filtration.

vii. Enzymatic processes

Enzymatic processes in omega-3 concentration are based on the use of specific enzymes, normally lipases, which are able to catalyse reactions such hydrolysis, ethanolysis or transesterification of triglycerides.

Due to the fatty acid distribution in the glycerol backbone found in several marine triglycerides (Ando and others 1992) and the stereospecifical activity of certain lipases (*Wong*, 2003), these methods are very useful both in omega-3 concentration from fish oil and in the production of structured lipids.

In the last years, a great amount of enzymatic methods followed by a separation process such membrane filtration, urea complexation or molecular distillation have been proposed in the literature to obtain omega-3 concentrates, especially EPA and DHA, as different forms such free fatty acids, ethyl esters or 2-acylglycerides (Oliveira-Carvalho and others 2003; Shahidi and Wanasundara, 1998). Among these procedures, both enzymatic hydrolysis and enzymatic esterification or transesterification it may be distinguished.

- Enzymatic hydrolysis

Enzymatic hydrolysis has been proposed by several authors as an interesting way to obtain omega-3 concentrates as free fatty acids from fish oil.

Linder et al. developed a method to increase the amount of PUFA in salmon oil from 39.20 mol % to 43.05 mol % throughout an enzymatic hydrolysis catalyzed by Novozym® SP398, followed by a filtration step in a flat membrane device. In addition, they proposed a final esterification step with glycerol using an immobilized 1,3-specific lipase to slightly increase the amount of PUFA up to 43.29 mol % (Linder and others 2002).

Gámez-Meza et al. studied the concentration of omega-3 from sardine oil coupling hydrolysis reaction and urea complexation. Comparing enzymatic hydrolysis with different *Pseudomona* lipases with the chemical hydrolysis using KOH, ethanol and hexane, they concluded that the lipase from *Pseudomona cepacia* immobilized on chemically modified ceramic with a 10 % protein is the best enzymatic system to obtain the highest purity of omega-3 fatty acids (86.58 %) with an acceptable yield (78.0 %), while chemical hydrolysis enabled to obtain a higher omega-3 recovery (90.5 %) but with a lower purity (83.13 %). In addition, they pointed out that the enzymatic method is more advantageous since the separation of the products is easier and the process can be developed in continuous packed-bed reactors (Gámez-Meza and others 2003).

Kojima et al. designed a process to concentrate alternatively DHA or EPA from a mixture of natural fish oil through an enzymatic method using HU-lipases (which show a high reactivity for any fatty acid with 20 atoms of carbon) or AK-lipases (which shows a poor reactivity for fatty acids with 20 atoms of carbon and a Δ5 unsaturated bond), followed by urea complexation to increase the purity. They concluded that, using this method with HU-lipase, it is possible to selectively enrich EPA from 12.2 % to 43.1 %, while the amount of DHA is practically constant. On the other hand, if the same method was repeated using AK-lipase, a selective enrichment of DHA from 16.3 % to 44.6 % was obtained, while the amount of EPA was hardly altered (Kojima and others 2006).

- Enzymatic esterification

Enzymatic esterification or transesterification processes are very useful in the production of lipids derived from omega-3 PUFA that present different properties than the corresponding free fatty acids. For instance, omega3 ethyl or methyl esters are easily separated by SFF or SFC, as mentioned in section 0, triacylglycerides are more attractive in the food industry since they are well absorbed by the human organism (Lawson and Hughes, 1988), and phospholipids (Lyberg and others 2005) or wax esters (Gorreta and others 2002) are important as a stabilization strategy because they are the most stable lipid forms against oxidation.

In the last decade, several studies about enzymatic esterification and transesterification of fish oil with microbial lipases have been also reviewed in the literature (Oliveira-Carvalho et al., 2003; Shahidi and Wanasundara, 1998). Recently, a method has been patented by Le Goffic et al., which combines chemical and enzymatic transesterification of fish oil with short path distillation steps to achieve a fraction rich in DHA (more than 90 %) and poor in EPA (less than 5 %), besides to another fraction rich in EPA (more than 50 %) and poor in DHA (less than 2 %) (LeGoffic and others 2000). However, the main drawback of this method is the use of high temperatures (above 100 ºC) during the distillation steps, which may be related with a high omega-3 oxidation.

From then until now, many scientists have continued investigating on the improvement of the omega-3 concentration processes, to achieve higher yield and purity at lower cost. Among the new trends, it is worth to noting the enzymatic processes involving the use of supercritical fluids as reaction media, which are described in section 0.

2.1.4. Fish Oil Formulation and Stabilization

One of the major drawbacks of oils containing a high amount of omega-3 PUFA, such as fish oils, is their high susceptibility to oxidation, which involve the formation of toxic products as peroxides or volatile compounds relative to non-desirable off-flavors.

Omega-3 oxidation is carried out by a complex mechanism that depends on the type of lipids and their presentation (bulk oil, water-in-oil emulsion or oil-in-water emulsion, encapsulation or microencapsulation), and can be catalyzed by other parameters as temperature, exposure to light and oxygen or presence of trace metals (*see* Figure 5).

Therefore, optimum processing, storage and packaging of fish oils are essential to preserve omega-3 PUFA from oxidation. In addition, other strategies to improve fish oil stability and prolong its shelf-life are necessary (Kamal-Eldin and Yanishlieva, 2002).

viii. Addition of Antioxidants

The use of antioxidants is one of the most common methods to prevent fish oil oxidation. A great amount of antioxidants, as BHA, BHT, EDTA, tocopherols, ascorbic acid, ascorbyl palmitate, propyl gallate, gallic acid, lactoferrines, etc., has been studied to prevent lipid oxidation both in bulk fish oil (Kamal-Eldin and Yanishlieva, 2002) and in fish oil-in-water emulsions (Jacobsen and others 2008).

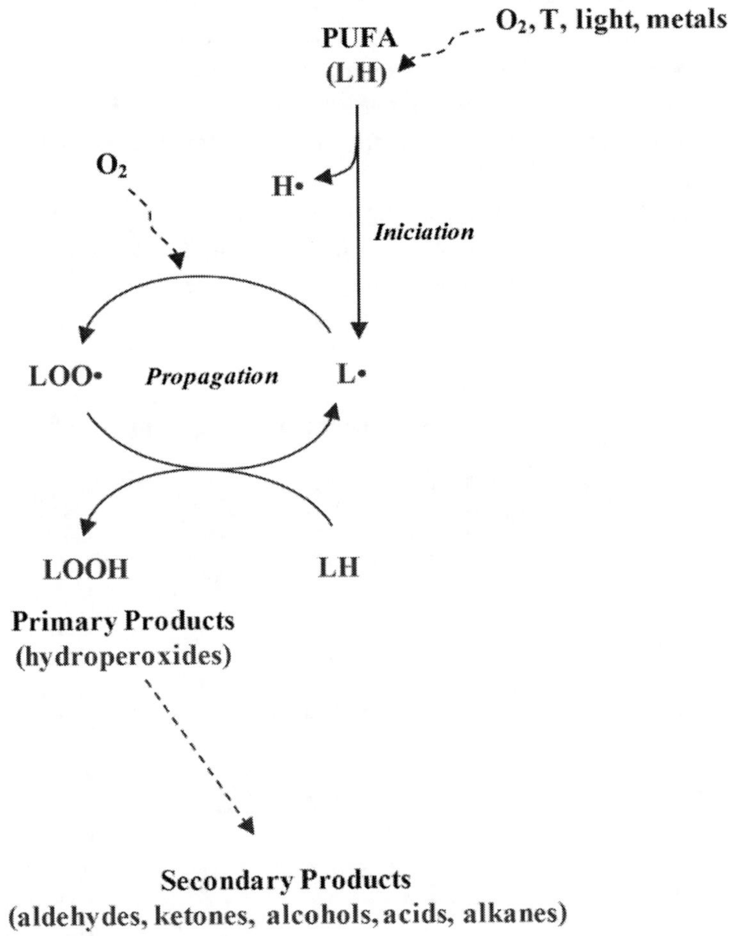

Figure 5. Mechanism of PUFA oxidation (*adapted from* (*FAO*, 1995)).

In the last decade, the use of natural antioxidants instead of synthetic compounds has acquired great relevance and several studies regarding the efficiency of plant extracts, as oregano, rosemary, parsley or olive mill wastewaters, on the stabilization of bulk fish oil and fish oil-in-water emulsions have been developed (Bhale and others 2007; Frankel and others 1996; Wada and Fang, 1992; Jiménez-Álvarez and others 2008).

In addition, several studies about the effect of adding natural antioxidants in omega-3 enriched foods, as meat products (Valencia and others 2008) or frozen surimi (Pérez-Mateos and others 2006), have been published.

ix. Encapsulation or Microencapsulation

Encapsulation or microencapsulation with a coating material has also been proposed as strategy to retard lipid auto-oxidation and enzyme hydrolysis, improve the oil stability and control off-flavors (Matsuno and Adachi, 1993). In addition, it has been proved that the use of fish oil microcapsules offers good results in the design of functional foods as cream to fill sandwich cookies (Borneo and others 2007), instant foods (soups, cocoa drinks…) (Kolanowski and others 2007a), dairy products (yoghurt, fresh cheese, butter…) (Kolanowski and others 2007b) or pasta (Iafelice and others 2008).

Nowadays, a great amount of physical and chemical processes using several wall materials have been developed to encapsulate and stabilize active compounds as fish oil (Desai and Park, 2005) and several companies produce and commercialise powder fish oil and fish oil concentrated formulas especially designed for bakery, baby food, beverage or dairy industry (*see* Table 10).

Among the methods used, spray-drying is the most common and cheaper (Gharsallaoui and others 2007), although other processes as freeze drying (Heinzelmann and others 2000) or ultrasonic atomization (Klaypradit and Huang, 2008) have also been developed recently as alternative to reduce omega-3 oxidation since they avoid the use of high temperatures during the drying step.

Table 10. Commercial fish oil microencapsulated aimed to food industry

Company	Product	Applications
Lipid Nutrition	MarinolTM Omega-3 HS MarinolTM DHA HS	Backery Baby food
The Wright Group	O-3 Complete®	Backery Baby food Beverages
NuMega	Driphorm HiDHA®	Backery Baby food Beverages
Ocean Nutrition	MEG-3®	Backery Dairy Sauces
BASF	Dry n-3® 5:25 C Dry n-3® 18:12	Dairy Baby food
DSM	ROPUFA®	Backery Dairy Baby food

2.2. Production Processes Based on Supercritical Fluid Technology

2.2.1. Introduction to Supercritical Fluids

The use of supercritical fluids technology in the production of natural compounds has acquired an enormous interest in the last years, especially when the final products is, as occurs with omega-3 fatty acids, a high value product aimed to food and pharmaceutical industries.

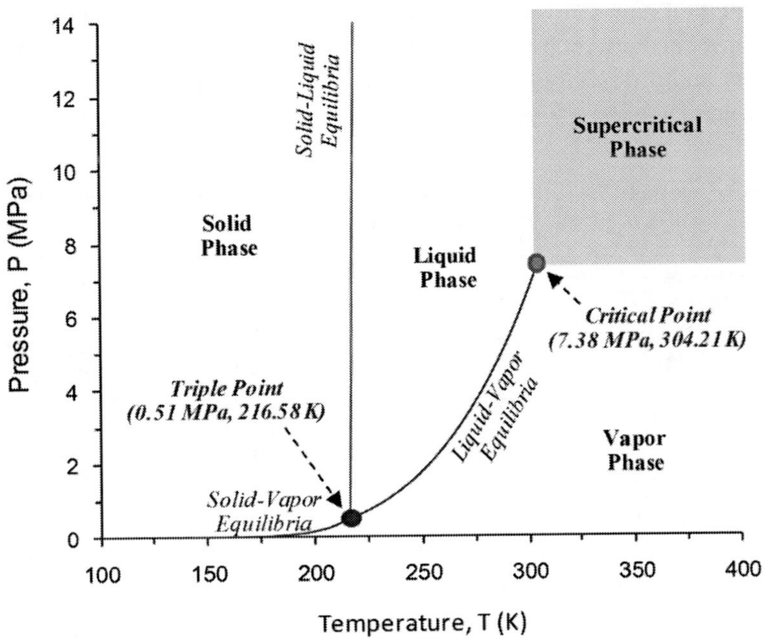

Figure 6. Phase diagram of carbon dioxide illustrating the supercritical region above the critical pressure (P_c) and temperature (T_c).

Supercritical fluids are considered to be any fluid at a reduced pressure, temperature and density, defined as (0.1), (0.2) and (0.3) respectively, above unity, pressure being below the necessary to solidify the fluid.

$$P_r = \frac{P}{P_c} \quad (0.1)$$

$$T_r = \frac{T}{T_c} \quad (0.2)$$

$$\rho_r = \frac{\rho}{\rho_c} \quad (0.3)$$

Table 11. Comparison of physical properties of gases, liquids and SCF. Adapted from Brunner (*Brunner*, 1994)

Physical State	Pressure & Temperature conditions [T (K) / P (MPa)]	Density (kg/m^3)	Viscosity (Pa s)	Diffusivity (m^2/s)	Surface Tension (mN/m)
Gas	[0.1 / 298]	0,5 – 2	10^{-5}	10^{-5}	0
SCF	[P_c, T_c]	200-500	$1.3 \cdot 10^{-5}$	$0.7 \cdot 10^{-7}$	0
	[4P_c, T_c]	40-900	$3.9 \cdot 10^{-5}$	$0.2 \cdot 10^{-7}$	0
Liquid	[0.1 / 298]	600 – 1600	10^{-3}	10^{-9}	25-80

In the region above its critical point, characterized by one only phase (*see* Figure 6) the fluid possesses intermediate properties between a gas and a liquid, i.e.: liquid-like density and gas-like viscosity and diffusivity (*see* Table 11). Therefore supercritical fluids (SCF) have at the same time a good solvent power and good transport properties (*Brunner*, 1994).

Table 12. Critical properties of different solvents. Adapted from Cengel et al., (Cengel and Boles, 2002)

Solvent		T_c (K)	P_c (MPa)	ρ_c (g/cm^3)
Carbon dioxide	CO_2	304.1	7.38	0.469
Water	H_2O	647.1	22.06	0.322
Metane	CH_4	190.4	4.60	0.162
Ethane	C_2H_6	305.3	4.87	0.203
Propane	C_3H_8	369.8	4.25	0.217
Ethylene	$H_2C{=}CH_2$	282.4	5.04	0.215
Propylene	$CH_3CH{=}CH_2$	364.9	4.60	0.232
Methanol	CH_3OH	512.6	8.09	0.272
Ethanol	CH_3CH_2OH	513.9	6.14	0.276
Acetone	CH_3COCH_3	508.1	4.70	0.278

In the last decades, different SCF have been proposed (*see* Table 12), being supercritical carbon dioxide, SC-CO_2 the most widely used since it is considered a green solvent, non toxic, cheap and non flammable; has mild critical conditions (T_c = 304.15 K and P_c= 7.38 MPa) that allow to process thermolabile compounds, as omega-3 PUFA, and makes operation costs not too expensive. In addition, CO_2 is gaseous under ambient conditions, which means that it is easy to separate from the processed products after processing.

2.2.2. Historical development of the Supercritical Fluids Technology

The first reported observations of the supercritical phase phenomenon were carried out by Baron Cagniard de la Tour in 1822, who reported that, when the temperature of some substances was increased by heating in a closed vessel, the gas-liquid boundary disappears (*Tour*, 1822). From this starting point, the critical point of a substance was defined.

Years later, authors like Hannay & Hogarth, who studied the solubility of different inorganic salts in supercritical ethanol (Hannay and Hogarth, 1879); or Buchner, who studied the solubility of non-volatile organic compounds in supercritical carbon dioxide (*Buchner*, 1906), demonstrated that the solvating power of supercritical fluids were much higher than would be expected from the vapour pressure of the solid, and, moreover, this was tunable according to the supercritical fluid pressure. During 1930 and 1940 different phases equilibria were studied, which aimed to design a deasphalting process for refining lubricants oils, although the most significant development in supercritical fluid technology was carried out from 1960 when Zosel described and patented more than 80 extraction processes using supercritical fluids, the most important related to the decaffeination of green coffee with supercritical carbon dioxide (*Zosel*, 1982).

Table 13. Current industrial processes based on supercritical fluid extraction

Process	Manufacturer	Country
Coffee / tea decaffeination	Kaffee HAG AG Hermsen Jacobs Suchard	Germany
	SKW-Trostberg	Italy
	General Foods	USA
Hops Extraction	Pfizer Hops Extraction	Australia
	Hopfenextraktion, HVG, Barth, Raiser & Co. SKW Trostberg Barth & Co. SKW-Trostberg	Germany
	Carlton, United Breweries Pauls & White	United Kingdom
	Hops Extraction Corp. of America J.I. Haas, Inc. Pitt-Des Moines, Inc.	USA
	NORAC	Canada
	Nan Fang Flour Mill	China
	Natal Cane By-Products Ltd.	South Africa
Flavors/Aromas/Spices	Flavex GmbH Raps & Co.	Germany
	Camilli Albert & Louie,	France
	Soda Flavor Co.	Japan
	Guangxia Toothpaste Shaanxi Jia De Agriculture Eng. Co., Ltd.	China
	Mohri Oil Mills Fuji Flavor	Japan
Nicotine extraction	Philip Morris	USA
	Nippon Tobacco	Japan
Color Extraction / Red Pepper	Sumitomo Seiko Yasuma (Mitsubishi Kokoki facility) Hasegawa Koryo Takasago Foods (Mitsubishi Kokoki facility)	Japan

Since 1980, the development of supercritical fluid extraction has increased noticeably, and several extraction plants have been built all over the world to extract different natural compounds on commercial scale by using supercritical carbon dioxide as solvent (*see* Table 13).

Nowadays, a great amount of processes involve the use of supercritical fluids as solvents, such as supercritical fluid extraction (SFE), fractionation (SFF), chromatography (SFC); whereas other procedures are based in the use of supercritical fluid as a media for enzymatic reaction or particle formation. The main processes related to the use of supercritical fluid technologies in fish oil extraction, refining, omega-3 concentration or formulation are reviewed below.

2.2.3. Supercritical Fluid Extraction of Fish Oil

Fish oil is a natural mixture of different lipid compounds, liquid at room temperature, soluble in non-polar solvents, as hexane or petroleum ether, and insoluble in polar solvents as water.

SC-CO_2 has been also shown to be a good solvent of natural fish oil: Imanishi et al. measured the solubility of fish oil from sardine in SC-CO_2 in a pressure range of 20 to 35 MPa at four different temperatures (313, 333, 343 and 353 K). They observed that, at constant temperature, fish oil solubility increased significantly with pressure, whereas, at constant pressure, oil solubility decreased with temperature up to a pressure value from which oil solubility began to increase as temperature increased (Imanishi and others 1989).

This crossover behaviour has also been observed in other natural fish oils from sand eel (Borch-Jensen and Mollerup, 1997), orange roughy, spiny dogfish liver or cod liver (Catchpole and others 1998). It is explained considering that, at constant pressure, a temperature increase has a double effect: the density of the solvent decreases, which would make solubility to decrease, and the vapour pressure of the solute increases, which would make the solubility to increase. At low pressures the first effect predominates and at high pressures is the solute vapour pressure effect which becomes stronger (*Brunner*, 1994). It has been also observed that fish oil solubility increases by adding polar co-solvents such as ethanol (Catchpole et al., 1998).

The experimental determination of phase equilibrium data of mixtures formed by the different components of fish oil, and its derivatives, and SC-CO_2 has acquired more relevance in the last years because phase equilibrium data are essential to design fish oil processes such as supercritical fluid extraction (SFE), fractionation (SFF) or supercritical fluid chromatography (SFC), which are technologies involved in oil refining and omega-3 concentration.

Staby & Mollerup summarized most of the published phase equilibrium data involving SC-CO_2 and fish oil components or derivatives. Their paper includes reference data for the main lipid compounds, pure or mixtures, such as glycerides, free fatty acids, fatty acid methyl or ethyl esters, and other minority components such as cholesterol, β-carotene or α-tocopherol (Staby and Mollerup, 1993).

Güçlü-Üstündağ & Temelli published a compilation of solubility data for the main pure lipid classes such as fatty acids, fatty acid esters and mono-, di- and triglycerides (Güçlü-Üstündağ and Temelli, 2000) and for other minor lipids as β-carotene, α-tocopherol, stigmasterol and squalene in SC-CO_2 (Güçlü-Üstündağ and Temelli, 2004). In both reviews, they used the Chrastil's solubility model to quantify the influence on solubility, not only of the equilibrium pressure and temperature, but also of the physical properties of the solute such as molecular weight, polarity or vapour pressure.

Based on the good solubility of fish oil, and its individual components, in SC-CO_2, abundant research dealing with fish oil extraction using SC-CO_2 as solvent has been made. Raventós et al. (Raventós and others 2002) made a general overview of the possibilities of SC-CO_2 as an extracting solvent in the food industry, including the extraction of lipids and cholesterol from fish. Staby & Mollerup, besides reviewing the solubility or phase equilibrium data of typical components of fish oil in supercritical fluids, also made an overview of the supercritical fluid extraction, fractionation and/or chromatography of these compounds, especially acylglycerides, free fatty acids, fatty acid methyl or ethyl esters, cholesterol, α-tocopherols, squalene or phospholipids (Staby and Mollerup, 1993).

Some recent studies about SC-CO_2 extraction of oil from fish, and some not so recent studies that have not been considered in previous reviews (Dunford and others 1998; Dunford and others 1997; Esquível and others 1997; Letisse and others 2006; Rubio-Rodríguez and others 2008) are detailed next: Esquível et al. studied the extraction of sardine oil with SC-CO_2, concluding that it is possible to find the conditions to recover most of the oil (95 %) without degradation of the omega-3 PUFA (Esquível et al., 1997). Dunford et al. studied the effect of moisture on mackerel oil extractability using SC-CO_2. They concluded that the extraction yield increased with decreasing moisture content and proposed a mathematical model to explain this extraction behaviour (Dunford et al., 1998; Dunford et al., 1997). Some fish by-products have also been considered as raw material to obtain omega-3 rich oil by using supercritical carbon dioxide: Letisse et al. looked for the optimum extraction conditions to obtain an oil rich in omega-3 PUFA from freeze dried sardine heads (Letisse et al., 2006). Rubio-Rodriguez et al. studied the oil extraction from hake by-products, specifically from hake skin, by using SC-CO_2. They studied the influence of all the important process parameters to search the most efficient extraction conditions regarding oil yield and quality (Rubio-Rodríguez et al., 2008).

Nowadays, SFE is generally considered a useful technology to replace traditional extraction processes as steam distillation or solvent extraction. Therefore, SFE is a promise technology to be scaled up to indusial scale in order to produce good quality fish oil, suitable as raw material to produce n-3 concentrates.

2.2.4. Fish Oil Refining Using Supercritical Fluids

Supercritical fluid technology, together with membrane and enzymatic processes, are some of the most recent technologies proposed as alternative to oil refining with chemical products or high temperatures.

Several studies have been recently reported dealing with the application of these technologies, both in degumming or bleaching (Čmolík and Pokorný, 2000), and in deacidification (Bhosle and Subramanian, 2005) of different seed oils, as well as in fish oil refining.

Jakobsson et al. proposed a semi-continuous extraction process using SC-CO_2 with and without ethanol for removing dioxins and free fatty acids from cod liver oil. They found that it is difficult to lower the free fatty acid content at a level of 0.5 %-1 % and, at the same time, to remove a great amount of dioxins, due to the different polarity of both types of compounds. However, they found possible to separate dioxins from deacidified oil by using pure SC-CO_2 at low pressures (Jakobsson and others 1991). Subsequently, the same authors (Jakobsson and others 1994) proposed a counter-current extraction process to improve the contact between oil and SC-CO_2 and increase the amount of dioxins to be removed. Their results showed that 80 % of the dioxins can be extracted together with the first 17 % of the oil.

Catchpole et al. developed a method for removing impurities as peroxides, fatty acids or odour components, from different crude fish oils as orange roughy oil, deep sea shark liver oil, spiny dogfish oil and cod liver oil, by using SC-CO_2. They used a pilot plant with a countercurrent fractionation column with two separation vessels. Additionally, they proved the effect of using ethanol as co-solvent in the supercritical CO_2 fractionation, concluding that a mixture of CO_2-ethanol (5 % by mass) enabled to obtain a product (raffinate) lower in acidity (aprox. 0.5 %) and with a negligible fishy odor compared to the raffinate obtained using pure SC-CO_2 under the same experimental conditions (Catchpole and others 2000).

Yuqian et al. also proposed a method for refining crude fish oil by combining supercritical fluid extraction (SFE) with CO_2 or propane and a physical adsorption step (Yuqian and Huashi, 2001).

Kawashima et al. proposed combining extraction with SC-CO_2 and adsorption on activated carbon to remove polychlorinated biphenyls (PCB), polychlorinated dibenzo-p-dioxins (PCDD), and polychlorinated dibenzofurans (PCDF) from fish oil. They found the SFE process to be effective for removal of PCB and the adsorption method for removal of PCDD / DF. By combining both methods they could achieve a reduction of the total toxicity of about 100 % (Kawashima and others 2006).

As a conclusion, it can be said that traditional oil refining is being revised to explore new technologies, mainly supercritical fluid technologies that have been shown to produce high quality oil.

2.2.5. Supercritical Fluids in Omega-3 Concentration

In the last years, the use of supercritical fluids in omega-3 concentration from fish oil has acquired a great interest and several processes have been developed based on supercritical fluid fractionation (SFF), supercritical fluid chromatography (SFC) or enzymatic reaction under supercritical media.

x. Supercritical Fluid Fractionation (SFF)

During the 1980ties, several authors proposed some of the first methods to fractionate fish oil ethyl esters by using supercritical fluids (Pettinello and others 2000; Snoey-Elich, 2001) and take advantage of their previously mentioned attractive features (*see* Section 0). Since then, several authors have continued exploring this field. In many cases, the research has included the study of the phase equilibrium of the mixtures involved in the processes, because it is essential for the design of an extraction or fractionation process. Nowadays, most of the fractionation studies using SCF are performed over omega-3 ethyl esters and, therefore, phase equilibria involving this type of esters has been also the most widely studied.

Fleck et al. designed an automated countercurrent column for fractionation of FAEE by using SC-CO_2. Only adding automation to the column caused a significant improvement in the separation efficiency, very important for the development of SFF processes at industrial scale (Fleck and others 1998).

Riha & Brunner studied phase equilibria between SC-CO_2 and many fatty acid ethyl esters (FAEE) derived from fish oil, proving that it is possible to fractionate them according to their carbon number (Riha and Brunner, 1999). Based on these results, the same authors developed a method to separate FAEE from fish oil by countercurrent multistage extraction with CO_2 in a pilot scale column (Riha and Brunner, 2000). They also proposed a thermodynamic model that enabled to calculate the optimal conditions to separate FAEE by this process that resulted to be 14.5 MPa and 333 K. Finally, they proved that the application of the optimized method at industrial scale produced a concentration of EPA, DHA and DPA higher than 90 %. Moreover, the use of a theoretical model also enabled to reduce the operation cost and increase the profitability of the process (*Brunner*, 2000).

Espinosa et al. studied phase equilibria between a mixture of FAEE and SC-CO_2 based in a Group Contribution Equation of State (GC-EOS). From these results, they performed a simulation of the extraction process, and optimized the experimental conditions. Finally, they proposed a method to obtain a high yield of high purity fractions of EPA and DHA respectively, using a high pressure countercurrent system with three columns, which enabled to obtain an EPA fraction with a purity of 60.46 mol % and a yield of 98.18 %; and a DHA fraction with a purity of 80.09 mol % and a yield of 80.34 %. Alternatively, to increase the purity of the product, they proposed a previous step based on urea complexation (Espinosa and others 2002).

Perreti et al. have recently confirmed the possibility of modifying the FAEE concentration of a mixture by using SC-CO_2 and optimizing the fractionation process in terms of pressure, temperature, and flow rate of this selective solvent (Perretti and others 2007).

Gironi & Maschietti proposed a thermodynamic model that assumed the oil to be composed of five ethyl esters (EE), each of them representing a specific acid chain length. They validated this model with some experimental data obtained in a semicontinuous single-stage fractionation process and then applied it to simulate a multistage continuous process. They demonstrated that this process enables to produce a raffinate with 95% by weight of EE-EPA and EE-DHA, together with 95% recovery of these compounds (Gironi and Maschietti, 2006). However, the scale-up of this process at industrial scale has not been reported yet.

Martin & Cocero developed a comprehensive mathematical model for the SFF of liquids with SC-CO_2 by including the differential mass and energy balances in the column, and the coupled mass and heat transfer in the interface between the two fluid phases. Phase equilibrium and volumetric and thermal properties, were described by using a consistent equation of state and transport properties and mass transfer coefficients were estimated applying suitable correlations. They validated this model for the SFF of fish oil ethyl esters mixtures and found it to be able to predict the trends of variation of the composition of extract and raffinate with the different operating parameters (Martín and Cocero, 2007).

Antunes-Corrêa et al. focused their work towards obtaining concentrates of omega-3 PUFA in their natural form instead of their ethyl esters. They measured natural fish oil solubility by the dynamic method and determined the composition of both, the original oil and the collected fraction. These data allowed them to calculate the distribution coefficients of several of the oil components. The distribution coefficients they found were very close to unity giving little expectation to SFF of the natural triacylglycerides to concentrate omega-3 PUFA (Antunes-Corrêa and others 2008). Similar conclusions were reached also by other authors (Davarnejad and others 2008).

Research on fish oil SFF is still open with the aim of achieving production at large scale. The main limitations for scaling up the process is the knowledge of phase behaviour of the mixtures involved on SFF and models to describe it. As has been detailed previously, models to describe SFF are well developed once phase equilibria can be well described.

xi. Supercritical Fluid Chromatography (SFC)

Because of the physical properties of supercritical fluids, they can be used as a mobile phase along with packed or capillary columns filled with a suitable stationary phase. This technique is named supercritical fluid chromatography (SFC), and is an attractive alternative to traditional chromatographic techniques as gas chromatography (GC) or high pressure liquid chromatography (HPLC) for analytical, preparative or production purposes (Kiran and others 2000) due to the SCF properties mentioned at the beginning of this section.

SFC is especially suitable for the separation of omega-3 PUFA since it combines the high selectivity of both, the supercritical fluid and the stationary phase. Therefore, several methods based on SFC have been developed to obtain omega-3 PUFA with a high purity and recovery not only in the laboratory but also at large scale. As for SFF, most of the research and production of omega-3 concentrates deals with the ethyl esters. The most interesting works on this subject are reviewed next.

Perrut et al. patented a method to isolate EPA and DHA from a mixture of fatty acid ethyl esters obtained from fish oil, coupling preparative supercritical chromatography and simulated countercurrent moving bed chromatography with several columns placed in series. In both cases, octadecyl silica gel is used as column stationary phase whereas SC-CO_2 is the solvent eluent. Following this method, they obtained EPA and DHA fractions with a high yield (99 %) and purity (92 % and 85 % respectively) (Perrut and others 1998).

Brunner & Reichmann also patented a SFC method to isolate unsaturated fatty acids with at least 16 carbon atoms from a mixture of fatty acids or their derivatives using SC-CO_2 as eluent and aluminium oxide as stationary phase (Fleck et al., 1998).

Alternatively, other studies about SFC of omega-3 fatty acids have been found in the literature.

Alkio et al. reported a systematic study in order to find the optimal conditions to purify DHA-EE and EPA-EE from esterified tuna oil. They found that using SC-CO_2 at 65 ºC and 145 bar and octadecyl silane as stationary phase, it was possible to obtain simultaneously a DHA-EE production of 0.85 g/(kg stationary phase × h) with a purity of 90 %, and an EPA-EE production of 0.23 g/(kg stationary phase × h) with a purity of 50 % (Alkio and others 2000).

Pettinello et al. studied the enrichment on bench-scale and on pilot-scale of an ester mixture from fish oil with 68 % of EPA-EE using supercritical chromatography with SC-CO_2 as mobile phase and silica gel as stationary phase. They concluded that, on bench-scale production, using a column of 25 mm × 200 mm, the highest EPA-EE purity (90 %) and recovery (49 %) was obtained at a temperature of 70 ºC with a pressure programme between 180 and 220 bar and a SC-CO_2 flow rate of 13.5 g/min. However, on semi-industrial scale using a column of 100 mm × 520 mm, the optimal conditions involved the use of the same temperature and pressure, but a higher CO_2 flow rate (15-25 kg/h), which enabled to process a total amount of 300 g fish oil per cycle and obtain an EPA-EE purity of 93 % with a yield of 24.6 % (Pettinello et al., 2000).

A recent method patented by Snoey-Elich has been also proposed to concentrate EPA-EE from fish oil, from a purity of 50 % to more than 95 %, using an industrial column of 50-60 cm × 260-280 cm filled with a porous silicon oxide impregnated with (3-aminopropyl)-triethoxysilane as stationary phase and SC-CO_2 as mobile phase working at a pressure of 100-150 bar, a temperature of 40-60 ºC and a flow rate between 4000-7000 kg/h (*Snoey-Elich*, 2001).

Other authors, as Yang et al., have continued the researches about SFC to isolate both EPA-EE and DHA-EE from fish oil with a high purity and yield (Yang and others 2004).

This process is already installed at production scale, and companies as KD-Pharma or Solutex, produce a combination of omega-3 PUFA in a proportion over 90 %, EPA up to a concentration of 95 % and DHA up to 80 % by applying this technology.

xii. Enzymatic Reactions in Supercritical Fluids

Supercritical CO_2 has also been proposed as a good medium to carry on enzymatic reactions, since it is considered a green solvent, nontoxic and easily removed from the reaction products. In addition, SC-CO_2 presents interesting physical properties such density, diffusivity or viscosity, which can be changed by changing pressure or temperature. Moreover, enzymatic reactions under supercritical fluids may be easily coupled with other processes such SFE, SFF, SFC or microencapsulation procedures using SC-CO_2, which has an enormous interest in the production of microencapsulated omega-3 concentrates directly from the raw material, minimising the oil manipulation and, therefore, preventing its oxidation.

In last years, several studies have been published by Gunnlaugsdottir et al. about the influence of experimental conditions, as pressure (Gunnlaugsdottir and Sivik, 1995)or solvent flow rate (Gunnlaugsdottir and Sivik, 1997) on the ethanolysis of cod liver oil with an immobilized lipase (Novozym 435). The same authors have also studied the phase behaviour of the reaction mixture in SC-CO_2 (Gunnlaugsdottir and others 1997) and a coupled process with supercritical fluid extraction and enzymatic ethanolysis to produce omega-3 ethyl esters from cod liver oil in a continuous mode (Gunnlaugsdottir and others 1998).

Another recent procedure, proposed by Lin et al., enables an omega-3 enrichment of fish oil through an enzymatic transesterification with an immobilized 1,3-specific lipase (Lipozyme IM-60) in a supercritical CO_2 medium (5 h, 323 K and 10.34 bar). They reported that under supercritical conditions, enzymatic transesterification was 40 % higher than under conventional solvents, proving that coupled processes with supercritical fluids and biotechnological methods may be an interesting strategy to produce omega-3 structured lipids from fish oil under mild conditions and with a high yield (Lin and others 2006).

A recent review shows all the possibilities of SCF technology to perform enzymatic reactions, including oil hydrolysis and transesterification (*Knez*, 2009). As observed, enzymatic methods by themselves, do not lead to omega-3 concentrates but further concentration is needed. Pretreatments using supercritical fluids present advantages regarding the non use of chemicals and the high yields obtained.

2.2.6. Supercritical Fluids in Omega-3 Formulation

Microencapsulation processes using supercritical fluids have also been proposed recently as a good alternative to protect active compounds as fish oil using mild temperatures in an inert atmosphere. Among them, encapsulation and co-precipitation processes as Rapid Expansion of Supercritical Solutions (RESS), Supercritical Solvent Impregnation (SSI), Particles from Gas Saturated Solutions (PGSS), Supercritical Anti Solvent precipitation (SAS) or Supercritical Fluid Extraction of Emulsions (SFEE) (Cocero and others 2009). These methods are still under investigation and no studies about supercritical fluid microencapsulation of fish oil have been found in the literature.

3. Production of Omega-3 Fatty Acids from Alternative Sources To Fish Oil

Abstract

As it has been previously treated (see Section 0), fish and fish by-products are the most important sources of omega-3 fatty acids, especially EPA and DHA. However, it is known that global fish stocks are in danger and marine fish production may decrease in the future.

Thus, searching for alternative sources of omega-3 PUFA is required, being marine microalgaes, algaes or transgenic plants some of the most recent proposal.

3.1. Omega-3 Production from Marine Algae and Microalgae

Marine microalgae, or phytoplankton, provide the food base that supports the entire animal population in open seas. Human application of microalgaes has been made in Asia since ancientness, although microalgae biotechnology has been developed in the last century. Nowadays, commercial applications of microalgaes are extended all over the world.

Spolaore et al. have reviewed some of the actual commercial applications of microalgaes in human and animal nutrition and in the cosmetic industry (Spolaore and others 2006).

Cardozo et al. have also reviewed the most recent researches on microalgae production of high-value compounds having economic relevance in food science, pharmacology or human health, as PUFA, sterols or carotenoids, among others (Cardozo and others 2007).

Conchillo et al. have published a study comparing microalgae oil and fish oil. They concluded that both oils presents a similar amount of omega-3, although microalgae oil has the advantage of presenting neither an unpleasant odour nor a high amount of cholesterol, and contains squalene and phytosterols, which offer additional benefits to human health. In addition to this, microalgaes are easily cultivated, which avoid differences in seasonal production and enables increasing the productivity of PUFA from an industrial point of view (Conchillo and others 2006). Several reviews have been published about the metabolism of PUFA in different types of marine microorganisms and the strategies to cultivate them (Guschina and Harwood, 2006; Sijtsma and Swaaf, 2004; Ward and Singh, 2005; Wen and Chen, 2003).

Ratledge has also reviewed the application of the biotechnology in the production of single cell oils, using arachidonic acid (ARA) and DHA as main source of PUFA (*Ratledge*, 2004). In the last years, many researches have also been made to optimize the technical design of bioreactors for microalgae production at industrial scale (Carvalho and others 2006).

Regarding the methods of oil extraction from algae or microalgae, Robles Medina et al., (Robles-Medina and others 1998) examined the recovery and purification of microalgae derived PUFA. They discussed the two main techniques used at the time for obtaining highly pure PUFA: urea fractionation and HPLC, and detailed “potentially useful techniques” such as supercritical fluid extraction and lipase-catalyzed processing.

Table 14. PUFA extraction processes from natural sources different than fish oil (since 1998)

Raw material	Technology	Product	Reference
Subtropical red seaweed (*H. charoides*)	SC-CO_2 extraction	Lipid extract	(*Cheung*, 1999)
Diatom (*P. tricornutum*) Green alga (*M. subterraneous*)	Extraction-transesterification Chromatography Decolorization	Pure EPA-EE	(Belarbi and others 2000)
Red algae filaments	SC-CO_2 extraction	Lipid extract rich in EPA	(Chen and Chou, 2002)
Microalgaes	SC-CO_2 extraction SC-CO_2 + ethanol extraction	Lipid extract rich in GLA	(Mendes and others 2003)
Microalgae (*Nannochloropsis sp.*)	SC-CO_2 extraction	Lipid extract	(Andrich and others 2005)
Cyanobacterium (*A. Spirulina maxima*)	SC-CO_2 extraction SC-CO_2 + ethanol extraction	Lipid extract rich in GLA	(Mendes and others 2006; Mendes and others 2005)

From then to now, several authors have proposed new PUFA extraction methods from different microorganisms, many of them using supercritical fluid technology, similar to the fish oil extraction processes described in Section 0 (Andrich et al., 2005; Belarbi et al., 2000; Chen and Chou, 2002; Cheung, 1999; Mendes et al., 2003; Mendes et al., 2006; Mendes et al., 2005) (*see* Table 14).

3.2. Omega-3 Production from Transgenic Plants

Transgenic plants have been also proposed as an alternative source of omega-3 fatty acids.

Napier et al. have recently published a review with the last advances in the production of enriched vegetables species through genetic modifications (*Napier*, 2006).

Robert et al., have also compiled the most recent studies about production of transgenic seed oils and their use in human and aquaculture nutrition (*Robert*, 2006).

In any case, nowadays the use of transgenic plants in agriculture is not well-accepted in many parts of the world, especially in Europe

References

Aidos I, Kreb N, Boonman M, Luten JB, Boom RM & van-der-Padt A. 2003. Influence of production process parameters on fish oil quality in a pilot plant *Journal of Food Science* 68:581-587.

Aidos I, van-der-Padt A, Boom RM & Luten JB. 2001. Upgrading of Maatjes Herring Byproducts: Production of Crude Fish Oil. *Journal of Agricultural and Food Chemistry* 49:3697-3704.

Al-Sayed-Mahmoud K, Linder M, Fanni J & Parmentier M. 2008. Characterisation of the lipid fractions obtained by proteolitic and chemical extractions from rainbow trout (*Oncorhynchus mykiss*) roe. *Process Biochemistry* 43:376-383.

Alkio M, González C, Jäntti M & Aaltonen O. 2000. Purification of polyunsaturated fatty acid esters from tuna oil wtih supercritical fluid chromatography. *JAOCS, Journal of the American Oil Chemists' Society* 77(3):315-321.

Ambring A, Johansson M, Axelsen M, Gan L, Strandvik B & Frieberg P. 2006. Mediterranean-inspired diet lowers the ratio of serum phospholipid n-6 to n-3 fatty acids, the number of leukocytes and platelets and vascular endothelial growth factor in healthy subjects. *American Journal of Clinical Nutrition* 83:575-581.

Ando Y, Nishimura K, Aoyanagi N & Takagi T. 1992. Stereospecific Analysis of Fish Oil Triacyl-*sn*.glycerols. JAOCS, *Journal of the American Oil Chemists' Society* 69(5):417-424.

Andrich G, Nesti U, Venturi F, Zinnai A & Fiorentini R. 2005. Supercritical fluid extraction of bioactive lipids from the microalga *Nannochloropsis* sp. *European Journal of Lipid Science and Technology* 107:381-386.

Antunes-Corrêa AP, Arantes-Peixoto C, Guaraldo-Gonçalves LA & Cabral FA. 2008. Fractionation of fish oil with supercritical carbon dioxide. *Journal of Food Engineering* 88:381-387.

Ariza-Ariza R, Mestanza-Peralta M & Cardiel MH. 1998. Omega-3 fatty acids in rheumatoid arthritis: An overview. *Seminars in Arthritis and Rheumatism* 27 (6):366-370.

Belarbi E-H, Molina E & Chisti Y. 2000. A process for high yield and scaleable recovery of high purity eicosapentaenoic acid esters from microalgae and fish oil. *Process Biochemistry* 35:951–969.

Bhale SD, Xu Z, Prinyawiwatkul W, King JM & Godber JS. 2007. Oregano and rosemary extracts inhibit oxidation of long-chain n-3 fatty acids in menhaden oil *Food Chemistry and Toxicology* 72:504-508.

Bhosle BM & Subramanian R. 2005. New approaches in deacification of edible oils - a review. *Journal of Food Engineering* 69:481-494.

Biscione F, Pignalberi C, Totteri A, Messina F & Altamura G. 2007. Cardiovascular Effects of Omega-3 Free Fatty Acids. *Current Vascular Pharmacology* 5(2):163-172.

Borch-Jensen C & Mollerup J. 1997. Phase equilibria of fish oil in sub- and supercritical carbon dioxide. *Fluid Phase Equilibria* 138(1-2):179-211

Borneo R, Kocer D, Ghai G, Tepper BJ & Karwe MV. 2007. Stability and Consumer Acceptance of Long-Chain Omega-3 Fatty Acids (Eicosapentaenoic Acid, 20:5, n-3 and Docosahexaenoic Acid, 22:6, n-3) in Cream-Filled Sandwich Cookies. *Journal of Food Science* 72:49-54.

BP. 2008. Omega-3-Marine Triglycerides. London (UK): *British Pharmacopoeia Commission 2007, Volume 1.*

Brunner G. 1994. *Gas extraction. An Introduction to Fundamentals of Supercritical Fluids and the Application to Separation Processes New York* (USA): Ed. Steinkopff Darmstadt Springer.

Brunner G. 2000. Fractionation of fats with supercritical carbon dioxide. *European Journal of Lipid Science and Technology*:240-244.

Buchner EG. 1906. Die beschrankte Mischbarkeit von Flussigkeiten das System Diphenyamin und Kohlensaure. *Zeitschrift für Physikalische Chemie* 56:257-260.

Calviello G, Serini S & Piccioni E. 2007 n-3 Polyunsaturated Fatty Acids and the Prevention of Colorectal Cancer: Molecular Mechanisms Involved. *Current Medicinal Chemistry* 14(29):3059-3069.

Cardozo KHM, Guaratini T, Barros MP, Falcão VR, Tonon AP, Lopes NP, Campos S, Torres MA, Souza AO, Colepicolo P & Pinto E. 2007. Metabolites from algae with economical impact. *Comparative Biochemistry and Physiology, Part C* 146:60-78.

Carvalho AP, Meireles LA & Malcata FX. 2006. Microalgal reactors: A review of enclosed system designs and performances. *Biotechnology Progress* 22:1490-1506.

Catchpole OJ, Grey JB & Noermark KA. 1998. Solubility of fish oil components in supercritical CO_2 and CO_2 + ethanol mixtures. *Journal of Chemical & Engineering Data* 43(6):1091-1095

Catchpole OJ, Grey JB & Noermark KA. 2000. Fractionation of fish oils using supercritical CO_2 and CO_2+ethanol mixtures. *Journal of Supercritical Fluids* 19(1):25-37.

Cengel YA & Boles MA. 2002. *Thermodynamics: An Engineering Approach,4 th ed.* ed. New York (USA): McGraw-Hill. .

Clayton EH, Hanstock TL, Garg ML & Hazell PL. 2007. Long chain omega-3 polyunsaturated fatty acids in the treatment of psychiatric ilnesses in children and adolescents. *Acta Neuropsychiatrica* 19:92-103.

Čmolík J & Pokorný J. 2000. Physical refining of edible oils. *European Journal of Lipid Science and Technology* 102:472-486.

Cocero MJ, Martín A, Mattea F & Varona S. 2009. Encapsulation and co-precipitation processes with supercritical fluids: Fundamentals and applications. *Journal of Supercritical Fluids* 47:546-555.

Conchillo A, Valencia I, Puente A, Ansorena D & Astiasarán I. 2006. *Componentes funcionales en aceite de pescado y alga Nutrición Hospitalaria* 21:369-373.

Cunnane S, A.Drevon C, Harris B, Sinclair A & Spector A. 2004. Recommendations for Dietary Intake of Polyunsaturated Fatty Acids in Healthy Adults. *International Society for the Study of Fatty Acids and Lipids Report on Dietary Intake of Essential Fatty Acids, ISSFAL.*

Chang SS, Bao Y & Pelura TJ, inventors. 1989. *Purification of fish oil.*

Chantachum S, Benjakul S & Sriwirat N. 2000. Separation and quality of fish oil from precooked and non-precooked tuna heads. *Food Chemistry* 69:289-294.

Chen CY & Chou HN. 2002. Screening of red algae filaments as potential alternative source of eicosapentaenoic acid. *Marine Biotechnology* 4:189-192.

Chen YQ, Edwards IJ, Kridel SJ, Thornburg T & Berquin IM. 2007. Dietary fat - gene interaction in cancer. *Cancer Metastasis Rev* 26:535-551.

Cheung PCK. 1999. Temperature and pressure effects on supercritical carbon dioxide extraction of n-3 fatty acids from red seaweed. *Food Chemistry* 65:399-403.

Chow CK. 2000. *Fatty Acids in Foods and their Health Implications,* Second Edition, Revised and Expanded ed. New York - Basel: Marcel Dekker, Inc.

Das UN. 2008. Beneficial Actions of Polyunsaturated Fatty Acids in Cardiovascular Diseases: But, How and Why? *Current Nutrition & Food Science* 4(1):2-31.

Daukšas E, Falch E, Šližyte R & Rustad T. 2005. Composition of fatty acids and lipid classes in bulk products generated during enzymic hydrolysis of cod (*Gadus morhua*) by-products. *Process Biochemistry* 40:2659-2670.

Davarnejad R, Kassim KM, Zainal A & Sata SA. 2008. Extraction of Fish Oil by Fractionation through Supercritical Carbon Dioxide. *Journal of Chemical & Engineering Data* 53:2128–2132.

Desai K & Park HJ. 2005. Recent developments in microencapsulation of food ingredients. *Drying Technology* 23:1361-1394.

Diamond IR, Sterescu A, Pencharz PB & Wales PW. 2008. The rationale for the use of parenteral omega-3 lipids in children with short bowel syndrome and liver disease. *Pediatric Surgery International* 24:773-778.

Domingo JL, Bocio A, Falcó G & Llobet JM. 2007. Benefits and risks of fish consumption I. A quantitative analysis of the intake of omega-3 fatty acids and chemical contaminants. *Toxicology* 230:219-226.

Dunford NT, Goto M & Temelli F. 1998. Modelling of oil extraction with supercritical CO_2 from Atlantic mackerel (*Scomber scombrus*) at different moisture contents. *Journal of Supercritical Fluids* 13(1-3):303-309.

Dunford NT, Temelli F & Leblanc E. 1997. Supercritical CO_2 extraction of oil and residual proteins from atlantic mackerel (*Scomber scombrus*) as affected by moisture content *Journal of Food Science* 62(2):289-294

Dyerberg J. 1986. The Eskimo experience. n-3 News 1:1-4.

EC. 2006. Commision Regulation of 19 December 2006 setting the maximun levels for certain contaminants in foodstuffs. . *Official Journal of the European Union* L364:5-24.

Espinosa S, Diaz S & Brignole EA. 2002. Thermodynamic Modeling and Process Optimization of Supercritical Fluid Fractionation of Fish Oil Fatty Acid Ethyl Esters. *Industrial & Engineering Chemistry Research* 41(6):1516-1527

Esquível MM, Bandarra NM, Fontan I, Bernardo-Gil MG, Batista I, Nunes ML & Empis JA. 1997. Supercritical Carbon Dioxide Extraction of *Sardine Sardina pilchardus* Oil. *Food Science and Technology* 30(7):715-720

FAO FaAD. 1995. *Quality and quality changes in fresh fish*. Rome (Italy): FAO.

FAO FID. 1986. *The production of fish meal and oil.* Rome (Italy): FAO.

Fernández-SanJuan PM. 2000. Fatty acid composition of commercial Spanish fast food and snack food. *Journal of Food Composition and Analysis* 13:275-281.

Fleck U, Tiegs C & Brunner G. 1998. Fractionation of fatty acid ethyl esters by supercritical CO_2: high separation efficiency using an automated countercurrent column *Journal of Supercritical Fluids* 14:67-74.

Fournier V, Destaillats F, Juanéda P, Dionisi F, Lambelet P, Sébédio JL & Berdeaux O. 2006. Thermal degradation of long-chain polyunsaturated fatty acids during deodorization of fish oil. *European Journal of Lipid Science and Technology* 108:33-42.

Frankel EN, Huang SW, Prior E & Aeschbach R. 1996. Evaluation of antioxidant activity of rosemary extracts, carnosol and carnosic acid in bulk vegetable oils and fish oil and their emulsions. *Journal of the Science of Food and Agriculture* 72:201-208.

Gámez-Meza N, Noriega-Rodríguez JA, Medina-Juárez LA, Ortega-García J, Monroy-Rivera J, Toro-Vázquez FJ, García HS & Angulo-Guerrero O. 2003. Concentration of eicosapentaenoic acid and docosahexaenoic acid from fish oil by hydrolysis and urea complexation *Food Research International* 36:721-727.

Gbogouri GA, Linder M, Fanni J & Parmentier M. 2006. Analysis of lipids extracted from salmon (Salmo salar) heads by commercial proteolytic enzymes. *European Journal of Lipid Science and Technology* 108:766–775.

Gharsallaoui A, Roudaut G, Chambin O, Voilley A & Saurel R. 2007. Applications of spray-drying in microencapsulation of food ingredients: An overview. *Food Research International* 40: 1107–1121.

Gironi F & Maschietti M. 2006. Separation of fish oils ethyl esters by means of supercritical carbon dioxide: Thermodynamic analysis and process modelling. *Chemical Engineering Science* 61:5114-5126.

GOED. 2006. Global Organization for EPA and DHA. *Voluntary Monograph, v.3.*

Gorreta F, Bernasconi R, Galliani G, Salmona M, Tacconi MT & Bianchi R. 2002. *Wax esters of n-3 polyunsaturated fatty acids: a new stable formulation as a potential food supplement. 1 - Digestion and absorption in rats. Lebensmittel-Wissenschaft und-Technologie, LWT* 35:458-465.

Güçlü-Üstündağ Ö & Temelli F. 2000. Correlating the Solubility Behaviour of Fatty Acids, Mono-, Di-, and Triglycerides, and Fatty Acid Esters in Supercritical Carbon Dioxide. *Industrial & Engineering Chemistry Research* 39:4756-4766. .

Güçlü-Üstündağ Ö & Temelli F. 2004. Correlating the solubility behaviour of minor lipid components in supercritical carbon dioxide. *Journal of Supercritical Fluids* 31 235–253.

Gunnlaugsdottir H, Järemo M & Sivik B. 1998. Process parameters influencing ethanolysis of cod liver oil in supercritical carbon dioxide. *Journal of Supercritical Fluids* 12:85-93.

Gunnlaugsdottir H, Karlsson AA & a BS. 1997. Lipase-Catalyzed Alcoholysis with Supercritical Carbon Dioxide Extraction 2: Phase Behavior. JAOCS, *Journal of the American Oil Chemists' Society* 74:1491-1494.

Gunnlaugsdottir H & Sivik B. 1995. Lipase-Catalyzed Alcoholysis of Cod Liver Oil in Supercritical Carbon Dioxide. JAOCS, *Journal of the American Oil Chemists' Society* 72:399-405

Gunnlaugsdottir H & Sivik B. 1997. Lipase-Catalyzed Alcoholysis with Supercritical Carbon Dioxide Extraction 1: Influence of Flow Rate. *JAOCS, Journal of the American Oil Chemists' Society* 74:1483-1490.

Guschina IA & Harwood JL. 2006. Lipids and lipids metabolism in eukaryotic algae. *Progress in Lipid Research* 46:160-186.

Hannay JB & Hogarth J. 1879. On the solubility of solids in gases. . *Chemical News* 40:256.

Heinzelmann K, Franke K, Velasco J & Mařquez-Ruiz G. 2000. Microencapsulation of fish oil by freeze-drying techniques and influence of process parameters on oxidative stability during storage *European Food Research and Technology* 211 (4):234-239

Horrobin DF, Manku MS, Hillman J, Iain A & Glen M. 1991. Fatty acid levels in the brains of schizophrenics and normal controls *Biological Psychiatry* 30:795-805.

Iafelice G, Caboni MF, Cubadda R, Criscio TD, Trivisonno MC & Marconi E. 2008. *Development of functional spaghetti enriched with long chain omega-3 fatty acids Cereal Chemistry* 85 146-151

Imanishi N, Fukuzato R, Furuta S & Ikawa N. 1989. Supercritical fluid extraction of fish oil with carbon dioxide. *R & D Kobe Engineering Reports* 39(3):29-32.

Jacobsen C, Let MB, Nielsen NS & Meyer AS. 2008. Antioxidant strategies for preventing oxidative flavour deterioration of foods enriched with n-3 polyunsaturated lipids: a comparative evaluation. *Trends in Food Science & Technology* 19:76-93.

Jakobsson M, Sivik B, Bergqvist PA, Strandberg B, Hjelt M & Rappe C. 1991. Extraction of dioxins from cod liver oil by supercritical carbon dioxide. *Journal of Supercritical Fluids* 4:118-123.

Jakobsson M, Sivik B, Bergqvist PA, Strandberg B & Rappe C. 1994. Counter-current extraction of dioxins from cod liver oil by supercritical carbon dioxide. *Journal of Supercritical Fluids* 7:197-200.

Jiménez-Álvarez D, Giuffrida F, Golay PA, Cotting C, Lardeau A & Keely BJ. 2008. Antioxidant Activity of Oregano, Parsley, and Olive Mill Wastewaters in Bulk Oils and Oil-in-Water Emulsions Enriched in Fish Oil. *Journal of Agricultural and Food Chemistry* 56:7151-7159.

Kamal-Eldin A & Yanishlieva NV. 2002. *N-3* fatty acids for human nutrition: stability considerations. *European Journal of Lipid Science and Technology* 104:825-836.

Kamei M, Ki M, Kawagoshi M & Kawai N. 2002. Nutritional evaluation of Japanese take-out lunches compared with Western-style fast foods supplied in Japan *Journal of Food Composition and Analysis* 15:35-45.

Kawashima A, Iwakiri R & Honda K. 2006. Experimental study on the removal of dioxins and coplanar polychlorinated biphenils (PCBs) from fish oil. *Journal of Agricultural and Food Chemistry* 54:10294-10299.

Kiran E, Debenedetti PG & Peters CJ. 2000. Supercritical fluids: *Fundamentals and Aplications*. Kluwer Academica Publishers, Netherlands:31-68.

Klaypradit W & Huang YW. 2008. *Fish oil encapsulation with chitosan using ultrasonic atomizer*. Lebensmittel-Wissenschaft und-Technologie, LWT 41:1133-1139.

Knez Z. 2009. Enzymatic reactions in dense gases. *Journal of Supercritical Fluids* 47:357–372.

Kojima Y, Sakuradani E & Shimizu S. 2006. Different Specificity of Two Types of *Pseudomonas* Lipases fo C20 Fatty Acids with D5 Unsaturated Double Bond and Their Application for Selective Concentration of Fatty Acids. *Journal of Bioscience and Bioengineering* 101(6):496-500.

Kolanowski W, Jaworska D, Laufenberg G & J.Weißbrodt. 2007a. Evaluation of sensory quality of instant foods fortified with omega-3 PUFA by addition of fish oil powder. *European Food Research and Technology* 225:715-721.

Kolanowski W, Jaworska D, Weibbrodt J & Kunz B. 2007b. Sensory Assement of Microencapsulated Fish Oil Powder *JAOCS, Journal of the American Oil Chemists' Society* 84:37-45.

Kolanowski W & Laufenberg G. 2006. Enrichement of food products with polyunsaturated fatty acids by fish oil addition. *European Food Research and Technology* 222:472-477.

Koletzko B, Cetin I & Brenna JT. 2007. for the Perinatal Lipid Intake Working Group - Dietary fat intakes for pregnant and lactating women (Consensus Statement). *British Journal of Nutrition*:1-5.

Kris-Etherton PM, Harris WS & Appel LJ. 2002. FIsh consumption, fish oil, omega-3 fatty acids and cardiovascular disease. *Circulation*, . American Heart Association Nutrition Committee. 106:2747-2757.

Kromann N & Green A. 1980. Epidemiological studies in the Upemavik district, Greenland. *Acta Medica Scandinavica* 208:401-406.

Lands B. 2008. A critique of paradoxes in current advice on dietary lipids. *Progress in Lipid Research* 47 77-106.

Lawson LD & Hughes BG. 1988. Human absorption of fish oil fatty acids as triacylglicerols free fatty acids or ethyl esters. *Biochemical and Biophysical Research Communications* 152:328-335.

LeGoffic F, Nguyen A & Khayat-Frydman C, inventors. 2000. *Concentration and purification of polyunsaturated fatty acid esters by distillation enzimatic transesterification coupling.*

Letisse M, Rozieres M, Hiol A, Sergent M & Comeau L. 2006. Enrichment of EPA and DHA from sardine by supercritical fluid extraction without organic modifier. I. Optimization of extraction conditions. *Journal of Supercritical Fluids* 38(1):27-36.

Liaset B, Julshamn K & Espe M. 2003. Chemical composition and theoretical nutrition evaluation of the produced fractions from enzyme hydrolysis of salmon with Protamex™. *Process Biochemistry* 38:1747-1759.

Lin T-J, Chen S-W & Chang A-C. 2006. Enrichment of n-3 PUFA contents on triglycerides of fish oil by lipase-catalyzed trans-esterification under supercritical conditions. *Biochemical Engineering Journal* 29:27–34.

Linder M, Fanni J & Parmentier M. 2005. Proteolytic Extraction of Salmon Oil and PUFA Concentration by Lipases. *Marine Biotechnology* 7(1):70-76

Linder M, Matouba E, Fanni J & Parmentier M. 2002. Enrichment of salmon oil with n-3 PUFA by lipolysis, filtration and enzymatic re-esterification. *European Journal of Lipid Science Technology* 104:455–462.

Liu S, Zhang C, Hong P & Ji H. 2006. Concentration of docosahexaenoic acid (DHA) and eicosapentaenoic acid (EPA) of tuna oil by urea complexation: optimization of process parameters. *Journal of Food Engineering* 73:203-209.

Lyberg A-M, Fasoli E & Adlercreutz P. 2005. Monitoring the oxidation of docosahexaenoic acid in lipids. *Lipids* 40:969-979

MacLean CH, Newberry SJ, Mojica WA, Khanna P, Issa AM, Suttorp MJ, Lim YW, Traina SB, Hilton L, Garland R & Morton SC. 2006. Effects of omega-3 fatty acids on cancer risk. A systematic review. *Journal of American Medical Association* 295:403-416.

Maes J, De-Meulenaer B, Van-Heerswynghels P, De-Greyt W, De-Pauw E & Huyghebaert A. 2005. Removal of dioxins and PCB from fish oil by activated carbon and its influence on the nutritional quality of the oil. *Journal of the American Oil Chemists' Society, JAOCS* 82:593-597.

Martín A & Cocero MJ. 2007. Mathematical modeling of the fractionation of liquids with supercritical CO_2 in a countercurrent packed column. *Journal of Supercritical Fluids* 39:304–314.

Massaro M, Scoditti E, Carluccio MA, Montinari MR & DeCaterina R. 2007. Omega-3 fatty acids, inflammation and angiogenesis: Nutrigenomic effects as an explanation for anti-atherogenic and anti-inflammatory effects of fish and fish oils. *Journal of Nutrigenetics and Nutrigenomics* 1:4-23.

Mataix J & Gil A. 2005. *Libro Blanco de los Omega-3 - Los ácidos grasos poliinsaturado Omega-3 y monoinsaturados tipo oleico y su papel en la salud.* Granada (España): Puleva Food.

Matsuno R & Adachi S. 1993. Lipid encapsulation technology - techniques and applications to food. *Trends in Food Science & Technology* 4 256-261.

Mazza M, Pomponi M, Janiri L, Bria P & Mazza S. 2007. Omega-3 fatty acids and antioxidants in neurological and psychiatric diseases: An overview. *Progress in Neuro-Psychopharmacology & Biological Psychiatry* 31 12-26.

McNamara RK. 2006. The emerging role of omega-3 fatty acids in phychiatry. *Prostaglandins, Leukotriens and Essential Fatty Acids* 75:223-225.

Mendes RL, Nobre BP, Cardoso MT, Pereira AP & Palavra AF. 2003. Supercritical carbon dioxide extraction of compounds with pharmaceutical importance from microalgae. *Inorganica Chimica Acta* 356:328-334.

Mendes RL, Reis AD & Palavra AF. 2006. Supercritical CO_2 extraction of g-linolenic acid (GLA) from the cyanobacterium *Arthrospira (Spirulina) maxima*: Comparison with organic solvent extraction. *Food Chemistry* 99:57-63.

Mendes RL, Reis AD, Pereira AP, Cardoso MT, Palavra AF & Coelho JP. 2005. Supercritical CO_2 extraction of g-linolenic acid (GLA) from the cyanobacterium *Arthrospira (Spirulina) maxima*: *Experiments and modeling Chemical Engineering Science* 105:147-152.

Mishra VK, Temelli F & Ooraikul B. 1993. Extraction and purification of w-3 fatty acids with an emphasis on supercritical fluid extraction-A review. *Food Research International* 26:217 -226.

Napier JA. 2006. The production of n-3 long chain polyunsaturated fatty acids in transgenic plants. *European Journal of Lipid Science and Technology* 108:965-972.

Nishimoto Y & Nagagawa M, inventors. 1996. Method for refining fish oil.

Okada T & Morrissey MT. 2007. Recovery and characterisation of sardine oil extracted by pH adjustment. *Journal of Agricultural and Food Chemistry* 55:1808-1813.

Oliveira-Carvalho P, Bueno-Campos PR, D'Addio-Noffs M, Oliveira JG, Tsunezi-Shimizu M & Silva DMd. 2003. Aplicação de lipases microbianas na obtenção de concentrados de ácidos graxos poliinsaturados. *Quimica Nova* 26(1):75-80.

Oterhals A, Solvang M, Nortvedt R & Berntssen MHG. 2007. Optimization of activated carbon-based decontamination of fish oil by response surface methodology. European *Journal of Lipid Science and Technology* 109:691-705.

Pérez-Mateos M, Lanier TC & Boyd LC. 2006. Effects of rosemary and green tea extracts on frozen surimi gels fortified with omega-3 fatty acids. *Journal of the Science of Food and Agriculture* 86:558-567.

Perretti G, Motori A, Bravi E, Favatic F, Montanari L & Fantozzi P. 2007. Supercritical carbon dioxide fractionation of fish oil fatty acid ethyl esters. *Journal of Supercritical Fluids* 40:349-353.

Perrut M, Nicoud RM & Breivik H, inventors. 1998. *Processes for chromatographic fractionation of fatty acids and their derivatives.*

Pettinello G, Bertucco A, Pallado P & Stassi A. 2000. Production of EPA enriched mixtures by supercritical fluid chromatography: from the laboratory scale to the pilot plant. *Journal of Supercritical Fluids* 19:51–60.

Ratledge C. 2004. Fatty acid biosynthesis in microorganism being used for Single Cell Oil production. *Biochimie* 86:807-815.

Raventós M, Duarte S & Alarcón R. 2002. Application and Possibilities of Supercritical CO_2 Extraction in Food Processing Industry: An Overview. *Food Science and Technology International* 8(5):269 -284.

Razack R & Seidner DL. 2007. Nutrition in inflammatory bowel disease. *Current Opinion in Gastroenterology* 23:400-405.

Reisman J, Schachter HM, Dales RE, Tran K, Kourad K, Barnes D, Sampson M, Morrison A, Gaboury I & Blackman J. 2006. Treating asthma with omega-3 fatty acids: where is the evidence? A systematic review. *BMC Complementary and Alternative Medicine* 6:26-34.

Riha V & Brunner G. 1999. Phase equilibrium of fish oil ethyl esters with supercritical carbon dioxide. *Journal of Supercritical Fluids* 15(1):33–50.

Riha V & Brunner G. 2000. Separation of fish oil ethyl esters with supercritical carbon dioxide. *Journal of Supercritical Fluids* 17:55-64.

Robert SS. 2006. Production of eicosapentaenoic and docosahexaenoic acid-containing oils in transgenic land plants for human and aquaculture nutrition. *Marine Biotechnology* 8:103-109.

Robles-Medina A, Molina-Grima E, Gimenez-Gimenez A & Ibanez-Gonzalez MJ. 1998. Downstream Processing of Algal Polyunsaturated Fatty Acids. *Biotechnology Advances* 16(3):517-580.

Rolle RS. 1998. Review: Enzyme applications for agro-processing in developing countries: an inventory of current and potential aplications. *World Journal of Microbiology & Biotechnology* 14:611-619.

Ross BM, Seguin J & Sieswerda LE. 2007. Omega-3 fatty acids as treatments for mental illness: Which disorder and which fatty acid? *Lipids in Health and Disease* 6:21.

Rubio-Rodríguez N, Beltrán S, Jaime I, S.deDiego, Sanz MT & Rovira J. 2010. Production of omega-3 polyunsaturated fatty acid concentrates: A review. *Innovative Food Science and Emerging Technologies* 11 1–12.

Rubio-Rodríguez N, de-Diego-Rupérez S, Beltrán S, Jaime I, Sanz MT & Rovira J. 2008. Supercritical fluid extraction of the omega-3 rich oil contained in hake (*Merluccius capensis – Merluccius paradoxus*) byproducts: study of the influence of process parameters on the extraction yield and oil quality. *Journal of Supercritical Fluids* 47:215-226.

Ruxton CHS, Calder PC, Reed SC & Simpson MJA. 2005. The impact of long-chain n-3 polyunsaturated fatty acids on human health. *Nutrition Research Reviews* 18:113-129.

Shahidi F & Wanasundara UN. 1998. Omega-3 fatty acid concentrates: nutritional aspects and production technologies. *Trends in Food Science & Technology* 9:230-240.

Shaikh SR & Edidin M. 2008. Polyunsaturated fatty acids and membrane organization: elucidating mechanisms to balance immunotherapy and susceptibility to infection. *Chemistry and Physics of Lipids* 153 24-33.

Sijtsma L & Swaaf ME. 2004. Biotechnological production and applications of the ω-3 polyunsaturated fatty acid docosahexaenoic acid. *Applied Microbiology and Biotechnology* 64(2):146-153.

Simopoulos AP. 1991. Omega-3 fatty acids in health and disease and in growth and development. *American Journal of Clinical Nutrition* 54:438-463.

Snoey-Elich H, inventor. 2001. *Nuevo procedimiento de preparación del éster etílico del ácido eicosapentaenoico.* Spain patent.

Song C & Zhao S. 2007. Omega-3 fatty acid eicosapentaenoic acid. A new treatment for psychiatric and neurodegenerative diseases: a review of clinical investigations. *Expert Opinion on Investigational Drugs* 16(10):1627-1638.

Spolaore P, Joamis-Cassan C, Duran E & Isambert A. 2006. Comercial Applications of Microalgae. *Journal of Bioscience and Bioengineering* 101(2):87-96.

Staby A & Mollerup J. 1993. Separation of constituents of fish oil using supercritical fluids: a review of experimental solubility, extraction, and chromatographic data. *Fluid Phase Equilibria* 91(2):349-386.

Stancík R, Rovenský J & Stančíková M. 2006. Diet in the rheumatoid arthritis and the omega-3 fatty acids *Rheumatologia* 20:159-166.

Stillwell W & Wassall SR. 2003. Docosahexaenoic acid: membrane properties of a unique fatty acid. *Chemistry and Physics of Lipids* 126:1-27.

Tour C. 1822. Exposé de quelques resultats obtenus par l'action combinée de la chaleur et de la compression sur certains liquides, tels que l'eau, l'alcool, l'éther sulfurique et l'essence de pétrole rectifiée. *Annales de Chimie et de Physique* 21:127-132.

Turner D, Zlotkin SH, Shah PS & Griffiths AM. 2008 Omega 3 fatty acids (fish oil) for maintenance of remission in Crohn's disease. *Cochrane Database of Systematic Reviews* 89:2070S-2084S.

Tziomalos K, Athyros VG & Mikhailidis DP. 2007. Fish Oils and Vascular Disease Prevention: An Update. *Current Medical Chemistry* 14:2622-2628.

Valencia I, O'Grady MN, Ansorena D, Astiasarán I & Kerry JP. 2008. Enhancement of the nutritional status and quality of fresh pork sausages following the addition of linseed oil, fish oil and natural antioxidants. *Meat Science* 80:1046-1054.

von-Schacky C & Harris WS. 2007. Cardiovascular benefits of omega-3 fatty acids *Cardiovascular Research* 73:310-315.

Wada S & Fang X. 1992. The synergistic antioxidant effect of rosemary extract and α-tocopherol in sardine oil model system and frozen-crushed fish meat *Journal of Food Processing and Preservatives* 195:95-98

Ward OP & Singh A. 2005. Omega-3/6 fatty acids: Alternative sources of production. *Process Biochemistry* 40:3627-3652.

Wen ZY & Chen F. 2003. Heterotrophic production of eicosapentaenoic acid by microalgae *Biotechnology Advances* 21:273-294.

WHO/FAO. 1994. *Fats and oils in human nutrition.*

Wong DWS. 2003. *Lipase.* New York Marcel Dekker, cop. .

Yang YW, Wu CJ, Wang XD, Huang M & Ren QL. 2004. Purification of EPA-EE and DHA-EE with supercritical fluid chromatography. *Journal of Chemical Engineering of Chinese Universities* 18:293-296.

Yoshikazu T, Hirosi Y, Kazuko H & Satoru K, inventors. 1997. *Method for refining and manufacturing fats and oils containing polyunsaturated fatty acids.*

Yuqian H & Huashi G, inventors. 2001. *Preparation of high-grade fish smell-eliminating fish oil.*

Zosel K, inventor. 1982. *Process for the direct decaffeination of aqueous coffee extract solutions*

Zulfakar MH, Edwards M & Heard CM. 2007. Is there a role for topically delivered eicosapentaenoic acid in the treatment of psoriasis? *European Journal of Dermatology* 17:284-291.

In: Fish Oil: Production, Consumption and Health Benefits
Editors: Matthias Van Dijk and Jürgen Vitek
ISBN: 978-1-61470-963-3

Chapter XIV

Dietary Fish Oil, the Central Control of Food Intake and Obesity Prevention

Regina L. H. Watanabe, Juliane C. S. Zemdegs, Cláudia M. O. Nascimento, Lila M. Oyama and Eliane B. Ribeiro
Universidade Federal de São Paulo, São Paulo, SP, Brasil

I. Introduction

The last decades of human history saw an expressive modification in both the amount and the composition of dietary fat, with increased intake of saturated, trans, and omega-6 polyunsaturated fats, and a concomitant substantial reduction in the consumption of omega-3 sources. Intake of saturated and trans fatty acids have long been recognized to impair metabolic control while polyunsaturated fatty acids (PUFAs) in general have been thought to be less harmful (Albuquerque et al. 2006; Buettner et al. 2007; Innis 2007).

The importance of intake of adequate amounts of the essential fatty acids linoleic acid (LA, 18:2ω-6) and α-linolenic acid (ALA, 18:3ω-3) is well established. The long-chain ω-3 fatty acids, particularly eicosapentaenoic acid (EPA, 20:5ω-3) and docosahexaenoic acid (DHA, 22:6ω-3), are essential constituents of cell membranes and are highly concentrated in neuronal membrane phospholipids, playing important roles in aspects as relevant as membrane stability, neuroplasticity, neurotransmission and signal transduction (Innis 2007).

The current ratio of ω-6 to ω-3 total intake is estimated to be in the range of 10-25 to 1, an imbalance that has been suggested to contribute to the deleterious health consequences culminating in the current worldwide epidemic of obesity and co-morbidities (Connor 2000; Simopoulos 2011). There have been reports linking high intake of ω-6 PUFAs to increased adipogenesis rate in children and adults. Studies conducted in either experimental animals or human subjects have shown high ω-6 PUFA intake to be positively linked to insulin resistance and obesity. On the other hand, intake of ω-3 PUFA, which are highly enriched in fish oils, have been inversely related with body adiposity and have thus been ascribed a protective role (Ruzickova et al. 2004; Ailhaud et al. 2006; Kabir et al. 2007; Phillips 2010; Oliver et al. 2010).

Obesity results from the disequilibrium between energy intake and expenditure, parameters that are regulated by complex central nervous system mechanisms. Disruption of this control results in hyperphagia and/or inadequation of food intake to energy requirements. Food intake is a complex behavior controlled by the interaction of homeostatic and hedonic influences, mainly processed in hypothalamic and mesocorticolimbic sites, respectively. While the homeostatic component of this control system aims at promoting body energy and nutrient equilibrium, the hedonic pathway operates under the command of motivational and reward aspects associated with eating.

The hypothalamus is a key site in the central nervous system control of energy balance. Under the influence of the peripheral adiposity and satiety signals, the activity of anabolic and catabolic neurons of various hypothalamic nuclei modulates food intake and energy expenditure. Several hypothalamic sites are implicated in the feeding regulatory circuitry, mainly the arcuate nucleus (ARC), the ventromedial nucleus (VMH), the paraventricular nucleus (PVN), the dorsomedial nucleus (DMH) and the lateral area (LHA). The proper balance between the orexigenic and the anorexigenic influences exerted by the mediators produced in these nuclei is essential for energy homeostasis and the disruption of this equilibrium plays a prominent role in the pathogenesis of obesity (Ribeiro et al. 2006; Velloso et al. 2006; Ribeiro 2009).

The hypothalamus is importantly impacted by the hedonic influences as the LHA receives inputs from the nucleus accumbens (NAc), an important center of the hedonic component of feeding control, whose dopaminergic, opioid, and endocannabinoid innervations are stimulated by motivation- and reward- related signals. Orexigenic mediators at the LHA are thus influenced by these signals (Erlanson-Albertsson et al. 2005).

Fish oil intake has been shown to be able to interact with the central control of food intake and some potential mechanisms underlying the fish oil effects have been examined. The purpose of the present review is to summarize recent findings linking dietary consumption of fish oil, or of its ω-3 fatty acid constituents, to the central control of feeding. Although the majority of studies focusing on the mechanisms targeted by fish oil have been performed in animals, their examination provide valuable insights into the processes by which these nutrients may modify food intake in the context of feeding disorders like obesity and anorexia.

II. The Homeostatic and the Hedonic Components of the Central Control of Food Intake

The brief exposition presented below, of the main pathways and mediators, is intended to guide the reader through the mechanisms targeted by fish oil.

II.a. Homeostatic Control: Interaction of Acute and Long-Term Aspects

The hypothalamus is the site of convergence and integration of information on body energy and nutrient status, of both peripheral and central origin and comprised of neural, endocrine, nutritional or metabolic signals. Essential efferent commands from this cerebral region are then aimed at maintaining homeostasis by matching food intake and energy expenditure to the needs.

The afferent inputs reaching the hypothalamus from the periphery are related to either the acute states of hunger and satiety or to the long-term control of body energy stores, represented by adipose tissue size. The latter aspect integrates the concept known as the adipostatic hypothesis of energy homeostasis control, which proposes that the control mechanisms operate around the maintenance of body adiposity, through variations of energy intake and expenditure.

The adipocyte hormone leptin and the pancreatic β-cell hormone insulin constitute the main peripheral signals of body adiposity to the CNS. Their circulating levels are directly proportional to body fat stores and their interaction with hypothalamic neurons initiates responses which culminate with inhibition of feeding and/or stimulation of energy expenditure. The ARC is their primary target (Ahima et al. 2000; Flier, 2004).

The factors which communicate hunger and satiety to the CNS include the gastrointestinal hormones ghrelin, cholecystokinin (CCK), and glucagon-like peptide (GLP-1), among others, whose secretion varies as a function of the presence of food in the tract. They are able to relay information directly to the ARC or to the area postrema (AP) of the brainstem, but they do so, for the most part, via the vagus nerve to the nucleus of the solitary tract (NST) of the brainstem. The information proceeds to the hypothalamus through the NTS neurons innervating the ARC.

Ghrelin is orexigenic, i.e., it stimulates food intake, acting as a hunger signal to the CNS. The adiposity signals, as leptin and insulin, as well as the satiety signals, as CCK and GLP-1, are anorexigenic, i.e., they inhibit food intake. It is important to point out that, besides modifying feeding, some of these hormones may also affect energy expenditure. The term anabolic is used to designate those mediators whose actions favor energy deposition, through stimulating feeding and/or inhibiting energy expenditure. In contrast, those that inhibit food intake and/or stimulate energy expenditure are named catabolic mediators.

Leptin and insulin are the main adiposity hormones reaching the hypothalamus, where they interact mainly with ARC neurons, which show abundant expression of OB-Rb, the long form of leptin receptor, and of insulin receptors. Their activation triggers stimulation of catabolic neurons and inhibition of anabolic neurons at the ARC, producing inhibition of food intake and stimulation of energy expenditure. Either deficiency of adiposity signals or resistance to their actions is interpreted by as low adiposity, triggering the responses aimed at restoring body fat stores (Niswender and Schwartz 2003; Gerozissis 2004).

The ARC contains two distinct subpopulations of neurons, which produce either the anabolic mediators neuropeptide Y (NPY) and *agouti*-related protein (AgRP) or the catabolic mediators proopiomelanocortin (POMC) and cocaine-and amphetamine-regulated transcript (CART). ARC neurons innervate the other hypothalamic nuclei, PVN, DMH, VMH, and LHA, which, in turn, express other catabolic and anabolic mediators. The POMC released at the PVN/VMH is cleaved to produce the catabolic α-melanocyte-stimulating hormone (α-

MSH) which, stimulating receptors of the melanocortin family (MC-4R), inhibits feeding. The AgRP released at the PVN/VMH blocks MC-4R, an action that stimulates feeding by preventing receptor activation by α-MSH.

The LHA neurons express the anabolic mediators melanin concentrating hormone (MCH) and orexins. The PVN neurons express, besides the MC-4R, the anorexigenic factors thyrotropin-releasing hormone (TRH), corticotropin-releasing hormone (CRH) and ocitocin. The brain-derived neurotrophic factor (BDNF), produced following MC-4R activation, participates in the stimulation of the anorexigenic mediators (Xu et al. 2003; Morton et al. 2006).

The adiposity signaling performed by leptin and insulin interacts with the hunger and satiety signaling performed by the gastrointestinal hormones, whose actions affect aspects as important as amount of food ingested in each meal, the duration of this meal, as well as post-prandial satiety, that determines the intermeal interval. The so called satiety hormones are stimulated by food entering the tract and inhibit intake, performing an acute meal regulation. They include CCK, GLP-1 and PYY. Ghrelin has the opposite effect, i.e., it stimulates feeding, and it is secreted by the empty stomach (Wynne et al. 2005).

Once released, they may communicate hunger/satiety to the CNS by interacting directly with receptors at the ARC or at the AP. Their main mechanism, however, occurs via stimulation of vagal receptors, with the signal then reaching the NTS via vagus nerve. These acute signals are integrated with the long-term adiposity signals at the ARC (Chaudhri et al. 2008).

Recent animal studies have pointed out that circulating nutrients may also act directly at the CNS sites that control food intake. Long chain fatty acids have been particularly involved, as they may be sterified upon penetrating the CNS. The fatty acyl-Coenzime A accumulated in the cytosol has been suggested to function as a nutrient abundance signal and hence inhibit food intake, at least in part through inhibition of NPY and AgRP expression. The hypophagia induced by intracerebroventricular injection of DHA in rats could depend on this mechanism. Cytosolic fatty acyl-CoA accumulation has also been proposed to mediate signaling for glucose-induced hypophagia (Lam et al. 2005; Schwinkendorf et al. 2011).

One important component of the CNS control of feeding is represented by the monoaminergic systems. Norepinephrine (NOR) and dopamine (DA) effects depend on their site of release and receptor type. NOR produced in the locus coeruleus and is anorexigenic when stimulating α-1 e β-2 receptor subtypes. DA is anorexigenic at D1 or D2 receptors and it has an important participation in food reward circuits acting at D5 receptors. Serotonin (5-HT) is produced in the raphe nuclei and innervate all brain promoting satiety and hence inhibiting feeding through hypothalamic interaction with melanocortin, NPY, and orexins neurons. The receptor subtypes 5-HT1B and 5-HT2C are the main mediators of serotonin hypophagia (Barnes and Sharp 1999; Dalton et al. 2006; Lam and Heisler 2007; Garfield and Heisler 2009).

II.b. Hedonic Control

Despite the complex system of homeostatic control described above, body nutrient and energy needs are not the only aspects affecting food intake. The hedonic value of food, i.e., the aspects relating to the pleasure associated with eating, is a relevant part of the central control mechanisms and has been attributed a prominent role in hyperphagia.

Food palatability, which plays a critical role in the modulation of food reward, is influenced by features as taste, texture, appearance, smell, and consistency. Additionally, the hedonic value attributed to food is largely influenced by subjective aspects related to memory and personal experiences. Food rich in fat and/or sugar are considered to be palatable. The hedonic aspect of feeding is believed to play a relevant part in the current obesity epidemic since, by overriding the homeostatic control, it leads the individual to consuming food in excess of nutrient and energy requirements.

The nucleus accumbens (NAc) is highly involved in the motivation and reward mechanisms related food intake. It is interesting that the NAc also participates in reward related to drug abuse. Dopamine released in the NAc and other prosencephalic areas as striatum and cortex, plays a pivotal role in the motivation and reward circuits. It has recently been demonstrated that obese individuals have low dopamine receptor density and dopaminergic activation in these areas when consume food, which leads to higher intake. Endogenous opioids as ß-endorphin, encephalin, and dinorphin, also released at the NAc among other CNS sites, are involved in the acquisition of the hedonic experience. Opioids receptor activation in NAc stimulates feeding by disinhibition of orexigenic neurons in the LHA. Interacting with the dopaminergic and opioid systems, the endocannabinoids anandamide and 2- arachidonylglycerol (2-AG) are orexigenic, increasing the satisfaction brought by palatable food. Reciprocal connections between NAc and LHA are important for integrating homeostatic and hedonic influences of feeding. The LHA also receives impulses from the amigdala, thalamus, and cortex, regions that modulate feeding behavior (Erlanson-Albertsson et al. 2005; Kelley et al. 2005).

III. Interaction of Dietary Fish Oil with the CNS Mechanisms of Feeding Regulation

There have been few published studies that have directly examined the effects of prolonged intake of diets enriched with fish oil or ω-3 PUFAs upon aspects of the hypothalamic control of feeding.

In hypothalamic nuclei of mice, the intake of fish oil diet for six weeks reportedly failed to modify c-Fos-immunereactivity, a method used to estimate the status of neuronal activation. In the ARC of mice, in situ hybridization studies have shown that those diet protocols also failed to affect the expressions of NPY, AGRP and POMC (Wang et al. 1999 and 2002). However, ω-3 feeding for seven weeks has been demonstrated to decrease rat gene expression of the orexigenic mediators MCH and prepro-orexin in the LHA and of NPY in the ARC while POMC expression was stimulated. These effects have been found to respond to fat amount, being more pronounced in the rats receiving a high-fat fish-oil diet than in those fed a normolipidic fish-oil diet (Dziedzic et al. 2007).

We have recently studied in rats the effect of long-term high-fat feeding with fish oil-enriched diet on neuronal activation in hypothalamic feeding-regulatory areas. Using c-Fos immunereactivity, we found no alteration in the fish-fed rats when they were evaluated in the fasted state. However, their acute response to refeeding was strongly modified in comparison to the rats fed control balanced diet. Upon refeeding, the fish-diet rats showed neuronal activation in PVN, DMH, VMH, and ARC, all hypothalamic nuclei associated with the production of anorexigenic mediators. These findings indicated that the high intake of fish oil led to alterations in the hypothalamic circuitry, favoring the catabolic over the anabolic activity, and creating a pattern able to protect against the hyperphagia and/or low energy expenditure which could follow high-fat feeding. Interestingly, the rats fed with a soy oil-rich diet showed a potentially obesogenic profile, with high LH and low VMH/PVN activation after refeeding (Watanabe et al. 2009).

It is noteworthy that the hypothalamic consequences of fish oil intake seem to be influenced by the metabolic status. In rats with cancer cachexia, in which the catabolic anorexia state had been induced by tumor cells inoculation, EPA and DHA supplementation reverted the alterations induced by the tumor, stimulating NPY protein expression and food ingestion while it decreased the expressions of α-MSH and of the serotonergic 5-HT1B receptor. The same ω-3 food supplement had divergent effects in the normal rats, decreasing NPY and α-MSH production while failing to modify 5-HT1B levels (Ramos et al. 2005). In the same line of evidence are the findings of normalization of satiety and hedonic mediators by fish oil supplementation in mice severely undernourished to reproduce the alterations of anorexia nervosa. Restoration by fish oil of 2- arachidonylglycerol, dopamine and serotonin levels, diminished during food restriction in hypothalamus and hippocampus, was accompanied by better survival rates and cognitive function (Avraham et al. 2010).

An adequate offer of dietary ω-3 PUFAs is known to be important for the function of brain monoaminergic systems (Zimmer et al. 2000; Chalon 2006). However, the exact nature of its effects are not yet elucidated. Intrauterine deficiency of α-linolenic acid led to decreased content of ω-3 PUFAs in hippocampal membrane phospholipids and increased serotonin release, as measured by microdialysis in this brain region of the adult rats (Kodas et al. 2004). Dietary deficiency of ω-3 PUFAs has been shown to induce increased 5-HT2 receptor density in the prefrontal cortex and low basal and stimulated serotonin levels in the hippocampus (Chalon 2006; Su 2009). On the other hand, dietary supplementation with ω-3 PUFA for 7 weeks in mice did not affect tissue levels of serotonin and 5-HIAA in the frontal cortex and striatum, but decreased 5-HIAA content in hippocampus (Vancassel et al. 2008). These studies focused on aspects related to the dysfunctions of serotonin transmission in mood disorders, since low ω-3 PUFAs status has been reported in diseases such as depression.

There are limited data available about the influence of dietary ω-3 PUFAs on the serotonergic inhibition of feeding. Fish oil supplementation for 20 days prevented the cancer-induced anorexia and up-regulation of 5-HT1B receptor density in the supra-optical nucleus of rats (Ramos et al. 2005). In normal rats, 5 to 8 weeks on fish oil diet failed to modify the hypophagia induced by a SR-2C agonist and the density of SR-2C and serotonin transporter in hypothalamic feeding regulatory nuclei (Rice and Corwin 2002; du Bois et al. 2006). On the other hand, we have recently demonstrated in rats that high-fat fish oil diet for 9 weeks since weaning impaired serotonin-induced hypophagia and hypothalamic serotonin turnover, and protein levels of serotonin transporter and 5-HT2C receptor. Despite the serotonergic impairment, the rats failed to show feeding disturbances, indicating that the serotonergic impairment was either compensated by other factors or not of a sufficient extent to affect feeding. However, we did see increased fat pad weight, what could represent a consequence of a serotonergic deficit in energy expenditure stimulation (Watanabe et al. 2010).

Some of the effects of fish oil feeding on the central regulation of energy balance could be secondary to actions modifying adipose tissue metabolism, inflammatory status, or adipokines secretion. Variable consequences of fish oil consumption on leptin levels and sensitivity have been reported (Puglisi et al. 2011). Increased plasma leptin has been found to accompany either normal or decreased body fat after fish oil consumption (Cha et al. 1998; Peyron-Caso et al. 2002; Rossi et al. 2005; Perez-Matute et al. 2007). Additionally, reduced body fat and leptinemia have also been observed (Hun et al. 1999; Wang et al. 2002; Ruzickova et al. 2004). On the other hand, elevated leptin levels and body adiposity, indicating leptin resistance, have been seen with high-fat fish oil feeding (Wohlers et al. 2005; Watanabe et al. 2010) and associated with reduced leptin transport into the CNS (Oh-I et al. 2005).

Increased adiponectin levels have been found after fish oil intake. Low adiponectin levels are usually found in obese animals and humans, correlating with insulin resistance, glucose intolerance, dislipidemia and cardiovascular risk (Puglisi et al. 2011). Adiponectin receptors are widely distributed in the brain and their activation induce fat oxidation and body mass loss (Ahima and Lazar 2008). On the other hand, we have demonstrated that mice receiving fish oil-enriched diet for 2 months had unchanged adiponectin gene expression and plasma levels while diet intake for 2 days or the treatment of 3T3-L1 adipocytes for 2 days with EPA or DHA led to decreased gene expression and adiponectin secretion (Bueno et al. 2008). In rats submitted to sleep deprivation stress, we have shown that fish oil intake failed to correct the stress-induced low adiponectin expression and protein levels (de Mattos et al. 2008). However, it is possible that fish oil does exhibit beneficial effects on adiponectin activity, as we have observed stimulation of adiponectin R2 receptor protein levels in mice exposed to foot shock stress, along with improvement of glucose tolerance, although adiponectin levels were unchanged (Eguchi et al. 2011).

We have recently demonstrated that hypothalamic insulin signaling was affected by high-fat fish oil diet in a beneficial way. We have found insulin hypophagia to be abolished and hypothalamic signaling after central injection to be highly impaired by the consumption of high-fat diets enriched with either lard or soy oil, sources of saturated and poliunsaturated ω-6 fats, respectively. On the other hand, the high-fat fish oil diet produced decreased body and fat pads weight, low leptin and corticosterone levels, and improved serum lipid profile, with preservation of insulin hypophagia and hypothalamic signaling. As all diets were equally hyperlipidic, our results show that the fish oil prevented the deleterious effects of high-fat feeding with other fat types (Pimentel et al. 2011; Dornellas et al. unpublished data).

Hypothalamic inflammation has been attributed a great importance in the disturbances of obesity, leading to insulin and leptin resistance and hyperphagia. High consumption of saturated fats have been particularly associated with this central deleterious action. The toll like 4 receptors (TLR4) have been shown to be activated by saturated fatty acids, thus triggering the NFκB inflammatory pathway, leading to impairment of insulin and leptin signaling (Velloso et al. 2008; Posey et al. 2009).

We have examined the hypothalamic inflammatory status induced by high-fat diets rich in soy or fish oil. The fish-diet group had reduced protein levels of the inflammatory cytokines TNF-α, and IL-6, and TRAF6, an intermediary participant of NFκB pathway, while levels of the anti-inflammatory cytokine IL-10 were decreased. The soy oil had opposite effects, stimulating inflammatory parameters. These results suggested that high-fat fish diet improved the hypothalamic inflammatory profile via reduction of intracellular inflammatory mediators, protecting against central insulin resistance and obesity (Pimentel et al. unpublished data). Our data agree with previous studies showing that diet supplementation with EPA and DHA reduced expression of TNF-α in ARC and PVN in normal but not tumor-bearing rats (Ramos et al. 2004). The beneficial effects of fish oil on insulin central actions have also been suggested to rely on protection against the cytotoxic properties of TNF-α (Das et al. 2003).

Although fish oil is assumed to have anti-obesity effects, only a few studies have examined their central effects on the mechanisms that control food intake and energy expenditure. The data seem to indicate the effects to be dependent on diet composition and metabolic status. Furthermore, some conflicting findings might be explained by different ω-3 PUFA products and the ratio of EPA to DHA content of the different oils used. Neuropeptides, neurotransmitters and cytokines have been found to be affected by fish oil consumption, explaining part of its effects in the control of food intake. However, more studies are necessary to elucidate the mechanisms targeted by fish oil that modify energy balance.

References

[1] Ahima RS, Lazar MA. Adipokines and the peripheral and neural control of energy balance. *Mol Endocrinol* 2008; 22(5):1023-31.

[2] Ahima RS, Saper CB, Flier JS, Elmquist JK. Leptin regulation of neuroendocrine systems. *Front Neuroendocrinol* 2000; 21(3):263-307.

[3] Ailhaud G, Massiera F, Weill P, Legrand P, Alessandri J-M, Guesnet P. Temporal changes in dietary fats: role of n-6 polyunsaturated fatty acids in excessive adipose tissue development and relationship to obesity. *Prog Lipid Res* 2006; 45:203-36.

[4] Albuquerque KT, Sardinha FL, Telles MM *et al.* Intake of *trans* fatty acid-rich hydrogenated fat during pregnancy and lactation inhibits the hypophagic effect of central insulin in the adult offspring. *Nutrition* 2006; 22:820-9.

[5] Avraham Y, Saidian M, Burston JJ, Mevorach R, Vorobiev L, Magen I, Kunkes E, Borges B, Lichtman AH, Berry EM. Fish oil promotes survival and protects against cognitive decline in severely undernourished mice by normalizing satiety signals. *J Nutr Biochem* 2010 Nov 24 [Epub ahead of print].

[6] Barnes NM, Sharp T. A review of central 5-HT receptors and their function. *Neuropharmacology* 1999; 38(8):1083-152.

[7] Bueno AA, Oyama LM, de Oliveira C, Pisani LP, Ribeiro EB, Silveira VL, Oller do Nascimento CM. Effects of different fatty acids and dietary lipids on adiponectin gene expression in 3T3-L1 cells and C57BL/6J mice adipose tissue. *Pflugers Arch* 2008; 455(4):701-9.

[8] Buettner R, Schölmerich J, Bollheimer LC. High-fat diets: modeling the metabolic disorders of human obesity in rodents. *Obesity* 2007; 15:798-808.

[9] Cha MC, Jones PJ. Dietary fat type and energy restriction interactively influence plasma leptin concentration in rats. *J Lipid Res* 1998; 39(8):1655-60.

[10] Chalon S. Omega-3 fatty acids and monoamine neurotransmission. *Prostaglandins Leukot Essent Fatty Acids* 2006; 75(4-5):259-69.

[11] Chaudhri OB, Salem V, Murphy KG, Bloom SR. Gastrointestinal satiety signals. *Annu Rev Physiol* 2008; 70:239-255

[12] Connor WE. Importance of n-3 fatty acids in health and disease. *Am J Clin Nutr*. 2000; 71(1 Suppl):171S-5S.

[13] Dalton GL, Lee MD, Kennett GA, Dourish CT, Clifton PG. Serotonin 1B and 2C receptor interactions in the modulation of feeding behaviour in the mouse. *Psychopharmacology* 2006; 185(1):45-57.

[14] Das UN, Ramos EJ, Meguid MM. Metabolic alterations during inflammation and its modulation by central actions of omega-3 fatty acids. *Curr Opin Clin Nutr Metab Care* 2003; 6(4):413-9.

[15] de Mattos AB, Pinto MJ, Oliveira C, Biz C, Ribeiro EB, do Nascimento CM, Andersen ML, Tufik S, Oyama LM. Dietary fish oil did not prevent sleep deprived rats from a reduction in adipose tissue adiponectin gene expression. *Lipids Health Dis* 2008; 7:43-9.

[16] du Bois TM, Deng C, Bell W, Huang XF. Fatty acids differentially affect serotonin receptor and transporter binding in the rat brain. *Neuroscience* 2006; 139(4):1397-40.

[17] Dziedzic B, Szemraj J, Bartkowiak J, Walczewska A. Various dietary fats differentially change the gene expression of neuropeptides involved in body weight regulation in rats. *J Neuroendocrinol* 2007; 19(5):364-73.

[18] Eguchi R, Scarmagnani FR, Cunha CA, Souza GIH, Pisani LP, Ribeiro EB, Nascimento CMO, Spadari-Bratfisch R, Oyama LM. Fish oil consumption prevents glucose intolerance and hypercorticosteronemy in footshock-stressed rats. *Lipids Health* Dis 2011, 10:71.

[19] Erlanson-Albertsson C. How palatable food disrupts appetite regulation. *Basic Clin Pharmacol Toxicol* 2005; 97(2):61-73.

[20] Flier JS. Obesity wars: molecular progress confronts an expanding epidemic. *Cell* 2004; 116(2):337-50.

[21] Garfield AS, Heisler LK. Pharmacological targeting of the serotonergic system for the treatment of obesity. *J Physiol* 2009; 587(Pt 1):49-60.

[22] Gerozissis K. Brain insulin and feeding: a bi-directional communication. *Eur J Pharmacol* 2004; 490 (1-3):59-70.

[23] Hun CS, Hasegawa K, Kawabata T, Kato M, Shimokawa T, Kagawa Y. Increased uncoupling protein2 mRNA in white adipose tissue, and decrease in leptin, visceral fat, blood glucose, and cholesterol in KK-Ay mice fed with eicosapentaenoic and docosahexaenoic acids in addition to linolenic acid. *Biochem Biophys Res Commun* 1999; 259(1):85-90.

[24] Innis SM. Dietary (n-3) fatty acids and brain development. *J Nutr* 2007; 137(4):855-9.

[25] Kabir M, Skurnik G, Naour N, Pechtner V, Meugnier E, Rome S, et al. Treatment for 2 mo with n3 polyunsaturated fatty acids reduces adiposity and some atherogenic factors but does not improve insulin sensitivity in women with type 2 diabetes: a randomized controlled study. *Am J Clin Nutr* 2007; 86:1670-9.

[26] Kelley AE, Baldo BA, Pratt WE, Will MJ. Corticostriatal-hypotalamic circuitry and food motivation: integration of energy, action and reward. *Physiol Behav* 2005; 86:773-95.

[27] Kodas E, Galineau L, Bodard S, Vancassel S, Guilloteau D, Besnard JC, Chalon S. Serotoninergic neurotransmission is affected by n-3 polyunsaturated fatty acids in the rat. *J Neurochem* 2004; 89(3):695-702.

[28] Lam DD, Heisler LK. Serotonin and energy balance: molecular mechanisms and implications for type 2 diabetes. *Expert Rev Mol Med* 2007; 9(5):1-24.

[29] Lam TK, Schwartz GJ, Rossetti L. Hypothalamic sensing of fatty acids. *Nat Neurosci* 2005; 8(5):579-84.

[30] Morton GJ, Cummings DE, Baskin DG, Barsh GS, Schwartz MW. Central nervous system control of food intake and body weight. *Nature* 2006; 443:289-95.

[31] Niswender KD, Schwartz MW. Insulin and leptin revisited: adiposity signals with overlapping physiological and intracellular signaling capabilities. Front *Neuroendocrinol* 2003; 24(1):1-10.

[32] Oh-I S, Shimizu H, Sato T, Uehara Y, Okada S, Mori M. Molecular mechanisms associated with leptin resistance: n-3 polyunsaturated fatty acids induce alterations in the tight junction of the brain. *Cell Metab* 2005; 1(5):331-41.

[33] Oliver E, McGillicuddy F, Phillips C, Toomey S, Roche HM, et al. The role of inflammation and macrophage accumulation in the development of obesity-induced type 2 diabetes mellitus and the possible therapeutic effects of long-chain n-3 PUFA. *Proc Nutr Soc* 2010; 69:232-43.

[34] Pérez-Matute P, Pérez-Echarri N, Martínez JA, Marti A, Moreno-Aliaga MJ. Eicosapentaenoic acid actions on adiposity and insulin resistance in control and high-fat-fed rats: role of apoptosis, adiponectin and tumour necrosis factor-alpha. *Br J Nutr* 2007; 97(2):389-98.

[35] Peyron-Caso E, Taverna M, Guerre-Millo M, Véronèse A, Pacher N, Slama G, Rizkalla SW. Dietary (n-3) polyunsaturated fatty acids up-regulate plasma leptin in insulin-resistant rats. *J Nutr* 2002; 132(8):2235-40.

[36] Phillips CM, Goumidi L, Bertrais S, Field MR, Ordovas JM, Cupples LA, et al. Leptin receptor polymorphisms interact with polyunsaturated fatty acids to augment risk of insulin resistance and metabolic syndrome in adults. *J Nutr* 2010; 140:238-44.

[37] Pimentel GD, Dornellas APS, Rosa JC, Lira FS, Cunha CA, Boldarine VT, de Souza GIH, Hirata AE, Nascimento CMO, Oyama LM, Watanabe RLH, Ribeiro EB. High-fat diets rich in soy or fish oil distinctly alter hypothalamic insulin signaling in rats. *J Nutr Biochem* 2011, *In Press*.

[38] Posey KA, Clegg DJ, Printz RL, Byun J, Morton GJ, Vivekanandan-Giri A, Pennathur S, Baskin DG, Heinecke JW, Woods SC, Schwartz MW, Niswender KD. Hypothalamic proinflammatory lipid accumulation, inflammation, and insulin resistance in rats fed a high-fat diet. *Am J Physiol Endocrinol Metab.* 2009; 296(5):E1003-12.

[39] Puglisi MJ, Hasty AH, Saraswathi V. The role of adipose tissue in mediating the beneficial effects of dietary fish oil. *J Nutr Biochem* 2011; 22(2):101-8.

[40] Ramos EJ, Middleton FA, Laviano A, Sato T, Romanova I, Das UN, Chen C, Qi Y, Meguid MM. Effects of omega-3 fatty acid supplementation on tumor-bearing rats. *J Am Coll Surg* 2004; 199(5):716-23.

[41] Ramos EJ, Romanova IV, Suzuki S, Chen C, Ugrumov MV, Sato T, Goncalves CG, Meguid MM. Effects of omega-3 fatty acids on orexigenic and anorexigenic modulators at the onset of anorexia. *Brain Res* 2005; 1046(1-2):157-64.

[42] Ribeiro EB, Telles MM, Oyama LM, Silveira VLF, Nascimento CMO. Hypothalamic serotonin in the control of food intake: physiological interactions and effect of obesity. In: *Focus on Nutrition Research*. ISBN 1-59454-768-8. Editor:Tony P. Starks, pp. 121-148. 2006 Nova Science Publishers, Inc.

[43] Ribeiro EB. Studying the central control of food intake and obesity in rats. *Rev Nutr* 2009; 22(1):163-171.

[44] Rice HB, Corwin RL. mCPP-induced hypophagia in rats is unaffected by the profile of dietary unsaturated fatty acids. *Pharmacol Biochem Behav* 2002; 73(3):545-50.

[45] Rossi AS, Lombardo YB, Lacorte JM, Chicco AG, Rouault C, Slama G, Rizkalla SW. Dietary fish oil positively regulates plasma leptin and adiponectin levels in sucrose-fed, insulin-resistant rats. *Am J Physiol Regul Integr Comp Physiol* 2005; 289(2):R486-R494.

[46] Ruzickova J, Rossmeisl M, Prazak T, Flachs P, Sponarova J, Veck M, Tvrzicka E,Bryhn M, Kopecky J. Omega-3 PUFA of marine origin limit diet-induced obesity in mice by reducing cellularity of adipose tissue. *Lipids* 2004; 39(12):1177-85.

[47] Schwinkendorf DR, Tsatsos NG, Gosnell BA, Mashek DG. Effects of central administration of distinct fatty acids on hypothalamic neuropeptide expression and energy metabolism. *Int J Obes* 2011; 35(3):336-44.

[48] Simopoulos AP. Evolutionary Aspects of Diet: The Omega-6/Omega-3 Ratio and the Brain. *Mol Neurobiol*. 2011 Jan 29 [Epub ahead of print].

[49] Su K-P. Biological mechanism of antidepressant effect of omega-3 fatty acids: how does fish oil act as a ‘mind-body interface’? *Neurosignals* 2009; 17:144-152.

[50] Vancassel S, Leman S, Hanonick L, Denis S, Roger J, Nollet M, Bodard S, Kousignian I, Belzung C, Chalon S. n-3 polyunsaturated fatty acid supplementation reverses stressinduced modifications on brain monoamine levels in mice. *J Lipid Res* 2008; 49:340-348.

[51] Velloso LA, Araújo EP, de Souza CT. Diet-induced inflammation of the hypothalamus in obesity. Neuroimmunomodulation 2008; 15(3):189-93.

[52] Velloso LA. The hypothalamic control of feeding and thermogenesis: implications on the development of obesity. *Arq Bras Endocrinol Metabol* 2006; 50(2):165-76.

[53] Wang H, Storlien LH, Huang XF. Effects of dietary fat types on body fatness, leptin, and ARC leptin receptor, NPY, and AgRP mRNA expression. *Am J Physiol Endocrinol Metab* 2002; 282(6):E1352-9.

[54] Wang H, Storlien LH, Huang XF. Influence of dietary fats on c-Fos-like immunoreactivity in mouse hypothalamus. *Brain Res* 1999; 843:184-92.

[55] Watanabe RL, Andrade IS, Telles MM, Albuquerque KT, Nascimento CM, Oyama LM, Casarini DE, Ribeiro EB. Long-term consumption of fish oil-enriched diet impairs serotonin hypophagia in rats. *Cell Mol Neurobiol* 2010; 30(7):1025-33.

[56] Watanabe RL, Andrade IS, Zemdegs JC, Albuquerque KT, Nascimento CM, Oyama LM, Carmo MG, Nogueira MI, Ribeiro EB. Prolonged consumption of soy or fish-oil-enriched diets differentially affects the pattern of hypothalamic neuronal activation induced by refeeding in rats. *Nutr Neurosci* 2009; 12(6):242-8.

[57] Wohlers M, Xavier RAN, Oyama LM, Ribeiro EB, Nascimento CMO, Casarini DE, Silveira VLF. Effect of fish or soybean oil-rich diets on bradykinin, kallikrein, nitric oxide, leptin, corticosterone, and macrophages in carrageenan stimulated rats. *Inflammation* 2005; 29(2-3):81-9.

[58] Wynne K, Stanley S, McGowan B, Bloom S. Appetite control. *J Endocrinol* 2005; 184(2):291-318.

[59] Xu B, Goulding EH, Zang K, Cepoi D, Cone RD, Jones KR, Tecott LH, Reichardt LF. Brain-derived neurotrophic factor regulates energy balance downstream of melanocortin-4 receptor. *Nat Neurosci* 2003; 6(7):736-42.

[60] Zimmer L, Delion-Vancassel S, Durand G, Guilloteau D, Bodard S, Besnard JC, Chalon S. Modification of dopamine neurotransmission in the nucleus accumbens of rats deficient in n-3 polyunsaturated fatty acids. *J Lipid Res* 2000; 41(1):32-40.

In: Fish Oil: Production, Consumption and Health Benefits
Editors: Matthias Van Dijk and Jürgen Vitek
ISBN: 978-1-61470-963-3

Chapter XV

Omega-3 Fatty Acids: Current State in Cardiovascular Disease

John H Lee*[*a], *James H O'Keefe*[b], *Richard Milani*[a] *and Carl J Lavie [a]

[a] John Ochsner Heart and Vascular Institute, Ochsner Clinical School-
The University of Queensland School of Medicine, New Orleans, LA, U. S.
[b] Mid America Heart Institute and University of Missouri, Kansas City, MO, U. S.

Abstract

Due to the weight of prior evidence, the American Heart Association has endorsed the use of omega-3 fatty acids for the secondary prevention of cardiovascular(CV) events in patients with known coronary artery disease. This recommendation was based on a large number of epidemiologic studies as well as a few large randomized control studies. In particular, the GISSI-Prevenzione illustrating significant reductions in both sudden cardiac death and CV events and the JELIS trial illustrating significant reductions in CV events contributed to these recommendations. However, more recent trials such as the OMEGA trial, the Alpha Omega Trial, and Kowey et al.'s study of omega-3 supplementation in atrial fibrillation(AF) patients have shown some conflicting results. The OMEGA trial evaluated supplementing 1g/d for one year and was unable to show a significant difference in CV outcomes in post myocardial infarction patients. This discrepancy could have potentially been from the improvements in medical therapy from the decade older trials which resulted in a lower number of events. The Alpha Omega trial investigated the supplementation of omega-3 in the form of 18.8 g of margarine per day and also showed no significant differences in CV events in patients with a history of myocardial infarctions. The patients in this trial were also on a modern regimen of CV medications and only received a small supplement of omega-3 which may have not been enough to exert an effect. In Kower et al.'s trial of AF patients, omega-3 supplementation did not reduce the recurrence of AF in the 6 month study period. On the other hand, the omega-3 arm of the GISSI heart failure (HF) trial showed an 8% reduction of mortality

* Address for correspondence: 1514 Jefferson Highway, New Orleans, LA 70121, Email: johlee@ochsner.org, Phone: 504-842-4135, Fax: 504-842-4465

and CV admissions in patients supplemented with omega-3 fatty acids. Although more recent trials have not shown the robust benefits that were seen in the earlier ones, the balance of evidence still favor the beneficial effects of omega-3 fatty acids. We would recommend the continuation of omega-3 fatty acids in patients with CV disease and in particular HF.

Keywords: Omega-3 fatty acids, EPA, DHA, eicosapentaenoic acid, docosahexaenoic acid, alpha linolenic acid, coronary disease prevention, fish oils

Introduction

Due to the weight of prior evidence, the American Heart Association (AHA) has endorsed the use of omega-3 fatty acids for the secondary prevention of cardiovascular (CV) events in patients with known coronary heart disease(CHD). This recommendation was based on a large number of epidemiologic studies as well as a few large randomized control studies. The AHA recommends 1 g/d of omega-3 fatty acids with a mixture of docosahexaenoic acid (DHA) and eicosapentaenoic acid (EPA). The preferential source is oily fish but fish oil (in capsules or liquid form) is considered an acceptable option as well [1]. This recommendation is based on an extensive and growing body of evidence supporting the CV benefits and triglyceride-lowering effects of the omega-3 oils. In addition, the Food and Drug Administration (FDA) has approved an omega-3 fatty acid ethyl ester formulation for the treatment of very high triglycerides at a dose of 4 g/d. This review will summarize current scientific data on omega-3 fatty acids and CV health including the more recently published trials which offer some conflicting data as well as discuss the sources and sustainability of fish oil production.

Background

Over the past several decades there has been an abundance of epidemiological, observational, experimental and randomized controlled studies that have been published on the CV effects of omega-3 fatty acids [2]. Aside from the more recent studies, they have document clear CV protective effects [3]. DHA and EPA are the two specific omega-3 fatty acids that have been associated with CV benefit and triglyceride lowering. DHA and EPA are present in various ratios in oily fish [4]. Commonly consumed fish such as salmon contain DHA and EPA in a ratio of about 2:1. DHA can, to be a limited extent, be retro-converted to EPA [5]; but EPA supplementation does not raise tissue or blood levels of DHA [6]. A meta-analysis [7] pooling the results of prospective clinical trials and epidemiologic studies suggests that the majority of reduction in risk of CHD death is conferred with modest omega-3 fatty acid consumption: 250 to 500 mg/d of DHA + EPA. (Figure 1) This corresponds to approximately 1-2 servings/wk of oily fish.

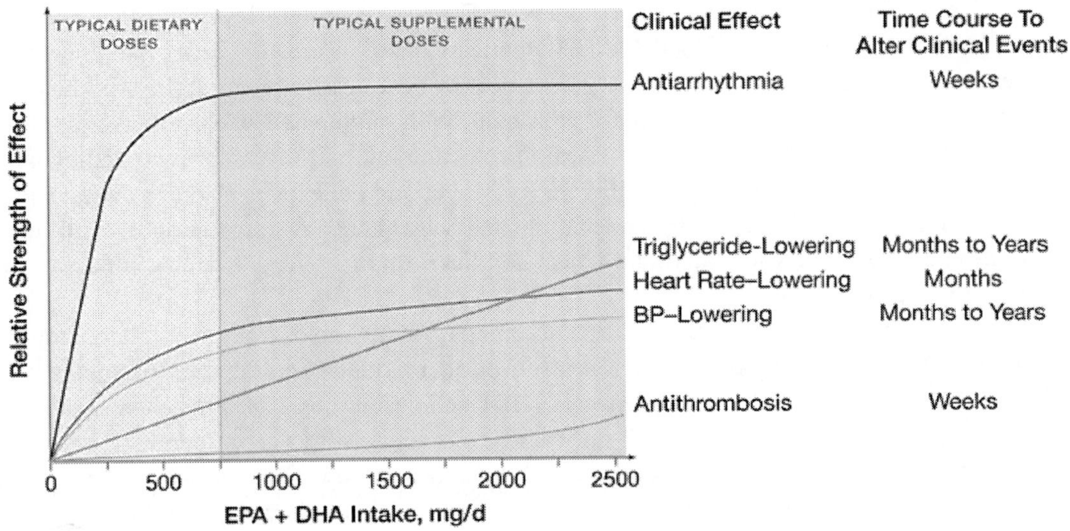

Figure 1. Potential dose responses and time courses for altering clinical events of physiologic effects of fish or fish oil intake [7].

Alpha-linolenic acid (ALA) is another form of omega-3 that is found in flaxseed, nuts, and in trace amounts in green leafy vegetables. Humans convert less than 5% of ALA to EPA (and less to DHA) [8] so ALA is inadequate as the sole dietary source of omega-3 fatty acids. ALA intake has been inversely associated with CV events in some epidemiological studies but conflicting data remains [3].

Omega-3 fatty acids appear to confer CV benefits largely through DHA and EPA enrichment of membrane phospholipids [9] which can increase arrhythmic thresholds [10],reduce blood pressure [11,12], improve arterial and endothelial function [13], reduce platelet aggregation [14], and favorably impact autonomic tone [11,15]. Omega-3 fatty acid intake has also been shown to be inversely related to the development of type 2 diabetes in woman from a large population study of over 100,000 subjects [16]. A meta-analysis by Geleijnse and colleagues evaluated 22 double blind studies showing that omega-3 fatty acid intakes of about 4 g/d was associated with a significant 1.7 and 1.5 mm Hg reduction in systolic and diastolic pressures, respectively [17]. This effect was noted to be more pronounced in older patients and in those with higher blood pressures. Lowering systolic blood pressure as little as 2 mm Hg can yield mortality reductions of up to 4% from CHD [18]. The anti-platelet, anti-inflammatory, and triglyceride-lowering effects of omega-3 fatty acids are seen with higher doses of DHA + EPA (e.g., 3 to 4 g/d), where the reduction in sudden cardiac death (SCD) risk can be achieved at lower intakes (0.5 to 1.0 g/d) [19-21]. Omega-3 fatty acids have been shown to suppress production of pro-inflammatory cytokines such as interleukin-6, interleukin-1β, and tissue necrosis factor-α [22]. In a study by Noori et al. of 145 patients on hemodialysis, they found that a higher omega-6 fatty acid to omega-3 fatty acid ratio was associated with higher C-reactive protein (CRP) levels [23]. Additionally, it has been shown that when EPA is administered to obese individuals there is an increase in the levels of adiponectin, which may reduce inflammation and improve insulin sensitivity [24]. Very high doses of omega-3 fatty acids (i.e., 8 g/d) have anti-inflammatory effects and can improve body composition in heart failure(HF) patients [25]. However, omega-3 fatty acids have not been consistently shown to lower C-reactive protein levels [26]. A dose of DHA + EPA (810 mg/d) given to stable CHD patients decreases resting heart rate, increases post-exercise heart rate recovery, and increases beat-to-beat heart rate variability (in the high frequency band) [11]. These changes are consistent with augmented vagal tone, suggesting that omega-3 fatty acids may confer cardio-protection in part by improving autonomic sympatho-vagal balance [11,15]. Recent work by Moyer and colleagues also corroborated the effects of omega-3 fatty acid supplementation and vagal tone by illustrating a significant association between omega-3 fatty acid levels and heart rate recovery, exercise capacity and exercise time [27].

Some of the cardio-protective effect of omega-3 fatty acids may be related to the favorable effects on the lipid profile. Davidson et al. reported the additional reductions in triglycerides and non-high density lipoprotein (HDL) cholesterol by 29% and 9% respectively with the addition of 3.4 g/d of omega-3 fatty acids to baseline simvastatin therapy. There was also a small but significant increase in HDL [28] . In a review of 25 trials by Harris and colleagues, they found that the risk of CHD events was related to vivo omega-3 fatty acid levels [20]. The risk of CV events was inversely related to the amount of DHA in plasma and cellular phospholipids which correlates closely with the amount of DHA in the myocardium [20,29].

Omega-3 and CV Disease

Omega-3 fatty acid supplementation has as a profound effect on patient survival and CVevents [21]. Starting from the early randomized trials conducted, it was apparent that omega-3 fatty acids, either in the form of oily fish or fish oil capsules, reduced all-cause mortality in post-myocardial infarction (MI) patients [30]. Subsequently, 2 major randomized controlled trials examined the effects of supplemental omega-3 fatty acids on CHD risk. The Gruppo Italiano per lo Studio della Sopravvivenza nell'Infarto Miocardico (GISSI)-Prevenzione study randomized 11,323 post-MI patients to omega-3 acid ethyl esters (1 capsule/d providing 850 mg of DHA + EPA) or usual care. Treatment with omega-3 fatty acids significantly reduced the risk of death from any cause by 28%. By 4 months, the risk for SCD was decreased by 45%. [19] (Figure 2) The other major randomized controlled trial was the Japan EPA Lipid Intervention Study (JELIS) [31] which studied 18,645 hypercholesterolemic patients who were randomly assigned to either statin alone or statin + pure EPA (1.8 g/d). By the end of the 5-year follow up period, the patients who received EPA had 19% lower major adverse CV events (Figure 3).

Among the older trials, several studies have not had positive outcomes. Of which, the most commonly discussed are the randomized trials reported by Burr et al. [32] and by Nilsen et al. [33]. In Burr's study, patients with angina who were given fish oil capsules had higher rates of sudden death than untreated controls. This study was criticized as being "well designed" but sub-optimally "conducted and reported" and thus its results are questionable [34]. The Nilsen study is thought to be flawed because of the high background intake of fish oils in the Norwegian subjects possibly masking the treatment effects.

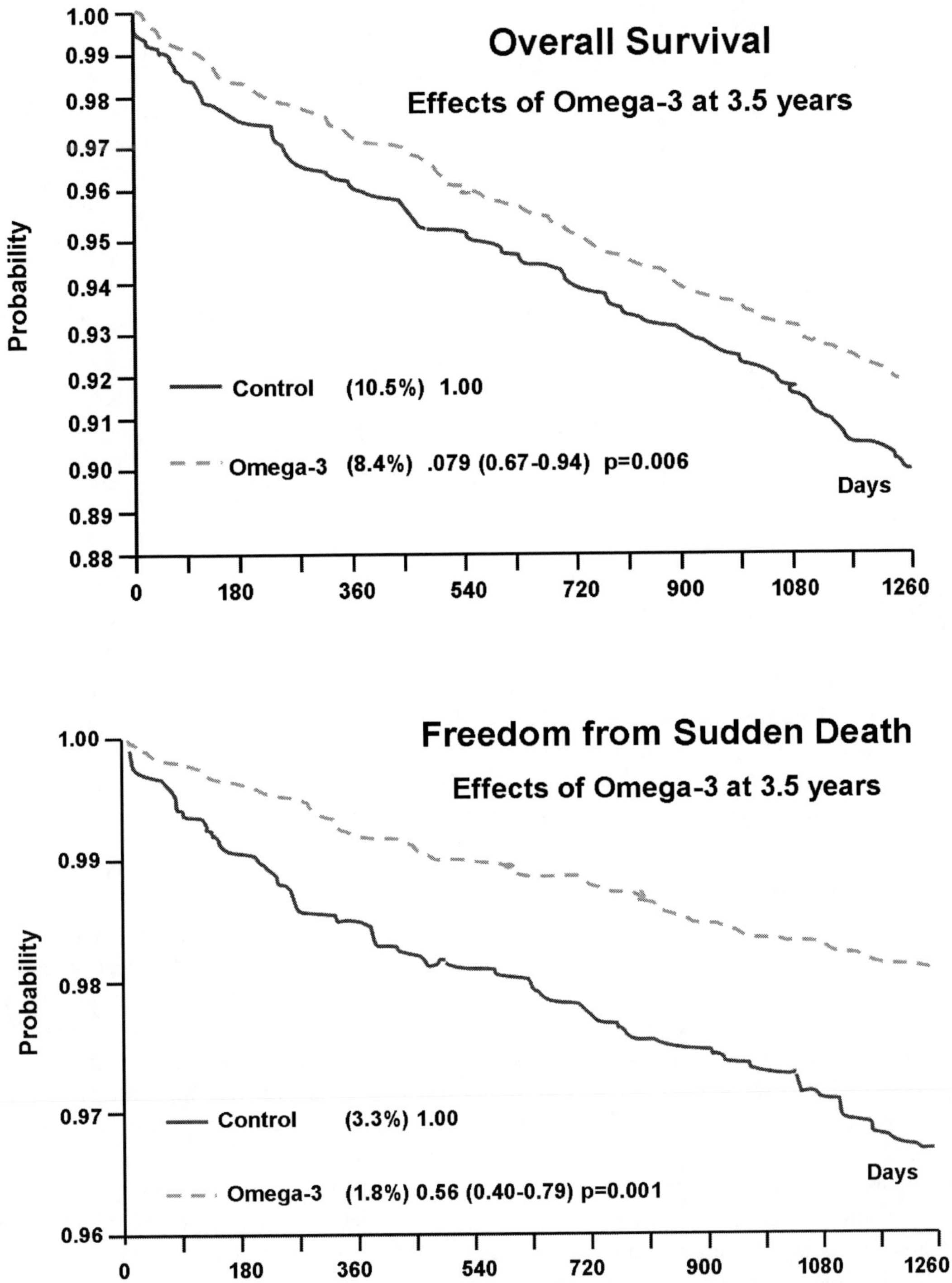

Figure 2. Time Course of Clinical Events in the Gruppo Italiano per lo Studio della Sopravvivenza nell'Infarto Miocardico (GISSI)-Prevenzione study.Treatment with 850 mg per day of omega-3 acid ethyl esters reduced total mortality (A) by 21% and the sudden death (B) by 44% [19].

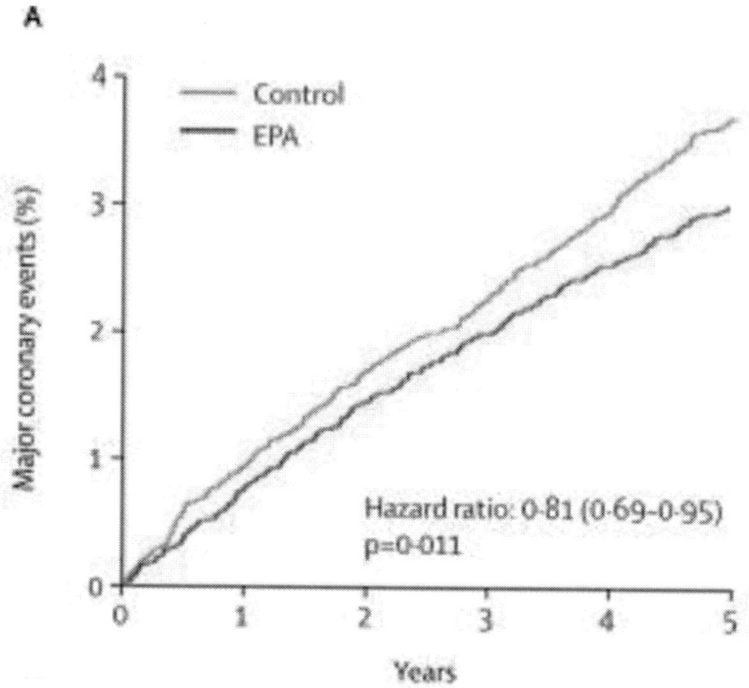

Numbers at risk						
Control group	9319	8931	8671	8433	8192	7958
Treatment group	9326	8929	8658	8389	8153	7924

Figure 3. EPA (1.8 gm per day) reduced the incidence of major adverse coronary events in the Japan EPA Lipid Intervention Study (JELIS) Study by 19% [31].

Of the more recent trials such as the OMEGA trial [35], the Alpha Omega Trial [36], and Kowey et al.'s [37] study of omega-3 supplementation in atrial fibrillation(AF) patients, here have been some conflicting results. The OMEGA trial [35] is a randomized controlled multi-center trial which enrolled 3851 patients and compared patients receiving 1 g/d of omega-3 fatty acids versus placebo for one year and was unable to show a significant difference in CV outcomes in post -MI patients. This discrepancy could have potentially been from the improvements in medical therapy and stent technology from the decade older trials which resulted in a lower number of events. In addition enrolled subjects had high levels of fish consumption that increased significantly during the course of the study in both arms. The Alpha Omega trial [37] enrolled 4837 patients into their randomized controlled trial which investigated the supplementation of omega-3 in the form of 18.8 g of margarine per day and also showed no significant differences in CV events is patients with a history of MI. The patients in this trial were also on a modern regimen of CV medications and only received a small supplement of omega-3 which may have not been enough to exert an effect. In Kowey et al.'s trial [37] of 663 AF patients, omega-3 supplementation did not reduce the recurrence of AF in the 6 month study period. On the other hand, the omega-3 arm of the GISSI HF trial which evaluated 7046 patients who were randomized to receive either 1g/d of omega-3 fatty acids or placebo showed an 8% reduction of mortality and CV admissions in patients supplemented with omega-3 fatty acids [38]. (Figure 4)

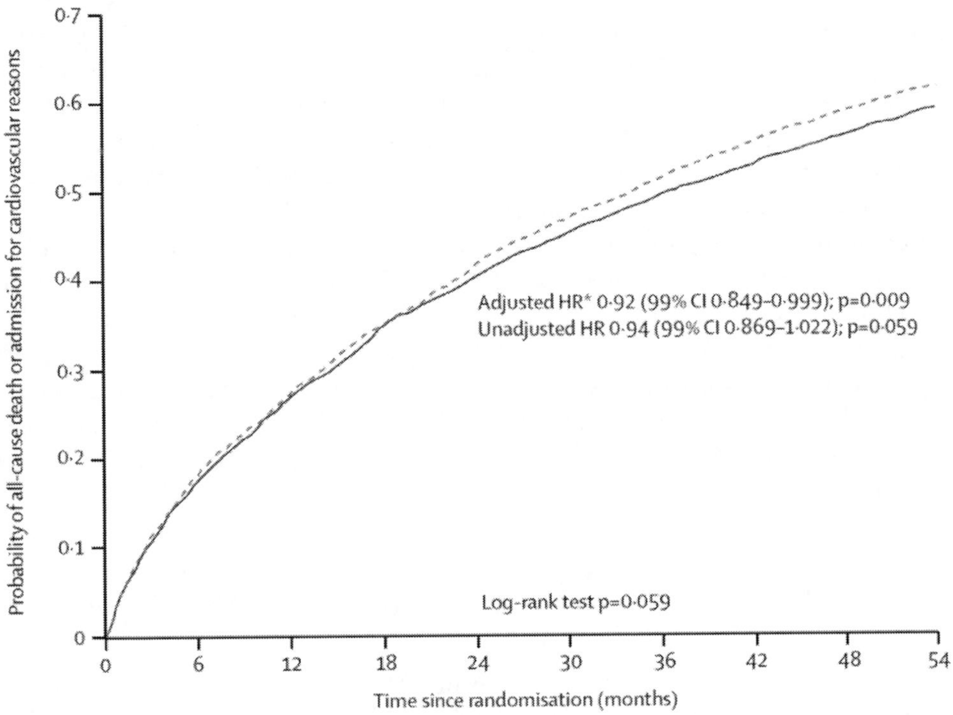

Patients at risk

n-3 PUFA	3494	2876	2543	2261	2066	1896	1718	1342	949	502
Placebo	3481	2846	2518	2251	1826	1826	1640	1254	876	446

Figure 4. Kaplan-Meier curve for all-cause death or admissions to the hospital for cardiovascular reasons [38].

Calo and colleagues showed a significant reduction of post-operative AF in CABG patients [39]. Others have described trends towards benefits in malignant ventricular arrhythmias [10,40-42]. Although omega-3 fatty acids appear to be effective for reducing SCD in the setting of CHD with reduced left ventricular systolic function [43], 3 trials using omega-3 fatty acids in implantable cardioverter defibrillator patients have shown mixed results [40-42]. The most recent trial looking at arrhythmic events was a substudy of the GISSI HF trial that showed fewer events in the omega-3 arm but was not statistically significant [44].

Levitan and colleagues further linked omega-3 fatty acids and CV disease by showing that moderate intake of fatty fish and marine omega-3 fatty acids in 39,367 middle-aged or older men was associated with lower rates of HF [45]. The Cardiovascular Health Study showed an inverse association in the intake of baked or broiled fish and incidence of HF [46,47]. Further evidence to support the benefit of omega-3 fatty acids in HF patients was reported in the Atherosclerosis Risk in Community study which showed an inverse relationship between omega-3 PUFA intake and incidence of HF in women [48]. The GISSI HF trial, mentioned previously, enrolled patients in NYHA class II to IV chronic HF who were then randomized to receive 1 g daily of omega-3 polyunsaturated fatty acids or matching placebo [38]. There were significantly lower mortality and combined mortality and admission for CV events in the arm which received omega-3 fatty acid supplementation. A recent randomized controlled trial in 133 patients with chronic HF secondary to non-ischemic cardiomyopathy showed significant improvements in many HF and cardiac parameters at 12 month follow up in the subjects who received 2 g/day omega-3 fatty acid supplementation versus placebo [49]. LV ejection fraction in the omega-3 arm was increased by 10.4% compared to a decrease of 5.0% in the placebo arm ($p<0.001$) [49]. Significant improvements in exercise capacity, New York Heart Association functional class, re-hospitalization rates, and inflammatory cytokines were also seen [49].

Certain blood levels of DHA + EPA have been reported to be a markers of cardio-protection [9]. Red blood cell membrane DHA + EPA levels of > 8% appear to be associated with the lowest risk for CHD death [9,50] and are associated with reduced risk for acute coronary syndromes [51]. On the other hand, individuals with DHA + EPA < 4% are considered to be at higher risk for CV events [51]. In addition, low blood omega-3 fatty acid levels are associated with increased risk of SCD [52]. Optimal membrane levels of omega-3 fatty acid usually are achieved with consumption of 1 to 1.5 g of DHA + EPA per day, which is an intake similar to that in Japan [50].

Best Source of Omega-3 Fatty Acids

The AHA recommends a total of 1 g/d of DHA and EPA preferably from oily fish but considers fish oil supplements in an acceptable option [1]. Oily fish is the preferred source of the AHA, but not all fish have the same amount or ratio of DHA and EPA. (**Table 1**) The question of whether fish or fish oils confer the same beneficial CV effects has been addressed in several studies evaluating the various modes of consumption. A recent study published in the Journal of Clinical Nutrition compared the effects of supplementing with walnuts versus fatty fish and found that walnut supplementation significantly lowered cholesterol while fatty fish significantly lowered triglycerides [53]. Another study of cod protein supplementation showed significant reductions in CRP when compared to diets containing similar quantities of other types of protein [54]. This would suggest that there may be other elements in a diet of fish intake that may contribute to the CV benefits. The fact that several important nutrients such as vitamin D, phospholipids, and naturally occurring antioxidants are missing in fish oil supplements have some experts advocating dietary sources of fatty fish as the main source of omega-3 fatty acids. However, there is much data from landmark omega-3 trials such as the GISSI-Prevenzione [19] and JELIS [31] trials that clearly indicate that fish oil supplements confer CV benefits . In addition, Harris and colleagues have illustrated that equivalent amounts of EPA and DHA from either a fish diet or a fish oil supplement enriches the omega-3 content of erythrocyte membranes equally well [55].

A potential drawback to fish consumption over fish oil supplements is that certain fish can contain environmental toxins such as mercury, PCBs(WRITE THIS OUT!!!), chlordane, dioxins, and DDT(SAME). Concentrations of these contaminants increase as they move up the food chain, so top predators (such as swordfish, shark, king mackerel, largemouth bass, and walleye) may not be safe to eat on a frequent basis. (**Table 2**) On the other hand, many of the most popular fish varieties such as salmon, shrimp, canned light tuna, pollock, and catfish are relatively low in these chemical contaminants and are safe to eat up to several times per week [56]. Unfortunately, except for salmon, they are relatively poor sources of EPA and DHA.

Table 1. Fish content of EPA + DHA [4,21]

Type	DHA (gm per 100 g)	EPA (gm per 100 g)	DHA+EPA	Ratio DHA:EPA
Tuna, Bluefin	1.141	0.363	1.504	3.1 : 1.0
Tuna, Light, canned-in water	0.223	0.047	0.27	4.8 : 1.0
Tuna, Albacore, canned-in water	0.629	0.233	0.862	2.7 : 1.0
Salmon, Atlantic, farmed	1.457	0.69	2.147	2.1 : 1.0
Salmon, Atlantic, wild	1.429	0.411	1.84	3.5 : 1.0
Salmon, Chinook	0.727	1.01	1.737	1.0 : 1.4
Salmon, Sockeye	0.7	0.53	1.23	1.3 : 1.0
Mackerel, Atlantic	0.699	0.504	1.203	1.4 : 1.0
Herring, Atlantic	1.105	0.909	2.014	1.2 : 1.0
Trout, rainbow, farmed	0.82	0.334	1.154	2.5 : 1.0
Trout, rainbow, wild	0.52	0.468	0.988	1.1 : 1.0
Halibut	0.374	0.091	0.465	4.1 : 1.0
Cod	0.154	0.004	0.158	38.5 : 1.0
Haddock	0.162	0.076	0.238	2.1 : 1.0
Catfish, channel, farmed	0.128	0.049	0.177	2.6 : 1.0
Catfish, channel, wild	0.137	0.1	0.237	1.4 : 1.0
Swordfish	0.681	0.087	0.768	7.8 : 1.0
Grouper	0.213	0.035	0.248	6.1 : 1.0
Shrimp	0.144	0.171	0.315	1.0 : 1.2

Table 2. Levels of Methyl Mercury in Commonly Consumed Fish [56]

Species	Range (ppm)	Average (ppm)
Domestic Samples		
Catfish	ND - 0.16	ND
Cod	ND-0.17	0.13
Crab	ND-0.27	0.13
Flounder	ND	ND
Hake	ND	ND
Halibut	0.12 - 0.63	0.24
Pollock	ND	ND
Salmon (canned)	ND	ND
Salmon (fresh or frozen)	ND	ND
Shark	0.30 - 3.52	0.84
Swordfish	0.36 - 1.68	0.88
Tuna (canned)	ND - 0.34	0.20
Tuna (fresh or frozen)	ND - 0.76	0.38
Import Samples		
Pollock	ND - 0.78	0.16
Shark	ND - 0.70	0.36
Swordfish	0.80 - 1.61	0.86
Tuna (canned)	ND - 0.39	0.14
Tuna (fresh of frozen)	ND - 0.75	0.27

Sustainability of Wild Fish Stocks

Reports have documented a rapid worldwide decline in fish stocks overthe past 50 years. Populations of some commercially popular fish species have collapsed to only 10% of their historic maximum, with over 100 confirmed cases of marine-species extinctions. It has been reported that worldwide fish stocks could be depleted within 40 years if harvest continues at the current rate [57,58]. This forecast, has however, been severely criticized [59] and may be overly pessimistic. With the current recommendations for omega-3 supplementation, there is increased pressure on fish stocks. Furthermore, there is increasing jeopardy with recommendations for higher levels of fish and/or fish oil consumption for the millions of Americans in the treatment of hypertriglyceridemia. Whether the demand for fish and fish oil supplements can be met a sustainable manner remains to be seen. Currently, close to 90% of Americans have suboptimal intake of omega-3 fatty acids [60]. Repletion of deficient omega 3 levels should be an important goal both for individual patient care and for public health but may seriously impact our fish sources. Major changes in the way we source omega 3 fatty acid supplements, such as aquaculture (fish farming), and bioengineering seem to be logical and increasingly practical solutions to this conundrum. Non-traditional sources of marine-based omega-3 fatty acids such as algae to produce DHA and yeast to produce EPA are being developed and may help to offload some of the burden of demand. Additionally, the plant-derived omega-3 fatty acid, alpha-linolenic acid (ALA), and stearidonic acid (the delta-6 desaturase product of ALA which can be produced by biotechnology in soybeans) might provide some of the benefits of DHA and EPA but that remains to be firmly established [61].

Conclusions

Although more recent trials have not shown the robust benefits that were seen in the earlier ones, the balance of evidence still favor the beneficial effects of omega-3 fatty acids. We would recommend the continuation of omega-3 fatty acids in patients with CV disease and the evidence is particularly strong for the prevention and treatment of HF.

References

[1] Kris-Etherton PM, Harris WS, Appel LJ. Fish consumption, fish oil, omega-3 fatty acids, and cardiovascular disease. *Circulation.* 2002;106:2747-2757.

[2] Lavie, J. C, Milani, et al. Omega-3 polyunsaturated fatty acids and cardiovascular diseases. *J Am Coll Cardiol.* 2009;54:585-594.

[3] Wang C, Harris WS, Chung M, et al. n-3 Fatty acid from fish or fish-oil supplements, but not alpha-linolenic acid, benefit cardiovascular disease outcomes in primary- and secondary-prevention studies: a systematic review. *Am J Clin Nutr.* 2006;84:5-17.

[4] Nutrient Data: USDA Nutrient Laboratory. Available at: *http://www.ars.usda.gov/nutrientdata;* 2006.

[5] Conquer JA, Holub BJ. Dietary docosahexaenoic acid as a source of eicosapentaenoic acid in vegetarians and omnivores. *Lipids.* 1997;323:341.

[6] Park Y, Harris WS. Omega-3 fatty acid supplementation accelerates chylomicron triglyceride clearance. *J Lipid Res.* 2002;44:455-463.

[7] Mozaffarian D, Rimm EB. Fish intake, contaminants, and human health: Evaluating the risks and the benefits. *JAMA.* 2006;296:1885-1899.

[8] Plourde M, Cunnane SC. Extremely limited synthesis of long chain polyunsaturates in adults: implications for their dietary essentiality and use as supplements. *Appl Physiol Nutr Metab.* 2007;32:619-637.

[9] Harris WS. Omega-3 fatty acids and cardiovascular disease: a case for omega-3 index as a new risk factor. *Pharmacol Res.* 2007;55:217-223.

[10] Anand RG, Alkadri M, Lavie CJ, Milani RV. The role of fish oil in arrhythmia prevention. *J Cardiopulm Rehabil.* 2007;In Press.

[11] O'Keefe JH, Abuissa H, Sastre A, Steinhaus DM, Harris WS. Effects of omega-3 fatty acids on resting heart rate, heart rate recovery after exercise, and heart rate variability in men with healed myocardial infarctions and depressed ejection fractions. *Am J Cardiol.* 2006;97:1127-1130.

[12] Ventura HO, Milani RV, Lavie CJ, et al. Cyclosporine-induced hypertension. Efficacy of omega-3 fatty acids in patients after cardiac transplantation. *Circulation.* 1993:II281-285.

[13] Thies F, Garry JM, Yaqoob P, et al. Association of n-3 polyunsaturated fatty acids with stability of atherosclerotic plaques: a randomized controlled trial. *Lancet.* 2003;361:477-485.

[14] Din JN, Harding SA, Valerio CJ, et al. Dietary intervention with oil rich fish reduces platelet-monocyte aggregation in man. *Atherosclerosis.* 2007;E-pub ahead of print.

[15] Abuissa A, O'Keefe JH, Harris WS, Lavie CJ. Autonomic function, omega-3 and cardiovascular risk. *Chest.* 2005;127:1088-1090.

[16] Villegas, R., Xiang, et al. Fish, shellfish, and long-chain n-3 fatty acid consumption and risk of incident type 2 diabetes in middle-aged Chinese men and women. *Am J Clin Nutr.*

[17] Geleijnse, M. J, Giltay, et al. Blood pressure response to fish oil supplementation: metaregression analysis of randomized trials. *J Hypertens.* 2002;20:1493-1499.

[18] Ueshima, H., Stamler, et al. Food omega-3 fatty acid intake of individuals (total, linolenic acid, long-chain) and their blood pressure: INTERMAP study. *Hypertension.* 2007;50:313-319.

[19] Marchioli R, Barzi F, Bomba E, et al. Early protection against sudden death by n-3 polyunsaturated fatty acids after myocardial infarction: time-course analysis of the results of the Gruppo Italiano per lo Studio della Sopravvivenza nell'Infarto Miocardico (GISSI)-Prevenzione. *Circulation.* 2002;105:1897-1903.

[20] Harris WS, Poston WC, Haddock CK. Tissue n-3 and n-6 fatty acids and risk for coronary heart disease events. *Atherosclerosis.* 2007;193:1-10.

[21] Lee, H. J, O'Keefe, et al. Omega3 fatty acids for cardioprotection. *Mayo Clin Proc.* 2008;83:324-332.

[22] Zhao, G., Etherton, et al. Dietary alpha-linolenic acid inhibits proinflammatory cytokine production by peripheral blood mononuclear cells in hypercholesterolemic subjects. *Am J Clin Nutr.* 2007;85:385-391.

[23] Noori, N., Dukkipati, et al. Dietary Omega-3 Fatty Acid, Ratio of Omega-6 to Omega-3 Intake, Inflammation, and Survival in Long-term Hemodialysis Patients. *Am J Kidney Dis.*

[24] Itoh, M., Suganami, et al. Increased adiponectin secretion by highly purified eicosapentaenoic acid in rodent models of obesity and human obese subjects. *Arterioscler Thromb Vasc Biol.* 2007;27:1918-1925.

[25] Mehra MR, Lavie CJ, Ventura HO, Milani RV. Fish Oils produce anti-inflammatory effects and improve body weight in severe heart failure. *J Heart Lung Transplant.* 2006;25:834-838.

[26] Madsen, T., Schmidt, B. E, Christensen, H. J. The effect of n-3 fatty acids on C-reactive protein levels in patients with chronic renal failure. *J Ren Nutr.* 2007;17:258-263.

[27] Moyers, B., Farzaneh-Far, et al. Relation of whole blood n-3 fatty acid levels to exercise parameters in patients with stable coronary artery disease (from the heart and soul study). *Am J Cardiol.*107:1149-1154.

[28] Davidson, H. M, Stein, et al. Efficacy and tolerability of adding prescription omega-3 fatty acids 4 g/d to simvastatin 40 mg/d in hypertriglyceridemic patients: an 8-week, randomized, double-blind, placebo-controlled study. *Clin Ther.* 2007;29:1354-1367.

[29] Metcalf RG, James MJ, Gibson RA, et al. Effects of fish-oil supplementation on

[30] Burr, L. M, Fehily, et al. Effects of changes in fat, fish, and fibre intakes on death and myocardial reinfarction: diet and reinfarction trial (DART). *Lancet.* 1989;2:757-761.

[31] Yokoyama M, Origasa H, Matsuzaki M, et al. Effects of eicosapentaenoic acid on major coronary events in hypercholesterolaemic patients (JELIS): a randomized open label, blinded endpoint analysis. *Lancet.* 2007;369:1090-1098.

[32] Ness, R. A, Hughes, et al. The long-term effect of dietary advice in men with coronary disease: follow-up of the Diet and Reinfarction trial (DART). *Eur J Clin Nutr.* 2002;56:512-518.

[33] Nilsen, W. D, Albrektsen, et al. Effects of a high-dose concentrate of n-3 fatty acids or corn oil introduced early after an acute myocardial infarction on serum triacylglycerol and HDL cholesterol. *Am J Clin Nutr.* 2001;74:50-56.

[34] Schacky v, C., Harris, S. W. Cardiovascular benefits of omega-3 fatty acids. *Cardiovasc Res.* 2007;73:310-315.

[35] Rauch, B., Schiele, et al. OMEGA, a randomized, placebo-controlled trial to test the effect of highly purified omega-3 fatty acids on top of modern guideline-adjusted therapy after myocardial infarction. *Circulation.*122:2152-2159.

[36] Kromhout, D., Giltay, J. E, Geleijnse, M. J. n-3 fatty acids and cardiovascular events after myocardial infarction. *N Engl J Med.*363:2015-2026.

[37] Kowey, R. P, Reiffel, et al. Efficacy and safety of prescription omega-3 fatty acids for the prevention of recurrent symptomatic atrial fibrillation: a randomized controlled trial. *JAMA.*304:2363-2372.

[38] Tavazzi, L., Maggioni, et al. Effect of n-3 polyunsaturated fatty acids in patients with chronic heart failure (the GISSI-HF trial): a randomised, double-blind, placebo-controlled trial. *Lancet.* 2008;372:1223-1230.

[39] Calo L, Bianconi L, Colivicchi F, et al. N-3 fatty acids for the prevention of atrial fibrillation after coronary artery bypass surgery: A randomized, controlled trial. *JACC.* 2005;45:1723-1728.

[40] Raitt MH, Conner WE, Morris C, al e. Fish oil supplementation and risk of ventricular tachycardia and ventricular fibrillation in patients with implantable defibrillators. *JAMA*. 2005;293:2884-2891.

[41] Brouwer IA, Zock PL, Camm AJ, al e. Effects of fish oil on ventricular tachyarrhythmia and death in patients with implantable cardioverter defibrillators. *JAMA*. 2006;295:2613-2619.

[42] Leaf A, Albert CM, Josephson M, et al. Prevention of fatal arrhythmias in high-risk subjects by fish oil n-3 fatty acid intake. *Circulation*. 2005;112:2762-2768.

[43] Macchia A, Levantesi G, Franzosi MG, Geraci E, Maggioni AP, al e. Left ventricular systolic dysfunction, total mortality, and sudden death in patients with myocardial infarction treated with n-3 polyunsaturated fatty acids. *Eur J Heart Fail*. 2005;7:904-909.

[44] Finzi, A. A, Latini, et al. Effects of n-3 polyunsaturated fatty acids on malignant ventricular arrhythmias in patients with chronic heart failure and implantable cardioverter-defibrillators: A substudy of the Gruppo Italiano per lo Studio della Sopravvivenza nell'Insufficienza Cardiaca (GISSI-HF) trial. *Am Heart J*.161:338-343 e331.

[45] Levitan, B. E, Wolk, A., Mittleman, A. M. Fish consumption, marine omega-3 fatty acids, and incidence of heart failure: a population-based prospective study of middle-aged and elderly men. *Eur Heart J*. 2009.

[46] Mozaffarian D, Bryson CL, Lemaitre RN, Burke GL, Siscovick DS. Fish intake and risk of incident heart failure. *J Am Coll Cardiol*. 2005;45:2015-2021.

[47] Lavie CJ, O'Keefe JH, Milani RV, Ventura HO, Mehra MR. New data on the clinical impact of exercise training, fish oils, and statins in heart failure. *Phys Sportsmed*. 2009;37:22-28.

[48] Yamagishi K, Nettleton JA, Folsom AR. Plasma fatty acid composition and incident heart failure in middle-aged adults: the Atherosclerosis Risk in Communities (ARIC) Study. *Am Heart J*. 2008;156:965-974.

[49] Nodari, S., Triggiani, et al. Effects of n-3 polyunsaturated fatty acids on left ventricular function and functional capacity in patients with dilated cardiomyopathy. *J Am Coll Cardiol*.57:870-879.

[50] Harris WS, VonSchaky C. The omega-3 index: a new risk factor for death from coronary artery disease? *Prev Med*. 2004;39:212.

[51] Block RC, Harris WS, Reid KJ, Sands SA, Spertus JA. EPA and DHA in blook cell membranes from acute coronary syndrome patients and controls. *Atherosclerosis*. 2007;In Press.

[52] Albert CM, Campos H, Stampfer MJ, et al. Blood levels of long-chain n-3 fatty acids and the risk of sudden death. *NEJM*. 2002;346:1113-1118.

[53] Rajaram, S., Haddad, et al. Walnuts and fatty fish influence different serum lipid fractions in normal to mildly hyperlipidemic individuals: a randomized controlled study. *Am J Clin Nutr*. 2009;89:1657S-1663S.

[54] Ouellet, V., Weisnagel, et al. Dietary cod protein reduces plasma C-reactive protein in insulin-resistant men and women. *J Nutr*. 2008;138:2386-2391.

[55] Harris WS, Pottala JV, Sands SA, Jones PG. Comparison of the impact of fish and fish oil capsules on the n-3 fatty acid content of blood cells and plasma phospholipids. *American Journal of Clinical Nutrition*. 2007 (In Press).

[56] Foulke JE. Mercury In Fish: Cause For Concern? : U.S. Food and Drug Administration; 1994.

[57] Jenkins, J. D, Sievenpiper, et al. Are dietary recommendations for the use of fish oils sustainable? *Cmaj.* 2009;180:633-637.

[58] Lee, H. J, O'Keefe, et al. Omega-3 fatty acids: cardiovascular benefits, sources and sustainability. *Nat Rev Cardiol.* 2009;6:753-758.

[59] Murawski, S., Methot, R., Tromble, G. Biodiversity loss in the ocean: how bad is it? *Science.* 2007;316:1281-1284; author reply 1281-1284.

[60] Sands, A. S, Reid, et al. The impact of age, body mass index, and fish intake on the EPA and DHA content of human erythrocytes. *Lipids.* 2005;40:343-347.

[61] Harris, S. W. Cardiovascular risk and alpha-linolenic acid: can Costa Rica clarify? *Circulation.* 2008;118:323-324.

In: Fish Oil: Production, Consumption and Health Benefits
Editors: Matthias Van Dijk and Jürgen Vitek
ISBN: 978-1-61470-963-3

Chapter XVI

The Consumption of the Fish Oil and Some Benefits in the Human Health

Rey Gutierrez Tolentino*[1], *Salvador Vega y León*[1], *Claudia Radilla Vázquez*[2], *María Radilla Vázquez*[2], *Rafael Díaz García*[1], *Jesús Pérez González*[1] and *María de Lourdes Ramírez Vega*[1]

[1] Department of Agricultural and Animal Production, Universidad Autónoma Metropolitana- Xochimilco, México City, México
[2] Médica Sur Hospital, Tlalpan, México City, Mexico

Abstract

Important benefits exists in the human health associated with the ingestion of fish and his oil, such as the prevention of cardiovascular diseases, immunological diseases, diabetes mellitus, colon´s cancer, beside serving like helpingly in the treatment of arthritis and taking part in the development of the brain and retina. The origin of marine oils perform at the present great importance in the supplies and in the human nutrition, due to it contained high place of polyunsaturated fatty acids (PUFA) specially, omega 3. The fished ones of deep and sweets waters called of meat blue or fished blue they are a source of omega-3 fatty acids as alpha - linolenic acid (ALA), eicosapentanoic acid (EPA) and docosahexaenoic acid (DHA). According to the database FAOSTAT 2007, in many countries such as China, Japan, United States and Mexico, per capita intake of fresh water fish was of 12.3, 4.9, 4.5 and 1.2 Kg respectively. It recommends to increase the consumption frequency of fish in quantities adapted in the populations with low ingestion, as the Mexican one, since this food constitutes a nutritional practical and cheap form to incorporate in the supply omega-3 fatty acids. The aim of the present work is to give updated information about the benefits in the human health that offers the consumption of fish oil.

Keywords: Fish oil, human health, Mexico

Introduction

The diet constitutes a key factor in the maintenance of a good health. The nutritional qualities of every diet come determined by the different types of components that integrate it. Nowadays there is recommended that the ingestion of fat should correspond between 30-35 % of the total energetic value contributed in the diet, where 15-20 %, corresponds to monounsaturated fatty acids (MFA), 7-8 % to saturated fatty acids (SFA) and 5 % to polyunsaturated fatty acids (PUFA).The polyunsaturated fatty acids (PUFA) turn out to be healthy due to the fact that they decrease cholesterol blood levels, mainly LDL (low-density lipoprotein)-cholesterol, acquiring a particular interest, the high molecular weight omega-3 fatty acids (ω-3), because they reduce the levels of triglycerides, the platelet aggregation and induce the immunological response, though the high benefit effect of this type of polyunsaturated fatty acids resides in his antiarritmic mechanism which improve the evolution of the cardiovascular diseases; besides the fact that recent studies have suggested that this one type of fatty acids also has a fundamental role in the decrease of derivated risks from diseases such as the diabetes type 2 or hypertension, The fish oil constitutes significant potential sources of ω -3 PUFA and therefore they can be considered to be functional ingredients capable of being used for the food development by beneficial health effects (Conchillo et al., 2006).

It has encouraged the habitants of the developing countries in the last years to increase his ingestion of fatty fish in 2 to 3 portions per week. The goal consists in consuming suitable quantities of polyunsaturated fatty acids type ω-3 like eicosapentaenoic acid (EPA) and docosahexaenoic acid (DHA), to achieve an ideal health and a major prevention of chronic diseases. Nowadays the sanitary agencies recommended a daily ingestion of 100mg/d of ω-3 fish oil; same that will have to increase to 100mg (2 portions of fatty fish) per week for the prevention of chronic diseases; in addition it has been suggested that quantities that range between 250mg/d up to 1000mg/d prepare coronary disease, and quantities between 2000-4000mg/d are recommended for the treatment of the levels of raised triglycerides (Jenkins et al., 2009).

The aim of the present work is to offer updated information about the importance of the fatty acids contained in the fish oil, his paper in the human nutrition and in the processes of health - disease.

Generalities of Lipids

The human body needs of approximately 50 nutriments which are indispensable for its functioning and development, such as the vitamins, the minerals, the amino acids, the carbohydrates and the lipids (Rodríguez et al., 2005). The importance of the lipids, also commonly called fats, in the nutrition and the human development is recognized for decades (Castro, 2002; Valenzuela et al., 2003; Molina de Salazar, 2009).

The fats constitute one of the most important components of the animal and vegetable kingdom. Inside the animal kingdom in big vacuoles that are formed in the cytoplasm of the adipose cells located in the subcutaneous and visceral tissue, and in the vegetable kingdom, in the seeds and flowers of numerous plants. In the human body they serve as sources of energy and are distributed in three regions of the body: the gluteofemoral, the subcutaneous and the intraabdominal, the last one is characterizes the obesity as a factor of risk of cardiovascular diseases (Nasiff-Hadad, 2003). The lipids are important constituent of the structure of the cellular membranes, and form the basic structure of some hormones and of the bile salts (Valenzuela et al., 2003). In addition some lipids have the character of essential due to the fact that they cannot be synthesized from precursor structures (Valenzuela et al., 2003; Rodríguez M et al., 2005).

The lipids are classified like: a) sterols, b) phospholipids, c) ephingomyelins, d) waxes, c) fats (Rodríguez et al., 2005). They are composed by monoglycerides, diglycerides and triglycerides and these in turn are constituted by a molecule of glycerol which join 1, 2 ó 3 fatty acids (FA) (Castro, 2002; Nasiff-Hadad, 2003). The phospholipids and cholesterol esters also contain FA (Nasiff-Hadad, 2003).

Fatty Acids

The FA is a group of organic compounds formed by a hydrocarbonated chain and a carboxylic group that give that a physicist - chemistry properties to the fats (Nasiff-Hadad, 2003). FA presents in the alive beings possesses in the main an even number of carbon atoms and qualifies in saturated, when they do not have double bonds and unsaturated, when they have double bonds, the above mentioned can be a monounsaturated or polyunsaturated, as present one o more double bond (Figure 1) (Castro, 2002; Nasiff-Hadad, 2003; Rodríguez, 2005).

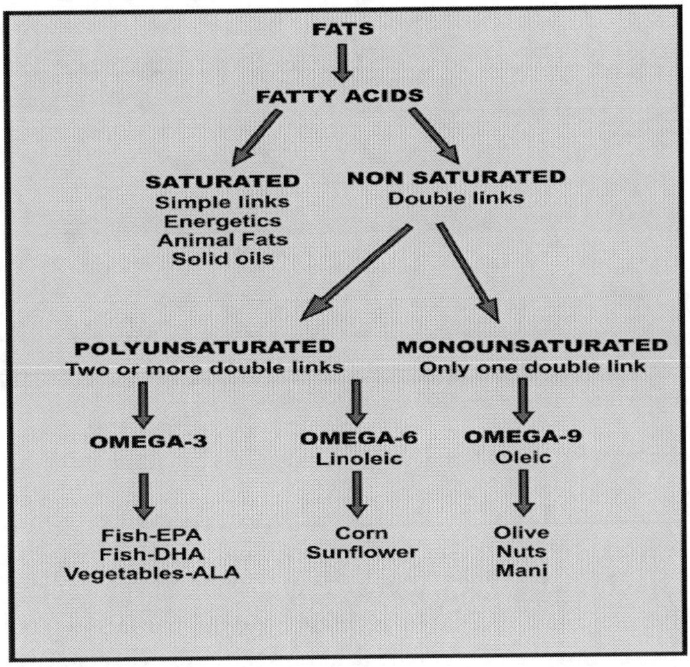

SOURCE: Modified of Sanchez, 2009.

Figure 1. Clinical importance of the omega-3 fatty acids.

As is observed in the Table 1, FA can qualify according to the number of carbon atoms.

Table 1. Classification of FA, according to the number of carbon atoms

Fatty acids	Number of carbon atoms
Short chain	Between 4 and 6
Medium chain	Between 8 and 10
Long chain	Between 12 and 18
Very long chain	Between 20 and 24

Source: Castro, 2002; Nasiff-Hadad, 2003.

Unsaturated Fatty Acids

The FA can also classified by families omega 3, 6 and 9 (Figure 2) (Nasiff-Hadad, 2003).

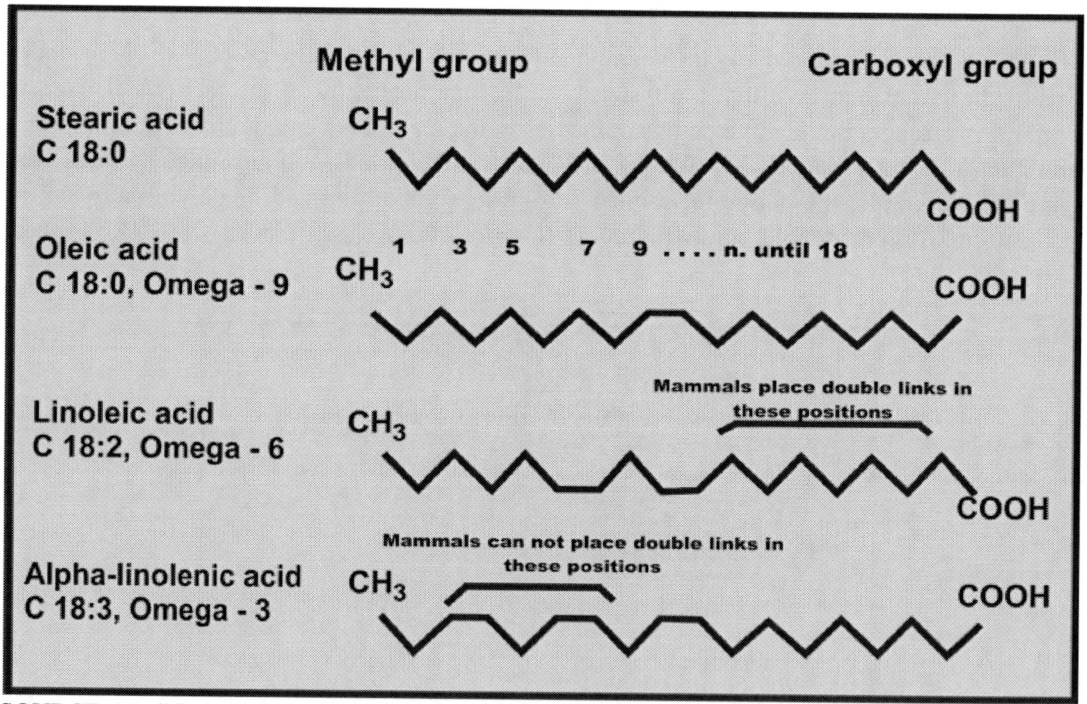

SOURCE: Modified of Valenzuela et al., 2003.

Figure 2. Families of omega-9, omega-6 and omega-3 fatty acids and its nomenclature.

For its pathogenic significance in the atherosclerosis, it groups them for the number of the carbon atoms where there locates the first double bond attended by the Greek letter omega (ω) (Castro, 2002; Nasiff-Hadad, 2003; Carrero et al., 2005). This way does identify omega-9 FA (ω-9) such as the oleic acid present in vegetable and animal fats, the omega-6 FA (ω -6), which principal representative is the linoleic acid present in the vegetable oils and the omega-3 FA (ω -3) which principal FA is α – linolenic acid present in the marine oils and in some vegetable oils (Innis, 2003; Nasiff-Hadad, 2003; Carrero et al., 2005).

The different numbers and positions of the double bonds of the chain, do they award to the fatty acids different physiological properties derived from its metabolism, which does that the relation among ω-3 and ω-6 FA of the diet be very important (Carrero et al., 2005). Unsaturated FA can be cis or trans, in dependence of the spatial configuration that they adopt. The cis form is produced when 2 carbons of the double bond place spatially of the same side and the trans when the carbons are placed in opposite direction. Trans FA conforms as consequence of the warming or the hydrogenation of FA and shows the same atherogenic power that saturated FA. The margarines obtained by hydrogenation of vegetable or marine oils, they can contain trans FA, condition that must appear in the labels of the packages of these products. Cis FA has not atherogenic properties (Nasiff-Hadad, 2003).

Some FA they qualify as " essential fatty acids " (Table 2), because they cannot be synthesized by the human body due to the fact that the mammals lack the necessary enzymes to insert double bonds beyond the carbon 9, and in addition they are necessary for the vital functions, these are those of the families ω-6 and ω-3 (Castro, 2002; Carrero et al., 2005; Sanchez, 2009).

Table 2. Nomenclature of the essential fatty acids

Common name	Systematic name	Abbreviation	Formula
ω-9 Family			
Oleic	Cis-9-octadecaenoic	18:1 ω-9	$C_{18}H_{34}O_2$
ω-6 Family			
Linoleic	Cis-9,12,-octadecadienoic (LA)	18:2 ω-6	$C_{18}H_{32}O_2$
γ-linolenic	Cis-6.9.12 octadecatrienoic	-18:3 ω-6	$C_{18}H_{30}O_2$
Dihomoglinoleic	Cis-8,11,14 -eicosatrienoic	20:3 ω-6	$C_{20}H_{34}O_2$
Arachidonic (AA)	Cis-5,8,11,14-eicosatetraenoic	20:4 ω-6	$C_{20}H_{32}O_2$
Adrenic	Cis-7,10,13,16-docosatetraenoic	22:4 ω-6	$C_{22}H_{36}O_2$
Osmond	Cis-4,7,10,13,16-docosapentaenoic	22:5 ω-6	$C_{22}H_{34}O_2$
ω-3 Family			
α-linolenic	Cis-9,12,15-octadecatrienoic (ALA)	18:3 ω-3	$C_{18}H_{30}O_2$
Estearidonic	Cis-6,9,12,15-octadecatetraenoic	18:4 ω-3	$C_{18}H_{28}O_2$
Timnodonic	Cis-5,8,11,14,17-eicosapentaenoic (EPA)	20:5 ω-3	$C_{20}H_{30}O_2$
Clupanodonic	Cis-7,10,13,16,19-docosapentaenoic (DPA)	22:2 ω-3	$C_{22}H_{34}O_2$
Cervonic	Cis-4,7,19,13,16,19-docosahexaenoic (DHA)	22:6 ω-3	$C_{22}H_{32}O_2$

SOURCE: Modified of Castro 2002.

Omega-6 and Omega-3 Polyunsaturated Fatty Acids (PUFA) Like Essential Nutrients in Human Diet

The proteins from the fish are considered of a high nutritional value, but in the last two decades emphasis has been done in the nutritional value of the fish in the diet for being one rich food in polyunsaturated fatty acids of long chain ω-3, of the type DHA (docosahexaenoic 22:6 ω-3) and EPA (eicosapentaenoic acid 20:5 ω-3) (Figure 3) (Sargent, 1997; Molina de Salazar, 2009).

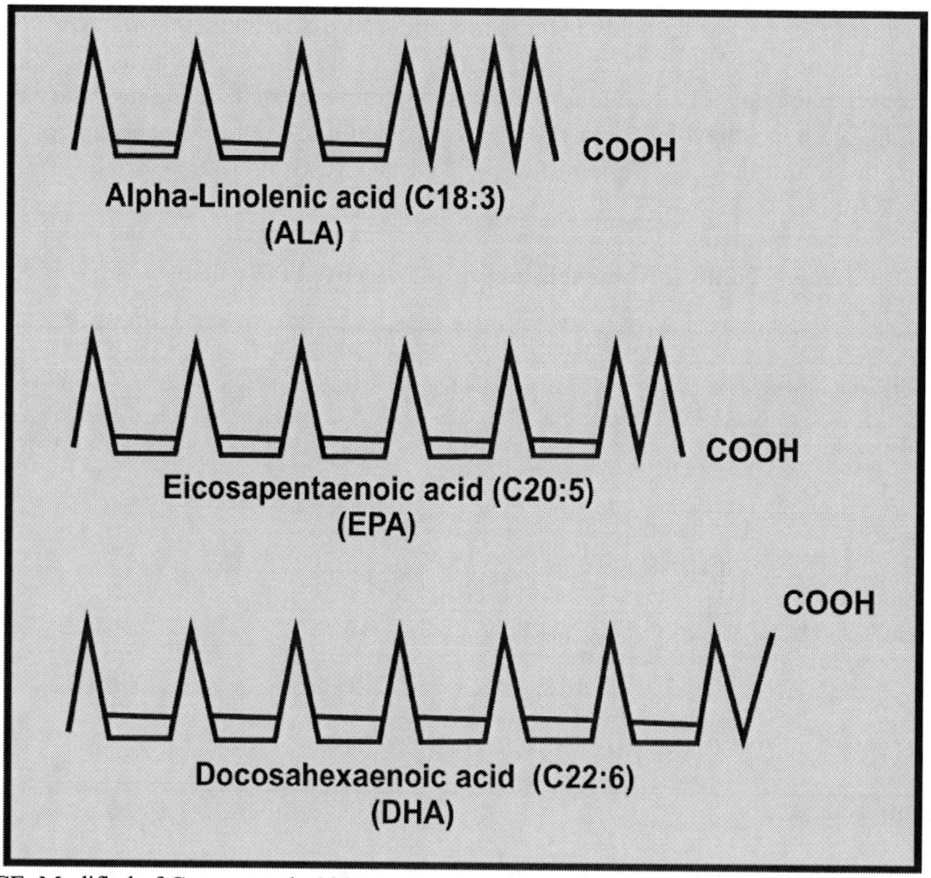

SOURCE: Modified of Carrero et al., 2007.

Figure 3. Chemical structure of the α-linolénic acid (ALA), ecosapentaenoic acid (EPA) and docosahexaenoic acid (DHA).

The long chain polyunsaturated fatty acids (PUFA) of the series ω-6 widely acquaintances as a essential constituent of the diet, specifically, the arachidonic acid (AA, 20:4 ω-6), and is considered to be essential for its numerous functions inside the human being metabolism, such as it can act like transcription factor bond (Sargent, 1997; Rodríguez et al., 2005). AA can be directly consumed in the diet or be synthesized in the organism from the linoleic acid (LA, 18:2 ω-6) (Sargent, 1997; Carrero et al., 2005; Gottrand, 2008). Whereas the AA is easily synthesized of the LA (the PUFA most abundant source in the natural food), the DHA experiences a longer and complicated synthesis route for what diverse authors affirm that the rate of ALA/DHA conversion is limited, principally in preterm born child (Figures 4) (Koletzko B, et al. 2001; Mc Gregor et al., 2003; Campoy et al., 2010).

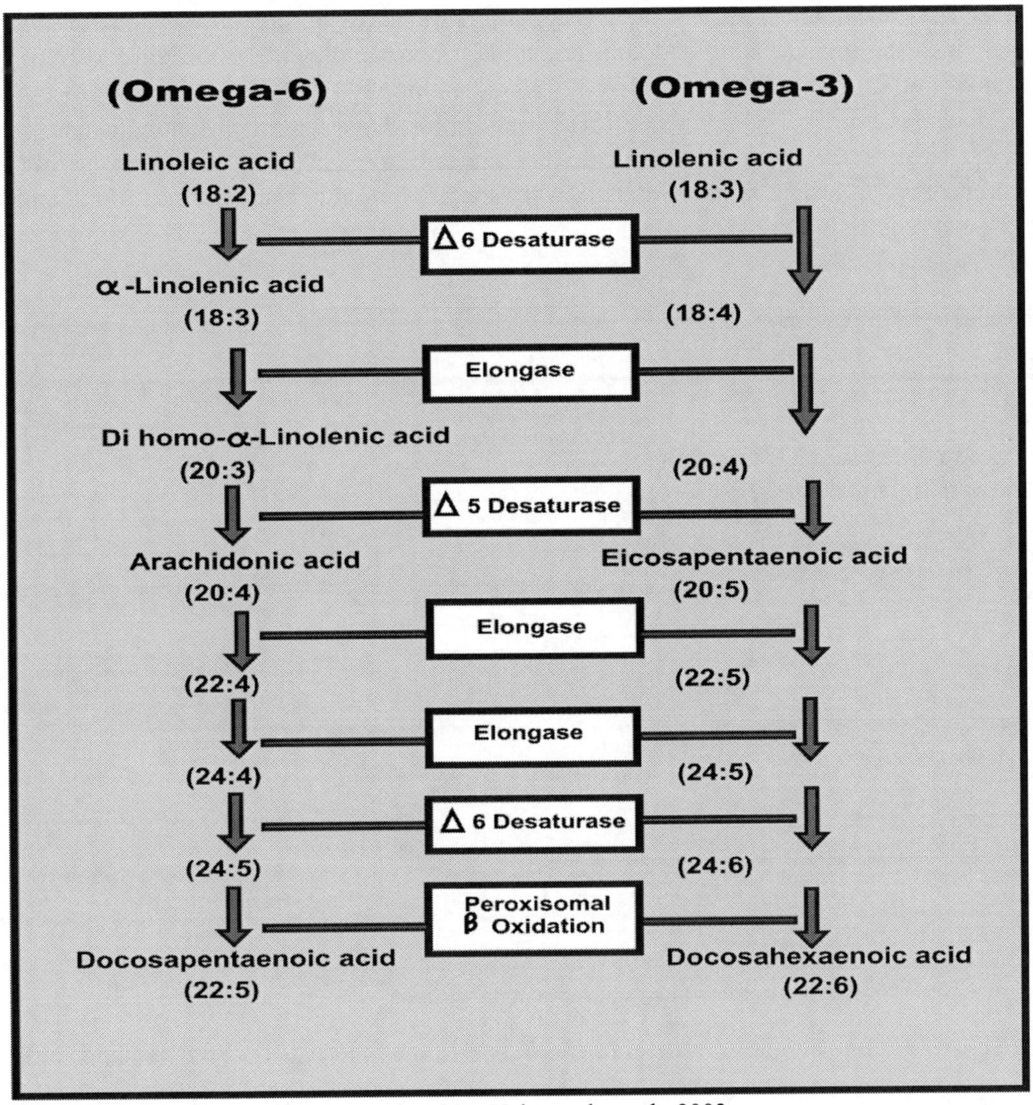

SOURCE: Modified for Valenzuela et al., 2001; Valenzuela et al., 2003.

Figure 4. Metabolic stages of the biosynthesis of fatty acids omega-6 and omega-3 from its predecessors.

The omega-3 fatty acids, not only are essential nutrients, but they also can modulate many diseases (Figure 5) (Castro, 2002; Cheatham et al., 2006). DHA is a vital component of the phospholipids of the cellular membranes (where they influences on the fluency, receptor functions, and enzymatical activity), and it is specially rich in the brain, retina and the sperms, since more than 60 % of its dry weight is constituted by lipids, phospholipids specially, considering that of 60-65 % of the total lipids in the brain are polyunsaturated fatty acids, and of this one percentage more than 85 % is constituting by DHA (35-40 %) and by the arachidonic (C20:4, AA) (40-50 %) of the total of fatty acids (Haschke-Becher et al., 2001;

Innis, 2003; Sanhueza et al., 2004; Adamkin, 2007; Sánchez, 2009; Campoy et al., 2010; Valenzuela et al., 2010). The ω-3 fatty acids are necessary for the conception from the pregnancy, the infancy and undoubtedly in the whole life (Sidhu, 2003; Rosenfeld et al., 2009). The development of the brain happens particularly during the last quarter of the gestation in the human being and finishes, though not completely, to the third year of life (Sanhueza et al., 2004; Cheatham et al., 2006; Adamkin, 2007). In this complex process the fatty acids, as principal components of the brain lipids, have important functions and in the specific case of the brain development, the omega-3 fatty acid docosahexaenoic (C22:6, DHA) it seems to have a fundamental and very specific role in the structure and functionality of the nervous tissue (Haschke-Becher et al., 2001; Sanhueza et al., 2004; Carrero et al., 2005; Adamkin, 2007).

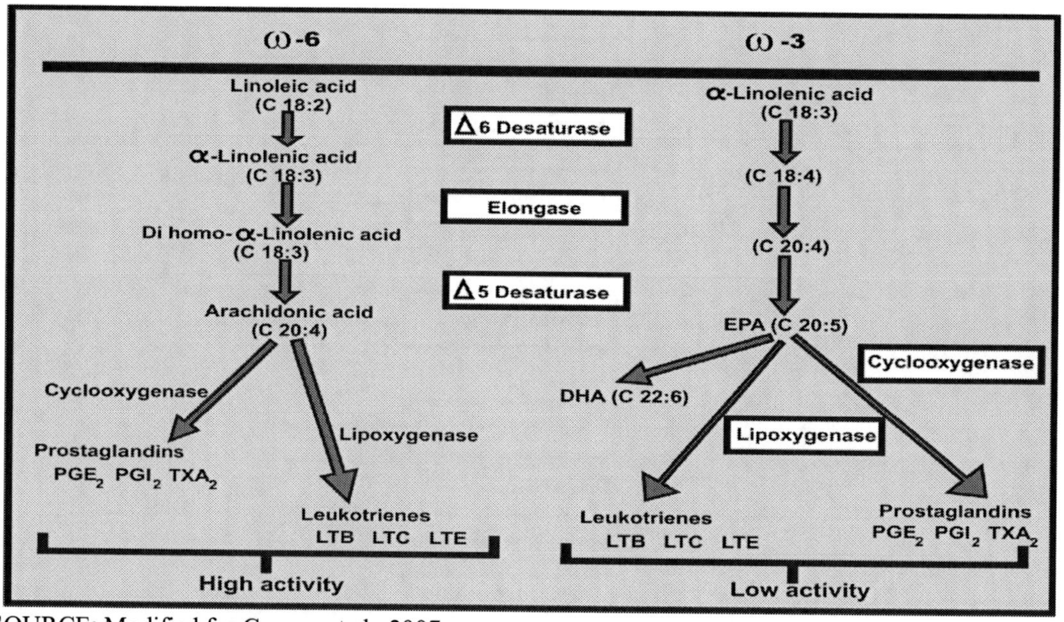

SOURCE: Modified for Carrero et al., 2007.

Figure 5. Series of polyunsaturated fatty acids and metabolic routes of eicosanoids.

Those are some important functions of polyunsaturated fatty acids in the human health:

1. Omega-3 fatty acids are essential for a suitable development and functioning of the brain and the nervous system. They center in the retina and the cerebral cortex, and have the aptitude to correct visual and cerebral problems in patients with demonstrated deficiency. Many aspects of anxiety, learning skills, memory, retinal function, does affected with the consumption of ω -3 FA (Castro, 2002; Carrero et al., 2007).
2. They are predecessors of hormonal compounds as the prostanoids (prostaglandins and thromboxanes) that facilitate the messages transmission in the central nervous system (CNS). (Figures 6) (Castro, 2002; Anderson, 2003).
3. When there exist DHA suitable levels in the brain there is improved the cerebral activity (Castro, 2002; Uauy et al., 2006).

4. Two third parts of the fatty acids in the membranes of the retina photoreceptors are ω-3, principally DHA (Castro, 2002).
5. Another relation among the DHA and the cerebral function has been found in the organization pattern of children dream. DHA low consumption results in fewer slow waves of dream, which serve as an indicator of the CNS ripeness and development (Castro, 2002).
6. Omega-3 FA are related to problems of depression and violence. There has been demonstrated that the intake of DHA has protective effects against the increase in the hostility in students under stress conditions (Castro, 2002).
7. DHA low concentrations are a useful indicator to predict major problems of children conduct to who has been diagnosed attention deficit hyperactivity disorder (ADHD). These problems can be reflex partly of the problems in the serotoninergic neurotransmission (Castro, 2002).

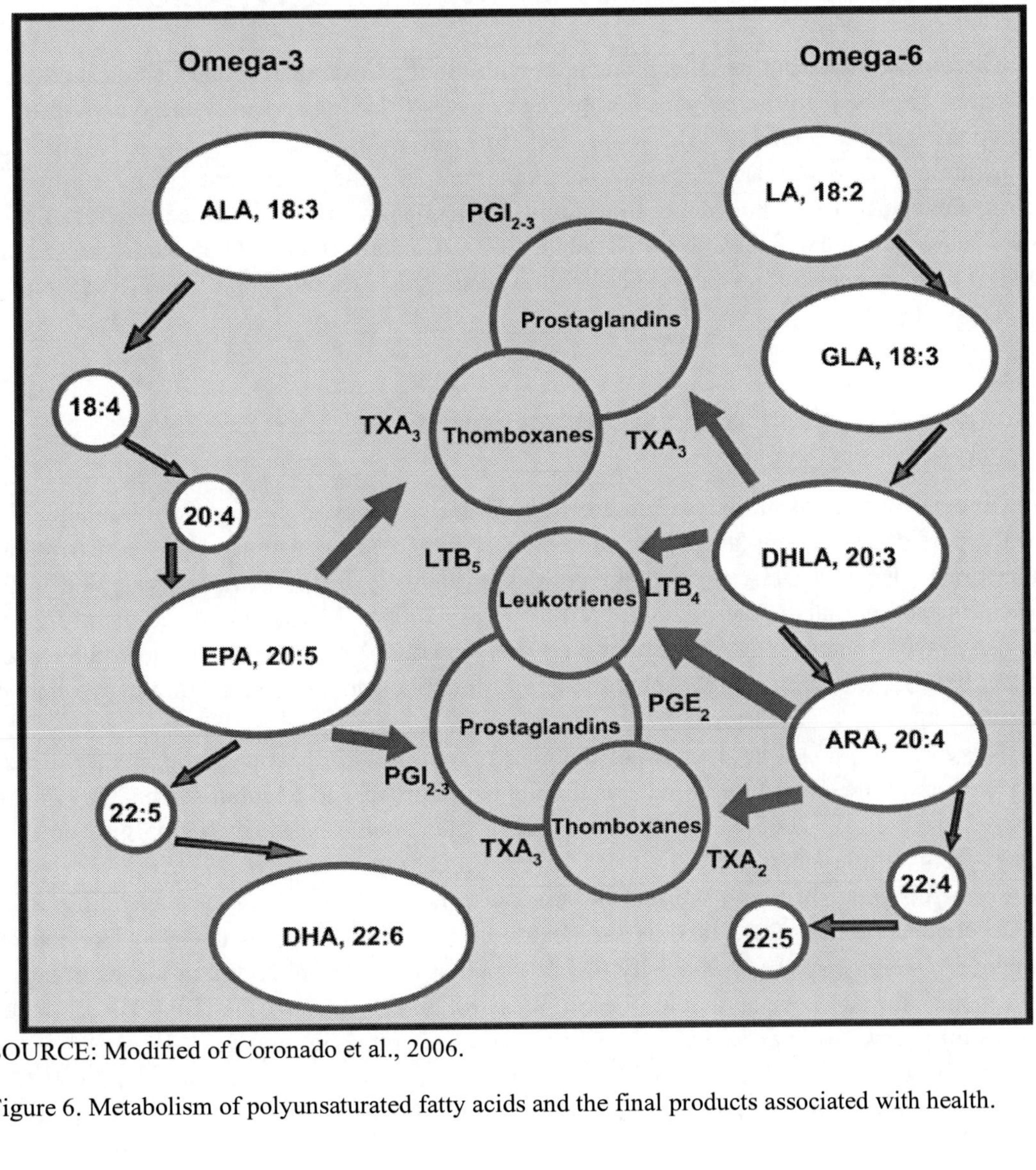

SOURCE: Modified of Coronado et al., 2006.

Figure 6. Metabolism of polyunsaturated fatty acids and the final products associated with health.

There exist two important considerations for fatty acids refer (Sargent, 2004):

In first place, which is the ideal relation of ω-6: ω-3 in the human being? The response is not completely known, but values of 5:1 are considered to be reasonable, whereas values that range in 50:1 are considered to be excessive (Sargent, 2004).

Secondly, since it is known that 18:2 ω-6 and 18:3 ω-3 can turn into the human body to its long chain homologues with C20 and C22, but will this conversion be able to be given efficiently to satisfy the tissues demands? With regard to this point, still the doubt exists of if these conversions are realized by the sufficient speed, mainly in those cases in which a high demand exists as for example during the growth and development in early stages of the life (Morris, 2000; Larqué et al., 2001; Innis, 2003; Sargent, 2004; Mc Namara et al., 2006; Mitmesser et al., 2006; Judge, 2007).

Food Sources of Omega 3 Fatty Acids

There exist important benefits associated with the ingestion of fish and fish oil, and these are narrowly related to the polyunsaturated fatty acids (PUFA), specially the omega-3 (ω-3) (Simopoulos, 1989; Sidhu, 2003).

α-linoleic acid (ω-3) it cannot be obtained of the diet, but from it derives eicosapentaenoic (EPA) and docosahexaenoic (DHA) acids who are in deep waters fishes, called also blue meat fishes (Nasiff-Hadad, 2003; Carrero et al., 2005; Rodríguez et al., 2005). Other sources of ω-3 fatty acids are the seeds, the nuts and some fruits (Rodríguez et al., 2005).

Fish Oil

Omega-3 PUFA of marine origin are formed in marine plant cloroplast, microalgae that form a part of the phytoplankton or macroalgae, which are consumed by the fish, which concentrate EPA and DHA as triacylglycerides, principally in the adipose tissue and in the muscle fat and entrails (Castro, 2002; Carrero et al., 2005). EPA accumulates mainly in the adipose tissue, whereas 90 % or more of the DHA, constitutes the nervous tissue and the brain of the fish, in the form of phosphatidylserine and phosphatidylethanolamine (Molina de Salazar, 2009).

The variation in ω-3 FA content of the marine food it will depend on the species of fish, the place, and time of capture, as well as the industrial process to which it surrenders (Castro, 2002; Carrero et al., 2005). The lipids content in the eatable parts of the marine food can change from a bit less than 0.5 % up to 25 % (Castro, 2002).

From this point of view, the marine animals can qualify in 4 groups depending on its lipidic content: loins (<2 % fat), as the seafood, the cod; low in fat (2-4 %) like the red grouper *(Epinephelus morio)*; half oily (4-8 %) such as the salmon; and high places in fats (> 8 %) such as the sardines, anchovies, herring (Castro, 2002). The ω-3 FA (EPA/DHA) richest species for every 100g of raw fish is: sardine 3.3g; macarela 2.5g; herring 1.7g; anchovy 1.4; salmon 1.4g and saber 2.5g; the cod oil is the most enriched since it contains 13.2 and 10.9 g/100g of oil EPA/DHA (Nasiff-Hadad, 2003; Rodríguez et al., 2005). The concentrates of fish oil with major content in EPA/DHA for every 100g of oil are: pro-omega 44.2g; Max EPA 29.4g; salmon oil 19.9g; livers cod oil 18.5g; and herring oil 11.4g (Table 3) (Nasiff-Hadad, 2003).

Table 3. Composition of fatty acids of several fish oil (g/100g total of fatty acids in the total lipids)

Fatty acid	*Salmon farm Meat*	*Farm Salmon fed on oils*	*Wild salmon meat*	*Herring*	*Capelin*	*Anchovies*
14:0	5	5	4	7	7	7
16:0	16	15	13	13	13	17
16:1 ω-7	7	6	4	7	10	9
18:0	3	2	3	1	1	4
18:1ω-9	13	10	19	10	14	12
18:2ω-6	3	3	1	1	2	1
18:3ω-3	2	2	1	1	1	1
18:4ω-3	3	5	1	3	4	-
20:1ω-9	9	9	12	13	16	2
20:5ω-3	7	9	7	6	8	17
22:1ω-11	10	15	11	23	15	2
22:6ω-3	12	12	10	6	6	9
Saturados	24	22	20	21	21	28
Mono insaturados	43	42	52	53	55	23
n-3 PUFA	28	30	24	16	19	31

PUFA: Polyunsaturated fatty acids
SOURCE: Modified of Rodríguez et al., 2005.

The place and time of capture produces big changes in the content of ω-3 of the fish oil still when it is the same fish. As the temperature of the water diminishes, increases the FA unsaturation degree of in the tissues to compensate the reduction of the fluency of the membranes owed to the low temperature. The opposite happens in the moderate regions, where the water temperature is major to 12°C, and the oil obtained after processing the fish can have a significant reduction of the content of ω-3. The condition for the conservation of the fish after the capture and the later industrial process does determine the ω-3 FA final content in the oil (Castro, 2002).

These profiles do that these oils are significant sources exceptionally natural of polyunsaturated fatty acids of high molecular weight, specially of ω-3 family, and therefore capable really being considered to be ingredients by healthy properties, marking that in relation with other PUFA, the fish oil presents a major percentage of essential fatty acids, linoleico and α-linolenic (Conchillo et al., 2006).

As for ingestion ω-3 FA the FAO/WHO recommends an ideal consumption from 1.1 to 1.5 g/day (0.8 to 1.1 g/day of TO, and 0.3 to 0.4g/day of EPA and DHA); the International Society for the Study of Fatty Acids and Lipids (ISS-FAL) suggests the quantity of 0.65g/day of DHA more 1g/day of AL (Carrero et al., 2005; Rodríguez et al., 2005).

On the other hand, the new recommendations of the American Heart Society (AHA) are: a) the adult persons have to consume fish at least twice a week, b) for patients with coronary disease the recommendations of consumption are 1 gram daily of EPA+DHA proceeding from fish oil or supplements and c) for patients with hypertriglyceridemia recommends supplement from 2 to 4 daily grams of EPA+DHA in order to diminish in 20-40 % the levels of triacylglycerides in plasma (Carrero et al., 2005). There is recommended that FA consumption in the diet should be in a proportion ω-3: ω-6 of 5-10:1 (Rodríguez et al., 2005). Some of supplements derived from marine oils are contained by them 180 mg of EPA and 120mg of DHA for capsule (Castro, 2002).

The supplements must be taken with precaution due to the high quantities of vitamins A and D that they contain (Table 4) (Castro, 2002).

Table 4. Random assignment clinical studies, with omega-3 pharmaceutical forms

Omega-3 fatty acids
Randomized controlled studies. Secondary prevention

Study/Year/n	OMEGA-3 Dosage	Year - according pathology	toRESULTS
Saks et al., (1) 1995/n=59	4,800mg/d EPA+DHA Olive oil	2,4 Ateroma Regression	Not effect in mortality, MI, CVS
Singh et al., (2) 1997/n=240	1,800mg/d EPA+DHA Placebo	1 Post MI	Questioned its results
Leng et al., (3) 1998/n=120	270mg/d EPA+DHA Sunflower oil	2 AD. Perifer	Not effect in mortality, MI, CVS
Von Schacky et al., (4) 1999/n=223	1,700mg/d EPA+DHA Placebo	2 Post MI	Not effect in mortality, MI, CVS
GISSI(6) 1999/n=11324	850mg/d EPA+DHA	3,5 Post MI	Coronary sudden total mortality
NORUEGO (5) 2001/n=300	3,500mg/d EPA+DHA Corn oil	1.5 Post MI	Not effect they consume fish
JELIS-Japonés (7) 2007/n=3664	1,800mg/d EPA Con/sin estatina	4,6 CD	MI, Unstable angor, revascularization, death.

MI: Myocardial infarction; AD: Arterial disease; CVS: Cerebrovascular stroke; CD: Coronary Disease
SOURCE: Modified of Merchán, 2009.

If is compared the essential fatty acids of the fish oil, in comparison with the vegetable eatable oils; it is possible to observe that the corn, sunflower or soy bean oils, have quantities of linoleic acid the order of 45-50mg/100g and olive oil the order of 7-11g/100g. As for the α-linolenic acid, its contribution on the part of fish oil can be even superior to that of some vegetable oils. This way, the olive or sunflower oils present quantities below 0.7g/100g. The stearic acid, considered predecessor of the oleic acid, is in major quantity in the oil of fish. The stearic acid (C18:0), unlike the rest of the saturated fatty acids (SFA) has undersized or no influence on the aptitude to increase the blood cholesterol levels. As for fraction SFA is observed a major presence of the principal acids of this fraction, palmitoleic and oleic, in the fish oil (Conchilla et al., 2006).

Consumption of Fish Oil in the World

The total of the world production of fish and fishing products rose from 140 million tons in 2007 to 145 million tons in 2009.

In 2008, the world consumed 115 million tons of fish, and there is foreseen that the demand increases, for the same year, the world exports of fish and fishing products reached the record number of 102 000 million US dollars, which supposes an increase of 9 % with regard to 2007. The fishing products continue being the most commercialized basic food ones, with a record value of 102 billion dollars in 2008, one 9.0 more per cent with regard to the previous year (FAO, 2010).

Table 5. Quantity of supply of fish oil in tons and two different types of fish rich in fatty acids in 2007

Countries	Fish oil	Sweet water fish	Marine fish, others
China	0	16453070.53	514134.60
Japon	62981.00	626983.49	876199.71
United States	0	1393782.58	4427.00
México	0	134013.27	231664.52

SOURCE: FAO, 2010.

Table 6. Per capita consume of fish oil and two different types of fish rich in fatty acids in 2007

Countries	Fish oil	Sweet water fish	Mariene fish, others
China	0	12.3	0.39
Japón	0.49	4.9	6.8
United States	0	4.5	0.01
México	0	1.2	2.1

SOURCE: FAO, 2010.

Omega-3 Fatty Acids in the Disease

Exist a variety of studies realized in human beings that shows the possible effects of ω-3 FA in different diseases (Tables 7 and 8) (Rodríguez et al., 2005). The majority of the researches have focused on the study of the consumption of the PUFA, in the diabetes, some types of cancers and cardiovascular diseases (Rodríguez et al., 2005).

Table 7. Some effects in the human health of the diet with omega-3 fatty acids

Study/Year	Relationship with health	Realized study	Results
Gylling and Miettinen, 2001.	Cardiovascular	Study of Lyon. Follow-up of 605 patients with coronary disease, for 46 months. Consumption of fewer cholesterol (217mg/día), fewer fat calories (30.5 %) more oleic acid (13 %) and three times more ALA and EPA (0.6 %), more fiber (19g/d)	Reduction of the total cholesterol (5 %), LDL (7%) and tryacilglycerides (14 %), HDL I increase 10 %. There diminished the risk of mortality and cardiac morbidity (73 %). The study suggests that it is possible to reduce the incident of heart diseases with this treatment.

Table 7. (continued)

Study/Year	Relationship with health	Realized study	Results
Hu et al., 2003.	Diabetes/cardiology	Prospective study to 18 years in 1503 women with diabetes type 2. Diet with fish source of EPA and DHA. There were vigilant the dietetic variants (fiber, fats with trans fatty acids, fruits, vegetables, etc.).	The ω-3 fatty acids can reduce the hearth diseases (incidence and mortality), in diabetics patients, due to it diminished the tryglycerides blood levels, platelet aggregation and the antiarrhythmic effects. Also low mortality was observed by not cardiac reasons. There were no adverse effects in the glycemic control.
Hardman, 2002.	Cancer	Study with 231 rats in 10 groups. Diet with 5 % or 2 % of corn oil, more 3 % of a product with ω-3 fatty acids. The tumor measured up three times a week to a caliper, from the 14th of initiating the diet and up to 46 days.	The analysis of linear regression show that the tumors of the animals fed on ω-3 fatty acids it was significantly minor that them of those fed only with corn oi ($p < 0.05$).
Mantzioris et al., 2000.	Inflammatory processes	Dietetic and clinical study, 15 healthy subjects between 31-43 years. Rich diet in omega-3 fatty acids and lower in omega 6 for 4 weeks. Ingestion of 1.8g/d of EPA+DHA and 9.0 g/d of ALA	The ω-3 fatty acids increased in plasma and the phospholipids of mononuclear cells. EPA 3 times. ALA 3-4 times. DPA 30 % and DHA 1-5 times. The ω-6 fatty acids did not diminish, LA 8 %, ARA 7 % and with it TXB_2, the PGE_2 and the IL-β (36%, 26%, and 20%) that are inflammatory mediators.
Stoll et al., 1999.	Bipolar disorder	30 subjects during four months with 6.2 g/d of EPA and 3.4 g/d of DHA	Longer periods of remission, significant reduction in Hamilton's scale of depression (HRSD)
De Busk et al., 2004.	Skin	13 persons with photodermatitis provided supplements with fish oil Another study with 40 subjects, with psoriasis administes medicine and supplements with EPA	They showed a significantly minor sensibility to the beams UV There were better results with regard to the controls. There is recommended also the linseed (omega-3) for the acne.
Sindelar et al., 2004	Physical intense activity (possible risk of sudden death)	12 trained runners in a study of four. Two of treatment with enriched egg (1/6d) with omega-3 (350mg of ω-3 c/u), and rest of four weeks and later the same subjects consumed for two weeks (1/6d) the conventional egg (60mg of ω-3 c/u)	Seric tryglycerides were kept in the recommended range. The LDL and the HDL cholesterol did not change in a significant way, independently of the daily consumption of egg. For it the use recommends those enriched with omega-3, because they increased the ingestion of ALA and DHA, which is helpful for the health.

SOURCE: Modified of Stoll, et al., 1999; Gylling and Miettinen, 2001; Hardman, 2002; Hu et al., 2003; De Busk et al., 2004; Sindelar, et al., 2004; Coronado et al., 2006.

Table 8. Effect of the consumption of the PUFA in different diseases in humans

Fatty acid	Consumption	Effect	Population
		Diabetes	
ADH AEP	Provided in capsules; 4g/d of ADH or AEP during 6 weeks	Reduction of the serum lipids and short-term adverse effects in glucose levels	39 men 12 women
PUFA	Content in the diet; 6.0± 1.9 g/d, men; 5.9± 1.9 g/d, women	Higher consumption of PUFA is associated with a lower concentration of glycated hemoglobin	Diabetics: 2,759 men, 3,464 women
PUFA	Content in the diet; 2 to 7 % of energy	Higher consumption of PUFA is associated with a lower risk of developing type 2 diabetes	84,204 women
EPA DHA	Provided in capsules 0.69/0.20 g/d to 5.40/2.30 g/d During 2 a 36 weeks	No changes are observed in the glucose nor in the concentration of glycated hemoglobin Reduction of triacylglycerols (-30%).	Meta-analysis of 26 studies
DHA EPA	Provided as fish oil 3 to 18 g/d during 12 weeks	No effect on the concentration of glucose Reduction of triacylglycerols by 0.56mmol/l Increase of LDL cholesterol by 0.21 mmol/l	823 women with type 2 diabetes
		Cáncer	
ω-3 PUFA	Provided as fish from <once/week, once/week and ≥ twice/week	Reduction of the risk of developing various types of cancer, especially of the digestive tract (esophagus, stoma and rectum)	7990 individuals
ω-3 PUFA	Fish from once/week, 1 to 2 days/week 3-4 days/week and almost daily	The higher the consumption of fish, the higher the content of ω-3 PUFA in serum. An inverse association is observed between the concentration of ω-3 PUFA in the serum and prostate cancer. This is not observed in other cancers (stomach, colon, rectum and breast).	297 men
		Cardiovascular diseases	
ALN	Provided in the diet (0.22 a 4.78 de ALN g/d)	Higher consumption is associated with a reduction in the formation of platelets in the arteries	1,575 adults (698 men, 877 women)
ALN	Dietary manipulation; increase in the consumption of foods rich in ALN such as nuts and nut oil (4.8 g of ALN + 2/1 for 6 weeks)	Inhibition of vascular inflammation and vascular activity	Adults 20 men y 3 women
ω-3 PUFA	Fish (once a week)	The consumption of fish is associated with a reduction in primary cardiac arrest	Cases of primary cardiac arrest 334 Controls 493
ω-3 PUFA	Fish (<once a month to ≥ 6 times a week	No reduction was observed in the risk of coronary disease by increasing the consumption of fish in individuals without antecedents of vascular disease	44,805 men
ω-3 PUFA	Fish (<once a month to ≥6 times a week	Higher consumption of fish is associated with a low risk of coronary disease	84,688 women
ω-3 PUFA	Fish (<once a month to ≥5 times a week)	Higher consumption of fish is associated with a lower incidence of cardiac disease and mortality from cardiac disease in diabetic women	5,103 women with type 2 diabetes
ω-3 PUFA	ω-3 PUFA of intermediate chain ≥ 1.08 g/d of sea or plant origin	Reduction by 50 % in risk of cardiac disease	45,722 individuals
PUFA	ω-3 PUFA of plant origin if the ingestion of ω-3 PUFA of sea origin is very low (< 0.1 g/d)	May reduce the risk of cardiovascular disease	45,722 individuals

SOURCE: Modified from Rodríguez-Cruz et al., 2005.

Omega-3 Fatty Acids in Diabetes

Omega-3 FA has provoked great interest due to the effects in the diabetics because this disease associates frequently to dislipidemy (Nasiff-Hadad, 2003). Have they proposed that ω-3 FA can have a benefit effect in the development or control of the diabetes across different mechanisms, for which multiple investigations have been reported in diabetics and not diabetics patients, in which ones the effect of ω-3 FA on the glycemia has been evaluated (Nasiff-Hadad, 2003; Rodríguez et al., 2005).

One of the mechanisms does refer to the capacity of omega-3 fatty acids to operate like bounds that activated PPARγ (Peroxisome Proliferator-activated Receptor γ), the PPARγ stimulate the differentiation of the preadipocites in adipocites, which generates in this cell an increase in the insulin receptors, reducing of this one way the resistance to the insulin (Rodríguez et al., 2005; Sánchez, 2009). Another ω-3 FA action mechanism is the protection of the beta pancreatic cells of the damage caused by the increase in free radicals produced during the diabetes (Rodríguez, et al., 2005; Sánchez, 2009).

Though not all the results agree, sufficient information exists at present to do some considerations. Since the administration of concentrates of fish oil (EPA/DHA) like dietetic supplement in diabetic patients will depend on the daily dose of the same one, one has indicated that high doses (7.5g/d) raise the glucose fasting; while low doses (4g/d) do not modify it; for what exists those who propose its use only in diabetics with hypertriglyceridemia (Nasiff-Hadad, 2003).

The American Diabetes Association recommends that the concentrate of fish oil in the diet of the diabetic patients with severe hypertriglyceridemia must do to with medical and dietetic supervision and not to must be established as a recommendation in general for diabetic patients (Nasiff-Hadad, 2003).

Omega-3 Fatty Acids and Plasmatic Lipids

Omega-3 fatty acids decrease the very low density lipoproteins (VLDLc) and the triglycerides of the plasma both in normal subjects and in the hypertriglyceridemic patients and suppress the postprandial lipidemia represented by the remaining kilomicron so much for the fat rich diets as for the carbohydrates rich ones, both considered atherogenic. The effects on the low density lipoproteins (LDLc) and the high density lipoproteins (HDLc) are variable (Nasiff-Hadad, 2003). It thinks that an approximate ingestion of 700mg/d decrease significantly the plasmatic levels of the low density lipoproteins (LDL) and of the very low density lipoproteins (VLDL) (Sidhu, 2003).

HDLc generally does not change. This effect is dose dependent in relation with the TG and with the VLDLc. The reduction of the hypertriglyceridemia will be major as major is the basal level of triglycerides, so much when they administer low doses of ω-3 FA during long time like when there offers the unique very high dose (Nasiff-Hadad, 2003).

The mechanism for which ω-3 FA reduces the hypetriglyceridemia it is multiple: decrease of the lipogenesis due to the reduction of TG hepatic synthesis, increase of plasmatic clearance and across the preoxisome proliferator-activated receptors (PPAR) (Nasiff-Hadad, 2003; Sanchez, 2009).

Omega-3 fatty acids also realize its effect in the lipids metabolism increasing the transcription of the uncoupling protein 3 (UCP3), inducing genes that they codify for proteins involved in FA oxidation such as carnitine palmitoyl transferase, diacylglycerol-acyltransferase and the acyl-CoA oxidase), and the same time it decreases the transcription of genes that they codify for proteins involved for synthesis of lipids (Rodríguez et al., 2005; Sánchez, 2009).

Omega-3 Fatty Acids and Obesity

Have they proposed different mechanisms for which ω-3 FA can be late or control the development of obesity. Omega-3 FA are negative regulators of the hepatic lipogenesis, which is half-full for the repression of SREBP-1(Rodríguez et al., 2005). Omega-3 FA improves the biochemical and metabolic alterations associated with the obesity, such as the hepatic estheatosis and insulin resistance, besides the ω-3 FA oxidizes faster that saturated FA since they have the special characteristic of increasing the thermogenesis and as consequence they reduce the efficiency of depositing the corporal fat (Clarke, 2001; Rodríguez et al., 2005).

Omega-3 Fatty Acids and Coronary Disease

There has been described that ω-3 FA present antiatherogenic and antithrombotic activity, due to its role in the decrease of cholesterol levels and triglycerides in plasma (Sidhu, 2003). The antithrombotic effects are to the inhibition of the thromboxan A_2 (TXA_2) production, the prostaglandin I2 (PGI2) preservation and the fibrinogen reductive action, close to the increase of the plasminogen (Sanchez, 2009).

It describes antisclerotic action on having improved the availability of the nitric oxide of endothelial origin and the decrease and synthesis of the cellular adhesion as well as that of the inflammatory activity of the atherosclerotic plate (Sanchez, 2009).

Has been observed that in patients who consume EPA and DHA proceeding of fish, the proportion of risk of fatal and no fatal heart attack, and of sudden death it was significantly lower for the consumption of these fatty acids, surely due to the impact that they have in the decrease of the arterial pressure, the platelet aggregation, the arrhythmias sensibility, the triglycerides levels and the variable effects on the HDL and LDL (Molina de Salazar, 2009).

Omega-3 Fatty Acids and High Blood Pressure

The omega-3 fatty acids effects in hypertense patients have been studied in several clinical essays (Nasiff-Hadad, 2003). On the cardiovascular system, they provide improvement in the ejection fraction of the left ventricle, decrease of the sensibility of the baro-receptors with lower hypertensive response and stabilization of the heart electrical activity which demonstrates as an antiarrhythmic property and of reduction of the sudden death risk (Sanchez, 2009).

Though ω-3 FA reduces the arterial moderate pressure, in occasions only associated in changes of life styles, one has indicated that in some individuals increases the risk of apoplexy for arterial hypertension for the consumption of concentrated fish oils, provoking a excessive vasopressor response mediated by catecholamines. It has been suggested that the fish oil produces increase of the arterial compliance and of the baroreceptors response, besides a major production of eicosanoids vasodilators and platelet antiaggregants. Omega-3 fatty acids contents in the concentrates of fish oil, can use in lower doses of 3g diaries as helping therapeutics to the medicaments to reduce the levels of arterial pressure in hypertense persons (Nasiff-Hadad, 2003).

Though the dietetic increase of the blue meat fish overcomes these benefits (Nasiff-Hadad, 2003). The American Heart Association informs as mechanisms of cardioprotección about the omega-3 fatty acids, the following functions:

- Diminution arrhythmias risk
- Diminution of thrombosis risk, which drives to offset the cerebro-vascular accident
- Reduction circulating levels of triglycerides and LDL lipoproteins
- Decrease of atherosclerotic plaque thickness
- Endotelial function improvement
- Increase of coagulation time
- Decrease of leukocytes polimorfonucleares chemotaxis
- Reduction of the inflammatory response (Molina de Salazar, 2009).

Omega-3 Fatty Acids and High Hemostasie

Does inverse relation exist among ω-3 FA consumption and the fibrinogen, VIII factor, and Von Willebrand's factor and does positive association with the protein C reactive, nevertheless the best ω-3 effect demonstrated in the hemostasie, it is like a regulator of the platelets in biochemical or physical damages and decreases the platelet aggregation for several mechanisms: modulation of platelet prostaglandin synthesis, inhibition of proliferative vascular response happened by macrophages or citoquines, and it increases the activity of endothelium relaxing factor, all that basically for the substitution of arachidonic acid for EPA and DHA in the membrane phospholipids (Nasiff-Hadad, 2003).

With the supplement of ω-3 there seems to be a reduction of some hemostatic factors and of the plasma protombotic activity; nevertheless, a proinflamatory activity increase has been detected expressed by increase of adhesion molecules and e-selectina and the cellular vacular adhesion molecule-1, result of the increase of the lipidic peroxidation, as well as also there has been verified increase of the IL6 and TNF-alpha, which increases the proinflamatory activity (Nasiff-Hadad, 2003).

Omega-3 Fatty Acids and Rheumatoid Arthritis

There has been demonstrated that ω-3 FA, can have a role inside the control of the artritis reumatoide (Sidhu, 2003).

Since patients treated with ω-3 FA supplements refers decrease and relief of their symptoms, beside presenting a decrease in the neutrofils chimiluminescence after the treatment (Sidhu, 2003).

Omega-3 Fatty Acids and Cancer

The quantity and the type of the diet fat can be important in the development of the human cancer. Epidemiological evidences suggest that ω-3 FA ingestion abundant ones in the fish oil, have benefit effects in the cancer. There are not known exactly the biochemical mechanisms for which ω-3 FA disable the cellular development in some tumors (Rodríguez et al., 2003).

Nevertheless studies realized in rodents and in tumour cells of the human being, they have proposed some hypotheses that involve different routes of signaling:

1. The DHA induces the arrest of the cellular cycle due to the dephosphorylation of the pRB1 protein, that is in active form and stops the cellular cycle. In addition, the DHA promotes the apoptosis of cellular human lines of pancreas cancer and leukaemia.
2. Omega-3 fatty acids are cytotoxic for certain tumour in vitro cells, this cytotoxic action can be related to the peroxidation of its double links, which generates a persistently oxidative stress due to the increase in the production of free radicals, which damage the DNA.
3. Omega-3 FA of the diet suppress the cellular growth of the tumor across the inhibition of the cyclo-oxygenase, enzyme that regulates the prostaglandins synthesis(PGs) (Rodríguez et al., 2003).

By there has been demonstrated that its consumption decreases the risk of beast, digestive tract (colon) and prostate cancer (Nasiff-Hadad, 2003; Rodríguez et al., 2003).

Other Effects of Ω-3 Fatty Acids

Omega-3 fatty acids have assumed antiarrhythmic effects, because indicated to cardiopathies it reduces the risk of heart failure. An increase of the seric aminotransferase activity has been observed during the supplement of fish oils, as well as airways antiinflammatory effect. The consumption of EPA/DHA high concentrations for a long period can drive to hypervitaminosis A or D (Nasiff-Hadadm 2003).

Toxicity Associated with the Consumption of Fish Oil

The potential risks against health associated with the consumption of fish oil (mainly in capsules) are in the following table:

Table 9. Side effects of fish oil

General	Gastrointestinal discomfort
Coagulation	Increase of bled time such as: epistaxis
Metabolism	It can raise theblood levels of cholestero with secondary hyperlipidemia
	It can increase the caloric ingestion with the consistent ponderal profit
Immune Response	Variable decrease of some parameters
Toxicity	Associated with the excess of vitamin A and D.
	Some types of fish oil can contain contaminants
Cost	Costlier in comparison with the ingestion of fish

SOURCE : Modificated for Sidhu, 2003.

The major health risks associated with the ingestion of fish oil are in first place the tisular damage due to a decrease of antioxidant as the vitamin E and the presence of profusely bled, demonstrating for example like epistaxis (Eritsland, 2000; Sidhu, 2003).

Environmental liposolubles contaminants exist, manage to concentrate inside the adipose fish tissue for bioaccumulation and biomagnification processes, hereby there exist potential health risks associated with the consumption of fish and its derivatives, these principally associated with carcinogenic environmental contaminants (DDT, dieldrin, heptachlor, PCBs, dioxines, etc.) and not carcinogenics (like methyl mercury) (Eritsland, 2000; Sidhu, 2003).

Conclusion

The information included in the present document, demonstrates that the consumption of fish oil is advisable for the human health, due to the fact that it helps to anticipate diverse diseases, for its content in omega 3 fatty acids, but in spite of the fact that diverse sources exist for the obtaining of this type of fatty acids as,like are the fish oil, the linseed and some nuts, the best omega 3 fatty acids are in the fish oil due to the fact that they are in the shape of 2 essential fatty acids for the human being like DHA and EPA. These acids fatty are key to help to anticipate the heart disease, cancer and other diseases, besides which the brain depends largely of one DHA good supply to avoid disorders such as depression, schizophrenia and alzheimer.

References

[1] Adamkin D. (2007). Controversias en nutrición neonatal: ácido docosahexanoico (DHA) y nucleótidos. *J Perinatology.,* 27: S79-S82.

[2] Anderson M., Fritsche K. (n-3) Fatty Acids and Infectious Disease Resistance. *J Nutr.* 2002;132: 3566-3576.

[3] Campoy C., Cabero L., Sanjurjo P., Serra-Majem L., Anadón A., Morán J., Fraga J. (2010). Actualización, recomendaciones y consenso sobre el papel de los ácidos grasos poli insaturados de cadena larga en la gestación, lactancia y primer año de vida. *Med Clin (Barc).* 135(2):75-82.

[4] Carrero J., Martín E., Baró L., Fonolla J., Jiménez J., Boza J., López E. (2005). Efectos cardiovasculares de los ácidos grasos omega-3 y alternativas para incrementar su ingesta. *Nutrición Hopsitalaria.* 20(1): 63-69.

[5] Castro M. (2002). Ácidos grasos omega 3: Beneficios y fuentes. *Interciencia.*27(3): 128-136.

[6] Cheatham C., Colombo J., Carlson S. (2006). N-3 Fatty acids and cognitive and visual acuity development: methodologic and conceptual considerations. *Am J Clin Nutr.* 83(suppl): 1458S-1466S.

[7] Clarke S. *2001.* Polyunsaturated Fatty Acid Regulation of Gene Transcription: A Molecular Mechanism to Improve the metabolic Syndrome. *J Nutr.* 131: 1129-1132.

[8] Conchillo A., Valencia I., Puente A., Ansorena D., Astiasarán L. (2006). Componentes funcionales en aceites de pescado y de alga. *Nutrición Hospitalaria.* 21(3): 369-373.

[9] Coronado M., Vega y León S., Gutiérrez R., García B., Díaz G. (2006). Los Ácidos grasos Omega-3 y Omega-6: Nutrición, Bioquímica y Salud. *REB.* 25(3): 72-79.

[10] De Busk R, Hart JA, Kracoff G, Ottariano S (2004) (Review). Maryland Medical Center Programs.

[11] Eritsland J. 2000. Safety considerations of polyunsaturated fatty acids. *Am J Clin Nutr.* 71 Suppl 1: 197S-201S.

[12] FAO State of World Fisheries and Aquaculture (2010).

[13] Gottrand E. Long-Chain Polyunsaturated Fatty Acids Influence the Immune System of Infants. *J Nutr.* 2008; 138(Suppl): 18907S-1812S.

[14] Gylling H, Miettinen T (2001) A review of clinical trials in dietary interventions to decrease the incidence of coronaryartery disease. *Curr Contr Trials C.* 2:123-128.

[15] Hardman WE (2002) Omega-3 fatty acids to augment cancer therapy. Symposium International Conference on food, nutrition & cancer July 11-12 Washington.

[16] Haschke-Becher E., Fazzolari-Noesci A., Minoli I., Räihä N., Carrié A-L., Haschke F., Bachman C., (2001). Perfiles de ácidos grasos en lactante alimentados con formulas suplmenmetadas con ácidos grasos poli insaturados de cadena larga. *Nestlé Nutrition Workshop Series. Pediatric Program.*, 47(S): 49-53.

[17] Hu F, Cho E, Rexrode K, Albert Ch, Manson J (2003) Fish and long chain w-3 fatty acid intake and risk of coronary heart disease and total mortality in diabetic woman. Circulation 107:1852-1857.

[18] Innis S (2003). Metabolismo lipídico del lactante prematuro. *Pediatrics in review en español.*24(7): 256-265.

[19] Innis S. (2003). Perinatal biochemistry and physiology of long-chain polyunsaturated fatty acids. *J Pediatr.* 143: S1-S8.

[20] Jenkins D., Sievenpiper J., Pauly D., Rashid U., Kendal C., Mowat F. (2009). Are dietary recommendations for the use of fish oils sustainable?. *CMAJ.*180(6): 633-637.

[21] Judge M., Harel O., Lammi-Keefe C (2007). Maternal consumption of a docosaheaenoic acid-containing functional food during pregnancy: benefit for infant performance on problem-solving but not on recognition memory tasks at age 9 mo. *Am J Clin Nutr.* 85: 1572-1577.

[22] Koletzko B., Agostoni C., Carlson S.E., Clandinin T., Hornstra G., Neuringer M., Uuay R., Yamashiro Y., Willatts. M. (2001). Long chain polyunsaturated fatty acids (LC-PUFA) and perinatal development. *Acta Pediatr.* 90: 460-464.

[23] Larqué E., Zamora S., Gil A.(2001). Dietary trans fatty acids in early life: a review. *Early Human Development.* 65 (Suppl): S31-S41.

[24] Mantzioris E, Cleland LG, Gibson R, Neumann M, Demasi M, James M (2000) Biochemical effects of a diet containing foods enriched with n-3 fatty acids. Amm J Clin Nutr 72:42-48.

[25] McGregor J., Carlson S., Hobel C., Mei S., Ogburn P.(2003). Nutritional roles of omega-3 fatty acids during pregnancy and neonatal development. *OBG Management.* Dowden Health Media Inc. (Suppl):S1-S12.

[26] Mc Namara R., Carlson S.(2006). Role of omega-3 fatty acids in brain development and function: Potential implications for the pathogenesis and prevention of psychopathology. Prostaglandins, Leukotrienes and Essential Fatty Acids. 75(4): 329-349.

[27] Merchán A. (2009). Evidencia clínica de las formas farmacéuticas de ácidos grasos omega-3 en prevención secundaria. *Revista Colombiana de Cardiología.* 16(Suppl 1). 14-17.

[28] Mitmesser S., Jensen C.(2006). Roles of Long-Chain Polyunsaturated Fatty Acids in the Term Infant: developmental Benefits. *Neonatal network: The Journal of Neonatal Nursing.* 26(4): 229-234.

[29] Molina de Salazar D. (2009). Evidencia clínica de los ácidos grasos omega-3 procedentes de los peces en prevención primaria y secundaria. *Revista Colombiana de Cardiología.* 16(Suppl 1). 9-11.

[30] Morris G., Moorcraft J., Mountjoy A., Wells J.C.K.(2000). A novel infant formula milk with added long-chain polyunsaturated fatty acids from single-cel sources: a study of growth, satisfaction and health. *European Journal of Clinical Nutrition.* 54: 883-886.

[31] Nasiff-Hadad A. (2003). Ácidos grados omega-3: Pescados de carne azul y concentrados de aceites de pescado. Lo bueno y lo malo. *Rev. Cubana Med.* 42(2). 49-55.

[32] Rodríguez M., Tovar A., del Prado M., Torres N. (2005) Mecanismos moleculares de acción de los ácidos grasos poli insaturados y sus beneficios en la salud. *Revista de Investigación Clínica.* 57(3). 157-172.

[33] Rosenfeld E., Beyerlein A., Hadders-Algra M., Kennedy K., Singhal A., Fewtrell M., Lucas A., Koletzko B., Von Kies R.(2009) IPD meta-analysis shows no effect of LC-PUFA supplementation on infant growth at 18 months. *Acta Paediatrica.* 98: 91-97.

[34] Sánchez G. (2009). ¿Qué son los ácidos grasos omega-3?. *Revista Colombiana de Cardiología.* 16(Suppl 1): 5-6.

[35] Sanhueza J., Nieto S., Valenzuela A.,(2004). Ácido docosahexaenoico (DHA), el desarrollo cerebral, memoria y aprendizaje: La importancia de la suplementación perinatal. *Rev Chil Nutr.,* 31(2): 1-15.

[36] Sargent R. (1997). Fish oils and human diet. *British Journal of Nutrition.* 78 (Suppl I): S5-S13.

[37] Sidhu K. (2003). Health benefits and potencial risks related to consumption of fish or fish oil. *Regulatory Toxicology and Pharmacology.*38: 336-344.

[38] Simopoulos A. (1989). Summary of the NATO Advance3d Research Workshop on Dietary ω· and ω6 Fatty Acids: Biological Effects and Nutritional Essentiality. *J Nutr.* 119: 521-528.

[39] Sindelar C, Scheerger S, Plugge Sh, Eskridge K, Wander R, Lewis N (2004) Serum lipids of physically active adults consuming omega-3 fatty acid enriched eggs or conventional eggs. Nut Res 24:731-739.

[40] Stoll AL, Locke CA, Marangell LB, Severus WE (1999) Omega-3 fatty acids and bipolar disorder: a review. Prostag Leukotr Ess 60:329-337.

[41] Uauy F.R., Dangour A.(2006). Nutrition in Brain Development and Aging: Role of Essential Fatty Acids. *Nutrition Reviews.* 64(5): S24-S33.

[42] Valenzuela A., Nieto S., Sanhueza J., Morgado N., Rojas I., Zañartu P., (2010). Supplementing female rats with DHA-lysophosphatidylcholine increases docosahexaenoic acid and acetylcholine contents in the brain and improves the memory and learning capabilities of the pups. *Grasas y aceites.* 61(1): 16-23.

[43] Valenzuela A., Nieto S. (2003). Ácidos grasos omega-6 y omega-3 en la nutrición perinatal: su importancia en el desarrollo del sistema nervioso y visual. *Rev., Chil. Pediatr.* 74(2): 149-157.

[44] Valenzuela A., Nieto S., (2001). Ácido dosahexaenoico (DHA) en el desarrollo fetal y en la nutrición materno-infantil. *Rev Med Chile.*, 129(10):1-14

In: Fish Oil: Production, Consumption and Health Benefits
Editors: Matthias Van Dijk and Jürgen Vitek
ISBN: 978-1-61470-963-3

Chapter XVII

The Role of Omega-3 in the Development of the Brain and Obesity

***Maria Luisa Forchielli**[*a] **and W. Allan Walker**[b]*
[a]Department of Pediatrics, University of Bologna, Italy
[b]Nutrition Division, Harvard Medical School, Boston, MA, U. S.

Abstract

The n-6 or omega 6 series [i.e. arachidonic acid (AA)] and the n-3 or omega-3 polyunsaturated fatty acids (n-3 PUFA), and particularly the long chain highly unsaturated ones (LC PUFA) [i.e. eicosapentaenoic and docosahexaenoic acid (EPA and DHA)], are essential for humans and work sometimes in synergy and sometimes in competition. Today, their role has been recognized as not only mere caloric, but with effects in cell differentiation and communication through a deep modulation to the cell core involved in gene regulation. These effects occur in all of the body systems and organs, but with different outcomes depending on local or systemic inputs. Therefore, during fetal and neonatal development, LC PUFA contribute to growth and evolution, while, during inflammation, they orchestrate various functions of cells. Many disease conditions develop from inflammation. Obesity and metabolic syndrome are two examples in which diet and the hormonal milieu may disrupt multiple cells with the release of cytokines. In the case of chronic stimuli, body metabolism changes. LC PUFA again, prove to be a potent tool to reverse or enhance these changes. In this chapter, we want to focus on the effects of n-3 PUFA with regard to brain development and obesity.

Keywords: obesity, omega-3, brain development.

* Corresponding author: Maria Luisa Forchielli, M.D., MPH, FACG, Assistant Professor of Pediatrics, Dept Pediatrics, University of Bologna, Italy, luisa.forchielli@unibo.it

Glossary

PUFA:	polyunsaturated fatty acids
LC PUFA:	long chain polyunsaturated fatty acids
AA:	arachidonic acid
EPA:	eicosapentaenoic acid
DHA:	docosahexaenoic acid
LNA:	alpha linolenic acid
LA:	linoleic acid
DPA:	docosapentaenoic acid
DHGLA:	homo-gammalinolenic acid
FADS1:	fatty acid desaturase 1
FADS2:	fatty acid desaturase 2
IQ:	intelligence quotient
COX:	cyclooxygenase
LO:	lipooxygenase
EFA:	essential fatty acid
PPAR:	peroxisome proliferator-activated receptor
BMI:	body mass index
TNF:	tumor necrosis factor

Introduction

The n-3 or omega-3 polyunsaturated fatty acids (n-3 PUFA), and particularly the long chain highly unsaturated ones (LC PUFA), i.e. eicosapentaenoic and docosahexaenoic acid (EPA and DHA), together with LC PUFA of the n-6 or omega 6 series [i.e. arachidonic acid (AA)], are found in appreciable concentrations in the structural membranes of highly specialized organs and systems. n-3 PUFA compounds, especially DHA, are particularly present in cell membranes endowed with highly developed functional activities (e.g. excitable and contractile cells). Through coordinated and sometimes antagonistic interactions with AA, n-3 PUFA modulate several key cellular functions (e.g., receptor activators, lipid mediators, ion channels, gene expression).

Unlike omega 6, omega 3 and especially EPA and DHA, are present in very low concentrations in our diets, being almost exclusively provided by fish and aquatic organisms, while their metabolic precursor Alpha Linolenic Acid (LNA) is present only in selected oils and plant food and is not effectively converted in the body to the LC n-3 PUFA. This is in contrast to the efficient conversion of the very abundant Linoleic Acid (LA) to AA in the omega 6 series.

The omega 3 series has been found to provide benefits in multiple diseases including heart disease, cystic fibrosis, some inborn errors of metabolism, Crohn's disease, metabolic syndrome and obesity, diabetes, arthritis, osteoporosis, and cognitive impairments such as attention deficit disorders, mood disorders, and senile dementia [1]. Finally, supplementation during pregnancy and especially during the perinatal period are two areas in which much intensive research is being devoted following a well-defined, positive correlation between an adequate preventive supplementation of omega 3 and appropriate mental, neurologic, and visual development of the offspring.

Overall, the beneficial role of omega 3 occurs through a direct incorporation into cell membranes and through the production of metabolites (prostaglandins and leukotrienes) which reduce the negative effects of stress-induced inflammation. The inflammatory response is modulated by both pro- or anti-inflammatory reactions depending on which LC PUFA form is supplemented. In particular, the omega 6 series preferentially reinforces inflammation, while the omega 3 series inhibits it [2]. From a biochemical perspective, prostaglandins, a derivative of LC PUFA, may play a critical role in adipocyte differentiation.

This paper intends to review the role of omega 3 during the neural development of children and its effects on inflammatory conditions such as obesity.

Omega-3 and the Human Brain

N-3 PUFA are present in all cell membranes but at different concentrations. For adequate development and function, high concentrations of DHA (without LNA and EPA) and PUFA's in general are stored in the cerebral cortex and retina [3].

The human fetal brain stores DHA exponentially in the last trimester [4,5] and at a lower rate until at least 2 years of age. The ratio of omega-6 to omega-3 is typically between 5-10:1, even if it is reckoned to be less than 4:1 recently. Based on dry weight of the human brain, it has been determined that 22% of the cerebral cortex and 24% of white matter are composed of phospholipids. In the presence of a lowered DHA level in the brain, a parallel increase in linoleic acid (18:2n-6) and docosapentaenoic acid (DPA, 22:5 n-6) occurs.

Breast milk shows relatively constant PUFA concentration in the first year of life with an AA:DHA ratio of 2:1. Colostrum has double quantities of AA and DHA with respect of mature milk: 1% and 0.5% (14-15 mg/dL) of AA, and 0.5% and 0.25% (7-8 mg/dL) of DHA, respectively. Later, in a group of Italian infants nursed by their mothers for 12 months, the median AA intake increased from 11.3 mg/kg in colostrum to 24 mg/kg at 1 month and decreased to 16 mg/kg at 3 months, while DHA intake was 6.8 mg/kg in colostrum at day 1, 11.7 mg/kg in mature hindmilk at 1 month, and 7.3 mg/kg at 3 months. During the first year of life in these infants, both AA and DHA levels remained constant, whereas LA and LNA along with total fat and total saturated fat, increased progressively [6]. In this cohort, the Mediterranean diet of mothers may have influenced the fatty acid profile through a generous oleic acid intake.

Historically, breast milk has been the perfect vehicle for DHA. In infants with sudden death who were divided into two groups based on the type of feeding received, those fed formula without DHA and AA showed a significantly lower mean weight content of DHA in their brain cortex and red blood cells than those fed human milk. No differences were found in the retina. Cortical DHA increased with age in breast-fed infants, while it remained constant in the formula-fed infants in whom the DHA homologues (22:4n-6 and 22:5 n-6) were more represented. The percentage of DHA in red blood cells was considered a marker for DHA brain content due to a high correlation. No differences were detected for AA content in the retina and brain in both groups. AA cortex concentration was dependent on age in a saturable hyperbolic manner, regardless of diet. The actual effect of diet, however, was likely to be underestimated due to the methodological choice of determining total lipids instead of phospholipids [7]. Today, most formulas are enriched with DHA resulting in levels similar to those of breast fed infants.

DHA content of human breast milk is influenced by several factors such as maternal diet, number of pregnancies, gestational age, smoking, and especially endogenous metabolism. Smoking mothers have lower total fat, PUFA and DHA content in their milk. The reduction of PUFA is also correlated to lower anthropometric measurements (length, head circumference), lower levels of DHA, AA, and homo-gammalinolenic acid (DHGLA), and higher LA and LNA levels in infants born to smokers for the entire pregnancy. The increase in LA and LNA stems from a decrease in the conversion of essential to bioactive PUFA: 18% for LA to AA, 50% for LNA to EPA, and 20% for LNA to DHA [8]. Inter-individual variation plays an important role in endogenous synthesis of LC PUFA. Genetic variants of the fatty acid desaturase 1 (FADS1) and fatty acid desaturase 2 (FADS2) gene cluster, encoding for the delta-5 and delta-6 desaturases (key enzymes in LC PUFA metabolism), influence omega-3 and omega-6 fatty acid status in mothers and children. Evidence that breast milk, produced by mothers on different nutritional regimens, showed analogous content of omega-3 and omega-6 [9] and suggests that the amount of dietary fat intake cannot accurately predict the levels of LC PUFA in serum, plasma or cell membrane phospholipids needed to achieve biological effects [10]. Thus, different combinations of minor genetic alleles may alter the LC PUFA plasma profile (e.g. lower AA and EPA levels along with higher LA or lower AA, EPA and DHA).

Omega-3 and Intellectual Development in Children

LNA and DHA, alone or in combination with LA, are implicated in the cognitive development of animals and humans in health and disease (11-16). Neurodegenerative diseases seem to lack DHA which, once restored to physiological levels, improves the patient's learning performance. In breast fed infants, many studies, including a meta-analysis of non-randomized trials, have shown a correlation between LC PUFA and an enhanced mental development with a 5-6 Intelligence Quotient (IQ) point increase (reduced by two points when significant variables were controlled for), improved visual acuity and attention span, and a better neural development during childhood and adolescence when compared to those fed formula devoid of LC PUFA [17-22]. After the marketing of formulas with DHA, the effects on visual acuity and development of full term infants receiving these formulas showed similar results although discrepancies existed [23-25]. In a prospective cohort of full term breast-fed infants, DHA levels were related to the development of visual acuity and the progression of language (34). This association was clearly demonstrated at 2 and 12 months of age. Consistent with the assumption that acuity precedes speech, those infants with higher DHA levels at 2 months were better able to differentiate syllables in both native and non-native languages at 6 and 8 months, and evolved toward a reorganization of their perceptions with recognition of their native language by 10-12 months. Growth was significantly and inversely correlated to the red-cell DHA level at 6 months, but not at 12 months. There was an inverse correlation between omega-3 fatty acids and growth at 6 months supporting the evidence that omega-3 may be involved with metabolic programming. A comment is needed on these studies and relates to the iron content present in all of the formulas. It is well known that iron has a high impact on cognitive performance. Although the association between iron status and cognitive performance has only been examined in anemic children, early supplementation is likely to have contributed to the observed outcomes.

Our knowledge on the effects of LC PUFA has improved after studies conducted during the perinatal period confirmed the benefits of DHA during the entire course of life. A study was conducted on children breast fed by mothers receiving either 10 ml/d cod liver oil (1183mg/10 ml DHA, 803 mg/10 ml EPA, and 2494 mg/ 10 ml total omega-3) or omega-6 (corn oil containing 4747 mg/10 ml LA, 92 mg/10 ml LNA) [27]. Those born to mothers receiving cod liver oil showed higher mental processing scores at 4 years of age. These mental processing scores correlated significantly with maternal intake of DHA and EPA during pregnancy, with head circumference at birth, but not with birth weight or length. The only variable that significantly mattered for children's IQ was the maternal intake of DHA during pregnancy. Breast milk of mothers receiving cod liver oil had 270% more DHA and 88% less AA than breast milk of mothers on corn oil. It should be mentioned, however, that some children spontaneously received cod liver oil at 3 months of age due to local feeding guidelines. This bias factor was apparently homogeneously distributed across both groups. In another study assessing the long-term effect on visual development of omega-3 exposure during pregnancy, the beneficial effects of DHA on visual acuity and color processing persisted in the Inuit children aged 11-13 years at no cost of higher exposure of contaminants typical of that area. Of note, visual acuity strongly correlated to cord DHA, which was higher than the mean maternal plasma DHA level, suggesting a preferential transfer of DHA to the fetus [28].

If reaching an appropriate DHA level is an issue for term infants, more DHA storage problems are expected in pre-term infants. A number of clinical trials have compared functional outcomes in pre-term infants fed diets with and without DHA and it is clear that pre-term infants need to be appropriately supplemented to favor a normal development of visual and mental functions. Of these studies, two are particularly relevant with regard to sample size and study design. In the first study, performed in 427 pre-term infants divided into three groups receiving (i) formula enriched with DHA (0.25% of total fat) and AA (0.4%) from egg phospholipids, (ii) DHA (0.25% of total fat) and AA (0.4%) from fungal oil, and (iii) control formula (DHA accounting for 0.15% of total fat), a visual acuity test was significantly better in the supplemented groups at 2, 4 and 6 months of age. No difference existed in other developmental performance tests in all three groups [29]. Supplemented pre-term infants in a birth weight category below 1250 g had better scores in mental development scales at 12 months of age. In the second similar study, pre-term infants were nourished by two different formulas (one supplemented by DHA from fish and AA from fungi, the second by DHA from alga and AA from fungi) and compared with controls on a standard formula. Those receiving either form of DHA showed an improved mental and psychomotor development at 18 months of age, even though the full term breast-fed infants had a higher DHA level [30]. Recently, in a study of fifty-one pre-term infants (gestational age range 24-36w) receiving breast milk until their term age or until they were one month of age, early development was negatively associated with omega-6 and mead acid while positively associated with omega-3 intake. Of note, increases in infants' plasma EPA levels seemed to confer autonomic stability. Increases in LA levels in mothers' plasma and AA in breast milk seemed to worsen the infants' orientation, whereas an increase in Mead acid in breast milk seemed to reduce general movement activity. In this group of infants, the longer they were breast fed, the higher was their level of EPA. This level, in turn, correlated with the DHA levels [31].

The issue of breast feeding variability with regard to IQ test scores has been investigated implicating a genetic variation in fatty acid metabolism. After identifying specific gene alleles involved in breast feeding, it was clear that infants may or may not be able to use supplemented LC PUFA in order to improve their IQ. That has to do with genetic imprinting. Therefore, it seem possible that those children, defined with single nucleotide polymorphism C-carrier linked to the major alleles of FADS1 and FADS2, are better able to metabolize fatty acids and achieve higher IQ [32].

Omega-3 and Obesity

Activities from the molecular to the clinical level of omega-3 have not yet been completely understood. However, LC PUFA have long been associated with obesity mainly through inflammation and gene regulation. During their chemical transformation, LC PUFA are metabolized by specific enzymes (cyclooxygenase or COX, lipooxygenase or LO, and monooxygenase-cytP450) and produce two by-product categories: eicosanoids from AA and docosanoids from DHA and EPA. Eicosanoids consist of prostaglandins (PG1, PG2, and PG3 series), leukotrienes, thromboxanes, all modulating an inflammatory response, and lipoxin with typical anti-inflammatory characteristics. DHA and EPA produce resolvins and protectins. Originally identified as neuroprotectins with paracrine action in the brain, protectins have been recognized to have systemic effects. Prostaglandins and leukotrienes seem to be involved in the early phases of inflammation, whereas resolvins, protectins, and lipoxins exist as second-line mediators to suppress active inflammation, to remove inflammatory cells and to restore tissue integrity. Lipoxins send inhibitory signals to leukocytes, promote resolution of damaged tissues and reduce fibrosis by acting on macrophages and monocytes [33]. All of the lipid mediators are functionally active in acute and chronic processes. Since omega-3 and omega-6 have common metabolic pathways, their ratio should be preserved through a balanced intake. Thus, the global burden of obesity and metabolic syndrome has to do in part with an omega-3 and omega-6 imbalanced intake. Diet in western countries has changed slowly shifting from higher intake of saturated and monounsaturated fatty acids from animal and plant fat to a higher intake of omega-6 from refined vegetable fat. It is also possible that LA requirements may have been overestimated by a need for more omega-6 assumed to prevent or correct essential fatty acid (EFA) deficiency than the amount specifically required to reintegrate a singular omega-6 fatty acid. This is even more evident in the presence of a concomitant lack of omega-3, which is protective toward the EFA deficiency [34]. Today, LC PUFA intakes consist almost entirely of LA (80-90%) and the remaining intake from EPA, DHA. This trend seems to have been continued onto new generations with fetal and infant blood and tissue lipid profiles mimicking that same ratio. Brain tissue of infants receiving a high quantity of omega-6, reverses its fat profile and predominantly stores LA and AA at the expenses of DHA. Adipose tissue also seems to be a LA repository within 7 weeks of starting a formula with an increased quantity of LA. Different was the time required by elderly people to reach a stable LA storage level. They required over 3 years after doubling their fat intake. From generation to generation, adipose tissue has tended to become hyperplastic and hypertrophic and loses its influence on metabolic and neuroendocrine pathways [35]. Four generations seem to be required to reach that level. AA more than short-chain or monounsaturated fatty acids, is a potent stimulator of adipogenesis both in pre-adipocytes and immature adipocytes via a surface prostacyclin receptor and the nuclear peroxisome proliferator-activated receptor gamma (PPARγ). Once stimulated, adipocytes are susceptible to altered programming. The fetal and neonatal periods are the most critical for altered programming. Diets, in which caloric and fat intakes have been inappropriate, change cells in various organs and expose infants to a higher risk of metabolic syndrome in adulthood [36]. Through interfering signals and angiogenetic dysfunctions, lower birth weight may lead to visceral obesity, while high birth weight correlates with higher body mass index (BMI) later in life [37,38]. Figure 1 summarizes this series of events.

Imbalanced Omega-6 omega-3 ratio intake (more AA than EPA and DHA)

↓

AA in preadipocytes and immature adipocytes

↓

Cytokines (IL1, IL6, TNF)

↓

Activation of surface prostacyclin receptor and nuclear peroxisome proliferator-activated receptor gamma

↓

Altered adipocyte programming

↓

Chronic inflammation and fibrosis

↓

High risk of metabolic syndrome

Figure 1. Summary of the main steps involved in adipogenesis.

Higher intake of omega-3, and in particular of EPA and DHA, may halt the metabolic derangements both in animal and in vitro studies and in human cell lines. These beneficial effects seem to be dose-dependent because the number of genes involved increases with the omega-3 dosage. High doses of EPA and DHA (1.8 gr/d), supplemented to elderly people for 26 weeks, were able to modify over a thousand genes responsible for the regulation of eicosanoid synthesis, interleukin and mitogen-activated protein kinase signaling, nuclear transcriptional factor function, toll-like receptors, cell adhesion, oxidative stress and liver retinoid receptors [39]. EPA and DHA can also reach the nucleus and bind to the peroxisome proliferator-activated receptor alpha (PPARα). PPARα functions in the upregulation of the genes devoted to lipid metabolism and the downregulation of the genes of inflammation. In murine cultured adipocytes, EPA was noted to reduce the pro-inflammatory cytokines released by adipocytes and was able to inhibit lipolysis improving insulin sensitization. It acted at the transcriptional level decreasing tumor-necrosis-factor(TNF)-alfa-induced nuclear factor-κβ and enhancing the AMP-kinase [40]. DHA also seems to inhibit adipogenesis via the blocking of prostaglandins' release by AA and the nuclear factor-κβ transcription of COX-2. Supplementations of 1.2 g/d DHA for 3 months to obese adolescents compared to a similar group receiving a placebo, led to an increase in the serum EPA by 191%, in the serum DHA by 34% with a general decrease in all of the omega-6 series. Following these increases, all of the major cytokines including IL6, IL1, TNF and c-reactive protein were reduced. Lymphocytes and monocytes and vascular function were ameliorated [41].

Interestingly, the same gene expression and regulation occurring in adipocytes with LC PUFA, can be obtained with a caloric restriction intervention in obese women [42]. Mechanisms seem to be analogous to EPA and DHA effect with the difference that genes regulating the synthesis of LC PUFA are suppressed by the restriction of energy supply. Again, these gene clusters involved in the LC PUFA synthesis are variants of the FADS1 and FADS2 genes. This observation may help us understand why animals on a low energy intake live longer.

One final thought is on the relation between DHA and EPA and animal proteins. DHA and EPA are made by aquatic plants and passed to fish and marine mammals. Fish is the main source of DHA and EPA for humans. Therefore, humans consume EPA and DHA, but, at the same time, also fish proteins. Pilon at al decided to verify whether different fish proteins had an influence on body weight, adiposity, inflammatory status and insulin sensitivity in high-fat-fed rats [43]. Rats were divided into five groups to receive proteins from casein, salmon, bonito, herring, mackerel. All of the fish groups had a reduction in inflammation (e.g. IL6, TNF) in visceral tissues, but the salmon group showed a lower weight gain and a better whole body insulin sensitivity compared to the other groups. The lower weight gain was attributed to the high content of salmon calcitonin, which appears to be an homolog of amylin, a pancreatic hormone regulating satiety and increasing weight loss. Inflammation, in turn, was believed to be blunted due to the rich content of taurine and glycine in fish protein. To further explain these results, the authors claimed that the omega-3 supplemented to these animals was almost insignificant as EPA and DHA were less than 0.8 and 1.2 mg/100g of diet, respectively. Thus if inflammation, obesity and metabolic programming are truly dependent on fish proteins, additional research will have to weight the benefits of a diet with more omega-3 or more fish protein or both.

A large body of evidence now exists to suggest that supplementation with LC PUFA is nutritionally feasible in all ages, although, as a word of caution, excessive intakes of Omega 3 can easily undergo oxidation due to their double bonds, which, in turn, may damage cellular membranes and tissues. Omega-3 and LC PUFA in general are necessary, but in nature, effects of one nutrient can rarely be often isolated as more than one contributor to that specific effect.

References

[1] Simopoulos AP. The importance of the omega-6/omega-3 fatty acid ration in cardiovascular disease and other chronic diseases. *Exp Biol Med* 2008;233:674-88.

[2] Serhan CN, Chiang N, Van dyke TE. Resolving inflammation: dual anti-inflammatory and pro-resolution lipid mediators. *Nature Reviews Immunology* 2008;8:349-61.

[3] Ballabriga A. Essential fatty acids and human tissue composition. An overview. *Acta Paediatr* 1994;402:S63-S68.

[4] Clandinin MT, Chappell JE, Leong S, Heim T, Swyer PR, Chance GW. Intrauterine fatty acid accretion rates in human brain: implications for fatty acid requirements. *Early Hum Dev* 1980;4:121–9.

[5] Martinez M. Developmental profiles of polyunsaturated fatty acids in the brain of normal infants and patients with peroxisomal diseases: severe deficiency of docosahexaenoic acid in Zellweger's and pseudo-Zellweger's syndromes. In Health Effects of Three Polyunsaturated Fatty Acids in Seafoods. *World Review on Nutrition Dietetics;* Simopoulos AP, Kifer RR, Martin RE, Barlow SM, Eds.; Karger: Basel 1991;Vol.66:87–102.

[6] Marangoni F, Agostoni C, Lammardo AM, Giovannini M, Gallli C, Riva E. Polyunsaturated fatty acid concentrations in human hindmilk are stable throughout 12-months of lactation and provide a sustained intake to the infant during exclusively breastfeeding: an Italian study. *Br J Nutr* 2000;84:103-9

[7] Makrides M, Neumann MA, Byard RW, Simmer K, Gibson RA. Fatty acid composition of brain, retina, and erythrocytes in breast- and formula-fed infants. *Am J Clin Nutr* 1994;60:189-94.

[8] Agostoni C, Riva E, Giovannini M, Pinto F, Colombo C, Rise' P, Galli C, Marangoni F. Maternal smoking habits are associated with differences in infants' long-chain polyunsaturated fatty acids in whole blood: a case-control study. *Arch Dis Child* 2008;93:414-8..

[9] Koletzko B, Mrotzek M, Bremer HJ. Fatty acid composition of mature human milk in Germany. *Am J Clin Nutr* 1988;47:954-9.

[10] Simopoulos AP. Genetic variants in the metabolism of omega-6 and omega-3 fatty acids: their role in the determination of nutritional requirements and chronic disease risk. *Exper Biol Med* 2010;235:785-95.

[11] Gamoh S, Hashimoto M, Sugioka K, Shahdat Hossain M, Hata N, Misawa Y, Masumura S. Chronic administration of docosahexaenoic acid improve reference memory-related learning ability in young rats. *Neuroscience* 1999;39: 237–241.

[12] Okaniwa Y, Yuasa S, Yamamoto N, Watanabe N, Kobayashi T, Okuyama H, Nomuras M, Nagata Y. A high linoleate and a high a-linolenate diet induced changes in learning behavior of rats. Effects of a shift and reversal of training stimuli. *Biol Pharm Bull* 1996;19:536–40.

[13] Carrie` I, Clement M, Javel A, Frances H, Bourre J-M. Phospholipid supplementation reverses behavioral and biochemical alterations induced by n-3 polyunsaturated fatty acid deficiency in mice. *J Lipid Res* 2000;41:473–80.

[14] Kalmjin S, Feskens EJM, Launer LJ, Kromhout D. Polyunsaturated fatty acids, antioxidants, and cognitive function in very old men. *Am J Epidemiol* 1997;145:33–41.

[15] Yehuda S, Rabinovitz S. Essential fatty acid preparations (SR-3) improves Alzheimer's patients quality of life. *Int J Neurosci* 1996; 87:141–149.

[16] Terano T, Fujishiro S, Ban T, Yamamoto K, Tanaka T, Noguchi Y, Tamura Y, Yazawa K, Hirayama T. Docosahexaenoic acid supplementation improves the moderately severe dementia from thrombotic cerebrovascular diseases. *Lipids* 1999;34 (suppl.):345–6.

[17] Fergusson DM, Beautrais AL, Silva PA. Breast feeding and cognitive development in the first seven years of life. *Soc Sci Med* 1982;16:1705-8.

[18] Rogan JM, Gladen BC. Breast feeding and cognitive development. *Early Hum Dev* 1993;31:181-93.

[19] Carlson SE, Ford AJ, Werkman SH, Peeples JM, Koo WWK. Visual acuity and fatty acid status of term infants fed human milk and formulas with and without docosahexaenoate and arachidonate from egg yolk lecithin. *Pediatr Res* 1996; 39:882–8.

[20] 20.Taylor B, Wadsworth J. Breast feeding and child development at five years. Dev *Med Child Neurol* 1984:26:73-80.

[21] Lanting CI, Fidler V, Huisman M, et al. Neurological differences between 9-year-old children fed breast-milk or formula-milk as babies. *Lancet* 1994;344:1319-22.

[22] Anderson JW, Johnston BM, Remley DT. Breast feeding and cognitive development: a meta-analysis. *Am J Clin Nutr* 1999;70:525-35.

[23] Birch EE, Hoffman DR, Uauy R, Birch DG, Prestidge C. Visual acuity and essentiality of docosahexaenoic acid in the diet of term infant. *Pediatr Res*1998;44:201-9.

[24] Lucas A, Stafford M, Morley R, Abbot R, Stephenson T, MacFayden U, et al. Efficacy and safety of long-chain polyunsaturated fatty acid supplementation of infant-formula milk: a randomized trial. *Lancet* 1999;354:1948-54.

[25] Makrides M, Neumann MA, Simmer K, Gibson RA. A critical appraisal of the role of dietary long-chain polyunsaturated fatty acids on neural indices of term infants: a randomized controlled trial. *Pediatrics* 2000;105:32-8.

[26] Innis SM, Gilley J, Werker J. Are human milk long-chain polyunsaturated fatty acids related to visual and neural development in breast-fed term infants? *J Pediatr* 2001;139:532-8.

[27] Helland IB, Smith L, Saarem K, Saugstad OD, Drevon CA. Maternal supplementation with very-long-chain n-3 fatty acids during pregnancy and lactation augments children's IQ at 4 years of age. *Pediatrics* 2003;111:e39-e44.

[28] Jacques C, Levy E, Muckle G et al. Long-term effects of prenatal omega-3 fatty acid intake on visual function in school-age children. *J Pediatr* 2011;158:83-90.

[29] O'Connor DL, Hall R, Admkin D, et al. Growth and development in pre-term infants fed long-chain polyunsaturated fatty acids: a prospective, randomized controlled trial. *Pediatrics* 2001;108:359-71.

[30] Clandinin MT, Van Aerde JE, Merkel KL, et al. Growth and development of pre-term infants fed infant formulas containing docosahexaenoic acid and arachidonic acid. *J Pediatr* 2005;146:461-8.

[31] Lundqvist-Persson C, Lau G, Nordin P, Strandvik B, Sabel KG. Early behavior and development in breast-fed premature infants are influenced by omega-6 and omega-3 fatty acid status. *Early Hum Development* 2010;86:407-12.

[32] Caspi A, Williams B, Kim-Cohen J, Craig IW, Milne BJ, Poulton R, Schalkwyk LC, Taylor A, Werts H, Moffitt TE. Moderation of breastfeeding effects on the IQ by genetic variation in fatty acid metabolism. *Proc Natl Acad Sci* 2007;104;18860-5.

[33] Serhan CN, Arita M, Hong S, Gotlinger K. Resolvins, docosatrienes, and neuroprotectins, novel omega-3 derived mediators, and their endogenous aspirin-triggered epimers. *Lipids* 2004;39;1125-32.

[34] Ailhaud G, Guesnet P, Cunnane SC. An emerging risk factor for obesity: does disequilibrium of polyunsaturated fatty acid metabolism contribute to excessive adipose tissue development? *Br J Nutrition* 2008;100:461-70.

[35] Massiera F, Barbry P, Guesnet P, Joly A, Luquet S, Moreilhon-Brest C, et al. A Western-like fat diet is sufficient to induce a gradual enhancement in fat mass over generation. *J Lipid Res* 2010;51:2352-61.

[36] Innis SM. Metabolic programming of long-term outcomes due to fatty acid nutrition in early life. *Maternal and Child Nutrtion* 2011;7:112-23.

[37] Sorensen HT, Sabroe S, Rothman KJ, Gilman M, Fischer P, Sorensen TI. Relation between weight and length at birth and body mass index in young adulthood. *BMJ* 1997;315:1137.

[38] Law CM, Barker DJ, Osmond C, Fall CH, Simmonds SJ. Early growth and abdominal fatness in adult life. *J Epidemiol Community Health* 1992;46:184-6.

[39] Bouswens M, van de Rest O, Dellschaft N, Bromhaar MG, de Groot LC, Geleijnse JM, Muller M, Afman LA. Fish oil supplementation induces anti-inflammatory gene expression profiles in human blood mononuclear cells. *Am J Clin Nutr* 2009;90:415-24.

[40] Lorente-Cebrian S, Bustos M, Marti A, Fernandez-Galilea M, Martinez JA, Moreno-Aliaga MJ. Eicosapentaenoic acid inhibits tumor necrosis factor-α-induced lipolisi in murine cultured adipocytes. *J Nutr Biochemistry* 2011;xx:xxx-xx. In press.

[41] Dangardt F, Osika W, Chan Y, Nilsson U, Gan L-M, Gronowitz E, Strandvik B, Friberg P. Omega-3 fatty acid supplementation improves vascular function and reduces inflammation in obese adolescents. *Atherosclerosis* 2010;212:580-5.

[42] Dahlman I, Linder K, Arvidsson Nordstrom E, Andersson I, Liden J, Verdich C, Serensen TI, Arner P. Changes in adipose tissue gene expression with energy-restricted diets in obese women. *Am J Clin Nutr* 2005; 81:1275-85.

[43] Pilon G, Ruzzin J, Rioux LE, Lavigne C, White PJ, Frøyland L, Jacques H, Bryl P, Beaulieu L, Marette A. Differential affects of various fish proteins in altering body weight, adiposity, inflammatory status, and insulin sensitivity in high-fat-fed rats. *Metabolism Clinical Experimental* 2011; doi:10.1016/2010.12.005. In press.

In: Fish Oil: Production, Consumption and Health Benefits
Editors: Matthias Van Dijk and Jürgen Vitek
ISBN: 978-1-61470-963-3

Chapter XVIII

Utilization of Marine Lipids for the Production of PUFA, Squalene, Wax Esters and Biodiesel for Commercial Application

***K.H. Sabeena Farvin*[*1] *and A. Surendraraj* [2]**
[1]Division of Industrial Food Research, National Institute of Food (DTU-Food), Technical University of Denmark, Lyngby, Denmark
[2]Department of Food Technology, Institute of Food and Dairy Technology, TANUVAS, Chennai, India

1. Introduction

The marine environment represents largely an untapped reservoir of novel and valuable bioactive compounds including lipids and lipid-soluble substance such as fatty acids, pigments, fat-soluble vitamins, terpenes, saponins, sterols, and glycolipids. Among them, marine long-chained polyunsaturated fatty acids fatty acids (LC-PUFA), specifically, docosahexaenoic acid [DHA, 22:6(n-3)] and eicosapentaenoic acid [EPA, 20:5(n-3)], have received considerable attention of researchers because of their beneficial biochemical and pharmacological effects on human health [1-3]. With growing public awareness of the clinical benefits of EPA and DHA, sale of marine oil supplements have grown almost ten folds over the last decade [4]. Most of these represent fish oil capsules made from various seafood sources including fish byproducts. In comparison with LC-PUFA, the other natural lipids from marine sources such as squalene and wax esters have received much less attention in spite of their proven potential as bioactive resources in promoting the human health and industrial applications. In addition, marine oils of inferior quality, which are not suitable for

* Corresponding author: Section of Seafood Research, National Institute of Food (DTU-Food), Technical University of Denmark, B. 221, Søltofts Plads, DTU, DK-2800 Kgs., Lyngby, Denmark.

human consumption can also be used as a starter material for biodiesel production to manage the eminent energy crisis of the world. This chapter mainly deals with composition of marine lipids and the different techniques for the production of LC-PUFA, squalene, wax esters and biodiesel from marine oils.

2. Composition of Marine Lipids

The term "marine oils" mainly represents fish oil even though krill oil, whale oil, algal oil and seal oil also included in this category. Compared with other oils or fats of vegetable origin, marine oils are more complex and contain not only a greater variety of fatty acids, but also considerable amount of long-chain poly unsaturated fatty acids (LC-PUFA) **(Table 1)** [5]. These PUFAs make up 30–40% of the total fatty acids, whereas ω-6 fatty acids constitute less than 10%. In contrast, PUFAs of vegetable oils are mainly ω-6 fatty acids, with less than 5% being ω-3. Saturated fatty acids comprise 20–35% of the total fatty acids in most fish oils, although herring oil may have up to 50% saturated [6]. Among the saturated fatty acids, the C16:0 content is between 10 and 25%, C14:0 is 3–13%, and that of C18:0 is 1–4%.

Table 1. List of unsaturated fatty acids found in marine lipids

Fatty acid name	Commercial Name	Chemical Name
Omega-3 fatty acids		
16:3 (n-3)		all-cis 7,10,13-hexadecatrienoic acid
18:3 (n-3)	Alpha-linolenic acid (ALA)	all-cis-9,12,15-octadecatrienoic acid
18:4 (n-3)	Stearidonic acid (STD)	All-cis-6,9,12,15-octadecatetraenoic acid
20:3 (n-3)	Eicosatrienoic acid (ETE)	All-cis-11,14,17-eicosatrienoic acid
20:4 (n-3)	Eicosatetraenoic acid (ETA)	All-cis-8,11,14,17-eicosatetraenoic acid
20:5 (n-3)	Eicosapentaenoic acid (EPA)	All-cis 5,8,11,14,17-eicosapentaenoic acid
22:5 (n-3)	Docosapentaenoic acid (DPA, Clupanodonic acid)	All-cis-7,10,13,16,19-docosapentaenoic acid
22:6 (n-3)	Docosahexaenoic acid (DHA	All-cis-4,7,10,13,16,19-docosahexaenoic acid
24:5 (n-3)	Tetracosapentaenoic acid	All-cis-9,12,15,18,21-tetracosapentaenoic acid
24:6 (n-3)	Tetracosahexaenoic acid (Nisinic acid)	All-cis-6,9,12,15,18,21-tetracosahexaenoic acid
Omega-6 fatty acids		
18:2 (n-6)	Linoleic acid	All-cis-9,12-octadecadienoic acid
18:3 (n-6)	Gamma-linolenic acid (GLA)	All-cis-6,9,12-octadecatrienoic acid
20:2 (n-6)	Eicosadienoic acid	All-cis-11,14-eicosadienoic acid
20:3 (n-6)	Dihomo-gamma-linolenic acid (DGLA)	All-cis-8,11,14-eicosatrienoic acid
20:4 (n-6)	Arachidonic acid (AA)	All-cis-5,8,11,14-eicosatetraenoic acid
22:2 (n-6)	Docosadienoic acid	All-cis-13,16-docosadienoic acid
22:4 (n-6)	Adrenic acid	All-cis-7,10,13,16-docosatetraenoic acid
22:5 (n-6)	Docosapentaenoic acid (Osbond acid)	All-cis-4,7,10,13,16-docosapentaenoic acid
Omega-9 fatty acids, mono and poly unsaturated		
18:1 (n-9)	Oleic acid[a]	Cis-9-octadecenoic acid
20:1 (n-9)	Eicosenoic acid[a]	Cis-11-eicosenoic acid
20:3 (n-9)	Mead acid	All-cis-5,8,11-eicosatrienoic acid
22:1 (n-9)	Erucic acid[a]	Cis-13-docosenoic acid
24:1 (n-9)	Nervonic acid[a]	Cis-15-tetracosenoic acid

[a]Monounsaturated

Proportions of fatty acids vary considerably between and within species. Herring oil is characterized by its high content of long-chain monoenes, usually about 30% or more. Menhaden oil has more C14:0 and less C22:6 than other fish oils. Monoenoic fatty acids, often present in significant quantities include C16:1, C20:1, and C22:1, the last two being mainly exogenous, originating as dietary components [7-9].

More than 90% of PUFAs present in fish oils are of the ω-3 configuration: an ethylene bond at the third carbon from the non-polar or at the ω-end of the molecule. Marine oils are characterized by ω-3 LC PUFAs with five or six ethylene bonds such as EPA and DHA. The contents of these fatty acids generally accounts for 10-35% of total fatty acids of most fish oils, although tuna oil may contain >35% ω-3 LC PUFAs [6]. Their presence reflects the composition of the diet, region and other environmental factors, especially water temperature. Fish from colder waters contain larger amounts of LC PUFAs, which allows more cell membrane flexibility. Considerable variation also occurs between and within species. For example, Pink salmon contains about 32% of total fatty acids as LC PUFAs, where as in sablefish the content is only about 7%. Moreover the relative levels of EPA and DHA also shows species variations and geographical variations. For example, the oils from menhaden, sardine, pilchard and anchovy are reported to contain greater EPA levels than DHA (EPA:DHA ratio of 3-4:1). In contrast, oils from tuna, mackeral and Atlantic salmon contains greater DHA levels than EPA levels (DHA:EPA ratio >3) [6]. Southern hemisphere (Australian) fishes generally reported to have higher relative levels of DHA than fish from northern hemisphere waters [10].

The basic pattern of fish triglycerides usually find polyenoic fatty acids preferentially bound in the middle (2nd) position, with monoenes at the ends (1 and 3 positions), although not all species conform to this pattern [11]. The fatty acid profile of seal oil can be distinguished from those of other marine oils by the presence of higher levels of docosapentaenoic acid (DPA, 22:5n-3). Moreover, in the case of seal oil the ω3-LC PUFA are located mainly at the sn-1 or 3 positions on the triglyceride molecules [6]. Features of krill oils are similar to conventional fish oils; it contains more EPA than DHA and also contains high levels of phospholipids and antioxidants such as astaxanthin. The fatty acid profile of krill varies markedly with the regions and season [12]. For example, reproductive male krill contained low oil content with a fatty acid profile closely resembling that of a typical phospholipid fraction [13]. Relative to fish oil, whale oil derived from the blubber is typically low in ω3-LC PUFA (3-5% of total PUFA) [14].

Recently, another source of marine oil produced commercially is algal oils. Conchillo, et al. [15] have published a study comparing microalgae oil and fish oil. They concluded that both oils contain similar amount of ω-3, although microalgae oil has the advantage of presenting neither an unpleasant odour nor a high amount of cholesterol. It also contains squalene and phytosterols, which offer additional benefits to human health. In addition to this, micro algae can be easily cultivated which avoid differences in seasonal production and is devoid of contamination problems from heavy metals and organic pollutants [16]. At present the algal oils which is produced commercially contains mainly DHA as sole LC PUFA. The dinoflagellates *Crypthecodinium cohnii* and *Schizochytrium sp* are reported to produce significantly higher amounts of DHA in the form of triacylglycerol (About 39 and 41% of total fatty acids respectively) [17]. Until recently, there is no useful microbial source of EPA as single LC PUFA oil that might be produced in the same way as DHA rich oil from *C.cohnii*. The best prospects for the production of a nearly EPA only oil would seems to be from the species of *Nanochloropsis* [18-19], *Navicula* [20], *Isochrysis galbana* and *Nitzchia* [21]. Some of the marine bacterial species such as *Shewanella, Alteramonas, Flexibactor, Psychroflexus* and *Vibro* may produce EPA as the sole LC-PUFA [21-23]. However, as these bacteria do not contain more than 5% lipids and must also be grown at very low temperature and in some cases, under high pressure [21], it is very difficult to obtain useful amounts of EPA rich oil from them. These bacteria would however be extremely useful as a source of the genes coding for EPA biosynthesis, which might then be introduced into plants or other micro organisms to achieve EPA production in a more amenable system.

Other minor components in marine oils are phospholipids, hydrocarbons, sterols, wax esters, vitamins, pigments, oxidation products and contaminants. Phospholipids are associated with cell membranes and, therefore, are scarce in oil produced as a byproduct of fish meal production. In phospholipids, approximately 50% lecithin and 25% cephalin, contribute to the total fatty acid [24]. Hydrocarbons are present at very low levels in most fish oils, but the liver oil of several species of shark may have up to 90% squalene with small amounts of pristine and zymene [25]. The properties and extraction methods of squalene are detailed later in this chapter. Sterols, almost all being cholesterol are always present in crude fish oils, with concentrations between 5 to 10% of total lipids [26]. Refining processing, however, can remove much free cholesterol and some cholesterol esters.

Wax esters, while present in certain species of fish (e.g., Orange roughy), are not found in liver oils or in marketed fillets as the esters occur just under the skin and are removed by deep cutting during fillet preparation [27]. The details of the wax esters are given later in this chapter. The fat-soluble vitamins A, D and E are always found as minor components, although levels present are subject to variation between and within the species. The body oils contain relatively low amounts of vitamin A and D, whereas liver oils are considerably rich in these vitamins [28]. Liver oils of halibut, shark and tuna are rich sources of vitamin D and Vitamin A [29].

Carotenoid pigments such as astaxanthin may be present as a result of dietary components in many crustacean oils and salmon oils. These pigments give an orange–red tint to the oil [30-31]. Oxidation and hydrolytic products such as free fatty acids, amines, peroxides, carbonyls, and volatile compounds will be present to various degrees depending upon the stability of the oil [32]. Contaminants occasionally found, depending on the source of crude oil, are pesticide residues and chlorinated biphenyls [33].

3. Production Technologies of PUFA

There are several rationales for producing concentrates of ω-3 fatty acids. For example, the individuals taking a pharmaceutical preparation or an ω-3 supplement, it is beneficial to reduce the volume of the capsules to be swallowed. In clinical applications, generally capsules containing fish oils, especially fish liver oils have been used. The dosage required to carry out the desired pharmacological effect carries the risk of vitamin A and D overdose and subsequent toxic effects as well as increase in the intake of cholesterol and other unwanted fatty acids [34]. Moreover, patients taking more concentrated formulations of ω-3 fatty acids (80%) have shown higher uptake and greater biological effects than formulations with lower concentrations [35]. In addition to this, for functional food applications, concentrates of ω-3 fatty acids will be more suitable for low fat applications than starting from fish oils. Achieving a high ω-3 concentrations can therefore be critical for developing convenient and practical therapeutic formulations.

Long chain ω-3 fatty acids in highly purified form are not easily prepared by any single fractionation technique due to the complex composition of marine oils as discussed previously. Usually a combination technique is used. The combination of which depends upon the fatty acid composition of the starting oil, the desired concentration and purity of the ω-3 fatty acids in the final product. This may typically be achieved by a combination of techniques which are selective on the basis of molecular size and the degree of unsaturation [36].

Studies have shown that the stability of ω-3 fatty acids against oxidation and their absorption in human organs are high when they are as acylglycerides than as esters [37-38]. Moreover, these effects will better when the fatty acid is bound to sn-2 position of glycerol structure than sn-1 and 3 positions [39]. Therefore, the production of acylglycerides concentrates with omega-3 in sn-2 position has acquired a great interest. Several methods have been reported for concentrating PUFAs in marine oils, with varied yields. Among methods that concentrate PUFAs as triglycerides, without prior hydrolysis, are solvent fractionation, winterization, and molecular distillation [5]. Concentrations of up to 30% EPA and DHA are feasible using these methods. However, higher levels (65% to 80%) are attainable by processes combining either hydrolysis or esterification with methods such as supercritical fluid extraction, urea complexation, and molecular distillation. Concentrations beyond 90% are possible with high-performance liquid chromatography (HPLC) [5].

Many scientists have continued investigating on the improvement of the omega-3 concentration processes, to achieve higher yield and purity at lower cost. Many of them utilized supercritical fluid fractionation [40- 44] or supercritical fluid chromatography [45-47] although other methods based on enzymatic reactions followed by urea complexation [48- 54] have also been proposed. These methods for omega-3 concentration are reviewed next.

3.1. Low Temperature Crystallization

Crystallization has been used in the study of the composition of fats and oils since early in the 19th century. Low-temperature crystallization was originally developed to separate certain fatty acids, triglycerides (TGs), esters and other lipids which are highly soluble in organic solvents at temperatures above 0°C, but become sparingly soluble at temperatures down to -80°C [55]. The solubility of fats in organic solvents decreases with increase in mean molecular weight and increases with increase in unsaturation [56]. The melting point of fatty acids changes considerably with the type and degree of unsaturation and thus separation of mixtures of saturated and unsaturated fatty acids may become possible [57]. Generally, the naturally occurring unsaturated acids are liquid at room temperature; as a rule, they have much lower melting points than the saturated acid of the same series. At low temperature saturated fatty acids which have higher melting point crystallize out and PUFA remain in the liquid form.

Low-temperature crystallization process may be carried out in the presence or absence of solvent/solvent mixture. Crystallization in the absence of a solvent occurs by Tirtiaux process, which involves slow cooling and slow agitation-, and by the hydrophilization process [4]. In this process, crystallization produces slurry of solid and liquid components, the latter being enriched with ω-3 fatty acids. An example for this is winterization. Cod-liver oil and other fish oils are winterized (cooled and filtered) before sale to avoid precipitation when refrigerated. This is to remove stearin and this process also slightly increases the content of PUFA in these oils. Fish body oils produced in this way typically declared to contain more EPA plus DHA [36].

Solvent crystallization of fatty acids is another method of concentrating poly unsaturated fatty acids. This method requires the least number of steps and the simplest equipment [58-29]. Briefly, the process consists of cooling the oil or fatty acids in a solvent, holding for a specified period of time, and removing the crystallized fraction by filtration. Most of the unsaturated acids are infinitely soluble in organic solvents at temperatures above 0°C, while the saturated acids are sparingly soluble at this temperature in solvents such as acetone, petroleum ether, and alcohol. In other solvents, such as ether and chloroform, the solubility differences are not so marked. The commonly used solvents are methanol and acetone and they have been employed to separate `stearic' and `oleic' fractions. Attempts have also been made to use other solvents such as hexane and methyl formate [60].

Yokochi et al. [61] reported that use of different organic solvents and temperatures affect the concentration of PUFA. The fungal oil extracted from *Mortierella* genus was used for concentration of γ-linolenic acid (GLA) by low-temperature crystallization [61, 62]. The concentration of GLA in different solvents was in the order of acetone (-20°C) > n-hexane (-20°C) > acetone (4°C) > petroleum ether (-20°C) at a solvent to oil ratio of 5:1 (v/v). Wanasundara, [63] reported the preparation of n3-PUFA concentrates from seal blubber oil by low-temperature fractional crystallization. In this study, seal blubber oil in the form of TGs or free fatty acids were subjected to solvent crystallization at different temperatures using hexane and acetone as solvents. They found that in triglyceride form, the content of ω-3 PUFA in the concentrate was increased with lowering of the crystallization temperature and under all temperature conditions; acetone afforded the highest concentration of total ω-3 PUFA. In the free fatty acid form, -60 and -70°C in hexane, resulted in total ω-3 PUFA content of up to 58.3 and 66.7% where as in acetone it is up to 56.7 and 46.8% in the preparation. Therefore, proper choice of solvent and temperature is necessary to achieve the optimum yield of the ω-3 PUFA.

Singleton [64] and Stout et al. [65] have determined the solubility of numerous fatty acids and esters in a variety of solvents at low temperature and revealed the following rules:

a) when the acids are saturated, long-chains are less soluble than short chains
b) saturated are less soluble than monoenoic and dienoic acids of equal chain length
c) trans isomers are less soluble than *cis* isomers and
d) normal acids are less soluble than branched acids.

Han *et al.* [66], have found that alkali salts of less unsaturated fatty acids crystallize more rapidly than those of PUFA containing four or more double bonds, when saponified solution was cooled. They also compared the cooling temperature and the rate of cooling on enrichment of ω-3 PUFA of alkali salts of sardine oil fatty acids. It was shown that EPA and DHA from sardine oil could be concentrated more than 2.3-fold with minimum yields of 87 and 91%, respectively and concluded that the cooling rate and temperature had little influence on the yield and contents of EPA and DHA. Therefore, use of ambient temperatures would offer a practical choice for large-scale separation and production of ω-3 PUFA concentrates.

Two important limitations in crystallization procedures are molecular association (compound formation in solution) and mixed-crystal formation. For example, palmitic acid was 2.5 times more soluble in carbon tetrachloride containing lauric acid than the pure solvent because of the formation of easily soluble compounds containing both acids. Similar compound formation was observed in chloroform, benzene, toluene, and nitrobenzene, but not in alcohol, ether, or ethyl acetate [67]. This type of association tends to increase the solubility of the more insoluble constituent, and would be likely to increase the tendency to mixed-crystal formation. Brocklesby [68] in a study of stearic, oleic, and linoleic acids has shown that association decreases with increase in unsaturation.

3.2. Urea Complexation

The principle of urea fractionation was first discovered by Bengen [69]. Under normal conditions urea crystallizes in tetragonal form with channels of 5.67 Å in diameter, however, in the presence of straight chain aliphatic compounds, it crystallizes in hexagonal prisms containing channels of 8-12 Å in diameter [70]. These channels formed in the presence of long straight chain molecules are sufficiently large to accommodate aliphatic chains. This principle works with all aliphatic compounds including hydrocarbons, alcohols, fatty acids and esters.

This method is favoured because complexation depends upon the configuration of the fatty acid due to presence of multiple bonds rather than pure physical properties like melting point or solubility. The stability of fatty acid-urea adducts parallels the geometry of the molecules involved. Any deviation from a straight chain arrangement weakens the stability of the adduct [4]. Therefore, formation of urea inclusion compounds depends on the degree of unsaturation of the fatty acids. The saturated fatty acids, because of the lack of steric irregularities, will be easily trapped into the channels of urea and thus form a stable crystalline complex. The presence of double bonds in the carbon chain increases the bulkiness of the molecule and reduces the likelihood of its complexation with urea [71]. Monoenes are more readily complexed as compared to dienes which, in turn, are more readily complexed than trienes. Thus the stability of adducts formed are in the order of saturated fatty acids > monounsaturated fatty acids > polyunsaturated fatty acids [72]. Linko and Karinkanta [73] found that the degree of formation of urea complexes of poly unsaturated fatty acids will increase with the length of the carbon chain, decrease with the number of double bonds and increase with the distance from the first double bond to the carbonyl group of the fatty acid ester commonly known as the Δ value. Accordingly, the tendency of incorporation of the long chain ω-3 fatty acids to form urea complexes are as follows 20:3n-3 (Δ11) > 20:4n-3(Δ8) > 22:5n-3(Δ7) > 21:5n-3(Δ6) > 20:5n-3 (Δ5, EPA) > 22:6n-3 (Δ4, DHA) [36].

Urea fractionation cannot be applied to triacyl glycerols but can be used for both free fatty acids and methyl or ethyl esters of fatty acids. When fractionating esters, it is common to transesterify the tri acylglycerols with alcohol and isolate the esters before the urea complexation step. However, combined in situ esterification and urea fractionation can also be performed [74]. There are advantages and drawbacks to each of these options. For example, fatty acids are more soluble in alcohol than their corresponding esters, hence they require much smaller volume of alcohol for processing. If the ester form of fatty acids is chosen, the re-esterification step of the concentrates can be eliminated. If the starting material for urea fractionation contains residual amounts of phospholipids or partial acylglycerols, the formation of urea complexes will be greatly reduced [75]. Hence in the process of urea complexation, first the oil (acylglycerol) is split into fatty acids using alcoholic KOH or NaOH. The unsaponifiables such as sterols, vitamins A and D and xenobiotics (e.g. PCB) as well as other undesirable components are removed from it. The free fatty acids thus obtained are then mixed with an alcoholic (methanol or ethanol) solution of urea and allowed to cool to a particular temperature depending on the desired degree of concentration. The saturated fatty acids, monoenes and, to a lesser extent, dienes are crystallized with urea and non-crystallized fatty acids in the solution can be separated by filtration. The liquid or non-urea complexing fraction is enriched with ω3-PUFA [76].

Urea complexes are formed not only with completely straight chain aliphatic compounds but also with unsaturated, branched chain and cyclyic compounds, provided that there is a sufficient long straight chain in the molecule and the branch or cycle is not too large. Almost all naturally occurring fatty acids and their corresponding n-alkyl esters are able to form crystalline urea complexes [71-72]. Due to this, urea fractionation does not concentrate all ω-3 fatty acids to the same degree. There will be residual amounts of all fatty acids in the urea complexes, the relative amounts differ among the different acids. For example, complete removal of saturated fatty acids by urea complexation may be impossible since some of the saturated fatty acids do not complex with urea during crystallization. Long chain monounsaturated fatty acids (MUFA), especially those of the C_{20} and C_{22}, form complexes with urea more readily than those of shorter chain saturated fatty acids (C_{14} and C_{16}). Thus the amount of MUFA in urea complex fraction may be increased up to 73% level under certain experimental conditions [76]. Different authors have reported that DHA is the major portion in the non-urea complexing fraction for urea complexation experiments carried out for cod liver, menhaden oil and seal blubber oil [76-78]. Although a major portion of EPA was recovered in the non-urea complexing fraction, the content of EPA in the non-urea complexing fraction was less than DHA in these studies. This might be due to the facts that, the content of EPA in the mixture of fatty acid is lower in these oils and EPA has a greater tendency to form a urea adduct than DHA. This means that small portions of EPA and DHA are also lost in the complexes.

Complex formation is exothermic, but requires dissolution of both urea and fatty acids. Methanol and ethanol are preferred solvents for small scale fractionation. Han et al. [79] have tested a series of solvents (ethanol, methanol, water, formamide and acetonitrile) as wetting agents for urea. They reported that all solvents tested served as appropriate wetting agents, but water may be the best choice of solvent for large scale operations because of its low cost and lack of toxicity.

The extent of crystallization also depends on the urea-to-fatty acid ratio and crystallization temperature. Generally, the enrichment of total ω 3-PUFA in the concentrate, and its overall recovery, varied inversely with increasing urea-to-fatty acid ratio as well as crystallization at lower temperatures. Therefore, these experimental variables should be carefully controlled in order to achieve maximum content of total ω3-PUFA in the concentrate with a reasonable recovery. Studies on marine oils, including cod liver oil [77], menhaden oil [76] and algal oil from *Crypthecodinium cohnii* [80] have reported an optimum urea to fatty acid ratio of 3:1 for the omega 3 enrichment. In general, at very lower temperatures the recovery efficiency of EPA was reduced. Wille et al. [81] reported that C18:4 ω3 and DHA were concentrated more efficiently in the filtrate when crystallization occurs at 5 °C, whereas total ω3 content and EPA maximize at 10 and 15 °C, respectively. Interestingly, urea complexation protects these ω3-PUFAs from autoxidation [81]. Some authors have reported optimal ratio of urea to fatty acid as 4:1 (w/w) for the algal oils such as *Isochrysis galbana* and *Porphyridum cruentum* [83-84] and the optimal crystallization temperature depends on the PUFA being isolated. For example, 28°C is the most suitable crystallization temperature for EPA, because at lower temperatures this fatty acid tends to make inclusion compounds.

Liu et al., [54] studied the process parameters in the concentration of EPA and DHA from tuna oil by urea complexation. They found that urea-to-fatty acid ratio and crystallization temperature were highly significant, but crystallization time was insignificant. The total DHA and EPA of 85.02% (with liquid recovery yield of 25.10%) were obtained from tuna oil at a urea-to-fatty acid ratio of 15 (mole/mole), a crystallization temperature of -5°C, and a crystallization time of 20 h. Urea fractionation will act differently for the various oxidation and isomerization products that can be formed from PUFA. Peroxides of fatty acids form urea complexes to a very limited degree [71]. However, *trans* fatty acids form urea complexes to a greater degree than the original *cis* fatty acids [85]. Polymeric oxidation products are not expected to form complexes with urea, and are concentrated by this fractionation step.

Advantages of urea complexation methods includes

a) Compared with the other methods of producing PUFA concentrates, urea fractionation allows handling of large quantities of materials in simple equipment.
b) In urea complexation, the complexed crystals are very stable and hence filtration at very low temperatures that used for solvent crystallization of fatty acids is not required [4].
c) Since the process requires only limited use of less toxic organic solvents such as ethanol, it is environment friendly.
d) It is also cost-effective because urea is relatively inexpensive.

Even though urea complexation has these advantages, the use of this method should be avoided if it is used for concentrating PUFA for human consumption because of the reported production of ethyl-carbamates [86]

$$EtOH + NH_2CONH_2 \text{ ----> } EtOCONH_2 \quad + \quad NH_3$$

(Ethanol) (Urea) (Ethyl carbamate) (Ammonia)

The formation of ethyl carbamate by the reaction of urea and ethanol was first reported by E. Wohler in 1845 [87]. Ethyl carbamate, also known as urethane, is an animal carcinogen [88-89] and has been an emerging health concern [90].

3.3. Silver Complexation

Complexation with a concentrated aqueous solution of silver ions represents another method for increasing the concentration of polyunsaturated fatty acids. This method works according to a different principle than by urea complexation. Urea complexation is a passive process in that sense the urea reacts with the less unsaturated fatty acids, while complexation with silver ions is a concentration process that interacts directly with the polyunsaturated fatty acids. If an ethyl ester mixture containing polyunsaturated fatty acids is stirred with a concentrated aqueous solution of silver nitrate, the most unsaturated fraction of the fatty acid esters (including EPA and DHA) will be brought into the aqueous solution by complexation with silver ions. Components with no polyunsaturated moiety will remain in the organic phase. After removal of the organic phase, the ethyl esters of the polyunsaturated fatty acids are easily separated by the addition of water to the aqueous solution. The added water breaks the strong bonding between the polyunsaturated fatty acids and the silver, and the ethyl esters of the polyunsaturated fatty acids form a separate organic phase [36].

The pattern of minor components will be very different in concentrates prepared by silver complexation than in those prepared using urea complexation. Concentrates from urea fractionation will contain traces of branched fatty acids and furan fatty acids [91], while such acids will be virtually absent from concentrates prepared by silver complexation [36]. Advantages of this method are that it is fast and efficient concentration method and lends itself to preparative separation purposes. Silver nitrate can be easily regenerated and complexation with silver ions does not lead to partial isomerization of poly unsaturated fatty acids or possibly toxic traces of silver in the product. The main disadvantage of this process is high initial investment for full scale production as large amounts of silver is required [36].

3.4. Formation of Iodolactones

This method is based on the principle that the unsaturated fatty acids reacts with potassium bicarbonate, iodine and potassium iodide to form Iodolactones. Acids with a Δ4 double bond such as DHA form an iodo γ-lactone whereas, acids with a Δ5 double bond such as arachidonic acid (AA) or EPA form an iodo δ-lactone. This reaction is reversible and five ring iodolactones are more stable than six ring iodolactones [36]. DHA forms iodolactone at a higher rate than EPA, while EPA reacts faster than DHA during the reverse reaction. The iodolactonization reaction depends on the solvent, reaction temperature, and on the ratio of iodine to iodide. For example, with ethanol as solvent and a reaction temperature of 25 °C, DHA gives a maximum yield of γ-iodolactone in 10 min, but EPA requires 90 min to produce the δ-iodolactone [92].

Wright et al., [93] used this method for the isolation of DHA from fish oil or concentrates of ω-3 fatty acids. After saponification of cod liver oil, unsaponifiable compounds such as waxes and sterols are removed by extraction. When most of the saturated and monounsaturated fatty acids are removed by precipitation of their lithium salts, a mixture concentrated in PUFA is obtained. To this PUFA mixture, 1.2 equivalents of iodine and potassium iodide (calculated according the amount of DHA present in the mixture) were added using aqueous tetrahydrofuran as solvent. The more stable five-ring iodo-γ-lactone of

DHA is selectively formed rather than the more labile six-ring iodo-δ-lactone of EPA. DHA is regenerated by treating the iodolactone with iodotrimethylsilane, generated in situ from chlorotrimethylsilane and sodium iodide. Then from the solution containing unreacted fatty acids from the first iodolactonization reaction, EPA can be purified through a second iodolactonization reaction using an excess of iodine and potassium iodide [94]. Now a mixture of the iodolactones derived from EPA and the residual amounts of DHA is obtained. When this mixture is treated with iodotrimethylsilane, selective cleavage of the iodo-δ-lactone of EPA occurs as a result of the greater stability of the iodo- γ -lactone of DHA. When most of the iodo-δ-lactone of EPA has reacted, the reaction mixture is worked up to yield purified EPA.

The iodolactone pathway has also been used for the production of several derivatives of DHA and EPA, including the introduction of hydrophilic substituents in the 4-position of DHA [95], for the conversion of EPA and DHA to related sulphur-and oxygen-containing fatty acids [96], for the production of unsaturated marine lipid hydrocarbons [97] and biologically active polyunsaturated trifluoromethyl ketones [98], as well as for the synthesis of omega-3 fatty acid octadecapentaenoic acid (18:5n-3) [99]. While studying the effect of varying solvent, temperature and ratio of components upon the rate of synthesis of several iodolactones, Gaiday et al. [100] pointed out that this reaction is useful for the synthesis of natural biostimulators 4-hydroxy DHA and 5-hydroxy EPA.

Although the iodolactone pathway represents a method to prepare pure DHA and EPA, it is unclear whether this method is currently being used for industrial scale production of these two acids. Moreover, arachidonic acid (20:4n-6), which is present in small amounts in fish oil, has a double bond in the 5-position can be expected to form iodolactone at the same rate as EPA, while the omega-6 form of docosapentaenoic acid (22:5n-6) which has a double bond in the 4-position may also be expected to form iodolactone at a similar rate as DHA.

3.5. Distillation Method

Distillation is rather an old technique used for partial separation of mixtures of fatty acids esters. This method takes advantage of the differences in the boiling point and molecular weight of fatty acids under reduced pressure. Separation by distillation depends on the volatility of different components in the mixture. For a mixture of fatty acids or fatty acid esters, the separation will depend upon the relative chain length of the fatty acids.

Generally, the oils are distilled as ethyl esters. Because of the absence of hydrogen bonding, fatty acid ethyl esters will distil at slightly lower temperature than the corresponding free fatty acids. As the molecular weight is lowered by 2 units for each introduction of a double bond to a fatty acid with a given chain length, in principle distillation can be used to separate long chain PUFA according to their degree of unsaturation. In theory, the following is the order of the ease of distillation for the long chain PUFA *viz:* EPA (20:5n-3) > 20:4n-3 =20:4n-6> 21:5n-3> DHA(22:6n-3) > 22:5n-3=22:5n-6 [36].

This technique requires high temperatures of approximately 250°C [101]. In the past, distillation was commonly performed at atmospheric pressure with large quantities of superheated steam. Today, fatty acids are distilled under vacuum [102]. Depending on the type of plant, still, flash, or film evaporation may be employed. In *still distillation,* the fatty acids are distilled from a large volume of liquid, and the residue remains completely or partially in the still. Because of high temperature and superheating in the still, the yield and quality of the distillate are affected adversely. In *flash evaporation,* the fatty acid undergoes forced circulation, and heating takes place outside the distillation zone, which is maintained under vacuum. In the distillation zone, the fatty acid evaporates and is cooled to its boiling point at the operating pressure. The internal heat is converted into heat of evaporation. In *film evaporation,* a thin film of fatty acid is formed. Evaporation takes place only from the surface of this film at operating pressure. The absence of hydrostatic pressure and liquid holdup, low temperature difference with respect to the heating medium (only 20 – 30°C) and few minutes residence time makes the film evaporation more suitable for distillation of fatty acids [102].

Distillation of marine oil esters is difficult since the separation of these components becomes less effective with increasing molecular weight. The large difference in molecular weight of vitamins A and D allows good separation of these two components in fish liver oils. Conversely, the small differences between many fatty acid components in oil make it difficult to accomplish effective separation or enrichment of a particular fatty acid [103]. Stout et al. [65] emphasized the practical difficulty of concentrating only ω3-PUFA from fish oil in the natural TGs form. The distillation of menhaden oil, as such, concentrated only EPA from an initial of 16.0 to 19.5%. However, distillation of its ethyl esters increased the EPA content from 15.9 to 28.4%. While, DHA doubled from 8.4 to 17.3% in the TGs form, and in the simple alkyl esters form it increased from 9.0 to 43.9%.

The most widely used distillation technique is fractional distillation under reduced pressure (0.1- 1mm HG). Even under these conditions moderately high temperatures are required, which is sufficient to cause oxidation, polymerization and isomerization of double bonds of ω-3 PUFA. Commonly used heated columns, packed with glass helices or metal packing have a disadvantage of significant hold up and pressure drop through the column. Spinning band column may be used to overcome these disadvantages [36]. Distillation at still lower pressures has been used in the isolation of some highly unsaturated acids, and is particularly valuable in polymerization studies to separate monomeric, dimeric and polymeric materials and in the separation of monoacylglycerols from di- and triacylglycerol mixtures. Marked decomposition of arachidonic acid was found when it was distilled slowly in a spinning band column [104-105]. Even when the catalytic effects of metal parts were eliminated by using an all-glass apparatus, high temperature and exposure to oxygen caused major losses of ω3-PUFA [106]. Therefore, for the preparation of ω-3 PUFA concentrates a method which involves low process temperature and time to minimize thermal damage is warranted.

Short-path distillation or molecular distillation is a distillation technique which uses lower temperatures and short heating intervals leading to the distillation of ω-3 PUFA without any apparent decomposition. However, the degree of fractionation that can be achieved by this method is limited, significant concentration effects can only be obtained at low yields [36]. Short path distillation is the economically viable option for concentration up to 65% of ω-3 fatty acid esters. Molecular distillation is normally performed as a two-step process. In the first distillation step, the shorter chain impurities are removed as distillate. The residue from this distillation is then transferred to a second distillation, where the bulk of the oil is distilled; the residue from this step, which contains heavy by products are discarded [36].

Brevick et al., [107] used short path distillation method for concentrating EPA and DHA from sardine oil after lipase hydrolysis. The acylglycerol/ethylester mixture was distilled in the short path distillation at 125°C, 0.005mbar pressure resulted in 47.4% distillate and 51.3% residue. The residue after short-path distillation contained as much as 47.39% EPA plus DHA, compared to 40.1% in the acylglycerol fractions. The distillation step resulted in 10.6% monoacylglycerol fraction in the distillate, which is predominantly of fatty acids with chain length below C_{20} and little or no EPA and DHA is lost into the distillate.

A limitation of short path distillation/distillation in general is limited degree of fractionation. This means that for esters from fish oil, which contain numerous fatty acids with similar volatility, molecular distillation can only give limited concentration effects. However, molecular distillation is an important tool in ensuring a constant ratio of EPA to DHA in the final product. So for the preparation of very high concentrates of ω-3 fatty acids, molecular distillation may be used as a first concentration step. The advantage of distillation technique is that it separates the fatty acids or fatty acid esters from oligomeric or polymeric material that might have been generated from oxidation of fish oil. If the starting fish oils have been stored for long time, ethylation or hydrolysis followed by molecular distillation will represent a quality assurance by removing heavy oxidation by products formed during storage [36].

3.6. Supercritical Fluid Extraction (SFE)

The conventional methods of n3 PUFA concentrations is having the disadvantages of requiring high-temperature processing which results in loss or decomposition of the thermally labile compounds and also leave the toxic residues of solvents in the n-3PUFA concentrates [108]. SFE may circumvent some of the problems associated with the use of conventional separation techniques.

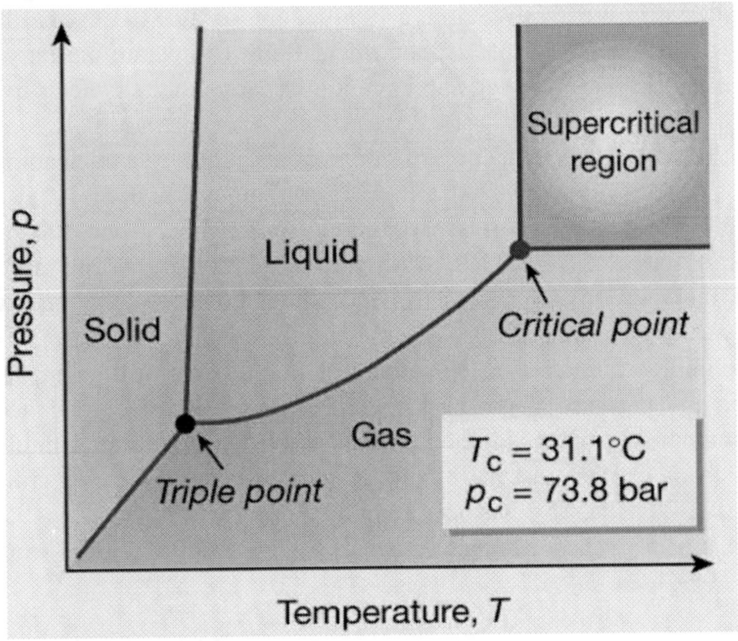

Figure 1. Pressure and temperature diagram of CO_2.

A number of gases are known to possess desirable selective solvent properties when raised to pressures above their critical values. The region in which a substance exists as a supercritical fluid is defined by its critical pressure (Pc) and critical temperature (Tc) (**Figure 1**). In the region above its critical point, the fluid possesses intermediate properties between a gas and a liquid, i.e., liquid-like density and gas-like viscosity and diffusivity. This means that supercritical fluids (SCF) have a good solvent power and good transport properties [109]. Since density depends on pressure and temperature, the solvent power of a SCF can be tuned to dissolve different types of solutes, which in the present chapter is interesting because fish oil can be fractionated to separate free fatty acids or to obtain concentrates of different components according to their molecular weight or degree of saturation. For food commodities, CO_2 is chosen because it has moderate critical temperature and pressure (Tc=304.15 K or 31.1°C and Pc=7.38 MPa or 73.8 bar) and is inert, inexpensive, non-inflammable, readily available, environment friendly and safe [110].

An abundance of work on the separation of fish oil related compounds using SFE have been done since Passino [111] described the solexol process for fractionation of fish oils using subcritical propane. Zosel [112] has described the use of supercritical ethane to extract and fractionate triglycerides from fish liver oil with a recirculation apparatus. The authour found that the molecular mass and the iodine value rose during the extraction and fractionation process. Eisenbach [113] utilized the same experimental procedure to separate EPA ethyl ester from a mixture of fatty acid ethyl esters derived from cod fish oil by means of supercritical carbon dioxide (SC-CO_2). In this study also the low molecular weight components were extracted preferentially, causing the high molecular weight components (like EPA ethyl ester) to be collected in some of the final fractions. After a two-step process of some of the fractions, a yield of 79.8% of the initial EPA content with a purity of 91.9% could be achieved. The impurities were mainly eicosenoic acid ethyl ester. Arai and Saito [114] have described the fractionation of a model mixture of fatty acids and fatty acid methyl esters from sardine oil by extractive urea crystallization using SC-CO_2, as the solvent. This method employs both the ability of a supercritical fluid to separate the fatty acids by chain length as well as the ability of urea crystallization to separate the fatty acids by their degree of unsaturation.

Lately, the interest in the extraction of components present in trace amounts in fish oil, such as vitamins or contaminations, has arisen. Thus, Yamaguchi et al. [115] have performed a series of SFEs of carotenoids from freeze-dried krill oil using carbon dioxide as the solvent in the temperature range of 313-353 K at a pressure of 25 MPa. Wong and Johnston [116] have measured the solubility of cholesterol in carbon dioxide in the temperature range of 308.2-333.2 K at the pressures of 10.1-27.9 MPa, while Ohgaki et al. [117] have published experimental solubility data of α -tocopherol in carbon dioxide at the temperatures of 298.2 and 313.2 K in the pressure range of 10.0- 18.3 MPa. Elvevoll [118] accomplished the extraction of components like ubiquinone, cholesterol, α-tocopherol, retinol, squalene, and cholecalciferol from codfish viscera oil at temperatures between 309 and 328 K in the pressure range of 8-28 MPa. SFE has been employed for the removal of contaminants such as polychlorinated biphenyls and pesticides from fish oil and fish tissue, respectively, using carbon dioxide (119-122).

Table 2. Concentration of ω-3 PUFA by using Enzymes

Enzymes used	Oils tested	Remarks	Yield/recovery	Reference
Thermomyces lanuginosus (TL), Pseudomonas cepacia(PC)	Nile perch viscera	*TL –lipase* discriminated DHA most, resulting in best DHA/DHA-EE enrichment *PC lipase* discriminated EPA most, resulting in best EPA/EPA-EE enrichment	DHA/DHA-EE recovery 76-84% EPA/EPA-EE recovery 79-92%	[140]
Candida Rugosa (CR), Candida cylindracea (CC), Mucor javanicus (MJ), and Aspergillus niger (AN)	Pacific sardines (Sardinops Sagax)	Non specific CR and CC lipases resulted in high n-3 PUFA, 1, 3 specific MJ and AN lipases resulted in low n -3 PUFA concentration	EPA increased from 26.86%to 33.74% in 1.5hr DHA increased13.62% to 29.94% in 9hr	[144]
Aspergillus oryzae (AO)	Salmon oil	1,3 specific lipase	Total PUFA increased from 41.6% in the crude oil to 46.5%, EPA 3.6% to 5.6% and DHA from 9.9%to 11.6%,.	[146]
AN, CC, Chromobacterium viscosum (CV), Geotrichum candidum (GC), Mucor Miehei (MM), Pseudomonas sp (PSL), Rhizopus oryzae (RO), and Rhizopus Niveus (RN).	Seal blubber oil(SBO) Menheden oil (MHO)	Non specific CC lipase gave highest content of total n-3 PUFA In both oils	CC lipase; total n-3 PUFA 43.5% in SBO [9.75% EPA, 8.61% DPA, and 24.0% DHA] and total n-3 PUFA 44.1% in MHO (18.5% EPA, 3.62% DPA, and 17.3% DHA) after 40 h of hydrolysis.	[149]
MM, CC, GC, *AN,* CR, CV, *RO, MJ, RN,* PSL, *C. antarctica* (CA), *Pseudomonas fluorescens* (PF), *Penicillium roqueforti* (PR), *Humicula lanuginosa* (HL), *Rhizopus delemar* (RD), *Penicillium camembertii* (PC), and *C. lipolytica* (CL).	Sardine oil	*Pseudomonas* lipases PF and PSLshowed highest activity toward the saturated and monounsaturated fatty acids lower activity toward EPA and DHA leaving n-3 PUFA in the mono,-di –tri acyglcerides in unreacted mixture	Residual mixtures contained 50% EPA + DHA. Total recovery of DHA >80% and EPA >90%	[164]
Esterification with Rhizomucor miehei	Tuna oil Chilean fish oil sardine oil	1,3 specific lipase	Chilean oil- residual FFA comprised 20.4% EPA and 15.8% DHA, Tuna oil: FFA residue contained only 2.9% EPA and 77.5% DHA, sardine oil: residual FFA comprised 13.2% EPA and 50.0% DHA	[133]

Table 2. (continued).

Enzymes used	Oils tested	Remarks	Yield/recovery	Reference
Lipase derived from *Bacillus licheniformis* MTCC 6824	Sardine oil	produced the highest degree of hydrolysis for SFAs and MUFAs	Lipase-catalyzed hydrolysis followed by urea complexation gave 55.4% EPA and 5.8% ARA,	[182]
Hydrolysis with PSL (Lipase-AK) and selective esterification by *RD lipase*	Tuna oil	1,3 specific *Rhizopus* lipase acted only weakly on DHA	DHA content in the unesterified FFA fraction could be raised from 24 to 72 wt% in an 83% yield	[134]
CC,AN,PSL,RD, RJ,CV -Lipases	Tuna oil	Non specific CC lipase enriched DHA 3 times than of original oil	Acylglycerols containing 53% DHA were obtained, But EPA levels were nearly unchanged	[141]
PSL, CC,CV-Lipases	Sardine oil	PSL was best enzyme to concentrate EPA and DHA	total % of EPA and DHA reached 65% in the giycerides	[165]
Pseudomonas fluorescens lipase	Tuna oil	Non specific and hydrolysed FA same manner regadless of their position	Gave 80% EPA and 70% DHA in free fatty acids	[135]
AN, RJ and *Penicillium solitum(PS)*	Salmon oil	*AN* lipase was the most effective in concentrating *n*-3 PUFA.	An increase in the DHA content from 14.4% in the original oil to 34.0%	[136]
Hydrolysis with CR, GC, RN, , Humicola lanuginosa (HL) CV and esterification with RM	Cod liver oil Refined fish oil	HL and CV lipases both enriched DHA in the TG fraction and that C. viscosum also enriched EPA. Most effective lipase for concentrating n-3 PUFA was CR lipase	> 95% TG can be synthesized from either long-chain n-3 FFA or long-chain n3 partial glycerides by using immobilized R. miehei lipase	[145]
AN, PF,CR,RO,MJ,PC-lipase	Atlantic salmon visera oil	CR and PC were effective in concentrating EPA and DHA	1g with 27.1% of EPA + DHA can be obtained from 4 g of viscera oil with 11.7% EPA + DHA by CR lipase.	[147]
Rhizomucor miehei lipase	Turkish anchovy oil	1,3 specific lipase	The level of PUFA in the glyceride mixture was raised to 40%. The individual TG and DG fractions contained 45 and 30% PUFA, respectively.	[150]

If the object of the supercritical fluid separation is to produce the essential fatty acids or triglycerides with a specific fatty acid composition, this cannot be accomplished by direct use of the naturally occurring triglycerides from crude fish oils due to their complex structure [123] and very low solubility. The separation of PUFA by SFE is dependent on the molecular size of the components involved rather than their degree of unsaturation therefore; a prior concentration step is needed to achieve a high concentration of PUFA in the final product [124]. Thus, most efforts are directed towards fractionating the free fatty acids or their esters. Esters are preferred as they are more soluble in supercritical fluids than the free fatty acids. Thus, oils to be used for n-3 PUFA concentration by SFE require preparation steps of extraction, hydrolysis and esterification by conventional methods [113,125]. Different authors stressed upon the importance of gaining knowledge on the solubilities, phase equilibria of the individual key components as well as natural mixtures in the super critical fluid and developing, testing them in theoretical thermodynamic models for achieving effective n-3 omega concentrate during the real time super critical fluid extraction[41,44, 126-127].

3.7. Enzymatic Methods

The use of enzymes in industrial processes is fairly recent but it has become a good alternative to traditional methods. Enzymes offer the following advantages over currently used chemical methods [128-129].

1) Catalytic efficiency is high, so a relatively low amount of enzyme is required.
2) Enzymes can be reused.
3) Wide range in fatty acid selectivity.
4) Enzymes offer mild treatments in terms of temperature, pH, and pressure.
5) Reduced energy cost.

Enzymes involved in the production of n-3 PUFA concentrates are lipases, which catalyze esterification, hydrolysis or exchange of fatty acids in esters [130]. The direction and the choice of the reaction can be influenced by the choice of experimental conditions [131]. The reaction is reversible and under low water activity conditions, the enzyme functions 'in reverse' ie., synthesis of an ester bond rather than its hydrolysis [132]. EPA and DHA can be enriched either as free fatty acids by selective esterification of fish oil free fatty acids with an alcohol or glycerol [133-135] or by hydrolysis of fish oil fatty acid ethyl esters [134]. Studies on the production of n-3 PUFA concentrates from marine oils using lipases are shown in the Table 2.

3.7.1. Lipase-Catalysed Hydrolysis

During the hydrolysis reaction, the lipases are expected to hydrolyze the bulk of saturated and monounsaturated fatty acid ethyl esters leaving behind the more resistant DHA and EPA in the residual fatty acid ethyl esters. The molecular conformation of *cis* carbon–carbon double bonds in PUFAs, particularly EPA and DHA, causes steric hindrance and subsequent bending of the fatty acid chains bringing the terminal methyl groups very close to the ester bonds. Because of this steric hindrance effect, enzymatic active sites cannot reach the ester-linkages of these fatty acids with their glycerol backbones, thereby protecting EPA and DHA from lipase-catalyzed hydrolysis. However, this does not occur with the relatively straight chains of saturated fatty acids and MUFAs, and therefore hydrolysis is not hindered [4,136]. Also, it has been suggested that triacylglycerides (TGs) without EPA and DHA are hydrolyzed in the first phase, and TGs with EPA and DHA are hydrolyzed later, indicating that the lipase recognizes the whole molecular structure, not only its ester bonds [137]. Thus, fatty acid selectivity of a lipase for EPA and DHA allows separation and concentration of these fatty acids from others in the remaining portion of marine oils [138].

The selectivity of lipases is however influenced by the distribution of fatty acids among the three positions of triglycerides and sometimes the glyceride structure [139-140].

Therefore one lipase may concentrate EPA and DHA in one kind of fish oil but not be effective in another depending on the distribution in the triglyceride molecule. For example, lipase from *Aspergillus niger* (AN) increased DHA concentration in cod liver oil and sardine oil [137], but did not increase it in menhaden oil [36] or tuna oil [141]. Lipase from *Thermomcyces lanuginosus* (TL) increased DHA and EPA contents in squid and menhaden oil [142-143] but was ineffective in enriching EPA in Nile perch oil [140]. The lipases also discriminate between EPA and DHA. Lipases from *Geotrichum candidum* (GC), *Candida rugosa* (CR), *Thermoyces lanuginosus* (TL) showing preference for EPA over DHA while lipases from *Pseudomonas* species showed DHA preference over EPA.

Studies have shown that hydrolysis with Non-specific lipases (*Candida rugosa* (CR) lipase and *Candida culindracea* (CC) lipase) resulted in improved total ω-3 PUFAs than 1,3-specific lipases (*Aspergillus niger* (AN) *and Mucor javanicus* (MJ) lipases) [141,144]. The reason for the high efficiency of the non-specific lipase in the production of an n -3 PUFA concentrate is due to its chainlength selectivity. CR and CC lipase are known to possess fatty acid chain length selectivity, showing higher activity with relatively short-chain fatty acids such as C_{18} or below [145]. Additional possible reasons for higher efficiency of non-specific lipases might be lipase regiospecificity and/or original fatty acid profiles of fish oil [137, 145]. Preferential fatty acid hydrolysis could also depend on fish species, which may have varied positional arrangements of PUFAs. For example, the non-specific CR and CC lipases were not able to increase EPA content in salmon oil [146], salmon viscera oil [147] or Brazilian sardine oil [148], but did cause an increase in EPA content in seal blubber oil [149] and in Pacific sardine oil [144]. Moreover 1,3-specific lipase, which was found to be ineffective at n -3 PUFA concentration from sardine oil [144] and tuna oil [141], increased EPA and DHA levels in anchovy oil [150] and menhaden oil [151]. In the case of fish oil, the second position of the glycerol moiety is usually more enriched with n-3 PUFAs [152], although this may vary depending on species [153]. For example, stereospecific analysis has revealed that EPA is preferentially located in position 3 of the glycerol backbone in sardine oil [154]. The 1,3-specific lipases possess stereo specificity with respect to the 1- and 3-positions of the acylglycerols, hydrolyzing the fatty acids at these positions easier than at the 2-position, resulting in 2-mono glycerides and a mixture of di glycerides and fatty acids [155]. If the 2-position is high in EPA and DHA, 1,3-specific lipase should be more effective at concentrating n-3 PUFAs; however, if saturated or monounsaturated are located at the 2-position and PUFAs are located at the 1- and 3-positions of triacylglycerols, hydrolysis with 1,3-specific lipase would most likely result in low n-3 PUFA levels in the final product [147]. This could partially explain why 1,3-specific lipase was less effective at n-3 PUFA concentration compared to non-specific lipases. Kotting and Eble [156] have reported that lipases from *Rhizopus* spp are 1,3-positional specific. In seal blubber oil, EPA is located mainly in sn-1 and sn-3 positions of the TGs; however, EPA in menhaden oil is equally distributed over the sn-2 and sn-3 positions and was present only in small amounts in the sn-1 position [151]. Therefore, the higher hydrolysis rate of EPA from seal blubber oil may reflect abundance of this fatty acid in the sn-1 and sn-3 positions which is highly vulnerable to 1,3-specific RO-lipase hydrolysis. Tanaka et al. [141] have also reported that EPA content of tuna oil was decreased upon hydrolysis by lipases from *Rhizopus spp, Rhuzopus delemer* (RD) and *Rhizopus javanicum* (RJ).

Kojima et al. [52] designed a process to concentrate alternatively DHA or EPA from a mixture of natural fish oil through an enzymatic method using HU-lipases (which show a high reactivity for any fatty acid with 20 atoms of carbon) or AK-lipases (which shows a poor reactivity for fatty acids with 20 atoms of carbon and a Δ5 unsaturated bond), followed by urea complexation to increase the purity. They concluded that, using this method with HU-lipase, it is possible to selectively enrich EPA from 12.2% to 43.1%, while the amount of DHA is practically constant. On the other hand, if the same method was repeated using AK-lipase, a selective enrichment of DHA from 16.3% to 44.6% was obtained, while the amount of EPA was hardly altered.

3.7.2. Lipase-Catalysed Esterification

The acylglycerol form of PUFA is considered to be nutritionally more favorable than methyl or ethyl esters of fatty acids due to the impaired intestinal absorption of alkyl esters of n-3 fatty acids observed in laboratory animals [37, 157-158]. It has also been shown that methyl and ethyl esters of unsaturated fatty acids hydrolyze at a slower rate than their corresponding acylglycerols [159]. From a marketing point of view, mono-, di-, and triacylglycerols are often promoted as being more "natural" than free fatty acids and their methyl or ethyl esters [160]. The preparation of homogeneous TGs that contain both EPA and DHA can be achieved by (a) direct esterification of glycerol with pure EPA and DHA as free acids or (b) by interesterification (ester ester interexchange) of tributyrin with ethyl esters (EE) of pure EPA and DHA [161]. PUFA can also be concentrated (c) by transesterification (the process of exchanging the organic group R″ of an ester with the organic group R′ of an alcohol) of fish oil triglycerides with ethanol [160].

a) Direct Esterification

```
CH2-OH                          Lipase      CH2-OOC-R
|                                           |
CH-OH      + 3RCOOH               →         CH- OOC-R + 3 H2O
|                                           |
CH2-OH                                      CH- OOC-R
```

Were RCOOH= EPA/DHA

b) Inter esterification

```
CH2-OOC-R                       Lipase      CH2-OOC-R'
|                                           |
CH- OOC-R   + 3R'COOH             →         CH- OOC-R'+ 3 RCOOH
|                                           |
CH2- OOC-R                                  CH- OOC-R'
```

Were R'COOH = EPA/DHA

c) Trans- esterification

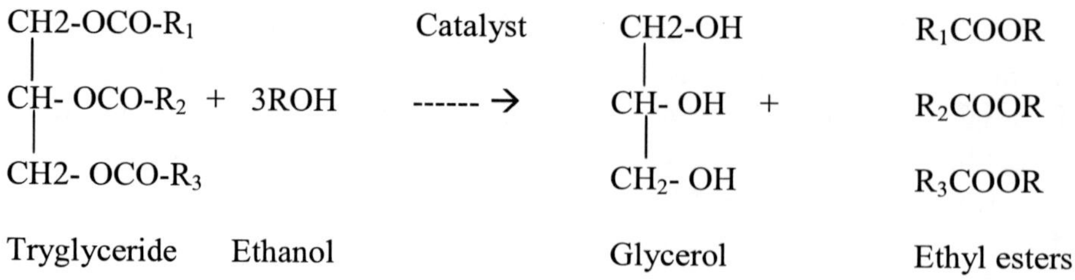

Water content in the reaction medium is a crucial factor that determines the extent of the esterification reaction. High water content in the reaction medium shifts the chemical equilibrium towards hydrolysis, whereas reduced water content shifts the equilibrium towards esterification. The optimum content of water in the esterification reaction should be kept to a minimum in order to discourage the partial hydrolysis of products and formation of glycerol as well as mono- and diacylglycerols.

Haraldsson et al., [160] concentrated n-3 PUFA by employing both direct esterification of glycerol and inter esterification of tributyrin with stoichiometric amount of 99 % pure EPA or DHA using yeast lipase from *Candida antarctica* (CA lipase). They obtained crude products with excellent yields (93 - 96 %) of very high purity (> 98 %). Similarly Osada et al. [162] found that in the direct esterification of glycerol with EPA and DHA, CV-lipase exhibited superiority over that of CC-lipase with a yield of 89-95%. Both these studies found that EPA is considerably a better substrate for CA-lipase compared to DHA. The reason for lower activity of the enzyme towards DHA is due to the fact that the carbon-carbon double bond in the nearest proximity of the carboxyl group is located one bond closer to the carboxyl group in DHA than EPA [163]. This affects its ability to fit properly into the active site of the enzyme.

In transesterification of fish oil with ethanol, Haraldsson et al., [164] found that, among the 17 lipases tested, *Pseudomonas* lipases had the highest activity toward the saturated and monounsaturated fatty acids in the fish oil and much lower activity toward EPA and DHA. Total recovery of DHA was over 80% and that of EPA 90%. Adachi et al. [165] also reported a similar finding while concentrating EPA and DHA from sardine oil by transesterification (acidolysis) with *Pseudomonas sp.* lipase. They found that acetone was more effective than n-hexane as a solvent for dissolving the reactants and concentrating the two fatty acids.

3.7.3. Chemical Interesterification

Another type of interesterification in use is chemical interesterification. Chemical interesterification has some advantages over enzymatic modification, which include lower catalyst cost, use of existing and more available industrial procedures and equipment, and shorter reaction times [166]. Interesterification can be carried out at 0–240°C depending on the type of catalyst used [167]. Klinkesorn et al., [168] studied the transesterification of tuna oil with n-3 fatty acid methyl ester (n-3 FAME) using sodium methoxide as catalyst. They found that, highest incorporation of EPA and DHA occurred after 5 h (at 80 °C), at a catalyst concentration of 1.5% w/w, and at a mole ratio of 1:4 (tuna oil: n-3 FAME). Sodium methoxide ($NaOCH_3$) is active at temperature around 50–90°C [130]. Addition of antioxidants or an inert atmosphere treatment should also be considered in order to prevent oxidative deterioration of oil especially fish oil due to the high level of polyunsaturated fatty acids.

3.7.4. Enzymatic Reactions in Supercritical Fluids

Supercritical carbon dioxide (SC-CO_2) has been proposed as a good medium to carry out enzymatic reactions since it is considered as a green solvent; nontoxic and easily removed from the reaction products. Gunnlaugsdottir and Sivik [169] studied the influence of experimental conditions such as pressure or solvent flow rate [170] on the ethanolysis of cod liver oil with an immobilized lipase (Novozym 435). The same authors have also studied the phase behavior of the reaction mixture in SC-CO_2 [171] and a coupled process with supercritical fluid extraction and enzymatic ethanolysis to produce omega-3 ethyl esters from cod liver oil in a continuous way [172]. Another recent procedure, proposed by Lin et al. [53], enables the ω-3 enrichment of fish oil through an enzymatic transesterification with an immobilized 1,3-specific lipase (Lipozyme IM-60) in a supercritical CO_2 medium (5 h, 323 K and 10.34 bar). They reported that under supercritical conditions, enzymatic transesterification was 40% higher than conventional solvents. A recent review shows all the possibilities of super critical fluid technology to perform enzymatic reactions, including oil hydrolysis and transesterification (Knez, 2009).

3.8. Chromatographic Methods

Using chromatographic methods it is possible to separate fatty acids according to their number of carbon and their degree of unsaturation by using appropriate adsorbents [55]. High performance liquid chromatography (HPLC) [173] and silver resin chromatography [174] have been used for the production of ω-3 PUFA concentrates. Solvent choice for separation of fatty acid esters depends on the desired purity of eluted fractions and their use as well as production requirements. Separation of n-3 PUFA from methyl esters of fish oil using tetrahydrofuran (THF)/methanol/water (25:55:20, v/ v/v) yielded fractions of EPA and DHA at 91.0 and 85.5% purity, respectively [175-176]. However THF is undesirable because it is potential explosive and its peroxides initiate oxidative decomposition of PUFA. Ethanol and water would be the solvents of choice if the end product is to be consumed by humans. Perrut [177] used methanol/ water (90:10, v/v) to separate ethyl esters of fish oil and obtained purities of 91-96% for EPA and 75-85% for DHA while methyl esters with the same solvent system yielded 86% purity for EPA and 83% DHA [81].

Teshima et al. [178] have used a silver nitrate-impregnated silica gel column to separate EPA and DHA from squid-liver oil after forming methyl esters. They were able to isolate 85-96% EPA and 95-98% DHA with a yield of 39 and 48%, respectively. Hayashi and Kishimura [179] have isolated 63-74% pure DHA from skipjack tuna eye orbital oil by stepwise elution with n-hexane, diethyl ether/n-hexane and diethyl ether on a silicic acid column. Adlof and Emiken [180] were able to enrich the ω-3 content of commercial n3-PUFA concentrates from 76.5 to 99.8% using silver resin column. In another study the same author's fractionated fish oil methyl esters containing 29.1% EPA and 20.5% DHA into fractions of 87.7% EPA and 95.4% DHA with increasing amounts of acetonitrile (0-30%) in methanol. They also fractionated non-enriched menhaden oil methyl esters and fatty acids, which contained about 12.5% EPA and 11.1% DHA. The separation was done isocratically using 40% acetonitrile in acetone; one of the eluted fractions contained approximately 69% of total EPA and DHA after being concentrated.

Guil-Guerrero *et al.*, [181] purified EPA and arachidonic acid (AA) from the red microalga *Porphyridium cruentum* by the urea inclusion method followed by silica gel column chromatography of the urea concentrate. They obtained AA and EPA with a purity of 97% for both fatty acids. Chakrabarthi and Raj [182] concentrated EPA derived from hydrolyzed sardine oil by a combination of urea fractionation and argentation neutral alumina column chromatography. They obtained EPA of high purity (99.6%) using 50% diethyl ether/n-hexane as eluting solvent.

Another chromatographic technique is simulated moving bed (SMB) chromatography. This is a continuous purification technique based on a flow of eluent moving counter-current to a constant flow of solid stationary phase. This technique is suited for the purification of EPA and DHA from a pre-concentrated feeds [183] by continuous injection of feed material for the separation as opposed to single injections in traditional batch chromatography [184].

3.8.1. Supercritical Fluid Chromatography (SFC)

As the recirculation of eluent represents a major part of the total cost of a preparative chromatographic process, the economy of such a process can be significantly improved if the organic eluent is substituted with a fluid in the supercritical state, preferably with carbon dioxide as the main component [185]. Perrut et al. [45] patented a method to isolate EPA and DHA from a mixture of fatty acid ethyl esters obtained from fish oil, coupling preparative supercritical chromatography and simulated countercurrent moving bed chromatography with several columns placed in series. In both cases, octadecyl silica gel is used as column stationary phase whereas SC-CO_2 is the eluent. Following this method, they obtained EPA and DHA fractions with a high yield (99%) and purity (92% and 85% respectively). The first pilot plant for supercritical fluid chromatography was built by Perrut and his group in Nancy, France [186]. They have shown that separation based on chain leghth can be combined with separation according to the degree of unsaturation, making supercritical fluid chromatography suitable for the production of purified ethyl esters of the two main omega 3-fatty acids, EPA and DHA [187-188]. Brunner and Reichmann [189] also patented a SFC method to isolate unsaturated fatty acids with at least 16 carbon atoms from a mixture of fatty acids or their derivatives using SC-CO_2 as eluent and aluminium oxide as stationary phase.

Alkio et al., [190] reported a systematic study in order to find the optimal conditions to purify DHA-EE and EPA-EE from esterified tuna oil. They found that using SC-CO_2 at 65°C and 145 bar and octadecyl silane as stationary phase, it was possible to obtain simultaneously a DHA-EE production of 0.85 g/ (kg stationary phase × h) with a purity of 90%, and an EPA-EE production of 0.23 g/(kg stationary phase × h) with a purity of 50%. Pettinello et al. [46] studied the enrichment on bench-scale and on pilot scale of an ester mixture from fish oil with 68% of EPA-EE using supercritical chromatography with SC-CO_2 as mobile phase and silica gel as stationary phase. They concluded that, on bench-scale production, using a column of 25 mm × 200 mm, the highest EPA-EE purity (90%) and recovery (49%) was obtained at a temperature of 70°C with a pressure program between 180 and 220 bar and a SC-CO_2 flow rate of 13.5 g/min. However, on semi-industrial scale using a column of 100 mm × 520 mm, the optimal conditions involved the use of the same temperature and pressure, but a higher CO_2 flow rate (15– 25 kg/h), which enabled to process a total amount of 300 g fish oil per cycle and obtain an EPA-EE purity of 93% with a yield of 24.6%. Snoey-Elich [47] has patented a method to concentrate EPA-EE from fish oil, from a purity of 50% to more than 95%, using an industrial column of 50–60 cm × 260–280 cm filled with a porous silicon oxide impregnated with (3-aminopropyl)- triethoxysilane as stationary phase and SC-CO_2 as mobile phase working at a pressure of 100–150 bar, a temperature of 40–60°C and a flow rate between 4000 and 7000 kg/h.

4. Squalene

Liver oils of some deep-sea sharks mainly *Centrophorus sp.* found at a depth of 300–3000 m in the Pacific, North Atlantic, and Indian Ocean contain about 85 to 90% unsaponifiable matter, which is essentially the hydrocarbon, squalene ($C_{30}H_{50}$, 2,6,10,15,19,23-hexamethyl, 2,6,10,14,18,22-tetracosahexaene) [191]. High content of low-density squalene (specific gravity 0.86 at 25°C) is believed to provide hydrostatic lift and enable the shark to maintain neutral buoyancy [192]. In basking shark (*Cetorhinus maximus*) about 7-45% of liver oil is composed of squalene and another hydrocarbon zamene [25]. A major species of shark *Centrophorus scalpratus* abundantly available in Indian Ocean, particularly off Andaman and Nicobar Islands, is one of the rich sources of squalene (80% of total unsaponifiable matter). Other species of sharks rich in squalene are Gulper shark (*Centrophorus granulosus*), Taiwan gulper shark (*Centrophorus niaukang*), Mandarian dogfish (*cirrhigaleus barbifer*), Kite fin shark (*Dalatias licha*), Bird peak dogfish (*Deania calcea*), Small-toothed sand tiger (*Carcharias ferox*) and Crocodile shark (*Pseudocarcharias kamoharai*) [193].

Squalene has been reported to possess antilipidemic, antioxidant and membrane stabilizing properties [194-196]. It has been found to be an efficient chemo preventive agent against variety of cancers, skin disorders, and liver diseases [197]. Its antiaging and detoxification properties have already been well studied [198-199]. In our own study, we found that squalene is able to mitigate the chemically induced myocardial infarction in experimental animals [200-205]. Squalene also has lots of industrial applications viz., used as bactericide, intermediate in the manufacture of pharmaceuticals, organic coloring matter, rubber chemicals, aromatics and surface-active agents [193].

4.1. Isolation of Squalene

Squalene can be isolated from the shark liver oil obtained from deep-sea sharks of the family squalidae. For the extraction of oil, the liver is removed immediately after the fish is landed. The chopped pieces of which are heated to 80°C in 2% caustic soda solution for 30-40 min. The floating oil is skimmed off and water is removed by filtration through anhydrous sodium sulphate and stored. The oil thus obtained can be fractionally distilled under vacuum (2 mbar) for isolation of squalene. A low boiling fraction distills out at 125-140°C is discarded and the major high boiling fraction distilled out at 240-245°C are collected separately. In low boiling fraction squalene accounts 3%, whereas the major high boiling fraction contains 85-90% squalene. The residue contains about 1-1.5% squalene. The pure squalene thus extracted is filled in bottles in inert atmosphere for storage [201]. Highly purified squalene or shark liver oil containing over 70% squalene is glassy-white in colour. The oil has a faint agreeable odor. On exposure to atmosphere squalene absorbs oxygen and colour starts changing to faint-yellow and finally brown due to oxidation. Oxidized squalene has very little biological properties [206].

5. Wax Esters

Wax esters are neutral lipids composed of long chain fatty alcohols esterified in equimolar amounts to long chain fatty acids. The chain lengths and the degree of unsaturation can vary in both the acid and alcohol moieties. A typical marine wax ester is palmitoyl oleate, 16: 0/18:1, consisting of palmitoyl alcohol (16: 0) esterified to oleic acid (18:1). Fatty acids in marine wax esters are typical of marine fatty acids, generally contains carbon chains ranging from C_{14} to C_{22}. The polyunsaturated fatty acids, 20:5 and 22:6, are prominent in marine wax esters from epipelagic zone [207]. Fatty acids of wax esters from meso- and bathypelagic organisms are generally deficient in polyunsaturated fatty acids. The fatty alcohols of all marine wax esters are invariably either saturated especially 16:0, or monounsaturated, especially 20:1 and 22:1. Organisms from the epipelagic zone are rich in 20:1 and 22:1 alcohols, whereas organisms from meso- and bathypelagic zones are rich in 16:0 alcohol. Thus, wax esters from epipelagic organisms generally have longer chain lengths than those from meso- and bathypelagic organisms [208].

Wax esters have been readily identified in many marine animals even though the sperm whale is the source of commercial wax. To date seven phyla, including *Coelenterata, Ctenophora, Chaetognatha, Mollusca, Annelida, Arthropoda and Chordata,* have species with wax esters as major neutral lipids, i.e., the wax esters account for more than 10% of the total lipid (Table 3). With the exception of the benthic corals and sea anemones, both of which contain substantial amounts of wax esters, most other marine animals rich in these lipids are pelagic [207]. The most studied groups are the crustaceans, especially the copepods that dominate the zooplankton biomass in most parts of the oceans. All the genera so far examined belonging to the calanoid copepod families Calanidae, Euchaetidae, Lucicutiidae, Heterorabdidae and Augaptilidae have wax esters accounting for more than 20% of their total lipid. An extreme example is the Arctic copepod *Calanus hyperboreus* that can contain nearly 80% of its dry mass as total lipid that is mostly wax esters [209].

Wax esters are synthesized *de novo* in the zooplanktons from carbohydrates, protein and fatty acid constituents of their phytoplankton diet. It accumulate in large amounts by those zooplankton that experience short periods of food abundance followed by prolonged periods of food shortage [210], especially in those living in polar regions. Thus the fundamental environment variable in determining the production of wax esters in copepods is the light regime, which is most extreme in high latitudes [211]. Wax esters are relatively stable metabolically in pre-adult and adult copepods but are rapidly consumed in developing eggs and nauplii [212]. Zooplankton eating fish such as the clupeoids convert dietary wax esters in their intestinal mucosa to triglycerides by a process whereby oxidation of fatty alcohol is coupled to reductive formation of triglyceride-glycerol from amino acids. In mid water or epipelagic fish, the wax esters are usually associated with the roe (mainly unsaturated) which function as energy reserves for developing fry, while in deep-water fishes wax esters are found mainly in the muscle and other tissues (both saturated and unsaturated) which helps to maintain buoyancy [208].

Table 3. Wax esters present in different marine organisms [a]

Species	Taxonomy	Wax esters as % of total lipids (Tissues)
Colelenterates		
Bolocera tuediae	P: Cnidaria, C:Anthozoa, O:Actiniaria, F:Actiniidae (sea anemons)	35 (Whole animal)
Condylactis giganta	P: Cnidaria, C:Anthozoa, O:Actiniaria, F:Actiniidae	40 (Whole animal)
Crustaceans		
Calanus helgolandicus	P: Arthropoda, C:Maxillipoda O:Calanoida, F:Calanidae	30-40 (Whole animal)
Gaussia principes	P: Arthropoda, C:Maxillipoda O:Calanoida, F:Metridiidae	73 (Whole animal)
Fishes		
Stenobrachius leucopsarus	P: Chordata, C: Actinopterygii, O:Myctophiformes F: Myctophidae (Lantern fishes)	90 (Muscle)
Triphoturus mexicanus	P: Chordata C: Actinopterygii, O:Myctophiformes F: Myctophidae	74 (Muscle)
Lampanyctus ritteri	P: Chordata, C: Actinopterygii, O:Myctophiformes F: Myctophidae	87 (Muscle)
Laemone mamorosum	P: Chordata, C: Actinopterygii, O:Gadiformes F: Moridae (deep sea cod)	50 (Muscle), >60 (Liver)
Holplostethus islandicus	P: Chordata, C: Actinopterygii O:Beryciformes F: Trachichthydae	90 (Muscle)
Mugil japonicus	P: Chordata, C: Actinopterygii O:Perciformes F: Mugilidae	70 (Roe or eggs)
Mugilcephalus	P: Chordata, C: Actinopterygii O:Perciformes F: Mugilidae	67 (Roe or eggs)
Ruvettus pretiosus	P: Chordata, C: Actinopterygii O:Perciformes F: Gempylidae	92 (Muscle)
Trichogaster cosby	P: Chordata, C: Actinopterygii O:Perciformes F: Osphrenomidae (Gauramis)	70(Roe or eggs)
Latimeria chalumnae	P: Chordata, C: Crossopterygii O:Coelacanthiformes F: Latimeridae (Celacanths)	93 (Muscle), 97 (Adipose tissue)
Birds		
Puffinus tenuirostris	P: 427Chordate, C: Aves, O:Ciconniiformes F: Procellariidae (Petrels)	90 (Stomach oil)
Mammals		
Berardius bairdii	P: 427Chordate, C: Mammalia O:Cetacea F: Ziphiidae (beaked whales)	80 (Blubber)
Hyperoodon ampullatus	P: 427Chordate, C: Mammalia O:Cetacea F: Ziphiidae	70 (Blubber)
Physester catodon	P: 427Chordate, C: Mammalia O:Cetacea F: Physeteridae (sperm whales)	66 (Blubber), 73 (Spermaceti organ)
Globicephala melaena	P: 427Chordate, C: Mammalia O:Cetacea F: Delphinidae (Dolphins and porpoises)	>30 (Head)
Tursiops truncatus	P: 427Chordate, C: Mammalia O:Cetacea F: Delphinidae	>35 (Jaw)

[a]: Data from Nevenzel et al. [207]

Wax esters have a variety of uses in many industries which includes as a high pressure lubricants, in the pharmaceutical, cosmetics, printing and leather industries, as well as in candles and polishes. It has been recently found that wax esters whose acidic moiety has been enriched in n-3 fatty acids are easily absorbed and metabolized by rats [213]. This result has a sound economic interest, since wax esters enriched in n-3 have interesting features when compared with traditional commercial products used as a source of n-3 fatty acids. Moreover, wax esters enriched in n-3 fatty acids have a low degree of susceptibility to oxidation, since they are not oils but in many cases waxy solids, and yet they are a good source of n-3 when they are ingested.

Marine wax esters as typically isolated are clear oils, fluid down to 0-2°C. Spermaceti from sperm whale oil is the only commercially extracted wax from marine sources and is extracted by crystallization of oil at 6°C by applying pressure and solution of caustic alkali. All the other works on isolation of wax esters are on laboratory scale. Wax esters can also be separated from neutral lipids by column chromatographic technique using silica gel with an eluent of 1:1 toluene/n-hexane, under a slight overpressure of nitrogen. Fractions containing esters were collected and evaporated under reduced pressure on a rotating evaporator [214].

6. Biodiesel

Biodiesel (monoalkyl esters) is considered as a renewable clean alternative fuel or fuel additive [215]. Biodiesel that is derived from animal fat, vegetable oil, or used cooking oil has noteworthy fuel characteristics, including a high flash point, outstanding biodegradability, excellent lubricity, and superior combustion efficiency in comparison with the fuel characteristics of petrodiesel. In addition, the burning of biodiesel does not produce polyaromatic hydrocarbons (PAH) which are carcinogenic in nature [216]. It has been well-reported that biodiesel obtained from canola, soybean, palm, sunflower oil and algal oil can be used as diesel fuel substitute [217]. It can also be prepared from used cooking oils and spent fish oils which would partly decrease the dependency on petroleum-based fuel. Several technologies are available to manufacture biodiesel, such as transesterification, amidation with diethylamine, catalyzing pyrolysis, and transesterification in supercritical methanol. Of these techniques, transesterification (Scheme) is the most widely applied in industrial biodiesel production [218].

CH2-OCO-R_1		Catalyst	CH2-H	R_1COOCH_3
CH- OCO-R_2 +	3 HOCH3	------ →	CH- OH +	R_2COOCH_3
CH2- OCO-R_3			CH_2- OH	R_3COOCH_3
Tryglyceride	**Methanol**		**Glycerol**	**Methyl esters (Biodiesel)**

Scheme: Transesterification process of biodiesel production.

A catalyst is required for transesterification reaction because the alcohol is sparingly soluble in the oil phase. The catalyst promotes an increase in solubility to allow the reaction to proceed at a reasonable rate. Three types of catalysts can be used in the transesterification process: a strong alkali, strong acid or enzyme. A strong alkali catalyst is most frequently used in the transesterification [219] reaction due to the following advantages:

- It does not require high temperature and pressure.
- Smaller amount of catalyst required
- It yields high conversion (98%) with minimal side reactions and reaction time.
- It allows a direct conversion into biodiesel with no intermediate compounds.
- It requires simple construction materials.

The base catalysts typically used are sodium hydroxide (caustic soda) or potassium hydroxide (caustic potash).

6.1. Production Process

Sodium hydroxide (1% wt), is dissolved in methyl alcohol using a standard agitator or mixer for 5 min to form sodium methoxide. This is then charged into a closed reactor and mixed with the fish oil by a mechanical homogenizer at a speed of 6000 rpm. Refined oil is the best starting material to produce biodiesel because the conversion of pure triglyceride into fatty acid methyl ester is high, and the reaction time is relatively short. The reaction mix is kept just below the boiling point of the methanol (63°C) in order to prevent the evaporation of methanol and to speed up the reaction. Recommended reaction time varies from 1 to 8 h, and optimal reaction time is about 2 h [220]. Lin and Li [221] reported a reaction time of 50 mins for the completion of transesterification reaction in marine oils. Excess alcohol is normally used to ensure total conversion of the fat or oil to its esters. After the reaction is completed, two major products *viz,* glycerin and biodiesel can be obtained, which contains substantial amount of the excess methanol that was used in the reaction. The reaction mixture is sometimes neutralized at this step if needed. The glycerin phase is much denser than the biodiesel phase and the two can be gravity separated, with glycerin simply drawn off the bottom of the settling vessel. In some cases, a centrifuge is used to separate the two materials faster. The crude biodiesel is then distilled at 70°C to collect the unreacted methanol. The biodiesel was then washed by adding 50% wt petroleum ether and then with cold distilled water (10°C) to remove other impurities. This was followed by a distillation at 105°C to remove the remaining water and unreacted reactant mixture to obtain good quality biodiesel [221]. The glycerin byproduct contains unused catalyst and soaps that are neutralized with sulfuric acid and sent to storage as crude glycerin. In most cases the salt is left in the glycerin. Water and alcohol are removed to produce 90% pure glycerin that is ready to be sold as crude glycerin [222-223].

The stoichiometric ratio for transesterification reaction requires three moles of alcohol and one mole of triglyceride to yield three moles of fatty acid ester and one mole of glycerol. Higher molar ratios result in greater ester production in a shorter time. The commonly accepted molar ratios of alcohol to oils are 3:1 to 6:1. Excess methanol (such as a 20:1 ratio) is generally necessary in batch reactors where water accumulates [222]. The cost of oils or fats directly affects the cost of biodiesel by as much as 70 to 80%. Crude oils contain some free fatty acids and phospholipids. The phospholipids are removed in a degumming step and the free fatty acids are removed in a refining step. For an alkali catalyzed transesterification, the triglycerides and alcohol must be substantially anhydrous [224] because water makes the reaction partially change to saponification, which produces soap. The soap lowers the yield of esters and renders the separation of ester and glycerol and the water washing difficult. Low free fatty acid content in triglycerides is required for alkali-catalyzed transesterification. If more water and free fatty acids are in the triglycerides, acid-catalyzed transesterification can be used [225].

6.2. Properties of Marine Biodiesel

Properties of the biodiesel make an important contribution to its efficiency. Lin and Li, [221] studied the fuel properties of biodiesel produced from the crude fish oil from the soapstock of marine fish. They found that, the marine fish-oil biodiesel contained as high as 37.07 % saturated fatty acids and 37.3% long chain fatty acids in the range between C_{20} and C_{22}. Oleic acid (C18:1) and palmitic acid (C16:0) were the two major components of the marine fish oil biodiesel.

Marine fish oil biodiesel was found to have higher cetane index (50.9) when compared to biodiesel from waste cooking oil (48.1) [221]. Biodiesel with larger cetane number may improve the engine performance and reduce pollutant emissions [226]. The acid number of a biodiesel can be used to indicate the content of free fatty acids of the fuel. The marine fish-oil biodiesel was found to have a larger acid number (1.17 mg/KOH) than that of the commercial biodiesel produced from waste cooking oil (0.69 mg/KOH) [221]. The reason for high acid value in their study is due to higher water content in the marine oil. The biodiesel produced from waste cooking oil is primarily composed of unsaturated fatty acids of C_{16}–C_{18} carbon chains whereas, the biodiesel from marine fish oil contained about 20% highly unsaturated fatty acids. This make them more prone to hydrolysis resulting in larger fraction of free fatty acids and larger acid number than that of the other biodiesel [221]. Biodiesel from marine sources have low oxidative stability as they contain polyunsaturated fatty acids with more than three double bounds which are prone to oxidation. Low oxidative stability can cause the precipitation of the biodiesel components in a fuel feeding system or combustion chamber [227].

Viscosity is a significant fuel property that affects the flow and atomization characteristics of a liquid fuel. Higher the viscosity, lower is the flow and atomization characteristics. In general, biodiesel from fish oil has a viscosity (7.2 cSt) greater than that of the biodiesel from vegetable oils and ASTM no.2Diesel (3.4cSt). Hence, it is inferred that the biodiesel fuels from crude marine fish oil and waste cooking oil (4.7cSt) which is having high viscosity than commercial diesel will have inferior injection and atomization performance, but offer lubrication and protection for the moving parts of an engine [221]. Reyes and Sepulveda [228] reduced the kinematic viscosity of the salmon-oil biodiesel from 4.96 cSt to 3.46 cSt at 70°C by removing some components at higher boiling points, which suggests that the kinematic viscosity of the marine fish-oil biodiesel could be decreased if the biodiesel were treated in similar processes. Knothe et al., [229] found that the values of kinematic viscosity vary with the kind of fatty acids in methyl esters. For example, larger proportions of saturated fatty acids with longer carbon chains cause kinematic viscosity to increase.

Distillation temperature is another characteristic which is strongly related with the boiling point of a liquid fuel and significantly affects the combustion characteristics of diesel engines. A higher distillation temperature may shorten the ignition delay of fuel and decrease the probability of the occurrence of knocking in diesel engines [230]. The biodiesel fuels from marine fish oil were reported to have higher distillation temperatures than of ASTM No. 2D diesel [221].

Another important burning characteristic of the biodiesel is the heating value. It is the enthalpy released after the complete combustion reaction of fuel at a constant pressure or volume. Monyem and Van Gerpen [231] found that a marine biodiesel had a heating value lower than that of ASTM No. 2D diesel by about 12.7–14.7%. The heating values of the biodiesel fuels from marine fish oil and commercial biodiesel from waste cooking oil and the ASTM No. 2D diesel fuel were 41.37 MJ/kg, 40.11 MJ/kg, and 46.16 MJ/kg, respectively. Hence, marine fish-oil biodiesel has a heating value higher than that of commercial biodiesel from waste cooking oil. However, the ASTM No. 2D diesel has a higher heating value than the other two biodiesel fuels. The higher the heating value, the lower is the fuel consumption rate.

The flash point of the marine fish-oil biodiesel was 103°C., However, the flash points of the biodiesel fuels from marine fish oil and waste cooking oil were much higher than the flash point of ASTM No. 2D diesel. Liquid fuel with a high flash point can prevent auto ignition and fire hazards at high temperatures during transportation and storage periods [221].

References

[1] Rambjor, G. S., Wålen, A.I., Windsor, S.L., & Harris, W.S. (1996). Eicosapentaenoic acid is primarily responsible for hypotriglyceridemic effect of fish oil in humans. *Lipids, 31S*, 545–S549.

[2] Simopoulos, A. P. (1991). Omega-3 fatty acids in health and disease and in growth and development. *Am. J. Clin. Nutr., 54,* 438–463.

[3] Connor, W. E. (2000). Importance of n -3 fatty acids in health and disease. *Am. J. Clin. Nutr., 71,* 171s–175s.

[4] Shahidi, F., & Wanasundara, U.N. (1998). Omega-3 fatty acid concentrates: nutritional aspects and production technologies. *Trend Food Sci. Technol., 9*, 230-240.

[5] Haraldsson, G. G., Gudmundsson, B. O., & Almarsson, O. (1995). Synthesis of homogeneous triglycerides of eicosapentaenoic acid and docosahexaenoic acid by lipase. *Tetrahedron, 51*, 941– 52.

[6] Nichols, P. D. (2007). Fish oil sources, In. Breivik, H. (Ed.) *Long chain omega 3 speciality oils*, pp 20-40, The Oil Press, PJ Barnes and associates, Bridgwater, England.

[7] Ackman, R.G., (1967). Characteristics of the fatty acid composition and biochemistry of some fresh water fish oil and lipids in comparison with marine oil and lipids. *Comp. Biochem. Physiol. 22*, 907–922.

[8] Sinclair, A. J., Murphy, K. J., Li, D. (2000). Marine lipids: overview "news insights and lipid composition of Lyprinol". *Allerg. Immunol. 32(7)*, 261-71.

[9] Stansby, M. E. (1967). *Fish oils: Their chemistry, technology, stability, nutritional properties and uses.* The Avi Publishing Company, Inc, Westport. p 440.

[10] Nichols, P. D., Mooney, B. D., Elliott, N. G., & Yearsley, G. K. (1998b). *Seafood the good food: The oil (fat) content and composition of Australian commercial fishes, shell fishes and crustaceans*, CSIRO marine research, Hobart, Tasmania, Australia.

[11] Brockerhoff, H., R. G., & Ackman, & Hoyle, R. J. (1963). Specific distribution of fatty acids in marine lipids. *Arch. Biochem. Biophy., 100*, 9-12.

[12] Phleger, C. F., Nelson, M. M., Mooney, B. D., & Nichols, P. D. (2002). Interannual and between species comparision in the lipids, fatty acids and sterols of Antartic krill from the US AMLR Elephant Island survey area:1997 and 1998. *Comp. Biochem. Physiol., 131B,* 733-747.

[13] Virtue, P., Nichols, P. D., Nicol, S., & Hosie, G. (1996). Reproductive trade off in male antartic krill. *Marine Biol, 126,* 521-527.

[14] Walters, A. (2005). *Long-finned pilot whales (G. melas)* (BSc Honors thesis), University of Tasmania, Hobart, Tasmania, Australia.

[15] Conchillo, A., Valencia, I., Puente, A., Ansorena, D., & Astiasarán, I. (2006). Componentes funcionales en aceite de pescado y alga. *Nutrición Hospitalaria, 21*, 369–373.

[16] Domingo, J. L., Bocio, A., Falcó, G., & Llobet, J. M. (2007). Benefits and risks of fish consumption I. A quantitative analysis of the intake of omega-3 fatty acids and chemical contaminants. *Toxicol., 230*, 219–226.

[17] Wynn, J. P. & Ratledge, C. (2007). Microbial oils: production, processing and markets for speciality long chain omega-3 polyunsaturated fatty acids. In: Breivik, H. (Ed.) *Long chain omega 3 speciality oil,* pp:43-76, The Oil Press, PJ Barnes and associates, Bridgwater, England.

[18] Seto, A., Kumasaka, K., Hosaka, M., Kojima, E., Kashiwakura, M., & Kato, M. (1992). Production of eicosapentaenoic acid by a mirine microalgae and its commercial utilization for aquaculture. In: Kyle, D. J., & Ratedge, C. (Eds). *Applications of single cell oils,* American oil Chemists' Society, IL,USA, pp 219-234.

[19] Zittelli, G. C., Pastorelli, R., & Tredici, M. R. (2000). A modular flat panel photobioreactor (MFPP) for indoor mass cultivation of *Nannochloropsis* sp. Under artificial illumination. *J. Appl. Phycol., 12*, 521-526.

[20] Tan, C. K., & Johns, M. R. (1996). Screening of diatoms for the heterotrophic eicosapentaenoic acid production. *J. Appl. Phycol., 8*, 59-64.

[21] Wen, Z. Y., & Chen F. (2005). Prospects of eicosapentaenoic acid production using micro organism. In. Cohen, Z., & Ratledge, C. (Eds.), *Single cell oils*, pp.138-160, AOCS press, IL,USA.

[22] Wen, Z. Y., & Chen, F. (2003). Heterotrophic production of eicosapentaenoic acid by micro algae. *Biotech. Adv. 21,* 273-294.

[23] Yazawa, K., Watanabe, K., Ishikawa, C., Kondo. K., & Kimura, S. (1992). Production of eicosapentaenoic acid from marine bacteria. In: Kyle, D. J., & Ratedge, C., (Eds.) *Industrial application of single cell oils*, pp 29-51, American oil Chemists' society, IL,USA

[24] Tocher, D. R., Bendiksen, E. A., Campbell, P. J., & Bell, J. G. (2008). The role of phospholipids in nutrition and metabolism of teleost fish. *Aquaculture*, *280,* 21–34.

[25] Lovern, J. A. (1962). The lipids of fish and changes occuring in them during processing and storage. In. Heen, E., & Kreuzer, R. (Eds.) *Fish in nutrition*, p 94, Fishing news (Books) Ltd. London.

[26] Njinkoue, J. M., Barnathan, G., Miralles, J., Gaydou, E. M., & Samb, A. (2002). Lipids and fatty acids in muscle, liver and skin of three edible fish from the Senegalese coast:

Sardinella maderensis, Sardinella aurita and Cephalopholis taeniops. Comp. Biochem. Physiol. 131B, 395–402.

[27] Takagi, T., Itabashi, Y., & Aso, S. (1985). Fatty acids and fatty alcohols of wax esters in the orange roughy: Specific textures of minor polyunsaturated and branched-chain components. *Lipids, 20,* 675-679.

[28] Green. J. (1951). Studies on the Analysis of Vitamins D 2. The analytical purification of vitamin d by differential solubility, precipitation reactions, and chromatography. *Biochem. J. 49,* 45.

[29] Bailey, B. E., Carter, N. M., & Swain, L. A., (1952). The chemistry and technology of marine oils with particular reference to those of Canada. *Fish. Res. Bd Can. Bull. No. 89.*

[30] Omara-Alwala, T. R., Chen, H. M., Ito, Y., Simpson, K. L., & Meyers, S. P. (1985). Carotenoid pigment and fatty acid analyses of crawfish oil extracts *.J. Agric. Food Chem., 33,* 260-263.

[31] Brinchmann, H. J. (1967). Technical University of Norway, Institute for Technical Biochemistry, Tronheim, 1967, pp 1-39 (translated by P. M. Jangaard, Fisheries and Marine Services, Environment Canada, Halifax, 1975).

[32] Frankel, E. N. (2005). *Lipid Oxidation,* 2nd ed. The Oily Press, Bridgwater.

[33] Breivik, H., & Thorstad, O. (2005). Removal of organic environmental pollutants from fish by short path distillation. *Lipid Technol., 17,* 55-58.

[34] Davidson, M. H., Burns, J. H., Subbaiah, P. Y., Conn, M. E., & Drennan, K. B. (1991) Marine Oil Capsule Therapy for the Treatment of Hyperlipidaemia, *Arch. Intern. Med. 151,* 1732-1740.

[35] Bryhn, M., Hansteen, H., Schanche, T., & Aakre, S.E. (2006). The bioavailability and pharmacodynamics of different concentrations of omega-3 acid ethyl esters. *Prostag. Leukotr. Essential Fatty Acids, 75,* 19–24.

[36] Breivik, H. (2007). Concentrates In: long chain Omega-3 speciality oil. Breivik, H. (Ed.) *The oil press* (pp 112), P J Barnes and Associates, Bridgwater, England.

[37] Lawson, L. D., & Hughes, B. G. (1988). Human absorption of fish oil fatty acids as triacylglycerols, free fatty acids or ethyl esters. *Biochem. Biophys. Res. Comm. 152,* 328-335.

[38] Boyd, L. C., King, M. F., & Sheldon, B. (1992). A rapidmethod for determining the oxidation of n−3 fatty acids. *J. Am. Oil Chem. Soc., 69,* 325−330.

[39] Wijesundera, C., Ceccato, C., Watkins, P., Fagan, P., Fraser, B., Thienthong, N., Patrick, P. ((2008). Docosahexaenoic acid is more stable to oxidation when located at the sn−2 position of triacylglycerol compared to sn-1. *J. Am. Oil Chem. Soc., 85,* 543−548.

[40] Fleck, U., Tiegs, C., & Brunner, G. (1998). Fractionation of fatty acid ethyl esters by supercritical CO2: High separation efficiency using an automated countercurrent column. *J. Supercrit. Fluids, 14,* 67−74.

[41] Brunner, G., & Riha, V. (2000). Separation of fish oil ethyl esters with supercritical carbon dioxide. *J. Supercri. Fluids, 17,* 55–64.

[42] Perretti, G., Motori, A., Bravi, E., Favatic, F., Montanari, L., & Fantozzi, P. (2007). Supercritical carbon dioxide fractionation of fish oil fatty acid ethyl esters. *J. Supercrit. Fluids, 40,* 349−353.

[43] Espinosa, S., Diaz, S., & Brignole, E. A. (2002). Thermodynamic modeling and process optimization of supercritical fluid fractionation of fish oil fatty acid ethyl esters. *Ind. Eng. Chem. Res. 41(6)*, 1516–1527.

[44] Gironi, F., & Maschietti, M. (2006). Separation of fish oils ethyl esters by means of supercritical carbon dioxide: Thermodynamic analysis and process modelling. *Chem. Eng. Sci., 61*, 5114–5126.

[45] Perrut, M., Nicoud, R. M. & Breivik, H. (1998). *Processes for chromatographic fractionation of fatty acids and their derivatives*. Patent US5719302.

[46] Pettinello, G., Bertucco, A., Pallado, P., & Stassi, A. (2000). Production of EPA enriched mixtures by supercritical fluid chromatography: From the laboratory scale to the pilot plant. *J. Supercrit. Fluids, 19,* 51–60.

[47] Snoey-Elich, H. (2001). *Nuevo procedimiento de preparación del éster etílico del ácido eicosapentaenoico*. Patent ES 2 159 257 A1. Spain.

[48] LeGoffic, F., Nguyen, A., & Khayat-Frydman, C. (2000). *Concentration and purification of polyunsaturated fatty acid esters by distillation enzymatic transesterification coupling*. WO 00/73254.

[49] Kulångs, E. & Breivik, H. (2001). *Recovery of polyunsaturated fatty acids from urea adducts*. Patent WO 01/10809.

[50] Linder, M., Matouba, E., Fanni, J., & Parmentier, M. (2002). Enrichment of salmon oil with n−3 PUFA by lipolysis, filtration and enzymatic re-esterification. *Eur. J. Lipid Sci. Technol., 104*, 455–462.

[51] Gámez-Meza, N., Noriega-Rodríguez, J. A., Medina-Juárez, L. A., Ortega-García, J., Monroy-Rivera, J., Toro-Vázquez, F. J., Garcia, H. S., & Angulo-Guerrero, O. (2003). Concentration of eicosapentaenoic acid and docosahexaenoic acid from fish oil by hydrolysis and urea complexation. *Food Res. Int., 36*, 721–727.

[52] Kojima, Y., Sakuradani, E., & Shimizu, S. (2006). Different specificity of two types of Pseudomonas lipases to C20 fatty acids with Δ5 unsaturated double bond and their application for selective concentration of fatty acids. *J. Biosci. Bioeng. 101(6),* 496–500.

[53] Lin, T. J., Chen, S. W., & Chang, A. C. (2006). Enrichment of n−3 PUFA contents on triglycerides of fish oil by lipase-catalyzed trans-esterification under supercritical conditions. *Biochem. Eng. J., 29*, 27–34.

[54] Liu, S., Zhang, C., Hong, P., & Ji, H. (2006). Concentration of docosahexaenoic acid (DHA) and eicosapentaenoic acid (EPA) of tuna oil by urea complexation: Optimization of process parameters. *J Food Eng.,* 73, 203–209.

[55] Brown, L. B., & Kolb, D. X. (1955). Application of low temperature crystallization in the separation of the fatty acids and their compounds. *Prog. Chem. Fats Lipids, 3*, 57-94.

[56] Chawala, P., & DeMan, J. M. (1990). Measurement of size distribution of fat crystals using a laser particle counter. *J. Am. Oil Chem. Soc.,76*, 329-332.

[57] Haraldsson, G. G. (1984). Separation of saturated/unsaturated fatty acids. *J. Am. Oil Chem. Soc., 61*, 219-222.

[58] Schlenk, H. (1961). Crystallization of fatty acids. *J. Am. Oil Chem. Soc., 38,* 728-736.

[59] Markley, K.S. (1964). Techniques of separation: Distillation, salt solubilities methods and low temperature crystallization. In. Markley, K. S., (Ed.). *Fatty Acids*, pp 1983-2123, Interscience Publishers, New York.

[60] Hixson, A. W., & Bockelmann, L. B. (1942). Liquid-liquid extraction employing solvents in the region of their critical temperatures. *Trans. Am. Inst. Chem. Eng., 38,* 891-930.

[61] Yokochi, T., Usita, M., Kamisaka, Y., Nakahara, T., Suzuki, O. (1990). Increase in the c-linolenic acid content by solvent winterization of fungal oil extracted from Mortierella genus. *J. Am. Oil Chem. Soc. 67,* 846–851.

[62] Kreulen, H. P. (1976). Tractionation and winterization of edible fats and oils. In. *J. Am. Oil Chem. Soc. 53*, 393-395.

[63] Wanasundara, U. N. (1996). *Marine oils: Stabilization, structural characterization and omega-3 fatty acid concentration*, Ph.D. thesis, Memorial University of Newfoundland, St. John's, NF, Canada.

[64] Singleton, W.S. (1960). Solution Properties, In. Mark- ley, K. S., (Ed.) Fatty acids, pp 609-678, Interscience Publishers, New York, NY, USA.

[65] Stout, V. F., Niisson, W. B., Krzynowek, J., & Schlenk, H. (1990). Fractionation of fish oil and their fatty acids, In. Stansby, M. E., (ed) *Fish oils in nutrition*, pp 73-119, Van Nostrand Rein- hold, New York, NY, USA.

[66] Han, D. S., Ahn, H. B., & Shin, H. K. (1987). Seperation of EPA and DHA from fish oils by solubility Differences of fatty acids salts in ethanol. Korean *J. Food Sci. Technol., 19*, 430-434.

[67] Brown, J. B. (1941). Low-temperature crystallization of the fatty acids and glycerides. *Chem. Rev., 29(2)*, 333–354.

[68] Brocklesby, H. N. (1936). Fatty acids and their esters: i. Some observations on the cryoscopy and ebullioscopy of fatty acids. *Can. J. Res., 14b(6)*, 222-230.

[69] Bengen, M. F. (1940). German patent application 3, 190, 197 IVd/12o (OZ 12438).

[70] Smith, A. E. (1952). Crystal Structure of the Urea-Hydrogen Complexes. *Acta Cryst. 5*, 224-235.

[71] Schlenk, H. (1954). Urea Inclusion Compounds of Fatty Acids. In Holman, R. T., Lundberg, W.O. and Malkin, T., (Eds.), *Progress in the Chemistry of Fats and Other Lipids*, pp 243-267, Pergamon Press, New York, NY, USA.

[72] Swern, D. (1963). Techniques of separation. E.Urea complexes. In. Markley, K. S. (Ed.) Fatty acids, Part 3, Interscience, New York, pp 2309-2358.

[73] Linko, R. R., & Karinkanta, H. (1970). Fractionation of baltic herring flesh oil fatty acids by urea adduct formation. *Suomen Kemistilehti B, 43,* 311-314.

[74] Breivik, H., Jøgensen, T. E., & Børretzen, B. (1985). *A refined fish oil concentrate and the production process of the same*. Patent application WO 87/03899.

[75] Hayes, D. G., Van Alstine, J. M., & Setterwall, F. (2000). Urea based fractionation of seed oil samples containing fatty acids and acylglycerols of polyunsaturated and hydrxyl fatty acids. *J. Am. Oil Chem. Soc., 77*, 207-213.

[76] Ratnayake, W. M. N., Olsson, B., Matthews, D., & Ackman, R. G. (1988). Preparation of omega-3 PUFA concentrates from fish oils via urea complexation. *Fat Sci. Technol., 90*, 381–386.

[77] Haagsma, N., Gent, C. M., Luten, J. B., Jong, R. W., & Doorn, E. (1982). Preparation of n-3 fatty acid concentrate from cod liver oil. *J. Am. Oil Chem. Soc., 59,* 117–118.

[78] Udaya, N., Wanasundara, X., & Shahidi, F. (1999). Concentration of omega 3-polyunsaturated fatty acids of seal blubber oil by urea complexation: Optimization of reaction conditions. *Food Chem., 65*, 41–49.

[79] Han, D., Shin, H. K., & Yoon, S. H. (1997) Separation of ω 3- polyunsaturated fatty acids from fish oils and stabilization of the oil against autoxidation. In. Shahidi, F., & Cadwallader, K.R., (Eds.) *Flavor and Lipid Chemistry of Seafood*, pp. 255-263, ACS Symposium Series 674, American Chemical Society, Washington, DC, USA.

[80] Senanayake, S. P. J. N., & Shahidi, V. (2000). Concentration of docosahexaenoic acid (DHA) from algal oil via urea complexation. J. Food Lipids, 7, 51 -61.

[81] Wille, H. J., Traitler, H. & Kelly, M. (1987). Production of polyenoic fish oil fatty acids by combined urea fractionation and industrial scale preparative high performance liquid chroma- tography. *Rev. Fr. Corps Gras., 34,* 69-74.

[82] Schlenk, H., & Holman, R. T. (1950). Separation and stabilization of fatty acids by urea complexes. *J. Am. Oil Chem. Soc., 27*, 5001-5004.

[83] Robles-Medina, A., Molina-Grima, E., Gimenez-Gimenez, A., & Ibanez-Gonzalez, M. J. (1998). Downstream processing of algal polyunsaturated fatty acids. *Biotechnol. Adv., 16*, 517–580.

[84] Guil-Guerrero, J. L., EI-Hassan Belarbi & Rebolloso-Fuentes. (2001). Eicosapentaenoic and arachidonic acids purification from the red microalga Porphyridium cruentum. *Bioseparation 9*: 299–306.

[85] Hayes, D. G. (2002). Free fatty acid fractionation via urea inclusion compounds. Inform, 13, 832-834.

[86] Canas, B. J., & Yurawecz, M. P. (1999). Ethyl carbamate formation during urea complexation for fractionation of fatty acids, *J. Am. Oil Chem. Soc., 76*, 537.

[87] Adams, P., & Baron, F. A. (1965). Esters of carbamic acid. *Chem. Rev., 65*, 567–602.

[88] Nettleship, A., Henshaw, P. S., & Meyer, H. L. (1943). Introduction of pulmonary tumors in mice with ethyl carbamate (Urethane), *J. Natl. Cancer Inst., 4*, 309–319.

[89] Mirvish, S. S., (1968). The carcinogenic action and metabolism of urethane and n-hydroxyurethane, *Adv. Cancer Res. 11*, 1–42.

[90] Food and Drug Administration, (1990). Urethane in alcoholic beverages, *Federal Register, 55,* 10816–10817.

[91] Odden, E. (2006). Analysis of minor fatty acids in omega 3 products. Abstract I-4, In. *Abstract Book, Nordic Lipidforum seminar on marine Oils, 21-22 September*, Bergen, Norway.

[92] Gunstone, F. D., Kates, M., & Harwood, J. L. (1994). Crystallisation. In: Gunstone, F. D., Harwood, J. L., & Padley, F. B. (Eds.) *The Lipid Handbook*, 2nd Edn, pp 225-226, Chapman and Hall, London.

[93] Wright, S. W., Kuo, E. Y., & Corey, E. J. (1987). An effective process for the isolation of DHA in quantity from cod liver oil. *J. Org.Chem., 52*, 4399-4401.

[94] Corey, E. J., & Wright, S. W., 1988. convenient method for the recovery of EPA from cod liver oil. *J. Org.Chem., 53,* 5980-5981.

[95] Ioth, T., Murota, I., Yoshikai, K.,Yamada, S., & Yamamoto, K. (2006). Synthesis of DHA derivatives designed as novel PPARγ agonists and antidiebetic agents. *Bioorg. Med. Chem., 14*, 98-108.

[96] Flock, S., Lundquist, M., & Skattebøl, L. (1999). Synthesis of some polyunsaturated sulphur aand oxygen containing fatty acids related to EPA and DHA. *Acta Chemica Scandinavia, 53*, 436-445.

[97] Holmeide, A. K., Skattebøl, L. & Sydnes, M. (2001). The synthesis of three highly unsaturated marine lipid hydrocarbons. *J. Chem. Soc. Perkin Trans., 1,* 1942-1946.

[98] Holmeide, A. K., & Skattebøl, L. (2000). Synthesis of some polyunsaturated trifluoromethyl ketones as potential phospholipase A2 inhibitors. *J. Chem. Soc. Perkin Trans. 1*, 2271-2276.

[99] Kuklev, D. V., Aizdaicher, N. A., Imbs, A. B., Bezuglov, V. V., & Latyshev, N. A. (1992). All-cis-3,6,9,12,15-octadecapentaenoic acid from the unicellular algae *Gymnodinium kowalevskii. Phytochem., 31,* 2401-2403.

[100] Gaiday, N. V., Imbs, A. B., Kuklev, D. V., & Latyshev, N. A. (1991). Separation of natural polyunsaturated fatty acids by means iodolactonisation. *J. Am. Oil Chem. Soc., 68,* 230-233.

[101] Berger, R., & McPherson, W. (1979). Fractional Distillation. *J. Am. Oil Chem. Soc., 56,* 743A-746A.

[102] Brockmann, R., Demmering, G., Kreutzer, U., Lindemann, M., Plachenka, J., Steinberner, U. (2005). *Separation of fatty acids in fatty acids*. pp.16-20, Wiley-VCH Verlag GmbH & Co. KGaA, Weinheim.

[103] Brevik, H. (1992). n-3 concentrates- A Scabdinavian viepoint. In: Ackman, R.G. (Ed.), *Compendium for AOCS short cource: Modern applications of marine oil*, May 8-9, Toronto, Canada, American Oil Chemists Society, Chapaign, Illinois, USA.

[104] Privett, O. S., Weber, R. P., & Nickell, E. C. (1959). Preparation and properties of methyl arachidonate from Pork liver. In. *J. Am. Oil Chem. Soc., 36,* 443-449

[105] Privett, O. S., & Nickell, E. C. (1963). Preparation of highly purified fatty acids via Liquid-Liquid Partition Chromatography. In. *J. Am. Oil Chem. Soc. 40,* 189-193.

[106] Ackman, R. G., Ke, P. L., & Jangaard, P. M. (1973). Fractional vacuum distillation of Herring oil methyl esters. *J. Am. Oil Chem. Soc., 50*, 1-8.

[107] Breivik, H., Haraldsson, G. G. & Kristinsson, B. (1997). The preparation of highly purified concentrates of EPA and DHA. *J. Am. Oil Chem. Soc., 74,* 1425-1429.

[108] Staby, A., & Mollerup, J. (1993). Separation of constituents of fish oil using supercritical fluids: A review of experimental solubility, extraction, and chromatographic data. *Fluid Phase Equilibria, 91(2)*, 349–386.

[109] Brunner, G. (1994). *Gas extraction. An introduction to fundamentals of supercritical fluids and the application to separation processes*. Springer, New York.

[110] Mishra, V. K., Temelli, F., & Ooraikul, B. (1993). Extraction and purification of w-3 fatty acids with an emphasis on supercritical fluid extraction-A review. *Food Res. Int., 26*, 217–226

[111] Passino, H. J. (1949). Drying Oils, The Solexol Process. *Eng. C & N. 41(Z)*: 280-287.

[112] Zosel, K., (1978). Praktische Anwendungen der Stofftrennung mit tiberkritischen *Gasen. Angew. Chem., 90(10),* 748-755.

[113] Eisenbach, W., (1984). Supercritical Fluid Extraction: A Film Demonstration. *Ber. Bunsenges. Phys. Chem. 88 (9)*, 882-887.

[114] Arai, K., & Saito, S. (1986). Fractionation of fatty acids and their derivatives by extractive crystallization using gas as a solvent. Paper presented at 'World Congress III of Chemical Engineering", Tokyo.

[115] Yamaguchi, K., & Murakami, M. (1986). Application of supercritical fluid extraction to aquatic organisms. *Yukagaku, 35(4),* 260-266.

[116] Wong, J. M., & Johnston, K. P., (1986). Solubilization of biomolecules in carbon dioxide based supercritical fluids. *Biotechnol. Prog., 2(1),* 29-39.

[117] Ohgaki, K., Tsukahara, I., Semba, K. & Katayama, T. (1987). A fundamental study of supercritical fluid extraction -solubilities of cr-tocopherol, pahnitic acid, and tripalmitin in compressed carbon dioxide at 25°C and 40°C. *Kagaku Kogaku Ronbunshu, 13(3)*, 298-303.

[118] Elvevoll, E. O., 1988. *Biokjemikalier fra Marint Fett.* Ph. D. Thesk, University of Trondheim, NTH, Norway.

[119] Krukonis, V. J., 1989. Supercritical fluid processing of fish oils: Extraction of polychlorinated biphenyls. *J. Am. Oil Chem. Soc., 66,* 818-821.

[120] Nam, K. S., Kapila, S., Viswanath, D. S., Clevenger, T. E., Johansson, J. & Yanders, A. F. (1989). Application of supercritical fluid extraction of biological tissue samples for the determination of polychlorinated organics. *Chemosphere, 19,* 33-38.

[121] Nam, K. S., Kapila, S., Yanders, A. F., & Puri, R. K., 1990. Supercritical fluid extraction and cleanup procedures for determination of xenobiotics in biological samples. *Chemosphere, 20,* 873-880.

[122] Nam, K. S., Kapila, S., Yanders, A. F., & Puri, R. K. (1991). A multiple sample extraction and on-line system for the analysis of chlorinated compounds. *Chemosphere, 23,* 1109-1116.

[123] Myher, J. J., Kuksis, A., & Yang, L. Y. (1990). Stereospecific analysis of menhaden oil triacylglycerols and resolution of complex polyunsaturated diacylglycerols by gas-liquid chromatography on polar capillary columns. *Biochem. Cell Biol., 68,* 336-344.

[124] Mishra, V. K., Temelli, F., & Ooraikul, B. (1993). Extraction and purification of omega 3 fatty acids with an emphisis on supercritical fluid extraction. *Food Res. Int. 26*, 217-227.

[125] Nilsson, W. B., Gauglitz, Jr., E. J., & Hudson, J. K. (1989). Supercritical fluid fractionation of fish oil esters using incremental pressure programming and a temperature gradient. *J. Am. Oil Chem. Soc., 66,* 1596-1600.

[126] Riha, V., & Brunner, G. (1999). Phase equilibrium of fish oil ethyl esters with supercritical carbon dioxide. *J. Supercrit. Fluids, 15*, 33−50.

[127] Brunner, G. (2000). Fractionation of fats with supercritical carbon dioxide. *Eur. J. Lipid Sci. Technol.,* 1, 240−244.

[128] Haraldsson, G. G., & Hjaltason, B. (1992). Using biotechnology to modify marine lipids, *Inform, 3*, 626–629.

[129] Haraldsson, G. G. (1989). the application of lipases for modification of fats and oils, including marine oils. In. Voigt, M. N., & Bhotta, R. (Eds.) *Advances in fisheries technology for increased profitability*, pp. 337–357, Technomic Publishing Co., Inc., Lancaster, Pennsylvania.

[130] Marangoni, A., and Rousseau, D. (1995). Engineering Triacylglycerol: the Role of Interesterification. *Trends Food Sci. Technol. 6*, 329-335.

[131] Yadwad, V. B., Ward, O. P., & Noronha, L. C. (1991). Application of lipase to concentrate the docosahexaenoic acid fraction of fish oil. *Biotech. Bioeng., 38, 956-959.*

[132] Miller, C., Austin, H., Posorske, L. & Gonzlez, J. (1988). Characteristics of an immobilized Lipase for the commercial synthesis of esters. *J. Am. Oil Chem. Soc. 65,* 927-931.

[133] Halldorsson, A., Kristinsson, B., Glynm, C., & Haraldsson, G. G. (2003). Separation of EPA and DHA in fish oil by lipasecatalyzed esterification with glycerol. *J. Am. Oil Chem. Soc., 80*, 915–921.

[134] Shimada, Y., Maruyama, K., Sugihara, A., Moriyama, S. & Tominaga, Y. (1997). Purification of docosahexaenoic acid from tuna oil by a two-step enzymatic method: Hydrolysis and selective esterification. *J. Am. Oil Chem. Soc., 74*, 1441– 1446.

[135] Rakshit, S. K., Vasuhi, R., Kosugi, Y. (2000). Enrichment of polyunsaturated fatty acids from tuna oil using immobilized Pseudomonas fluorescens lipase. *Bioprocess Eng., 23*, 251–255.

[136] Carvalho, P., Campos, P., Noffs, M., Fregolente, P., & Fregolente, L. (2009). Enzymatic hydrolysis of salmon oil by native lipases: Optimization of process parameters. *J. Br. Chem. Soc.*, *20*, 117–124.

[137] Hoshino, T., Yamane, T., & Shimuzu, S. (1990). Selective Hydrolysis of Fish Oil by Lipase to Concentrate ω 3-poly- unsaturated Fatty Acids. *Agric. Biol. Chem. 54,* 1459-1467.

[138] Bottino, N. R., Vandenberg, G. A., & Reiser, R. (1967). Resistance of certain long-chain polyunsaturated fatty acids of marine oils to pancreatic lipase hydrolysis. *Lipids, 2*, 489-493.

[139] Tanaka, Y., Funada, T., Hirano, J. & Hashizume, R. (1993). Triglyceride specificity of *Candida cylindracea* lipase-effect of docosahexaenoic acid on resistance of triglycerides to lipase. *J. Am. Oil Chem. Soc.*, *70*, 1031– 1034.

[140] Mbatia, B., Adlercreutz, D., Adlercreutz, P., Mahadhy, A., Mulaa, F., & Mattiassonet, B. (2010).Enzymatic oil extraction and positional analysis of omega-3 fatty acids in Nile perch and salmon heads. *Process Biochem., 45,* 815– 819.

[141] Tanaka, Y., Hirano, J., & Funada, T. (1992). Concentration of docosahexaenoic acid in glyceride by hydrolysis of fish oils with candida cylindracea lipase. In. *J. Am. Oil Chem. Soc. 69*, 1210-1214.

[142] Lyberg, A. M., & Adlercreutz, P., (2008a). Lipase-catalysed enrichment of DHA and EPA in acylglycerols resulting from squid oil ethanolysis. *Eur. J. Lipid Sci. Technol.*, *110*, 317– 324.

[143] Lyberg, A. M., & Adlercreutz, P., (2008b). Lipase specificity towards eicosapentaenoic acid and docosahexaenoic acid depends on substrate structure. *Biochim. Biophys. Acta*, *1784*, 343– 350.

[144] Okada, T. & Morrissey, M. T. (2007). Production of n-3 polyunsaturated fatty acid concentrate from sardine oil by lipase-catalyzed hydrolysis. *Food Chem. 103*, 1411–1419.

[145] McNeill, G. P., Moore, S. R., & Ackman, R. G. (1996). Lipase-catalyzed enrichment of long-chain polyunsaturated fatty acids. *J. Am. Oil Chem. Soc. 73*, 1403–1407.

[146] Linder, M., Fanni, J. & Parmentier, M., (2005). Proteolytic extraction of salmon oil and pufa concentration by lipases. *Marine Biotechnol., 15*, 70–76.

[147] Sun, T., Pigott, G. M., & Herwing, R. P. (2002). Lipase-assisted concentration of n 3 polyunsaturated fatty acids from viscera of farmed Atlantic salmon (*Salmo salar L.*). *J. Food Sci., 67,* 130–136.

[148] Carvalho, P. D. O., Campos, P. R. B., D'Addio Noffs, M., Bastos, D. H. M., & De Oliveira, J. G. (2002). Enzymic enhancement of n-3 polyunsaturated fatty acids content in Brazilian sardine oil. *Acta Pharma Boner., 21*, 85–88.

[149] Wanasundara, U. N., & Shahidi, F. (1998). Lipase-Assisted Concentration of n-3 Polyunsaturated Fatty Acids in Acylglycerols from Marine Oils, *J. Am. Oil Chem. Soc. 75,* 945–951.

[150] Ustun, G., Guner, S., Arer, G., Turkay, S., & Erciyes, A. T. (1997). Enzymatic hydrolysis of anchovy oil: Production of glycerides enriched in polyunsaturated fatty acids. *Appl. Biochem. Biotechnol. Part A. Enzyme Eng. Biotechnol., 68(3),* 171–186.

[151] Wanasundara, U. N., & Shahidi, F. (1997). Positional distribution of fatty acids in triacylglycerols of seal blubber oil. *J. Food Lipids, 4,* 51-64.

[152] Bornscheuer, U. T., (2000). Enrichment of lipids with EPA and DHA by lipase. In. Bornscheuer, U. T. (Ed.), Enzymes in lipid modification, (p. 170). Wiley-VCH Verlag GmbH, Weinheim.

[153] Gamez-Meza, N., Noriega-Rodriguez, J., Higuera-Ciapara, I., Calderon De La Barca, A. M., Vazquez-Moreno, L., & Angulo-Guerrero, O. (1999). Seasonal variation in the fatty acid composition and quality of sardine oil from Sardinops sagax caeruleus of the Gulf of California. *Lipids, 34 (6)*, 639–642.

[154] Ando, Y., Ota, T., Matsuhira, Y., & Yazawa, K. (1996). Stereospecific analysis of triacyl-sn-glycerols in docosahexaenoic acid-rich fish oils. *J. Am. Oil Chem. Soc.,73,* 483–487.

[155] Uhlig, H. (1998). Description of enzymes: ester cleavage. In. Linsmaier-Bednar, E. M., (Ed.), *Industrial enzymes and their applications*, pp 179–193, Wiley, Tronto.

[156] Kotting, J., & Elbl, H. (1994). Lipase and Phospholipase in Organic Synthesis. In. Woolley, P., & Petersen, S. B., (Eds.) Lipases, pp. 289-313, Cambridge University Press, Cambridge.

[157] Hamazaki, T., Hirai, A., Terano, T., Sajiki, J., Kondo, S., Fujita, T., Tamura, Y., & Kumagai, A. (1982). Effect of orally administrated ethyl ester of eicosapentaenoic acid on PGI-like substance production by rat aorta. *Prostaglandins*, *23*, 557-567.

[158] El-Boustani, S., Colette, C, Monnier, L., Descomps, B., Paulet, C. A., & Mendey, F. (1987). Eternal Absorption in Man of Eico- sapentaenoic Acid in Different Chemical Forms, *Lipids 22*, 711-714.

[159] Yang, L. Y., Kuksis, A., & Myher, J. J. (1989). Lumenal hydrolysis of menhaden and rapeseed oils and their fatty acid methyl and ethyl esters in the rats. *Biochem. Cell Biol.* 67, 192-204.

[160] Haraldsson, G. G., Gudmundsson, B., & Almarsson, O. (1993). The preparation of homogeneous triglycerides of eicosapentaenoic acid and docosahexaenoic acid by lipase. *Tetrahedron Lett., 34,* 5791-5794.

[161] Basheer, S., Mogi, K., & Nakajima, M. (1995). Interesterification kinetics of triglycerides and fatty acids with modified lipase in n-hexane. *J. Am. Oil Chem. Soc.,72*, 511–518.

[162] Osada, K., Nakamura, M., Nonaka, M., & Hatano, M. (1992). Esterification of glycerol with EPA and DHA by *Chromobacterium viscosum* and *Candida cylindracea* Lipases. *J. Jpn. Oil Chem. Soc., 41*, 39-43.

[163] Haraldsson, G. G., Höskuldsson, P. A., Sigurdsson, S. Th., Thorsteinsson, F., & Gudbjarnason, S. (1989). The preparation of triglycerides highly enriched with ω-3 polyunsaturated fatty acids via lipase-catalyzed interesterification. *Tetrahedron Lett. 30*, 1671–1674.

[164] Haraldsson, G. G., Kristinsson, B., Sigurdardottir, R., Gudmundsson, G. G., & Breivik, H. (1997). The preparation of concentrates of eicosapentaenoic acid and docosahexaenoic acid by lipase-catalyzed transesterification of fish oil with ethanol. *J. Am. Oil Chem. Soc., 74,* 1419–1424.

[165] Adachi,S. Okumura, K., Ota, Y., & Mankura, M. (1993). Acidolysis of sardine oil by lipase to concentrate eicosapentaenoic and docosahexaenoic acids in glycerides. *J. Ferment. Bioeng., 74 (4),* 259-264.

[166] Konishi, H., Neff, W. E., & Mounts, T. L. (1993). Chemical interesterification with regioselectivity for edible oils. *J. Am. Oil Chem. Soc. 70*, 411–415.

[167] Haumanm, B. F., (1994). Tools: hydrogenation, interesterification. *Inform*, *5*, 668–678.

[168] Klinkesorn, U., H-Kittikun, A., Chinachoti, P., & Sophanodora, P. (2004). Chemical transesterification of tuna oil to enriched omega-3 polyunsaturated fatty acids. *Food Chem., 87*, 415–421.

[169] Gunnlaugsdottir, H., & Sivik, B. (1995). Lipase-catalyzed alcoholysis cod liver oil in supercritical carbon dioxide. *J. Am. Oil Chem. Soc., 72*, 399-405.

[170] Gunnlaugsdottir, H., & Sivik, B. (1997). Lipase-catalyzed alcoholysis with supercritical carbon dioxide extraction 1: Influence of flow rate. *J. Am. Oil Chem. Soc., 74*, 1483−1490.

[171] Gunnlaugsdottir, H., Karlsson, A., & Sivik, B. (1997). Lipase-catalyzed alcoholysis with supercritical carbon dioxide extraction 2: Phase behavior. *J. Am. Oil Chem. Soc., 74*, 1491−1494.

[172] Gunnlaugsdottir, H., Järemo, M., & Sivik, B. (1998). Process parameters influencing ethanolysis of cod liver oil in supercritical carbon dioxide. *J. Supercrit. Fluids, 12(1),* 85−93.

[173] Beebe, L. M., Brown, P. R., & Turcotte, L.G. (1988) Preparative- scale-high-performance liquid chromatography of omega-3 polyunsaturated fatty acid esters derived from fish oil. *J. Chromatogr., 495*, 369-378.

[174] EH Belarbi, E Molina, Y Chisti. (2000) A process for high yield and scaleable recovery of high purity eicosapentaenoic acid esters from microalgae and fish oil. Enzyme and Microbial Technology 26 516–529.

[175] Tokiwa, S., Kanazawa, A., & Teshima, S. (1981). Preparation of eicosapentaenoic and docosahexaenoic acids by reversed phase high performance liquid chromatography. *Bull. Jap. Soc. Sci. Fish., 47,* 675

[176] Krzynowek, J., D'Entremont, D. L., Panuzio, L. J., & Maney, R. S. (1988) Purification of omega-3 fatty acids from fish oils using HPLC: An overview.*Proc. 12th Ann. Conf. Trop. Subtrop. Fish Technol. Soc.*, 74-77.

[177] Perrut, M. (1988). Purification of polyunsaturated fatty acid (EPA and DHA) ethyl esters by preparative high performance liquid chromatography. *LC-GC, 6*, 914-920.

[178] Teshima, S., Kanazawa, A., & Tokiwa, S. (1978) Separation of polyunsaturated fatty acids by column chromatography on silver nitrate-impregnated silica gel. *Bull. J. Soc. Sci. Fish., 44*, 927.

[179] Hayashi, K., & Kishimura, H. (1993). Preparation of n-3 PUFA ethyl ester concentrates from fish oil by column chromatography on silicic acid. *Nippon Suisan Gakkaishi, 59,* 1429.

[180] Adlof, R. O., & Emiken, E. A. (1985). The Isolation of omega-3 polyunsaturated fatty acids and methyl esters of fish oils by silver resin chromatography. *J. Am. Oil Chem. Soc., 62*, 1592-1595.

[181] Guil-Guerrero, J. L., Belarbi, E. H., & Rebolloso-Fuentes, M. M. (2000). Eicosapentaenoic and arachidonic acids purification from the red microalga Porphyridium cruentum. *Bioseparation*, *9*, 299- 306.

[182] Chakraborty, K., & Raj, R. P. (2007). Eicosapentaenoic Acid Enrichment from Sardine Oil by Argentation Chromatography. *J. Agric. Food Chem.*, *55*, 7586-7595.

[183] Nicoud, R. M., Perrut, M., & Breivick, H. (1993). *Process for chromatographic fractionation of fatty acids and other derivatieves*. US patent 5, 719, 302.

[184] Nicoud, R, M., Clavier, Y. J., & Breivick, H. (1997). Simulated moving bed chromatography for the preparation of highly purified concentrates of EPA and DHA. In: *1997 Annual meeting abstracts, American Oils Chemists' Society,* pp.85-86, Chamaign, Illinois, USA.

[185] Kiran, E., Debenedetti, P. G., & Peters, C. J. (2000). Supercritical fluids: Fundamentals and applications (pp. 31−68), Kluwer Academica Publishers, Netherlands.

[186] Perrut, M., & Jusforgues, P. (1989). A new fractionation process:Preparative chromatography with a supercritical eluent. *Int. Chem. Eng., 29,* 646-653.

[187] Breivick, H., & Perrut, M. (1988). *Process for the production of polyunsaturated (n-3) fatty acids and their derivatives*. Norwegian patent NO163139.

[188] Berger, C., & Perrut, M. (1990). Preparative supercritacal fluid chromatography. *J. Chromatogr.*, *505*, 37-43.

[189] Brunner, G., & Reichmann, F. (1998). Process for recovering unsaturated fatty acids and Canas BI, Yurawecz MP (1999) Ethyl carbamate formation during urea complexation for fractionation of fatty acids. *J. Am. Oil Chem. Soc., 76*, 537

[190] Alkio, M., González, C., Jäntti, M., & Aaltonen, O. (2000). Purification of polyunsaturated fatty acid esters from tuna oil with supercritical fluid chromatography. *J. Am. Oil Chem. Soc., 77,* 315−321.

[191] Summers, G. (1987). Squalene, a potential shark byproduct. *Catch., (Oct)*, pp 29.

[192] Hayashi, K., & Takagi, T. (1981). Distribution of squalene and diacyl glyceryl eters in the different tissue of deep sea shark, Dalatias licha. *B. Jpn. Soc. Sci. Fish., 47,* 281-288.

[193] Gopakumar, K., & Thankappan, T. K. (1986). Squalene: Its sources, uses and industrial applications. *Seafood Export Journal., 3*, 17-20.

[194] Ko, T. F., Weng, T. M., Chiou, R. Y. (2002). Squalene content and antioxidant activity of Terminalia catappa leaves and seeds. *J. Agric. Food Chem., 50,* 5343–8.

[195] Qureshi, A. A., Lehmann, J. W., Peterson, D. M. (1996). Amaranth and its oil inhibit cholesterol biosynthesis in six-week-old female chickens. *J. Nutr., 126,* 1972–8.

[196] Ivashkevich, S. P., Apukhovskaia, L. I., & Vendt, V. P. (1981). Effects of sterols having different chemical structure and squalene on osmotic resistance of erythrocytes. *Biokhimiia*, *46*, 1420–5.

[197] Xu, R. B., Liu, W. W., & Wang, M. Y. (2005). Progress of preparation and application in squalene. *Shandong Journal of Medicine, 45*, 69-70.

[198] Passi, S., De Pita, O., Puddu, P., & Littarru, G. P. (2002). Lipophilic antioxidants in human sebum and aging. *Free Radic Res., 36*, 471-477.

[199] Richter, E., & Schafer, S. G. (1982a). Effect of squalene on hexachlorobenzene (HCB) concentrations in tissue of mice. *J. Environ. Sci. Health., 17,* 195-203.

[200] Farvin, K. H. S., Anandan, R., Kumar, S. H. S., Shiny, K. S., Sankar, T. V., & Nair, P. G. V. (2006). Protective effect of squalene on changes in lipid profile in experimentally induced myocardial infarction in rats. *J. Med. Food, 9*, 531-536.

[201] Farvin, K. H. S., Anandan, R., Kumar, S. H. S., Shiny, K. S., Sankar, T. V., & Thankappan, T. K. (2004). Effect of squalene on tissue defense system in isoproterenol-induced myocardial infarction in rats. *Pharmacol. Res., 50*, 231-236

[202] Farvin, K. H. S., Anandan, R., Sankar, T. V., & Nair, P. G. V. (2005). Protective effect of squalene against isoproterenol-induced myocardial infarction in rats. *J. Clin. Biochem. Nutri.37*, 55-60

[203] Farvin, K. H. S., Kumar, S. H. S., Anandan, R., Suseela Mathew, Sankar, T. V., & Nair, P. G. V. (2007). Supplementation of squalene attenuates experimentally induced myocardial infarction in rats. *Food Chem. 105*, 1390-1395.

[204] Farvin, K. H. S., Surendraraj, A., & Anandan, R. (2009). Protective effect of squalene on endogenous antioxidant vitamins in experimentally induced myocardial infarction in rats, *Asian J. Biochem., 4*, 133-139

[205] Farvin, K. H. S., Surendraraj, A., & Anandan, R. (2010). Protective effect of squalene on certain lysosomal hydrolases and free amino acids in isoprenaline-induced myocardial infarction in rats. *Int. J. Pharmacol., 6*, 97-103.

[206] Gopakumar, K. (2002). Fish Products, In. GopaKumar, K., (Ed.), Text book of fish processing technology, pp.295-299, ICAR, New Delhi.

[207] Nevenzel, J. C. (1970). Occurrence, function and biosynthesis of wax esters in marine organisms. *Lipids, 5,* 308-319.

[208] Sargent, J. R., Gatten, R. R., & Mcintosh, R. (1977). Wax esters in the marine environment -- their occurrence, formation, transformation and ultimate fates. *Marine Chemistry, 5,* 573-584.

[209] Clarke, A., (1984). The lipid content and composition of some Antarctic macrozooplankton. *Br. Antarct. Surv. Bull., 63,* 57-70.

[210] Sargent, J. R., & Falk-Petersen, S. (1988). The lipid biochemistry of calanoid copepods. *Hydrobiologia, 167/168*, 101-114 .

[211] Lee, R. F., Nevenzel, J. C., & Puffenhofer, G. A. (1971). Importance of wax esters and other lipids in the marine food chain: phytoplankton and copepods. *Marine Biol., 9,* 99--108.

[212] Lee, R. F., Nevenzel, J. C & Lewis, A. G. (1974). Lipid changes during life cycle of marine copepod Euchaeta japonica Marukawa. *Lipids*, 9, 891-898.

[213] Gorreta, F., Bernasconi, R., Galliani, G., Salmona, M., Tacconi, M. T., & Bianchi, R. (2002). Wax esters of O-3 polyunsaturated fatty acids: a new formulation as a potential food supplement: digestion and absorption in rats. *Lebensmittel-Wissenschaft und Technologie*, *35*, 458–465.

[214] Bernasconia, R., Bolzacchinib, E., Gallianib, G., Gugliersib, F., Rindoneb, B., Rindoneb, M., Tacconia, M. T., & Terraneoc, A. (2007). Determination of the content of wax esters in some sea foods and their molecular composition. A comparison with ω-3 enriched wax esters. *LWT Food Sci. Technol.*, *40*, 569–573.

[215] Lin, C.Y., & Lin, H. A. (2007). Engine performance and emission characteristics of a three-phase emulsion of biodiesel produced by peroxidation. *Fuel Process Technol. 88*, 35–41.

[216] Dorado, M. P., Ballesteros, J. M., Arnal, J. & Gomez, F. J. (2003). Lopez, Exhaust emissions from a diesel engine fueled with transesterified waste olive oil, *Fuel*, *82,* 1311–1315.

[217] Fisheries Agency, (2007). *Fisheries production by years, Yearly Report of Fisheries in Taiwan*, Item No. 7, Council of Agriculture, ROC, Taiwan.

[218] Zhang, Y., Dube, M. A., McLean, D. D., Kates, M. (2003). Biodiesel production from waste cooking oil: 1. process design and technological assessment. *Bioresource Technol., 89,* 1–16.

[219] Wang, Y., Ou, S., Liu, P., & Zhang, Z. (2007). Preparation of biodiesel from waste cooking oil via two-step catalyzed process. *Energy Convers Mgmt, 48,* 184–188.

[220] Van Gerpen, J., Shanks, B., Pruszko, R., Clements, D., & Knothe, G. (2004). Biodiesel production technology. National Renewable Energy Laboratory. 1617 Cole Boulevard, Golden, CO. Paper contract No. DE-AC36-99-GO10337.

[221] Lin, C. Y., & Li, R. J. (2009). Fuel properties of biodiesel produced from the crude fish oil from the soapstock of marine fish. *Fuel Process Technol., 90*, 130–136.

[222] Ma, F., & Hanna, M. A. (1999). Biodiesel production: a review. *Bioresour Technol., 70*, 1–15.

[223] Demirbas, A. (2002). Biodiesel from vegetable oils via transesterification in supercritical methanol. *Energy Convers Management, 43,* 2349–56.

[224] Wright, H. J., Segur, J. B., Clark, H. V., Coburn, S. K., Langdon, E. E., DuPuis, R. N. (1944). A report on ester interchange. *Oil Soap, 21,* 145−148.

[225] Keim, G. I. (1945). *Process for treatment of fatty glycerides*. US Patent 2, 383−601.

[226] Lin, C.Y., & Lin, H. A. (2006). Diesel engine performance and emission characteristics of biodiesel produced by the peroxidation process, *Fuel*, *85*, 298–305.

[227] Office of Scientific and Technical Information, (2006). Biodiesel Handling and Use Guidelines, U.S. Department of Energy, USA.

[228] Reyes, J. F., Sepulveda, M. A. (2006). PM-10 emissions and power of a diesel engine fueled with crude and refined biodiesel from salmon oil. *Fuel, 85,* 1714–1719.

[229] Knothe, G., Dunn, R. O., & Bagby, M. O. (1997). Biodiesel: the use of vegetable oils and their derivatives as alternative diesel fuels. *Am. Chem. Soc. Symp. Ser., 666,* 172–208.

[230] Zheng, D., Hanna, M. A. (1996). Preparation and properties of methyl esters of beef tallow, Bioresource Technol., 57, 137–142.

[231] Monyem, A., & Van Gerpen, J. H., (2001). The effect of biodiesel oxidation on engine performance and emission. *Biomass and Bioenergy, 20,* 317–325.

Index

B

C

E

F

I

J

K

L

M

N

O

P

Q

R

S

T

U

V

W

Y

Z